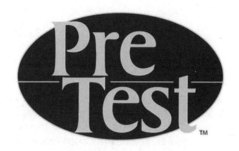

# Emergency Medicine

PreTest™ Self-Assessment and Review

## Notice

Medicine is an ever-changing science. As new research and clinical experience broaden our knowledge, changes in treatment and drug therapy are required. The authors and the publisher of this work have checked with sources believed to be reliable in their efforts to provide information that is complete and generally in accord with the standards accepted at the time of publication. However, in view of the possibility of human error or changes in medical sciences, neither the authors nor the publisher nor any other party who has been involved in the preparation or publication of this work warrants that the information contained herein is in every respect accurate or complete, and they disclaim all responsibility for any errors or omissions or for the results obtained from use of the information contained in this work. Readers are encouraged to confirm the information contained herein with other sources. For example and in particular, readers are advised to check the product information sheet included in the package of each drug they plan to administer to be certain that the information contained in this work is accurate and that changes have not been made in the recommended dose or in the contraindications for administration. This recommendation is of particular importance in connection with new or infrequently used drugs.

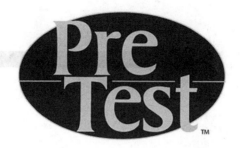

# Emergency Medicine
## PreTest™ Self-Assessment and Review
### Third Edition

**Adam J. Rosh, MD, MS, FACEP**
Clinical Assistant Professor
Department of Emergency Medicine
Wayne State University School of Medicine
Detroit Receiving Hospital
Detroit, Michigan

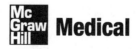 **Medical**

New York   Chicago   San Francisco   Lisbon   London   Madrid   Mexico City
Milan   New Delhi   San Juan   Seoul   Singapore   Sydney   Toronto

The McGraw

**Emergency Medicine: PreTest™ Self-Assessment and Review, Third Edition**

1 2 3 4 5 6 7 8 9 0   DOC/DOC   17 16 15 14 13 12

ISBN 978-0-07177310-2
MHID 0-07-177310-X

This book was set in Berkeley by Cenveo Publisher Services.
The editors were Kirsten Funk and Regina Y. Brown.
The production supervisor was Sherri Souffrance.
Project management was provided by Kritika Kaul, Cenveo Publisher Services.
The cover designer was Maria Scharf.
Cover Photo: Doctor defibrillating a patient.
RR Donnelley was printer and binder.

This book is printed on acid-free paper.

**Cataloging-in Publication Data is on file with the Library of Congress.**

McGraw-Hill books are available at special quantity discounts to use as premiums and sales promotions, or for use in corporate training programs. To contact a representative please e-mail us at bulksales@mcgraw-hill.com

# Contributors

### Keenan M. Bora, MD
Assistant Professor
Department of Emergency Medicine
Medical Toxicologist
Wayne State University School of Medicine
Detroit, Michigan
*Poisoning and Overdose*

### Richard D. Gordon, Jr., MD
Ultrasound Fellow
Georgia Health Sciences University
Augusta, Georgia
*Ultrasound in the Emergency Department*

### Sarkis R. Kouyoumjian, MD, FACEP
Medical Student Clerkship Director
Assistant Professor
Department of Emergency Medicine
Detroit Receiving Hospital
Wayne State University School of Medicine
Detroit, Michigan
*Chest Pain and Cardiac Dysrhythmias*

### Michelle Lall, MD, MHS
Assistant Resident Director
Sinai-Grace Hospital
Clinical Assistant Professor Department of Emergency Medicine
Wayne State University School of Medicine
Detroit, Michigan
*Musculoskeletal Injuries*
*Trauma, Shock, and Resuscitation*

### Matthew Lyon, MD, FACEP
Associate Professor
Director of Emergency and Clinical Ultrasound
Department of Emergency Medicine
Georgia Health Sciences University
Augusta, Georgia
*Ultrasound in the Emergency Department*

### Adam J. Rosh, MD, MS, FACEP
Clinical Assistant Professor
Department of Emergency Medicine
Wayne State University School of Medicine
Detroit Receiving Hospital
Detroit, Michigan

### Mark A. Saks, MD, MPH
Associate Program Director
Director of Undergraduate Education
Assistant Professor
Department of Emergency Medicine
Drexel University College of Medicine
Philadelphia, Pennsylvania
*Fever*
*Vaginal Bleeding*

### Lawrence R. Schwartz, MD, MEd, FACEP
Assistant Professor
Department of Emergency Medicine
Detroit Receiving Hospital
Wayne State University School of Medicine
Detroit, Michigan
*Chest Pain and Cardiac Dysrhythmias*

### Shereaf W. Walid, MD
Chief Resident
Department of Emergency Medicine
Detroit Receiving Hospital
Detroit, Michigan
*Prehospital, Disaster, and Administration*

### Ethan Wiener, MD, FAAP
Assistant Professor of Emergency Medicine
Mt. Sinai School of Medicine
New York, New York
Associate Director
Pediatric Emergency Medicine
Goryeb Children's Hospital
Morristown, New Jersey
*Pediatrics*

# Resident Reviewers

**Ayse M. Avcioglu, MD**
Resident
Department of Emergency Medicine
Detroit Receiving Hospital
Detroit, Michigan

**Brandon E. Cheppa, MD**
Chief Resident
Department of Emergency Medicine
Detroit Receiving Hospital
Detroit, Michigan

**Jeff Cloyd, MD**
Resident
Department of Emergency Medicine
Detroit Receiving Hospital
Detroit, Michigan

**Katie Jo Dobratz, MD**
Resident
Department of Emergency Medicine
Detroit Receiving Hospital
Detroit, Michigan

# Student Reviewers

**Annalee Baker, MD**
PGY-1 EM Resident
NYU School of Medicine
Bellevue Hospital Center
New York, NY

**Lee Donner, MD**
PGY-1 EM Resident
UMDNJ
The University Hospital
Newark, NJ

**Ambrose Wong, MD**
PGY-1 EM Resident
NYU School of Medicine
Bellevue Hospital Center
New York, NY

**Benjamin Chidester, MD**
PGY1 EM Resident
Eastern Virginia Medical School
Norfolk, VA

# Contents

# Introduction

*Emergency Medicine: PreTest Self-Assessment and Review, Third Edition,* is intended to provide medical students, as well as house officers and physicians, with a convenient tool for assessing and improving their knowledge of emergency medicine. The 500 questions in this book are similar in format and complexity to those included in Step 2 of the United States Medical Licensing Examination (USMLE). They may also be a useful study tool for Step 3 and clerkship examinations.

Each question in this book has a corresponding answer, a reference to a text that provides background for the answer, and a short discussion of various issues raised by the question and its answer. A listing of references for the entire book follows the last chapter. For multiple-choice questions, the **one best** response to each question should be selected. For matching sets, a group of questions will be preceded by a list of lettered options. For each question in the matching set, select **one** lettered option that is **most** closely associated with the question.

To simulate the time constraints imposed by the qualifying examinations for which this book is intended as a practice guide, the student or physician should allot about one minute for each question. After answering all questions in a chapter, as much time as necessary should be spent reviewing the explanations for each question at the end of the chapter. Attention should be given to all explanations, even if the examinee answered the question correctly. Those seeking more information on a subject should refer to the reference materials listed or to other standard texts in emergency medicine.

# Acknowledgment

A hearty thanks goes out to my family for their love and support, especially Ruby and Rhys; the dedicated medical professionals of the Emergency Departments at New York University/Bellevue Hospital and Wayne State University/Detroit Receiving Hospital; Catherine Johnson for giving me this opportunity, and my patients, who put their trust in me, and teach me something new each day.

—AJR

# Chest Pain and Cardiac Dysrhythmias

## Questions

**1.** A 59-year-old man presents to the emergency department (ED) complaining of new-onset chest pain that radiates to his left arm. He has a history of hypertension, hypercholesterolemia, and a 20-pack-year smoking history. His electrocardiogram (ECG) is remarkable for T-wave inversions in the lateral leads. Which of the following is the most appropriate next step in management?

a. Give the patient two nitroglycerin tablets sublingually and observe if his chest pain resolves.
b. Place the patient on a cardiac monitor, administer oxygen, and give aspirin.
c. Call the cardiac catheterization laboratory for immediate percutaneous coronary intervention (PCI).
d. Order a chest x-ray; administer aspirin, clopidogrel, and heparin.
e. Start a β-blocker immediately.

**2.** A 36-year-old woman presents to the ED with sudden onset of left-sided chest pain and mild shortness of breath that began the night before. She was able to fall asleep without difficulty but woke up in the morning with persistent pain that is worsened upon taking a deep breath. She walked up the stairs at home and became very short of breath, which made her come to the ED. Two weeks ago, she took a 7-hour flight from Europe and since then has left-sided calf pain and swelling. What is the most common ECG finding for this patient's presentation?

a. $S_1Q_3T_3$ pattern
b. Atrial fibrillation
c. Right-axis deviation
d. Right-atrial enlargement
e. Tachycardia or nonspecific ST-T–wave changes

**3.** A 51-year-old man with a long history of hypertension presents to the ED complaining of intermittent chest palpitations lasting for a week. He denies chest pain, shortness of breath, nausea, and vomiting. He recalls feeling similar episodes of palpitations a few months ago but they resolved. His blood pressure (BP) is 130/75 mm Hg, heart rate (HR) is 130 beats per minute, respiratory rate (RR) is 16 breaths per minute, and oxygen saturation is 99% on room air. An ECG is seen below. Which of the following is the most appropriate next step in management?

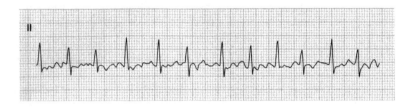

a. Sedate patient for immediate synchronized cardioversion with 100 J.
b. Prepare patient for the cardiac catheterization laboratory.
c. Administer warfarin.
d. Administer amiodarone.
e. Administer diltiazem.

**4.** A 54-year-old woman presents to the ED because of a change in behavior at home. For the past 3 years, she has end-stage renal disease requiring dialysis. Her daughter states that the patient has been increasingly tired and occasionally confused for the past 3 days and has not been eating her usual diet. On examination, the patient is alert and oriented to person only. The remainder of her examination is normal. An initial 12-lead ECG is performed as seen on the following page. Which of the following electrolyte abnormalities best explains these findings?

a. Hypokalemia
b. Hyperkalemia
c. Hypocalcemia
d. Hypercalcemia
e. Hyponatremia

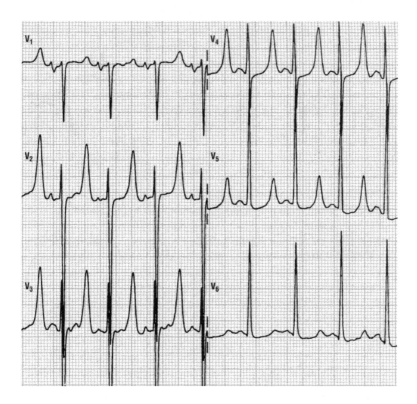

**5.** A 29-year-old tall, thin man presents to the ED after feeling short of breath for 2 days. In the ED, he is in no acute distress. His BP is 115/70 mm Hg, HR is 81 beats per minute, RR is 16 breaths per minute, and oxygen saturation is 98% on room air. Cardiac, lung, and abdominal examinations are normal. An ECG reveals sinus rhythm at a rate of 79. A chest radiograph shows a small right-sided (<10% of the hemithorax) spontaneous pneumothorax. A repeat chest x-ray 6 hours later reveals a decreased pneumothorax. Which of the following is the most appropriate next step in management?

a. Discharge the patient with follow-up in 24 hours.
b. Perform needle decompression in the second intercostal space, midclavicular line.
c. Insert a 20F chest tube into right hemithorax.
d. Observe for another 6 hours.
e. Admit for pleurodesis.

**6.** A 42-year-old man found vomiting in the street is brought to the ED by emergency medical services (EMS). He has a known history of alcohol abuse with multiple presentations for intoxication. Today, the patient complains of acute onset, persistent chest pain associated with dysphagia, and pain upon flexing his neck. His BP is 115/70 mm Hg, HR is 101 beats per minute, RR is 18 breaths per minute, and oxygen saturation is 97% on room air. As you listen to his heart, you hear a crunching sound. His abdomen is soft with mild epigastric tenderness. The ECG is sinus tachycardia without ST-T–wave abnormalities. On chest radiograph, you note lateral displacement of the left mediastinal pleura. What is the most likely diagnosis?

a. Aspiration pneumonia
b. Acute pancreatitis
c. Pericarditis
d. Esophageal perforation
e. Aortic dissection

**7.** A 65-year-old man with a history of chronic hypertension presents to the ED with sudden-onset tearing chest pain that radiates to his jaw. His BP is 205/110 mm Hg, HR is 90 beats per minute, RR is 20 breaths per minute, and oxygen saturation is 97% on room air. He appears apprehensive. On cardiac examination you hear a diastolic murmur at the right sternal border. A chest x-ray reveals a widened mediastinum. Which of the following is the preferred study of choice to diagnose this patient's condition?

a. Electrocardiogram (ECG)
b. Transthoracic echocardiography (TTE)
c. Transesophageal echocardiography (TEE)
d. Computed tomography (CT) scan
e. Magnetic resonance imaging (MRI)

**8.** A 47-year-old man with a history of hypertension presents to the ED complaining of continuous left-sided chest pain that began while snorting cocaine 1 hour ago. The patient states he never experienced chest pain in the past when using cocaine. His BP is 170/90 mm Hg, HR is 101 beats per minute, RR is 18 breaths per minute, and oxygen saturation is 98% on room air. The patient states that the only medication he takes is alprazolam to "calm his nerves." Which of the following medications is contraindicated in this patient?

a. Metoprolol
b. Diltiazem
c. Aspirin
d. Lorazepam
e. Nitroglycerin

**9.** A 32-year-old woman presents to the ED with a persistent fever of 101°F over the last 3 days. The patient states that she used to work as a convenience store clerk but was fired 2 weeks ago. Since then, she has been using drugs intravenously daily. Cardiac examination reveals a heart murmur. Her abdomen is soft and nontender with an enlarged spleen. Chest radiograph reveals multiple patchy infiltrates in both lung fields. Laboratory results reveal white blood cells (WBC) 14,000/μL with 91% neutrophils, hematocrit 33%, and platelets 250/μL. An ECG reveals sinus rhythm with first-degree heart block. Which of the following is the most appropriate next step in management?

a. Obtain four sets of blood cultures, order a TTE, and start antibiotic treatment.
b. Order a monospot test and recommend that the patient refrain from vigorous activities for 1 month.
c. Administer a nonsteroidal anti-inflammatory drug (NSAID) and inform the patient she has pericarditis.
d. Administer isoniazid (INH) and report the patient to the Department of Health.
e. Order a Lyme antibody and begin antibiotic therapy.

**10.** A 61-year-old woman was on her way to the grocery store when she started feeling chest pressure in the center of her chest. She became diaphoretic and felt short of breath. On arrival to the ED by EMS, her BP is 130/70 mm Hg, HR is 76 beats per minute, and oxygen saturation is 98% on room air. The nurse gives her an aspirin and an ECG is performed as seen below. Which of the following best describes the location of this patient's myocardial infarction (MI)?

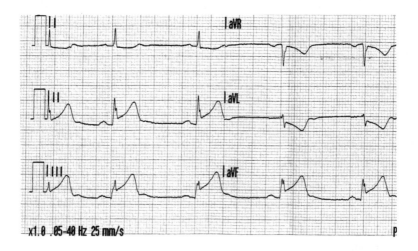

a. Anteroseptal
b. Anterior
c. Lateral
d. Inferior
e. Posterior

**11.** A 31-year-old man who works for a moving company presents to the ED because he thinks he was having a heart attack. He does not smoke, and jogs 3 days a week. His father died of a heart attack in his sixties. He describes a gradual onset of chest pain that is worse with activity and resolves when he is at rest. His HR is 68 beats per minute, BP is 120/70 mm Hg, and RR is 14 breaths per minute. On examination, his lungs are clear and there is no cardiac murmur. You palpate tenderness over the left sternal border at the third and fourth ribs. An ECG reveals sinus rhythm at a rate of 65. A chest radiograph shows no infiltrates or pneumothorax. Which of the following is the most appropriate next step in management?

a. Administer aspirin and send for a troponin.
b. Administer aspirin, clopidogrel, and heparin, and admit for acute coronary syndrome (ACS).
c. Administer ibuprofen and reassure the patient that he is not having a heart attack.
d. Inject corticosteroid into the costochondral joint to reduce inflammation.
e. Observe the patient for 6 hours.

**12.** A 21-year-old woman presents to the ED complaining of lightheadedness. Her symptoms appeared 45 minutes ago. She has no other symptoms and is not on any medications. She has a medical history of mitral valve prolapse. Her HR is 170 beats per minute and BP is 105/55 mm Hg. Physical examination is unremarkable. After administering the appropriate medication, her HR slows down and her symptoms resolve. You repeat a 12-lead ECG that shows a rate of 89 beats per minute with a regular rhythm. The PR interval measures 100 milliseconds and there is a slurred upstroke of the QRS complex. Based on this information, which of the following is the most likely diagnosis?

a. Ventricular tachycardia
b. Atrial flutter with 3:1 block
c. Atrial fibrillation
d. Lown-Ganong-Levine (LGL) syndrome
e. Wolff-Parkinson-White (WPW) syndrome

**13.** A 55-year-old man presents to the ED with worsening weakness, muscle cramps, and paresthesias. His past medical history is significant for hypertension and diabetes. He smokes one pack of cigarettes per day. On examination, the patient is alert and oriented and diffusely weak. An ECG is seen below. Which of the following is the most important next step in management?

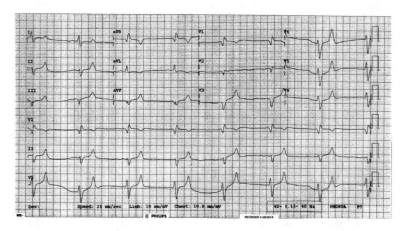

a. Administer calcium gluconate.
b. Administer insulin and dextrose.
c. Administer aspirin and call the catheterization laboratory.
d. Order an emergent head CT scan and get a neurology consult.
e. Collect a sample of his urine to test for ketones.

**14.** While eating dinner, a 55-year-old man suddenly feels a piece of steak "get stuck" in his stomach. In the ED, he complains of dysphagia, is drooling, and occasionally retches. On examination, his BP is 130/80 mm Hg, HR is 75 beats per minute, RR is 15 breaths per minute, and oxygen saturation is 99% on room air. He appears in no respiratory distress. Chest x-ray is negative for air under the diaphragm. Which of the following is the most appropriate next step in management?

a. Administer 1-mg glucagon intravenously while arranging for endoscopy.
b. Administer a meat tenderizer such as papain to soften the food bolus.
c. Administer 10-mL syrup of ipecac to induce vomiting and dislodge the food bolus.
d. Perform the Heimlich maneuver until the food dislodges.
e. Call surgery consult to prepare for laparotomy.

**15.** A 59-year-old man presents to the ED with left-sided chest pain and shortness of breath that began 2 hours prior to arrival. He states the pain is pressure-like and radiates down his left arm. He is diaphoretic. His BP is 160/80 mm Hg, HR 86 beats per minute, and RR 15 breaths per minute. ECG reveals 2-mm ST-segment elevation in leads I, aVL, and $V_3$ to $V_6$. Which of the following is an absolute contraindication to receiving thrombolytic therapy?

a. Systolic BP (SBP) greater than 180 mm Hg
b. Patient on Coumadin and aspirin
c. Total hip replacement 3 months ago
d. Peptic ulcer disease
e. Previous hemorrhagic stroke

**16.** A 67-year-old woman is brought to the ED by paramedics complaining of dyspnea, fatigue, and palpitations. Her BP is 80/50 mm Hg, HR is 139 beats per minute, and RR is 20 breaths per minute. Her skin is cool and she is diaphoretic. Her lung examination reveals bilateral crackles and she is beginning to have chest pain. Her ECG shows a narrow complex irregular rhythm with a rate in the 140s. Which of the following is the most appropriate immediate treatment for this patient?

a. Diltiazem
b. Metoprolol
c. Digoxin
d. Coumadin
e. Synchronized cardioversion

**17.** A 61-year-old woman with a history of congestive heart failure (CHF) is at a family picnic when she starts complaining of shortness of breath. Her daughter brings her to the ED where she is found to have an oxygen saturation of 85% on room air with rales halfway up both of her lung fields. Her BP is 185/90 mm Hg and pulse rate is 101 beats per minute. On examination, her jugular venous pressure (JVP) is 6 cm above the sternal angle. There is lower extremity pitting edema. Which of the following is the most appropriate first-line medication to lower cardiac preload?

a. Metoprolol
b. Morphine sulfate
c. Nitroprusside
d. Nitroglycerin
e. Oxygen

**18.** A 27-year-old man who is otherwise healthy presents to the ED with a laceration on his thumb that he sustained while cutting a bagel. You irrigate and repair the wound and are about to discharge the patient when he asks you if he can receive an ECG. It is not busy in the ED so you perform the ECG, as seen below. Which of the following is the most appropriate next step in management?

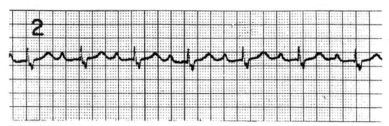

*(Reproduced, with permission, from Tintinalli J, Kelen G, Stapczynski J. Emergency Medicine: A Comprehensive Study Guide. New York, NY: McGraw-Hill, 2004:193.)*

a. Admit the patient for placement of a pacemaker.
b. Admit the patient for a 24-hour observation period.
c. Administer aspirin and send cardiac biomarkers.
d. Repeat the ECG because of incorrect lead placement.
e. Discharge the patient home.

**19.** A 61-year-old woman with a history of diabetes and hypertension is brought to the ED by her daughter. The patient states that she started feeling short of breath approximately 12 hours ago and then noticed a tingling sensation in the middle of her chest and became diaphoretic. An ECG reveals ST depression in leads II, III, and aVF. You believe that the patient had a non–ST-elevation MI (NSTEMI). Which of the following cardiac markers begins to rise within 3 to 6 hours of chest pain onset, peaks at 12 to 24 hours, and returns to baseline in 7 to 10 days?

a. Myoglobin
b. Creatinine kinase (CK)
c. Creatinine kinase-MB (CK-MB)
d. Troponin I
e. Lactic dehydrogenase (LDH)

**20.** A 27-year-old man complains of chest palpitations and light-headedness for the past hour. He has no past medical history and is not taking any medications. He drinks a beer occasionally on the weekend and does not smoke cigarettes. His HR is 180 beats per minute, BP is 110/65 mm Hg, and oxygen saturation is 99% on room air. An ECG reveals an HR of 180 beats per minute with a QRS complex of 90 milliseconds with a regular rhythm. There are no discernable P waves. Which of the following is the most appropriate medication to treat this dysrhythmia?

a. Digoxin
b. Lidocaine
c. Amiodarone
d. Adenosine
e. Bretylium

**21.** A 59-year-old man presents to the ED with left-sided chest pain and shortness of breath that began 1 hour ago. Initial vital signs are BP 85/45 mm Hg, HR 105 beats per minute, RR 20 breaths per minute, and oxygen saturation 94% on room air. An ECG is seen below. Which of the following is the most appropriate definitive treatment?

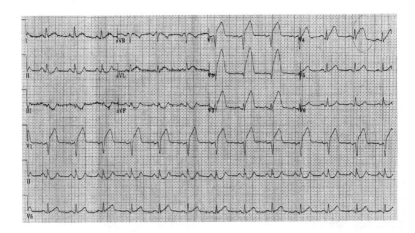

a. Administer metoprolol or diltiazem
b. Electrical cardioversion
c. Administer calcium gluconate
d. Thrombolytic therapy
e. Percutaneous angioplasty

**22.** A 55-year-old man presents to the ED at 2:00 AM with left-sided chest pain that radiates down his left arm. He takes a β-blocker for hypertension, a proton pump inhibitor for gastroesophageal reflux disease, and an antilipid agent for high cholesterol. He also took sildenafil the previous night for erectile dysfunction. His BP is 130/70 mm Hg and HR is 77 beats per minute. Which of the following medications is contraindicated in this patient?

a. Aspirin
b. Unfractionated heparin
c. Nitroglycerin
d. Metoprolol
e. Morphine sulfate

**23.** A 31-year-old kindergarten teacher presents to the ED complaining of acute-onset substernal chest pain that is sharp in nature and radiates to her back. The pain is worse when she is lying down on the stretcher and improves when she sits up. She smokes cigarettes occasionally and was told she has borderline diabetes. She denies any recent surgeries or long travel. Her BP is 145/85 mm Hg, HR is 99 beats per minute, RR is 18 breaths per minute, and temperature is 100.6°F. Examination of her chest reveals clear lungs and a friction rub. Her abdomen is soft and nontender to palpation. Her legs are not swollen. Chest radiography and echocardiography are unremarkable. Her ECG is shown below. Which of the following is the most appropriate next step in management?

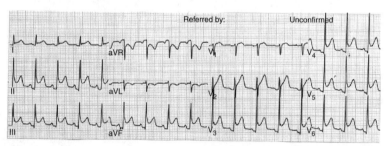

*(Reproduced, with permission, from Fuster V et al. Hurst's The Heart. New York, NY: McGraw-Hill, 2004: 304.)*

a. Anticoagulate and CT scan to evaluate for a PE.
b. Prescribe a NSAID and discharge the patient.
c. Aspirin, heparin, clopidogrel, and admit for ACS.
d. Administer thrombolytics if the pain persists.
e. Prescribe antibiotics and discharge the patient.

**24.** A 71-year-old man is playing cards with some friends when he starts to feel a pain in the left side of his chest. His fingers in the left hand become numb and he feels short of breath. His wife calls the ambulance and he is brought to the hospital. In the ED, an ECG is performed. Which of the following best describes the order of ECG changes seen in an MI?

a. Hyperacute T wave, ST-segment elevation, Q wave
b. Q wave, ST-segment elevation, hyperacute T wave
c. Hyperacute T wave, Q wave, ST-segment elevation
d. ST-segment elevation, Q wave, hyperacute T wave
e. ST-segment elevation, hyperacute T wave, Q wave

**25.** A 63-year-old insurance agent is brought to the ED by paramedics for shortness of breath and an RR of 31 breaths per minute. The patient denies chest pain, fever, vomiting, or diarrhea. His wife says he ran out of his "water pill" 1 week ago. His BP is 185/90 mm Hg, HR is 101 beats per minute, oxygen saturation is 90% on room air, and temperature is 98.9°F. There are crackles midway up both lung fields and 2+ pitting edema midway up his legs. An ECG shows sinus tachycardia. The patient is sitting up and able to speak to you. After placing the patient on a monitor and inserting an IV, which of the following is the most appropriate next step in management?

a. Obtain blood cultures and complete blood cell (CBC) count, and begin empiric antibiotic therapy.
b. Order a statim (STAT) portable chest x-ray.
c. Administer oxygen via nasal cannula and have the patient chew an aspirin.
d. Administer oxygen via non-rebreather, furosemide, nitroglycerin, and consider noninvasive respiratory therapy.
e. Rapid sequence endotracheal intubation.

**26.** Which of the following patients has the **lowest** clinical probability for the diagnosis of pulmonary embolism (PE)?

a. A 21-year-old woman 2 days after a cesarean delivery.
b. A 55-year-old woman on estrogen replacement therapy who underwent a total hip replacement procedure 3 days ago.
c. A 39-year-old man who smokes cigarettes occasionally and underwent an uncomplicated appendectomy 2 months ago.
d. A 62-year-old man with pancreatic cancer.
e. A 45-year-old man with factor V Leiden deficiency.

**27.** While playing a match of tennis, a 56-year-old man with a medical history significant only for acid reflux disease starts to feel substernal chest pain that radiates into his left arm and shortness of breath. His pain feels better after drinking antacid, but since it is not completely resolved, his partner calls 911. Upon arrival, EMS administers aspirin and sublingual nitroglycerin. After 20 minutes, the man's symptoms resolve. He is brought to the ED for further evaluation where his ECG shows sinus rhythm without any ischemic abnormalities. You order a chest radiograph and send his blood work to the laboratory for analysis. Which of the following statements regarding the diagnosis of acute MI is most accurate?

a. A normal ECG rules out the diagnosis of acute MI.
b. One set of negative cardiac enzymes is sufficient to exclude the diagnosis of MI in this patient.
c. Troponin may not reach peak levels for at least 12 hours.
d. Relief of symptoms by antacids essentially rules out a cardiac cause of his chest pain.
e. Epigastric discomfort and indigestion is a rare presentation of ACS.

**28.** A 62-year-old woman presents to the ED with general weakness, shortness of breath, and substernal chest pain that radiates to her left shoulder. Her BP is 155/80 mm Hg, HR is 92 beats per minute, and RR is 16 breaths per minute. You suspect that she is having an acute MI. Which of the following therapeutic agents has been shown to independently reduce mortality in the setting of an acute MI?

a. Nitroglycerin
b. Aspirin
c. Unfractionated heparin
d. Lidocaine
e. Diltiazem

**29.** A 22-year-old college student went to the health clinic complaining of a fever over the last 5 days, fatigue, myalgias, and a bout of vomiting and diarrhea. The clinic doctor diagnosed him with acute gastroenteritis and told him to drink more fluids. Three days later, the student presents to the ED complaining of substernal chest pain that is constant. He also feels short of breath. His temperature is 100.9°F, HR is 119 beats per minute, BP is 120/75 mm Hg, and RR is 18 breaths per minute. An ECG is performed revealing sinus tachycardia. A chest radiograph is unremarkable. Laboratory tests are normal except for slightly elevated WBCs. Which of the following is the most common cause of this patient's diagnosis?

a. *Streptococcus viridans*
b. Influenza A
c. Coxsackie B virus
d. Atherosclerotic disease
e. Cocaine abuse

**30.** A 51-year-old woman presents to the ED after 5 consecutive days of crushing substernal chest pressure that woke her up from sleep in the morning. The pain resolves spontaneously after 20 to 30 minutes. She is an avid rock climber and jogs 5 miles daily. She has never smoked cigarettes and has no family history of coronary disease. In the ED, she experiences another episode of chest pain. An ECG reveals ST-segment elevations and cardiac biomarkers are negative. The pain is relieved with sublingual nitroglycerin. She is admitted to the hospital and diagnostic testing reveals minimal coronary atherosclerotic disease. Which of the following is the most appropriate medication to treat this patient's condition?

a. Aspirin
b. Calcium channel blocker (CCB)
c. β-Blocker
d. $H_2$-Blocker
e. Antidepressant

**31.** A 23-year-old woman who is an elementary school teacher is brought to the ED after syncopizing in her classroom while teaching. Prior to passing out, she describes feeling light-headed and dizzy and next remembers being in the ambulance. There was no evidence of seizure activity. She has no medical problems and does not take any medications. Her father died of a "heart problem" at 32 years of age. She does not smoke or use drugs. BP is 120/70 mm Hg, pulse rate is 71 beats per minute, RR is 14 breaths per minute, and oxygen saturation is 100% on room air. Her physical examination and laboratory results are all normal. A rhythm strip is seen below. Which of the following is the most likely diagnosis?

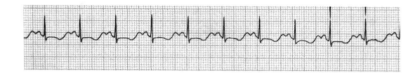

a. Wolff-Parkinson-White syndrome
b. Long QT syndrome
c. Lown-Ganong-Levine syndrome
d. Complete heart block
e. Atrial flutter

**32.** While discussing a case presentation with a medical student, a nearby patient who just returned from getting an ankle radiograph done yells out in pain. You walk over to him and ask what is wrong. He states that since returning from the radiology suite, his automatic implantable cardioverter-defibrillator (AICD) is discharging. You hook him up to the monitor and note that his rhythm is sinus. You observe a third shock while the patient is in sinus rhythm. Which of the following is the most appropriate next step in management?

a. Send the patient back to the radiology suite for another radiograph to desensitize his AICD.
b. Administer pain medication and wait until the device representative arrives at the hospital to power off the AICD.
c. Admit the patient to the telemetry unit to monitor his rhythm and find the cause of his AICD discharge.
d. Place a magnet over the AICD generator to inactivate it and thereby prevent further shocks.
e. Make a small incision over his chest wall and remove the AICD generator and leads.

**33.** A 55-year-old man presents to the ED with chest pain and shortness of breath. His BP is 170/80 mm Hg, HR is 89 beats per minute, and oxygen saturation is 90% on room air. Physical examination reveals crackles midway up both lung fields and a new holosystolic murmur that is loudest at the apex and radiates to the left axilla. ECG reveals ST elevations in the inferior leads. Chest radiograph shows pulmonary edema with a normalsized cardiac silhouette. Which of the following is the most likely cause of the cardiac murmur?

a. Critical aortic stenosis
b. Papillary muscle rupture
c. Pericardial effusion
d. CHF
e. Aortic dissection

**34.** An 82-year-old woman is brought to the ED by her daughter for worsening fatigue, dizziness, and light-headedness. The patient denies chest pain or shortness of breath. She has not started any new medications. Her BP is 140/70 mm Hg, HR is 37 beats per minute, and RR is 15 breaths per minute. An IV is started and blood is drawn. An ECG is seen below. Which of the following is the most appropriate next step in management?

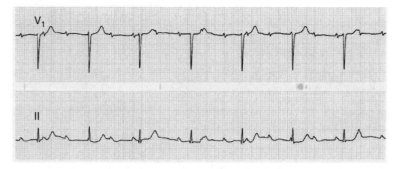

(Reproduced, with permission, from Fuster V et al. Hurst's The Heart. New York, NY: McGraw-Hill, 2004: 904.)

a. Bed rest for the next 48 hours and follow-up with her primary-care physician.
b. Administer aspirin, order a set of cardiac enzymes, and admit to the cardiac care unit (CCU).
c. Place a magnet on her chest to turn off her pacemaker.
d. Admit for Holter monitoring and echocardiogram.
e. Place on a cardiac monitor, place external pacing pads on the patient, and admit to the CCU.

**35.** A 22-year-old man presents to the ED with a history consistent with an acute MI. His ECG reveals ST elevations and his cardiac biomarkers are positive. He has been smoking half a pack of cigarettes per day for the last 3 months. He drinks alcohol when hanging out with his friends. His grandfather died of a heart attack at 80 years of age. The patient does not have hypertension or diabetes mellitus and takes no prescription medications. A recent cholesterol check revealed normal levels of total cholesterol, low-density lipoprotein (LDL), and high-density lipoprotein (HDL). Which of the following is the most likely explanation for his presentation?

a. Cigarette smoking
b. Family history of heart attack at age 80 years
c. Incorrectly placed leads on the ECG
d. Undisclosed cocaine use
e. Alcohol use

**36.** A 29-year-old man is brought to the ED by EMS for a syncopal episode that occurred during a basketball game. A friend states that the patient just dropped to the ground shortly after scoring a basket on a fast break. On examination, you note a prominent systolic ejection murmur along the left sternal border and at the apex. An ECG reveals left ventricular hypertrophy, left atrial enlargement, and septal Q waves. You suspect the diagnosis and ask the patient to perform the Valsalva maneuver while you auscultate his heart. Which of the following is most likely to occur to the intensity of the murmur with this maneuver?

a. Decrease.
b. Increase.
c. Remain unchanged.
d. Disappear.
e. The intensity stays the same, but the heart skips a beat.

**37.** A 57-year-old man complains of chest palpitations and light-headedness for the past hour. Five years ago he underwent a cardiac catheterization with coronary artery stent placement. He smokes half a pack of cigarettes daily and drinks a glass of wine at dinner. His HR is 140 beats per minute, BP is 115/70 mm Hg, and oxygen saturation is 99% on room air. An ECG reveals a wide complex tachycardia at a rate of 140 that is regular in rhythm. An ECG from 6 months ago shows a sinus rhythm at a rate of 80. Which of the following is the most appropriate medication to treat this dysrhythmia?

a. Digoxin
b. Diltiazem
c. Amiodarone
d. Adenosine
e. Bretylium

**38.** A 55-year-old man with hypertension and a one-pack-per-day smoking history presents to the ED complaining of three episodes of severe heavy chest pain this morning that radiated to his left shoulder. In the past, he experienced chest discomfort after walking 20 minutes that resolved with rest. The episodes of chest pain this morning occurred while he was reading the newspaper. His BP is 155/80 mm Hg, HR 76 beats per minute, and RR 15 breaths per minute. He does not have chest pain in the ED. An ECG reveals sinus rhythm with a rate of 72. A troponin I is negative. Which of the following best describes this patient's diagnosis?

a. Variant angina
b. Stable angina
c. Unstable angina
d. Non–ST-elevation MI
e. ST-elevation MI (STEMI)

**39.** A 58-year-old man is brought to the ED for a syncopal episode at dinner. His wife states that he was well until she found him suddenly slumping in the chair and losing consciousness for a minute. The patient recalls having some chest discomfort and shortness of breath prior to the episode. His rhythm strip, obtained by EMS, is shown below. Which of the following best describes these findings?

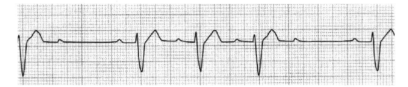

a. Mobitz type I
b. Mobitz type II
c. First-degree atrioventricular (AV) block
d. Atrial flutter with premature ventricular contractions (PVCs)
e. Sinus bradycardia

**40.** As you are examining the patient described in the previous question, he starts to complain of chest discomfort and shortness of breath and has another syncopal episode. His ECG is shown below. Which of the following is the most appropriate next step in management?

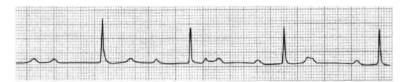

a. Call cardiology consult
b. Cardiovert the patient
c. Administer metoprolol
d. Administer amiodarone
e. Apply transcutaneous pacemaker

# Chest Pain and Cardiac Dysrhythmias

## Answers

**1. The answer is b.** (*Rosen, pp 948-952.*) The patient's presentation is classic for an ACS. He has **multiple risk factors** with T-wave abnormalities on his ECG. The most appropriate initial management includes **placing the patient on a cardiac monitor** to detect dysrhythmias, establish intravenous access, provide supplemental **oxygen**, and administer **aspirin.** If the patient is having active chest pain in the ED, sublingual **nitroglycerin** or **morphine** should be administered until the pain resolves. This decreases wall tension and myocardial oxygen demand. A common mnemonic used is **MONA** (Morphine, Oxygen, Nitroglycerin, Aspirin) greets chest pain patients at the door.

(**a**) Although nitroglycerin is one of the early agents used in ACS, it is prudent to first rule out a right ventricular infarct, which, if present, may lead to hypotension. Thirty percent of inferior myocardial infarctions have an associated right ventricular infarction. Patients with a right ventricular infarction rely on adequate preload to maintain their BP. Nitroglycerin will decrease preload, which will cause a critical drop in BP. Patients with an RV infarct need IV fluids to maintain preload and BP. (**c**) PCI is warranted if the patient's ECG showed ST-segment elevation. (**d**) The patient will require a chest x-ray and most likely receive clopidogrel and heparin; however, this is done only after being on a monitor with oxygen and chewing an aspirin. (**e**) β-Blockers are usually added for tachycardia, hypertension, and persistent pain and only given once the patient is evaluated for contraindications. Relative contraindications to the use of β-blockers include asthma or chronic obstructive lung disease, CHF, and third-trimester pregnancy.

**2. The answer is e.** (*Ouellette, 2011.*) The patient most likely has a **pulmonary thromboembolism (PE)** that embolized from a thrombus in her left calf. The diagnosis of PE is usually made with a CT angiogram, echocardiogram, or a ventilation-perfusion scan. The most common ECG abnormalities in the setting of PE are **tachycardia and nonspecific ST-T–wave**

**abnormalities.** Many other ECG abnormality may appear with equal likelihood, but none are sensitive or specific for PE. If ECG abnormalities are present, they may be suggestive of PE, but the absence of ECG abnormalities has no significant predictive value. Moreover, 25% of patients with proven PE have ECGs that are unchanged from their baseline state.

**(a, b, c, and d)** The finding of $S_1Q_3T_3$ pattern is nonspecific and insensitive in the absence of clinical suspicion for PE. The classic findings of right heart strain and acute cor pulmonale are tall, peaked P waves in lead II (P pulmonale), right-axis deviation, right bundle-branch block, a $S_1Q_3T_3$ pattern, or atrial fibrillation. Unfortunately, only 20% of patients with proven PE have any of these classic ECG abnormalities.

**3. The answer is e.** *(Rosen, pp 1010-1012.)* **Atrial fibrillation (AF)** is a rhythm disturbance of the atria that results in irregular, chaotic, ventricular waveforms. This chaotic activity can lead to reduced cardiac output from a loss of coordinated atrial contractions and a rapid ventricular rate, both of which may limit diastolic filling and stroke volume of the ventricles. Atrial fibrillation may be chronic or paroxysmal, lasting minutes to days. On the ECG, fibrillatory waves are accompanied by an irregular QRS pattern. The main ED treatment for stable atrial fibrillation is **rate control.** This can be accomplished by many agents, but the agent most commonly used is diltiazem, a CCB with excellent AV nodal blocking effects.

**(a)** If the patient was unstable, he should be immediately cardioverted. However, this patient is stable and asymptomatic; therefore, the goal in the ED is rate control. **(b)** Catheterization would be correct if the patient exhibited ST-segment elevations on the ECG. **(c)** If the patient is in atrial fibrillation for greater than 48 hours, he needs to be anticoagulated prior to cardioversion. Coumadin, along with heparin, are agents used for anticoagulation. In general, a patient with stable atrial fibrillation undergoes an echocardiogram to evaluate for thrombus. If there is a thrombus, patients are placed on Coumadin for 2 to 3 weeks and cardioversion takes place when their international normalized ratio (INR) is therapeutic. If no clot is seen on echocardiogram, heparin is administered and cardioversion can take place immediately. **(d)** Amiodarone is also used for rate control in atrial fibrillation; however, it is not a first-line agent and is recommended to be used selectively in patients with a low left ventricular ejection fraction.

**4. The answer is b.** *(Rosen, pp 1620-1625.)* Patients with end-stage renal disease, who require dialysis, are prone to electrolyte disturbances. This patient's clinical picture is consistent with **hyperkalemia**. The ECG can provide valuable clues to the presence of hyperkalemia. As potassium levels rise, **peaked T waves** are the first characteristic manifestation. Further rises are associated with progressive ECG changes, including **loss of P waves and widening of the QRS complex**. Eventually the tracing assumes a **sine-wave pattern**, followed by ventricular fibrillation or asystole.

(a) ECG manifestations of hypokalemia include flattening of T waves, ST-segment depression, and U waves. (c) Hypocalcemia manifests as QT prolongation, whereas hypercalcemia (d) manifests as shortening of the QT interval. (e) There are no classic ECG findings with hyponatremia.

**5. The answer is a.** *(Rosen, pp 393-396.)* The patient presents with a **primary spontaneous pneumothorax (PTX)**, which occurs in individuals without clinically apparent lung disease. In contrast, secondary spontaneous pneumothorax occurs in individuals with underlying lung disease, especially chronic obstructive pulmonary disease (COPD). For otherwise healthy, young patients with a small primary spontaneous PTX (<20% of the hemithorax), observation alone may be appropriate. The intrinsic reabsorption rate is approximately 1% to 2% a day and accelerated with the administration of 100% oxygen. Many physicians **observe these patients for 6 hours** and then **repeat the chest x-ray**. If the repeat chest x-ray shows no increase in the size of the PTX, the patient can be **discharged with follow-up in 24 hours**. Air travel and underwater diving (changes in atmospheric pressure) must be avoided until the PTX completely resolves.

(b) Needle decompression is a temporizing maneuver for patients with suspected tension PTX. (c) Tube thoracostomy is used in secondary spontaneous PTX, trauma PTX, and PTX greater than 20% of the hemithorax. (d) Unless there is a change in his status, the patient does not need to be observed for another 6 hours. (e) A pleurodesis is an operative intervention to prevent recurrence of PTX. It is performed on patients with underlying lung disease.

**6. The answer is d.** *(Rosen, pp 410-413, 1139-1140.)* **Esophageal perforation** (Boerhaave syndrome) is a potentially life-threatening condition that can result from any Valsalva-like maneuver, including childbirth, coughing, and heavy lifting. Alcoholics are at risk as a result of their frequent vomiting. The most common cause of esophageal perforation is from iatrogenic causes, such as a complication from upper endoscopy. The classic physical examination finding is **mediastinal or cervical emphysema**. This is noted by feeling air under the skin on palpation of the chest wall or by a **crunching** sound heard on auscultation, also known as **Hamman sign**. Radiographic signs of pneumomediastinum can be subtle. Lateral displacement of the mediastinal pleura by mediastinal air creates a linear density paralleling the mediastinal contour. On the lateral projection, mediastinal air can be seen in the retrocardiac space.

(a) Aspiration pneumonia is an inflammation of lung parenchyma precipitated by foreign material entering the tracheobronchial tree. Alcoholics are prone to aspiration pneumonia because of ethanol's sedating effect. This causes a decrease in the normal protective airway reflexes. Chest radiograph findings are often delayed with atelectasis typically being the first finding. (b) Alcoholics have a high incidence of pancreatitis and can present with epigastric tenderness; however, they usually do not have mediastinal air on radiography. (c) The physical examination hallmark of acute pericarditis is the friction rub. The rub may be caused by friction between inflamed or scarred visceral and parietal pericardium or may result from friction between the parietal pericardium and adjacent pleura. Aortic dissection (e) usually occurs in patients with chronic hypertension or connective tissue disorders. They should not have Hamman sign.

**7. The answer is c.** (Rosen, pp 1088-1092.) The patient's clinical picture of chronic hypertension, acute-onset tearing chest pain, diastolic murmur of aortic insufficiency, and chest x-ray with a widened mediastinum is consistent with an **aortic dissection**. The preferred study of choice is a **transesophageal echocardiogram (TEE)**, which is highly sensitive. It can be quickly performed at the bedside and does not require radiation or contrast.

(a) ECG changes that are consistent with an aortic dissection are ischemic changes, low-voltage complexes, and electrical alternans. However, this is suggestive but not diagnostic. (b) A TTE is limited in diagnosing aortic dissections because wave transmission is hindered by the overlying sternum. It can be useful to see pericardial fluid as a result of proximal dissection. (d) A CT scan is an excellent study with sensitivities that approach TEEs. It is the study of choice if a TEE is not readily available. However, it requires that the patient leave the ED and receive IV contrast. (e) An MRI has high sensitivity and specificity and has the benefit of identifying an intimal tear. However, the study requires that the patient leave the ED for an extended period of time. Currently, it is most useful for patients with chronic dissections.

**8. The answer is a.** (*Tintinalli, pp 384, 1236-1237.*) Patients with chest pain in the setting of cocaine use should be evaluated for possible myocardial ischemia. Patients suspected of ACS should be managed accordingly with oxygen, nitrates, morphine, aspirin, and benzodiazepines; however, β-adrenergic antagonist therapy is contraindicated. If β-adrenergic receptors are antagonized, α-adrenergic receptors are left unopposed and available for increased stimulation by cocaine. This may worsen into coronary and peripheral vasoconstriction, hypertension, and possibly ischemia. Therefore, benzodiazepines, which decrease central sympathetic outflow, are the cornerstone in treatment to relieve cocaine-related chest pain.

(b) Diltiazem, a CCB, can be used in patients with cocaine-related chest pain. It is used to lower HR. (c) Aspirin should be administered to all patients with chest pain, unless there is a contraindication. In patients with cocaine-related chest pain who also seize, aspirin may be held until a CT scan is performed to rule out an intracranial bleed. (d) Lorazepam, a benzodiazepine, is an excellent medication to use in cocaine-related chest pain as it reduces their sympathetic drive leading to a reduction in BP and HR. (e) Nitroglycerin should be administered to these patients if they have chest pain. Nitrates dilate the coronary arteries, increasing blood flow to the myocardium.

**9. The answer is a.** (*Tintinalli, pp 1042-1046.*) The incidence of endocarditis in the intravenous drug user (IVDU) is estimated to be 40 times that of the general population. Unlike the general population, endocarditis in IVDUs is typically right-sided with the majority of cases involving the tricuspid valve. Patients with IVDU-related endocarditis usually have no evidence of prior valve damage. Patients may present with fever, cardiac murmur, cough, pleuritic chest pain, and hemoptysis. Right-sided murmurs, which vary with respiration, are typically pathologic and more specific for the diagnosis. In patients with right-sided endocarditis and septic pulmonary emboli, pulmonary complaints, infiltrates on chest radiographs, and moderate hypoxia have been described in greater than 33% of patients; these symptoms and signs may mislead the physician to identify the lung as the primary source of infection. Blood cultures will be positive in more than 98% of IVDU-related endocarditis patients if 3 to 5 sets are obtained. Diagnosis generally requires microbial isolation from a blood culture or to demonstrate typical lesions on echocardiography. TTE is the most sensitive imaging modality for demonstrating vegetations and tricuspid valve involvement in IVDU-related endocarditis. Initial antibiotic treatment should be directed against *Staphylococcus aureus* and *Streptococcus* species.

(**b**) Mononucleosis presents with fever, sore throat, and lymphadenopathy. Patients may also have an enlarged spleen, which is more prone to trauma. However, mononucleosis does not cause a heart murmur or patchy infiltrates on chest radiograph. (**c**) Pericarditis can present with fever and chest pain, and NSAIDs are used for treatment. However, it does not cause valvular abnormalities leading to a murmur and pulmonary infiltrates. (**d**) Tuberculosis generally does not present with chest pain or cardiac murmur. (**e**) In Lyme disease, patients frequently have a bull's eye rash called **erythema migrans**. Although Lyme disease does not lead to valvular abnormalities, patients may present with cardiac conduction abnormalities, the most worrisome being complete heart block. Patients typically have risk factors for tick exposure, such as hiking in a wooded area.

**10. The answer is d.** (*Rosen, pp 956-958.*) The standard 12-lead ECG is the single best test to identify patients with acute MI upon presentation in the ED. It is important to identify the anatomic location of an acute MI to estimate the amount of endangered myocardium. The right coronary artery (RCA) supplies the AV node and inferior wall of the left ventricle in 90% of patients. **Inferior wall MIs** are characterized by **ST elevation in at least two of the inferior leads (II, III, aVF)**. Reciprocal ST changes (eg, ST depression) in the anterior precordial leads ($V_1$-$V_4$) in the setting of an inferior wall acute MI predict a larger infarct distribution, an increased severity of underlying coronary artery disease (CAD), more severe pump failure, and increased mortality. In general, the more elevated the ST segments and the more ST segments that are elevated, the more extensive the injury.

(**a**) The anteroseptal wall of the heart is supplied by the left anterior descending coronary artery (LAD). An acute MI is identified by ST elevation in leads $V_1$, $V_2$, and $V_3$. (**b**) The anterior wall of the heart is also supplied by the LAD and an infarct exhibits ST elevations in leads $V_2$, $V_3$, and $V_4$. (**c**) The lateral wall of the heart is supplied by the left circumflex coronary artery (LCA) and an infarct exhibits ST elevations in leads I, aVL, $V_5$, and $V_6$. (**e**) A posterior MI refers to the posterior wall of the left ventricle. It occurs in 15% to 20% of all MIs and usually in conjunction with inferior or lateral infarction. The following figure summarizes the distribution.

| I | aVR | V₁ | V₄ |
|---|---|---|---|
| **Lateral** | | **Septal** | **Anterior** |
| II | aVL | V₂ | V₅ |
| **Inferior** | **High Lateral** | **Septal** | **Lateral** |
| III | aVF | V₃ | V₆ |
| **Inferior** | **Inferior** | **Anterior** | **Lateral** |

**11. The answer is c.** *(Flowers, 2009.)* The patient has **costochondritis**, an inflammatory process of the costochondral or costosternal joints that causes **localized pain and tenderness**. Any of the seven costochondral junctions may be affected, and more than one site is affected in 90% of cases. The second to fifth costochondral junctions are most commonly involved. In contrast to myocardial ischemia or infarction, costochondritis is a benign cause of chest pain, often with an insidious onset, and is an important consideration in the differential diagnosis for chest pain. Of note, 5% to 7% of patients with cardiac ischemia also have chest wall tenderness. The onset is often insidious. Chest wall pain with a history of repeated minor trauma or unaccustomed activity (eg, painting, moving furniture) is common. The goal of therapy is to reduce inflammation. **NSAIDs** are typically prescribed.

(a) The patient has no cardiac risk factors, and his ECG and chest radiograph are normal. (b) This is a regime for ACS. (d) This is not a first-line therapy. Corticosteroid injection may lead to bone degradation. (e) The patient does not need to be observed.

**12. The answer is e.** *(Tintinalli, pp 138-140.)* **WPW syndrome** is caused by an **accessory electrical pathway (ie, bundle of Kent)** between the atria and ventricles. The primary significance of WPW syndrome is that it predisposes the individual to the development of reentry tachycardias. The classic ECG findings include a **short PR interval (< 120 milliseconds), widened QRS interval (> 100 milliseconds)**, and a **delta wave** (slurred upstroke at the beginning of the QRS). When conduction occurs antero-grade down the AV node and then retrograde up the accessory pathway (orthodromic), the ECG will appear normal. When the impulse occurs anterograde down the accessory pathway and retrograde up the AV node (antidromic), the QRS complex will be wide. In the presence of antidromic conduction (conduction first through the bypass tract), the normal slowing effect of the AV node is lost and rapid ventricular response rates (>200 beats per minute) can occur. The most dangerous circumstance is in atrial fibril-lation where impulses occur at a rate greater than 300 beats per minute. This can quickly lead to ventricular fibrillation. Procainamide is the drug most commonly associated with the acute treatment of WPW.

(a) Ventricular tachycardia may be difficult to distinguish from WPW. In a young patient with classic ECG findings, however, WPW is more likely. Nonetheless, it is prudent to avoid AV nodal blocking agents in any wide complex tachycardia. (b) Atrial flutter will have flutter waves that take on a sawtooth pattern. (c) Atrial fibrillation is an irregular rhythm. (d) LGL syndrome is classified as a preexcitation syndrome (similar to WPW) in which a bypass tract is present. LGL is characterized by an individual who is prone to tachydysrhythmias and has a PR interval less than 120 millisec-onds. Unlike WPW, the QRS complex is normal (no delta wave).

**13. The answer is a.** (*Rosen, pp 1620-1622.*) The patient has **life-threatening hyperkalemia**. His ECG shows a wide QRS complex, peaked T waves, and no P waves. At any moment the patient's rhythm can go into ventric-ular fibrillation or asystole. There are many symptoms of hyperkalemia that are often difficult to discern from those of the primary condition that precipitated the hyperkalemia. Patients may begin with lethargy and weakness and progress to paralysis and areflexia. If there are no ECG abnormalities in a patient with hyperkalemia, treatment can start with potassium-binding resins (eg, Kayexalate). However, this patient requires immediate administration of calcium because he has an unstable cardiac rhythm. **Calcium (gluconate or chloride)** antagonizes the effects of potassium in the myocardium and briefly stabilizes the cardiac mem-brane. However, calcium will not lower the potassium level; in order to promote transcellular shifts and removal from the body, other measures will also be required.

(b) Insulin works to redistribute excess potassium from the extra-cellular to the intracellular compartment, thereby lowering the serum concentration transiently. Dextrose is given to prevent hypoglycemia.

Sodium polystyrene sulfonate (Kayexalate) is a definitive treatment for hyperkalemia because it removes potassium from the body. However, the process is not immediate and takes between 30 minutes and 2 hours for the results to show. The other definitive treatment for hyperkalemia is dialysis. (c) Aspirin should be administered to all patients who are having coronary-related chest pain. Individuals with an ECG consistent with ST-elevation MI should be taken to the catheterization laboratory. (d) Though this patient presents with global weakness, his ECG is consistent with life-threatening hyperkalemia and needs to be addressed emergently. A head CT scan is not required at this time. (e) Checking urine ketones is an important step in this individual's workup to evaluate for diabetic ketoacidosis. However, it should wait until the patient is stabilized.

**14. The answer is a.** *(Rosen, pp 1137-1139.)* The patient most likely has a **partial or complete obstruction in his lower esophagus** secondary to the steak he ate. This usually occurs near the **gastroesophageal junction**. Administration of **glucagon** may cause enough **relaxation of the esophageal smooth muscle** to allow passage of the bolus in approximately 50% of patients. Its relaxant effect is limited to smooth muscle and therefore can only be used for impactions in the lower esophagus. If glucagon does not work, definitive management is with **endoscopy**.

Meat tenderizer **(b)**, once used for this situation, is now contraindicated secondary to the possibility of perforation as a result of its proteolytic effect on an inflamed esophageal mucosa. Syrup of ipecac **(c)** is used rarely in situations of toxic ingestions. Also, vomiting should be avoided in our patient to avoid risk of esophageal perforation. The Heimlich maneuver **(d)** can be a lifesaving procedure but is not necessary in this patient who is not in respiratory distress. Respiratory compromise may occur when a foreign body lodges in the oropharynx, proximal esophagus, or is large enough that it impinges on the trachea. Laparotomy **(e)** is not indicated for esophageal perforations.

**15. The answer is e.** *(Tintinalli, pp 376-377.)* Thrombolytic therapy (clotbusters) can be administered to patients having an acute ST-elevation MI that is within 12 hours from symptom onset. Contraindications to fibrinolytic therapy are those that increase the risk of hemorrhage. The most catastrophic complication is intracranial hemorrhage. Absolute contraindications include:

- Previous hemorrhagic stroke
- Known intracranial neoplasm
- Active internal bleeding (excluding menses)
- Suspected aortic dissection or pericarditis

(a) SBP greater than 180 mm Hg is a relative contraindication. However, if thrombolytics are going to be administered and the patient's SBP is greater than 180 mm Hg, antihypertensive medication can be administered to lower the SBP to below 180 mm Hg. (b) Anticoagulation is a relative contraindication. Many patients who suffer from an ST-elevation MI are on aspirin and other antiplatelet and anticoagulant therapies. (c) Major surgery less than 3 weeks prior to administration of thrombolytics is a relative contraindication. (d) Active peptic ulcer disease is a relative contraindication.

**16. The answer is e.** *(Rosen, pp 1010-1012.)* This patient is hypotensive and exhibits signs and symptoms of heart failure (dyspnea, fatigue, respiratory crackles, and chest pain) and is in atrial fibrillation (irregular, narrow complex). Any patient with **unstable vital signs** with a tachydysrhythmia should receive a dose of sedation and undergo **synchronized cardioversion** starting at 100 J.

(a) Diltiazem, a CCB, is used as a rate-control agent for patients in atrial fibrillation. If the patient was not hypotensive or exhibiting signs of heart failure, diltiazem is used to slow the ventricular response. (b) Metoprolol is sometimes used to control ventricular rate in atrial fibrillation; however, it is contraindicated in patients with acute heart failure. In addition, it has a greater negative inotropic effect than CCBs, thereby causing hypotension more often. (c) Digitalis is another option to control the ventricular response in atrial fibrillation; however, its relatively slow onset (ie, hours) precludes it from use in the acute setting. (d) Coumadin is an anticoagulant that is administered to a select group of patients in chronic atrial fibrillation to prevent thrombus formation. It is also used to anticoagulate stable patients who have been in atrial fibrillation for longer than 48 hours and are going to be pharmacologically or electrically cardioverted. Cardioversion of atrial fibrillation (if > 48 hours) carries the risk of thromboembolism.

**17. The answer is d.** *(Rosen, pp 1046-1048.)* This patient has **decompensated CHF with pulmonary edema**. **Nitroglycerin** is the most effective and most rapid means of **reducing preload** in a patient with CHF. Nitrates decrease myocardial preload and, to a lesser extent, afterload. Nitrates increase venous capacitance, including venous pooling, which decreases preload and myocardial oxygen demand. It is most beneficial when the patient who presents with CHF is also hypertensive. It is administered sublingually, intravenously, or transdermally.

(a) Metoprolol, a β-blocker is contraindicated in acute decompensated heart failure. (b) Morphine sulfate reduces pulmonary congestion through a central sympatholytic effect that causes peripheral vasodilation. This decreases central venous return and reduces preload. However, morphine sulfate is a respiratory depressant and may lead to hypoventilation. It does not act as rapidly or as effectively as nitroglycerin in preload reduction. (c) Nitroprusside is a mixed venous and arteriolar dilator; it reduces both pre- and afterload. It can be used in patients with acute pulmonary edema (APE) but is typically reserved for individuals with an SBP greater than 100 mm Hg who fail to respond to adequate doses of standard preload reducers (eg, nitroglycerin). (e) This patient is hypoxic with an oxygen saturation of 85% and requires supplemental oxygen. In the acute setting, this patient should be placed on a nonrebreather with 100% oxygen flowing through the mask.

**18. The answer is e.** *(Rosen, p 998.)* The patient's ECG shows a sinus rhythm at a rate of 70 with **first-degree heart block.** First-degree heart block is defined as prolonged conduction of atrial impulses without the loss of any impulse. On an ECG this translates to a **PR interval greater than 200 milliseconds** with a narrow QRS complex (<120 milliseconds). First-degree heart block is often a normal variant without clinical significance, occurring in 1% to 2% of healthy young adults. This variant requires no specific treatment.

(a) A pacemaker is considered in patients with a second-degree type II AV block or third-degree complete heart block. (b) An observation period is not required, as the prolonged PR interval is a normal variant in this individual. (c) Aspirin and cardiac biomarkers are sent for patients thought to have ACS. (d) There is no evidence that the ECG leads are placed incorrectly.

**19. The answer is d.** *(Tintinalli, pp 365-367.)* Serum cardiac markers are used to confirm or exclude myocardial cell death and are considered the gold standard for the diagnosis of MI. While there are many markers currently used; the most sensitive and specific markers are **troponin I** and **T.**

A rise in these levels, as seen in the figure, is diagnostic for an acute MI. Troponin levels **rise within 3 to 6 hours of chest pain onset, peak at 12 to 24 hours**, and **remain elevated for 7 to 10 days.**

(a) Myoglobin is found in both skeletal and cardiac muscle and released into the bloodstream when there is muscle cell death. It tends to rise within 1 to 2 hours of injury, peaks in 4 to 6 hours, and returns to baseline in 24 hours. (b) CK is an enzyme found in skeletal and cardiac muscle. Following acute MI, increases in serum CK are detectable within 3 to 8 hours with a peak at 12 to 24 hours after injury and normalize within 3 to 4 days. (c) CK-MB is an isoenzyme found in cardiac muscle and released into the bloodstream upon cell death. It rises 4 to 6 hours after acute MI, peaks in 12 to 36 hours, and returns to normal within 3 to 4 days. (e) LDH is an enzyme found in muscle and rises 12 hours after acute MI, peaks at 24 to 48 hours, and returns to normal at 10 to 14 days.

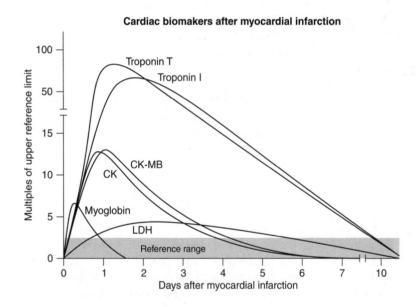

**Cardiac biomakers after myocardial infarction**

**20. The answer is d.** *(Tintinalli, pp 136-140.)* **Narrow-complex tachycardias** are defined as rhythms with a QRS complex duration less than 100 milliseconds and a ventricular rate greater than 100 beats per minute. Although virtually all narrow-complex tachydysrhythmias originate from a focus above the ventricles, the term **supraventricular tachycardia (SVT)** is conventionally used to denote those rhythms aside from sinus tachycardia, atrial tachycardia, atrial fibrillation, and atrial flutter (eg, atrioventricular nodal reentry tachycardia and atrioventricular reentry tachycardia). **Adenosine**, an ultrashort-acting AV nodal blocking agent, is typically used to treat SVTs. Because it is so fast-acting, it must be delivered through a large vein (eg, the antecubital fossa) with a rapid intravenous fluid bolus. In addition to adenosine, **maneuvers that increase vagal tone** have been shown to slow conduction through the AV node. Some of these maneuvers include carotid sinus massage, Valsalva maneuver, and facial immersion in cold water.

. **(a)** Digoxin is vagotonic, but it has a slow onset that may take several hours or more to work. It should be avoided if cardioversion is being considered because it can lead to a fatal dysrhythmia. **(b and c)** Lidocaine and amiodarone are effective in treating narrow-complex tachycardias, they are agents generally used to treat wide-complex or ventricular tachycardias. **(e)** Bretylium is no longer available in the United States as it has a poor safety profile.

**21. The answer is e.** *(Rosen, pp 956, 971-982.)* This ECG depicts an **acute anterior wall myocardial infarction with ST elevations in leads $V_1$ to $V_4$**. The patient is also hypotensive secondary to **cardiogenic shock**. The preferred treatment for an ST-elevation MI is primary PCI (eg, angioplasty, coronary stent). It has shown to improve long-term mortality over **(d)** thrombolytic therapy. As a stabilizing measure, the patient may require an intra-aortic balloon pump. This is a mechanical device that is used to decrease myocardial oxygen demand while at the same time increasing cardiac output. By increasing cardiac output, it also increases coronary blood flow and therefore myocardial oxygen delivery. It is inserted through the femoral artery.

**(a)** β-Blockers and CCBs are contraindicated in patients who are hypotensive. **(b)** The patient does not have a dysrhythmia and therefore should not be cardioverted. **(c)** Calcium gluconate is the agent of choice for individuals with ECG signs of potassium toxicity. It does not have a role in the management of acute MI.

**22. The answer is c.** *(Tintinalli, p 380.)* **Sildenafil (Viagra)** is a selective cyclic guanosine monophosphate (GMP) inhibitor that results in smooth-muscle relaxation and vasodilation by the release of nitric oxide. It is used in men for erectile dysfunction. It is **contraindicated to administer nitro-glycerin** to individuals who have taken sildenafil in the previous 24 hours. The combination of nitroglycerin and sildenafil can lead to hypotension and death. If nitrates are coadministered with sildenafil, the patient should be closely monitored for hypotension. Fluid resuscitation and pressor agents may be needed to restore BP.

(a) Aspirin is contraindicated in individuals with an anaphylactic allergy or active bleed. (b) Heparin is contraindicated in individuals with heparin-induced thrombocytopenia, and those who are actively bleeding. (d) Metoprolol is contraindicated in hypotensive individuals. (e) Morphine sulfate is contraindicated in patients with respiratory depression.

**23. The answer is b.** *(Rosen, pp 1054-1055.)* The classic presentation of **pericarditis** includes **chest pain, a pericardial friction rub, and ECG abnormalities.** A prodrome of fever and myalgias may occur. Pericarditis chest pain is usually substernal and varies with respiration. It is typically **relieved by sitting forward and worsened by lying down or swallowing.** The physical examination hallmark of acute pericarditis is the **pericardial friction rub.** The earliest ECG changes are seen in the first few hours to days of illness and include **diffuse ST-segment elevation** seen in leads I, II, III, aVL, aVF, and $V_2$ to $V_6$. Most patients with acute pericarditis will have concurrent **PR-segment depression.** The mainstay of treatment includes supportive care with **anti-inflammatory** medications (eg, NSAIDs). The use of corticosteroids is controversial. An echocardiogram should be performed to rule out a pericardial effusion and tamponade.

(a) PE can present with substernal chest pain that is sharp in nature and worse with inspiration. However, the patient does not exhibit any risk factors for a PE (c and d). It is very important to be able to differentiate an acute MI from acute pericarditis because thrombolytic therapy is contraindicated in pericarditis as it may precipitate hemorrhagic tamponade. Unlike the ECG in an acute MI, the ST elevations in early pericarditis are concave upward rather than convex upward. Subsequent tracings do not evolve through a typical MI pattern and Q waves do not appear. (e) Antibiotics are not routinely used to treat pericarditis.

**24. The answer is a.** *(Rosen, pp 953-956.)* The earliest ECG finding resulting from an AMI is the **hyperacute T wave**, which may appear minutes after the interruption of blood flow. The hyperacute T wave, which is short-lived, evolves to progressive **elevation of ST segments.** In general,

Q **waves** represent established myocardial necrosis and usually develop within 8 to 12 hours after an ST-elevation MI, though they may be noted as early as 1 to 2 hours after the onset of complete coronary occlusion.

**25. The answer is d.** *(Rosen, pp 1045-1049.)* The patient has acute **CHF exacerbation** with **APE.** Although not always apparent at presentation, it is important to find the cause of the exacerbation. This patient, for instance, has been noncompliant with his medications. Treatment begins by assessing the airway, breathing, and circulation (ABCs). Initial stabilization is aimed at maintaining airway control and adequate ventilation. Preload and afterload reduction is integral with **nitroglycerin** being the agent of choice if the patient is not hypotensive. Volume reduction with **diuretics** is also critical to lower BP and cardiac-filling pressures. **Noninvasive airway techniques (eg, bilevel positive airways pressure [BiPAP], continuous positive airway pressure [CPAP])** also aid in improving oxygen exchange, reducing the work of breathing, and decreasing left ventricular preload and afterload by raising intrathoracic pressure in the compromised but not agonal APE patients.

(**a**) It is important to first address the ABCs. If infection is thought to be the cause, obtaining a CBC and blood cultures and starting antibiotics should be performed after stabilization. (**b**) A chest x-ray is valuable, but initial stabilization takes priority. (**c**) Oxygen via nasal cannula is not sufficient for this patient who is hypoxic and tachypneic. If you are suspicious for ACS causing the CHF exacerbation, aspirin should be administered. (**e**) At this time, the patient does not require invasive airway control. If medication and noninvasive techniques fail and the patient's hypoxia worsens, endotracheal intubation may be necessary.

**26. The answer is c.** *(Tintinalli, pp 430-432.)* Risk factors for venous thromboembolism were first described by Virchow triad: **hypercoagulability, stasis, and endothelial injury**. Hypercoagulability can be broadly classified into malignancy-related or nonmalignancy-related. Malignancies of primary adenocarcinoma or brain malignancy are the most likely to cause thrombosis. Some causes of nonmalignancy-related thrombosis are estrogen use, pregnancy, antiphospholipid syndromes, factor V Leiden mutation, and protein C and S deficiencies. Immobility such as paralysis, debilitating diseases, or recent surgery or trauma also place patients at risk.

Another useful criteria in the Pulmonary Embolism Rule-out Criteria (PERC). If the patient is low-risk and meets criteria, there is less than a

2% risk that the patient has a PE and no further workup is needed. The criteria are

Age < 50
Pulse < 100 beats per minutes
$SaO_2 > 94\%$
No unilateral leg swelling
No hemoptysis
No recent trauma or surgery
No prior deep venous thrombosis (DVT) or PE
No hormone use

**27. The answer is c.** *(Tintinalli, pp 361-367.)* The patient's presentation is concerning for a cardiac cause of his chest pain. Chest pain radiating to the left arm that is associated with shortness of breath is a classic presentation of ACS. On arrival to the ED, the patient should be placed on a monitor, receive oxygen by nasal cannula, have an IV placed and blood sent to the laboratory, and an ECG performed. Any abnormalities in his vital signs should also be addressed. Serum cardiac markers are useful in detecting MI. Troponins T and I appear in the serum within 6 hours of symptom onset and remain elevated for 1 to 2 weeks. **Troponin I** is the **most specific cardiac marker** available (almost 100%) and **peaks between 12 and 18 hours.** However, the disposition of patients with suspected ACS should be based on the clinical examination and not the cardiac enzymes. Initial determination of these markers has a low sensitivity for detecting ischemia and cannot be used to reliably diagnose or exclude the presence of an ACS.

The ECG is the most important diagnostic test for assessing patients with suspected ACS. However, the initial ECG is diagnostic in only 25% to 50% of patients presenting with an acute MI. Therefore, a normal ECG **(a)** at presentation is not sufficient to rule out an acute MI. Detection of cardiac markers requires that sufficient myocardial cell damage has occurred and that enough time has passed for these markers to be released into the serum and subsequently detected. One set of cardiac enzymes **(b)** is typically insufficient to exclude the diagnosis of acute MI. It is well known that relief of symptoms after the administration of antacids or nitroglycerin **(d)** does not rule out ACS. Epigastric discomfort, indigestion, or nausea and vomiting **(e)** may be the only complaint in patients, particularly women, elderly, and diabetics with ACS. In addition, patients with an inferior wall MI often present this way.

**28. The answer is b.** *(Rosen, pp 973-977.)* **Aspirin** is an antiplatelet agent that should be administered early to all patients suspected of having an ACS, unless there is a contraindication. The ISIS-2 trial provides the strongest evidence that aspirin **independently reduces the mortality** of patients with acute MI. **(a)** Nitroglycerin provides benefit to patients with ACS by reducing preload and dilating coronary arteries. However, there is no mortality benefit with its use. **(c)** Unfractionated heparin acts indirectly to inhibit thrombin, preventing the conversion of fibrinogen to fibrin and thus inhibiting clot propagation. Heparin has not shown to have a mortality benefit. **(d)** Routine use of lidocaine as prophylaxis for ventricular arrhythmias in patients who have experienced an acute MI has been shown to increase mortality rates. **(e)** Use of CCBs in the acute setting has come into question, with some trials showing increased adverse effects.

**29. The answer is c.** *(Rosen, pp 1061-1063.)* The patient has **myocarditis.** The **enteroviruses**, especially the **coxsackievirus B**, predominate as causative agents in the United States. Coxsackie B virus usually causes infection during the summer months. Some other causes of myocarditis include adenovirus, influenza, human immunodeficiency virus (HIV), *Mycoplasma*, *Trypanosoma cruzi*, and steroid abuse. **Flu-like complaints**, such as fatigue, myalgias, nausea, vomiting, diarrhea, and fever, are usually the earliest symptoms and signs of myocarditis. **Tachycardia is common and can be disproportionate to the patient's temperature (ie, HR faster than what is expected).** This may be the only clue that something more serious than a simple viral illness exists. Approximately 12% of patients also complain of chest pain. Cardiac enzymes may be elevated and the CBC and erythrocyte sedimentation rate (ESR) are nonspecific. **(a)** *Streptococcus viridans* is a common cause of acute bacterial endocarditis, an infection of a cardiac valve. **(b)** The influenza virus rarely causes myocarditis. It is more commonly associated with myalgias, cough, diarrhea, and headache. The young and old are populations are greatest risk for pulmonary complications. **(d)** Myocarditis can masquerade as an acute MI because patients with either may have severe chest pain, ECG changes, elevated cardiac enzymes, and heart failure. Patients with myocarditis are usually young and have few risk factors for CAD. **(e)** Cocaine use can cause chest pain, tachycardia, and even a myocardial infarction. It does not lead to flu-like symptoms.

**30. The answer is b.** (*Wang, 2011.*) The patient's clinical presentation is consistent with **Prinzmetal** or **variant angina.** This condition is caused by focal **coronary artery vasospasm.** It **occurs at rest** and exhibits a **circadian pattern,** with most episodes occurring in the early hours of the morning. The pain commonly is severe. Distinguishing unstable angina related to coronary atherosclerosis from variant angina may be difficult and requires special investigations, including coronary angiography. Patients may also exhibit ST elevations on their ECGs. Nitrates and CCBs are the mainstays of medical therapy for variant angina. Nitroglycerin effectively treats episodes of angina and myocardial ischemia within minutes of administration, and the long-acting nitrate preparations reduce the frequency of recurrent events. CCBs effectively prevent coronary vasospasm and variant angina, and they should be administered in lieu of β-blockers.

(a) Aspirin is an antiplatelet agent that helps reduce progression of plaque formation in the coronary arteries. Aspirin will not treat the vasospasm that is responsible for variant angina. (c) β-Blockers can be beneficial in patients with fixed coronary artery stenosis and exertional angina. However, for variant angina, nonselective β-blockers may be detrimental in some patients because blockade of the β-receptors, which mediate vasodilation, allows unopposed β-receptor–mediated coronary vasoconstriction to occur, thus possibly causing an actual worsening of symptoms (d) $H_2$-blockers are used to treat acid reflux symptoms. (e) The etiology of the patient's symptoms will not be relieved by an antidepressant.

**31. The answer is b.** (*Sovari, 2010.*) **Long QT syndrome (LQTS)** is a **congenital disorder** characterized by a prolongation of the QT interval on ECG and a propensity to ventricular tachydysrhythmias, which may lead to syncope, cardiac arrest, or sudden death in otherwise healthy individuals. The QT interval on the ECG, measured from the beginning of the QRS complex to the end of the T wave, represents the duration of activation and recovery of the ventricular myocardium. In general, HR corrected QTc values above 440 milliseconds are considered abnormal. LQTS has been recognized as the **Romano-Ward syndrome** (ie, familial occurrence with autosomal dominant inheritance, QT prolongation, and ventricular tachydysrhythmias) or the **Jervell and Lang-Nielsen syndrome** (ie, familial occurrence with autosomal recessive inheritance, congenital deafness, QT prolongation, and ventricular arrhythmias). Patients with LQTS usually are diagnosed after a cardiac event (eg, syncope, cardiac arrest) already has occurred. In some situations, LQTS is diagnosed after sudden death in family members. Some individuals are diagnosed with LQTS based on an ECG showing QT prolongation. β-Blockers are drugs of choice for patients with LQTS. The protective effect of β-blockers is related to their adrenergic blockade diminishing the risk of cardiac arrhythmias. Implantation of **cardioverter-defibrillators** appears to be the most effective therapy for high-risk patients.

(a) WPW syndrome is characterized by a shortened PR interval (< 120 milliseconds), a slurred upstroke of the QRS complex (delta wave), and a wide QRS complex (> 120 milliseconds). It is caused by an accessory pathway (bundle of Kent) that predisposes individuals to tachydysrhythmias. (c) LGL syndrome is classified as a preexcitation syndrome (similar to WPW) in which a bypass tract is present. LGL is characterized by an individual who is prone to tachydysrhythmias and has a PR interval less than 120 milliseconds. Unlike WPW, the QRS complex is normal (no delta wave). (d) Complete heart block is characterized by the absent conduction of all atrial impulses resulting in complete electrical and mechanical AV dissociation. (e) Atrial flutter is distinguished by a sawtooth pattern seen on ECG. It is typically a transitional rhythm between sinus rhythm and atrial fibrillation.

**32. The answer is d.** (*Tintinalli, pp 244-246.*) Automatic implantable cardioverter-defibrillators (AICD) are placed in patients who are at high risk for fatal dysrhythmias (eg, ventricular tachycardia and fibrillation) and sudden death. In these patients, AICDs decrease the risk of sudden death from approximately 40% per year to less than 2% per year. Occasionally, it may become necessary to temporarily deactivate an AICD, as in the case of inappropriate shock in the setting of a stable rhythm (such as seen with the patient in question). The patient in this scenario is receiving a shock while he is in sinus rhythm. Some potential causes of inappropriate shock delivery include false sensing of SVTs, muscular activity (eg, shivering), sensing T waves as QRS complexes, unsustained tachydysrhythmias, and component failure. AICDs are generally inactivated by **placing a magnet over the AICD generator**. Although, there is some variability depending on the generation of the AICD, most EDs have a special donut magnet that is reserved for this function. If the patient subsequently experiences a dysrhythmia in the setting of having his or her defibrillator tuned off, the physician should use the bedside defibrillator to treat the patient.

Sending the patient back to the radiology suite (**a**) will not temporarily turn off the AICD. However, radiographs are important in detecting AICD lead fractures. Most patients carry a manufacturer card and it is often possible to contact the AICD company. However, it is not appropriate to wait for a representative (**b**) to arrive at the hospital to deactivate the AICD. (**c**) The patient will require that his AICD be interrogated to confirm that he was not having runs of a shockable rhythm. Either a cardiologist or company representative has the ability to do this. However, it is ill advised to let the AICD inappropriately deliver shocks to the patient while you administer pain medication. The AICD should not be removed (**e**) from the chest wall in the ED. If this procedure is required (if the device was a source of infection), it should be performed by a cardiothoracic surgeon in the operating room.

**33. The answer is b.** *(Rosen, pp 1072-1074.)* The patient's presentation is consistent with **acute mitral valve regurgitation** because of a **ruptured papillary muscle** in the setting of an AMI. Patients usually present with **pulmonary edema in the setting of an AMI.** Chest x-ray characteristically reveals pulmonary edema with a normal heart size. The characteristic murmur of mitral regurgitation is a **holosystolic murmur that is loudest at the apex.**

(**a**) Critical aortic stenosis produces a loud systolic murmur that is best heard at the second right intercostal space and radiates to the carotids. (**c**) The classic finding of a pericardial effusion is a pericardial friction rub. (**d**) CHF does not cause a murmur but rather an extra heart sound ($S_3$) from fluid overload. (**e**) Aortic dissection is associated with a murmur of aortic insufficiency.

**34. The answer is e.** *(Roberts and Hedges, pp 269-271.)* The patient's ECG reveals **third-degree complete heart block.** It is a disorder of the cardiac-conduction system, where there is no conduction through the AV node. This may occur secondary to MI, drug intoxication, infection, or infiltrative diseases. On the ECG complete heart block is represented by QRS complexes being conducted at their own rate and independent of the P waves. Individuals with second-degree type II or third-degree complete heart block are considered unstable. **External pacing pads** should be placed on them, followed by a transvenous pacer if their BP is unstable. They may require a permanent pacemaker for irreversible complete heart block.

(a) Clearly this patient has an unstable rhythm and should not be discharged home. (b) The patient should receive aspirin and have cardiac biomarkers obtained; however, the ABCs must be followed and the patient's rhythm is currently unstable. (c) Placement of the magnet over the pacemaker turns off the sensing function of the pacemaker and temporarily converts the pacemaker from the demand mode to a fixed-rate mode at a rate typically of 70. This assesses whether the pacing function is intact and the pacing stimulus can capture the myocardium. There is no evidence in this patient's medical history that she has a pacemaker. (d) Holter monitoring and echocardiogram are generally used to continuously monitor a patient's rhythm and cardiac function. This patient will likely undergo rhythm- and function-assessment as an inpatient.

**35. The answer is d.** *(Burnett, 2010.)* Often, young people are afraid to disclose a history of drug use. **Cocaine** is well known to cause **acute MI in young**, otherwise healthy individuals. Patients with cocaine-related MI often have fixed atherosclerotic lesions. Although these lesions may themselves be of clinical significance, cocaine-induced elevations in pulse and BP increase myocardial work. The additional metabolic requirements that result may convert an asymptomatic obstruction into one of clinical significance. Cocaine use combined with ethanol consumption produces cocaethylene, a longer-acting and more toxic by-product.

(a) Although cigarette smoking is a major risk factor for CAD, this individual would not develop enough plaque after only 3 months. The patient has no other cardiac risk factors. He puts himself at much greater risk if he continues to smoke cigarettes. (b) If his grandfather or father had a heart attack at age 40 or younger, there would be concern about his family history. A heart attack in a related family member at age 80 is not a risk factor. (c) The patient's cardiac biomarkers are also positive and consistent with the ECG. (e) Alcohol use at this age will not lead to an acute MI.

**36. The answer is b.** *(Tintinalli, pp 425-426.)* The patient has **hypertrophic cardiomyopathy**, which is characterized by left ventricular hypertrophy without associated ventricular dilation. The hypertrophy is usually asymmetric, involving the septum to a greater extent than the free wall. Patients are at increased risk of dysrhythmias and sudden death. Syncope is usually exertion-related and is caused by a dysrhythmia or a sudden decrease in cardiac output. The murmur associated with hypertrophic cardiomyopathy is a prominent **systolic ejection murmur** heard along the left sternal boarder and at the apex with radiation to the axilla. The murmur is a result of LV outflow obstruction and mitral regurgitation. It is **increased** with maneuvers that decrease left ventricular end-diastolic volume, such as the Valsalva maneuver, sudden standing, and exercise.

(a) The Valsalva maneuver will decrease the duration of all other murmurs except mitral valve prolapse and hypertrophic cardiomyopathy. (c, d, and e) are incorrect as described in the explanation above.

**37. The answer is c.** (Rosen, pp 988-994.) This patient has a **ventricular tachycardia** defined by a **QRS complex greater than 120 milliseconds** and a **rate greater than 100 beats per minute.** Ventricular tachycardia is the result of a dysrhythmia originating within or below the termination of the His bundle. Most patients with ventricular tachycardia have underlying heart disease. Treatment begins with assessing whether or not the patient is stable. If the patient shows signs of instability, such as hypotension or altered mental status, cardioversion should be performed. However, if the patient is stable, medications can be administered to treat the dysrhythmia. **Amiodarone**, a class III antidysrhythmic that has pharmacologic characteristics of all four classes, is considered a first-line agent in treating ventricular dysrhythmias. Other commonly used medications include procainamide and lidocaine.

(a) Digoxin, a cardiac glycoside, has positive inotropic effects on the heart and slows conduction through the AV node. It should not be used to treat ventricular dysrhythmias. (b) Diltiazem, a CCB, acts on the AV node to slow cardiac conduction and will not treat ventricular tachycardia. In addition, it can lead to hypotension in patients with ventricular tachycardia secondary to its peripheral dilatory effects. (d) Adenosine, an ultrashort-acting AV nodal blocking agent, is typically used to treat SVTs. (e) Bretylium is no longer available in the United States as it has a poor safety profile.

**38. The answer is c.** (Rosen, pp 948-949.) The patient exhibits **unstable angina**, which is defined as new-onset angina, angina occurring at rest lasting longer than 20 minutes, or angina deviating from a patient's normal pattern. Unstable angina is considered the harbinger of an acute MI and, therefore, should be evaluated and treated aggressively. Unstable angina is one of the three diagnoses that make up ACS, the other two being stable angina and acute MI (ST or non–ST elevation). Patients may be pain free and have negative cardiac biomarkers with unstable angina. In general, unstable angina is treated with oxygen, aspirin, clopidogrel, low-molecular-weight or unfractionated heparin, and further risk stratification in the hospital.

(a) Variant or Prinzmetal angina is caused by coronary artery vasospasm at rest with minimal coronary artery disease. It is sometimes relieved by exercise or nitroglycerin. It is generally treated with CCBs. Patients with Prinzmetal angina may have ST elevations on their ECG that are indistinguishable from an acute MI. (b) Stable angina is described as transient episodic chest discomfort resulting from myocardial ischemia. The discomfort is typically predictable and reproducible, with the frequency of attacks constant over time. The discomfort is thought to be caused by fixed, stenotic atherosclerotic plaques that narrow a blood vessel lumen and reduce coronary blood flow (d and e). Non–ST-elevation MI (NSTEMI) and ST-elevation MI (STEMI) result from myocardial necrosis with release of cardiac biomarkers (eg, troponin).

**39. The answer is b.** (*Tintinalli, pp 148-149.*) The rhythm strip shows **second-degree AV block type II or Mobitz type II.** Mobitz II presents with a prolonged PR interval (PR > 0.2 second) and random dropped beats (ie, P wave without QRS complex). The PR intervals are always the same duration. The block is below the level of the AV node, generally the His-Purkinje system. This heart block reflects serious cardiac pathology and may be seen with an anterior wall MI, which is the case with this patient.

Mobitz type I (a) (also called Wenckebach phenomenon) shows progressive prolongation of PR interval with each beat until AV conduction is lost causing a dropped beat. First-degree AV block (c) presents with prolonged PR interval (PR > 0.2 second) without loss of AV conduction. This block is asymptomatic. Atrial flutter (d) is a tachydysrhythmia with rapid atrial beat and variable AV block. It has a characteristic "sawtooth" appearance of atrial flutter waves. Sinus bradycardia (e) is similar to sinus rhythm except that the rate is less than 60 and generally greater than 45. There are several etiologies of sinus bradycardia; some are normal (eg, young person, well-trained athlete) and some pathologic (eg, β-blocker overdose, cardiac ischemia).

**40. The answer is e.** (*Tintinalli, p 149.*) The rhythm strip findings are consistent with **third-degree AV block**, also called **complete heart block**. It is characterized by absent conduction through the AV node, resulting in the dissociation of atrial and ventricular rhythms. The ECG shows independent P waves and QRS complexes. Mobitz type II often progresses to third-degree heart block, as seen in this case. The immediate step in managing complete heart block is applying a **transcutaneous pacemaker** for ventricular pacing as a temporizing measure. However, patients need **implantable ventricular pacemakers** for definitive management. In addition, the underlying cause of the block needs to be addressed.

Consulting cardiology (**a**) is a good choice as they will implant a permanent pacemaker and manage any underlying cardiac disease. However, the patient must first be stabilized. Cardioversion (**b**) is used to treat unstable patients with reentrant arrhythmias, such as atrial fibrillation. It is not helpful in a setting of conduction abnormality, such as heart block. Metoprolol (**c**), a β-blocker, is contraindicated in complete heart block. This agent prolongs AV nodal conduction. (**d**) Amiodarone is an antidysrhythmic used in patients with wide-complex tachycardias or atrial fibrillation.

# Shortness of Breath

## Questions

**41.** A 55-year-old woman with a past medical history of diabetes walks into the emergency department (ED) stating that her tongue and lips feel like they are swollen. During the history, she tells you that her doctor just started her on a new blood pressure (BP) medication. Her only other medication is a baby aspirin. Her vitals at triage are: BP 130/70 mm Hg, heart rate (HR) 85 beats per minute, respiratory rate (RR) 16 breaths per minute, oxygen saturation 99% on room air, and temperature 98.7°F. On physical examination, you detect mild lip and tongue swelling. Over the next hour, you notice that not only are her tongue and lips getting more swollen, but her face is starting to swell, too. What is the most likely inciting agent?

a. Metoprolol
b. Furosemide
c. Aspirin
d. Lisinopril
e. Diltiazem

**42.** A 45-year-old woman presents to the ED immediately after landing at the airport from a transatlantic flight. She states that a few moments after landing she felt short of breath and felt pain in her chest when she took a deep breath. Her only medications are oral contraceptive pills and levothyroxine. She is a social drinker and smokes cigarettes occasionally. Her BP is 130/75 mm Hg, HR is 98 beats per minute, temperature is 98.9°F, RR is 20 breaths per minute, and oxygen saturation is 97% on room air. You send her for a duplex ultrasound of her legs, which is positive for deep vein thrombosis. What is the most appropriate management for this patient?

a. Place patient on a monitor, provide supplemental oxygen, and administer unfractionated heparin.

b. Place patient on a monitor, order a chest computed tomography (CT) scan to confirm a pulmonary embolism (PE), and then administer unfractionated heparin.

c. Place patient on a monitor and administer aspirin.

d. Instruct the patient to walk around the ED so that she remains mobile and does not exacerbate thrombus formation.

e. Place the patient on a monitor, provide supplemental oxygen, and administer warfarin.

**43.** A tall, thin 18-year-old man presents to the ED with acute onset of dyspnea while at rest. The patient reports sitting at his desk when he felt a sharp pain on the right side of his chest that worsened with inspiration. His past medical history is significant for peptic ulcer disease. He reports taking a 2-hour plane trip a month ago. His initial vitals include an HR of 100 beats per minute, a BP of 120/60 mm Hg, an RR of 16 breaths per minute, and an oxygen saturation of 97% on room air. On physical examination, you note decreased breath sounds on the right side. Which of the following tests should be performed next?

a. Electrocardiogram (ECG)

b. D-dimer

c. Ventilation perfusion scan (V/Q scan)

d. Upright abdominal radiograph

e. Chest radiograph

**44.** A 30-year-old obese woman with no significant past medical history presents to the ED complaining of shortness of breath and coughing up blood-streaked sputum. The patient states that she traveled to Moscow a month ago. Upon returning to the United States, the patient developed a persistent cough associated with dyspnea. She was seen by a pulmonologist, who diagnosed her with bronchitis and prescribed an inhaler. However, over the following weeks, the patient's symptoms worsened, and she developed pleuritic chest pain. In the ED, she lets you know that she smokes half a pack per day. Her vitals include a temperature of 99°F, BP of 105/65 mm Hg, HR of 124 beats per minute, RR of 22 breaths per minute, and an oxygen saturation of 94% on room air. Physical examination is non-contributory, except for rales at the left-mid lung. Her ECG reveals sinus tachycardia with large R waves in $V_1$ to $V_3$ and inverted T waves. Given this patient's history and presentation, what is the most likely etiology of her symptoms?

a. *Mycoplasma pneumoniae* ("walking" pneumonia)
b. Q fever pneumonia
c. *Pneumocystis jiroveci* pneumonia (PCP)
d. PE
e. Acute respiratory distress syndrome (ARDS)

**45.** A 24-year-old woman is brought to the ED after being found on a nearby street hunched over and in mild respiratory distress. Upon arrival, she is tachypneic at 24 breaths per minute with an oxygen saturation of 97% on face mask oxygen administration. Upon physical examination, the patient appears to be in mild distress with supraclavicular retractions. Scattered wheezing is heard throughout bilateral lung fields. Which of the following medications should be administered first?

a. Corticosteroids
b. Magnesium sulfate
c. Epinephrine
d. Anticholinergic nebulizer treatment
e. $\beta_2$-Agonist nebulizer treatment

**46.** An 81-year-old woman presents to the ED with acute onset of shortness of breath just before arrival. She refuses to answer questions for the interview, but repeatedly states that she is feeling short of breath. Her initial vitals include an HR of 89 beats per minute, a BP of 168/76 mm Hg, and an RR of 18 breaths per minute with an oxygen saturation of 89% on room air. A portable chest x-ray appears normal. Her physical examination is unremarkable, except for a systolic ejection murmur. Intravenous (IV) access is successfully obtained. After placing the patient on oxygen and a monitor, which of the following should be performed first?

a. Evaluation of troponin level
b. Evaluation of D-dimer level
c. Rectal temperature
d. Repeat chest x-ray
e. ECG

**47.** As you evaluate a patient with shortness of breath, you appreciate decreased breath sounds at the left-lung base. You suspect the patient has a small pleural effusion. In which of the following views of the chest is this small pleural effusion most likely to be detected?

a. Supine
b. Lateral decubitus right-side down
c. Lateral decubitus left-side down
d. Lateral
e. Posterior-anterior (PA)

**48.** A 32-year-old firefighter presents to the ED in acute respiratory distress. He was taken to the ED shortly after extinguishing a large fire in a warehouse. His initial vitals include an HR of 90 beats per minute, a BP of 120/55 mm Hg, and an RR of 18 breaths per minute with an oxygen saturation of 98% on 2-L nasal cannula. An ECG shows a first-degree heart block. Upon physical examination, there are diffuse rhonchi bilaterally. The patient is covered in soot and the hairs in his nares are singed. Given this clinical presentation, which of the following may be responsible for this patient's respiratory distress?

a. Reactive airway disease
b. Foreign body aspiration
c. Decompression sickness
d. Thermal burns
e. Pneumothorax

**49.** A 76-year-old man presents to the ED in acute respiratory distress, gasping for breath while on face mask. Paramedics state that he was found on a bench outside of his apartment in respiratory distress. Initial vitals include an HR of 90 beats per minute, a BP of 170/90 mm Hg, and an RR of 33 breaths per minute with an oxygen saturation of 90%. Upon physical examination, the patient is coughing up pink, frothy sputum, has rales two-thirds of the way up both lung fields, and has pitting edema of his lower extremities. A chest radiograph reveals bilateral perihilar infiltrates, an enlarged cardiac silhouette, and a small right-sided pleural effusion. After obtaining IV access and placing the patient on a monitor, which of the following medical interventions is most appropriate?

a. Morphine sulfate only
b. Nitroglycerin only
c. Nitroglycerin and a loop diuretic
d. Aspirin
e. Antibiotics

**50.** A 67-year-old man is brought to the ED in respiratory distress. His initial vitals include an HR of 112 beats per minute, a BP of 145/88 mm Hg, and an RR of 18 breaths per minute with an oxygen saturation of 92% on room air. He is also febrile at 102°F. After obtaining IV access, placing the patient on a monitor, and administering oxygen via nasal cannula, a chest radiograph is performed and shows patchy alveolar infiltrates with consolidation in the lower lobes. On review of systems, the patient tells you that he had five to six watery bowel movements a day for the last 2 days with a few bouts of emesis. Which of the following infectious etiologies is most likely responsible for the patient's presentation?

a. *Streptococcus pneumoniae*
b. *Haemophilus influenzae*
c. *Mycoplasma pneumoniae*
d. *Chlamydophila pneumoniae*
e. *Legionella pneumophila*

**51.** A 32-year-old woman presents to the ED with a 1-month history of general malaise, mild cough, and subjective fevers. She states that she is human immunodeficiency virus (HIV) positive and her last CD4 count, 6 months ago, was 220. She is not on antiretroviral therapy or any other medications. Initial vitals include an HR of 88 beats per minute, a BP of 130/60 mm Hg, and an RR of 12 breaths per minute with an oxygen saturation of 91% on room air. Her chest radiograph shows bilateral diffuse interstitial infiltrates. Subsequent laboratory tests are unremarkable except for an elevated lactate dehydrogenase level. Given this patient's history and physical examination, which of the following is the most likely organism responsible for her clinical presentation?

a. *Coccidioides immitis*
b. *Mycobacterium tuberculosis*
c. *Pneumocystis jiroveci*
d. *Mycoplasma pneumoniae*
e. *Haemophilus influenzae*

**52.** A 27-year-old woman presents to the ED complaining of an intensely pruritic rash all over her body, abdominal cramping, and chest tightness. She states that 1 hour ago she was at dinner and accidentally ate some shrimp. She has a known anaphylactic allergy to shrimp. Her BP is 115/75 mm Hg, HR is 95 beats per minute, temperature is 98.9°F, RR is 20 breaths per minute, and oxygen saturation is 97% on room air. She appears anxious, and her skin is flushed with urticarial lesions. Auscultation of her lungs reveals scattered wheezes with decreased air entry. Which of the following is the most appropriate next step in management?

a. Administer oxygen via non-rebreather, place a large-bore IV, begin IV fluids, and administer methylprednisolone intravenously.
b. Administer oxygen via non-rebreather, place a large-bore IV, begin IV fluids, and administer methylprednisolone and diphenhydramine intravenously.
c. Administer oxygen via non-rebreather, place a large-bore IV, begin IV fluids, administer methylprednisolone and diphenhydramine intravenously, and give intramuscular epinephrine.
d. Administer oxygen via non-rebreather, place a large-bore IV, begin IV fluids, and start aerosolized albuterol.
e. Administer oxygen via non-rebreather, place a large-bore IV, begin IV fluids, and start aerosolized epinephrine.

**53.** A 72-year-old man presents to the ED with worsening dyspnea. His initial vitals include an HR of 93 beats per minute, BP of 110/50 mm Hg, and RR of 20 breaths per minute with an oxygen saturation of 88% on room air. The patient appears thin and anxious. He is using accessory muscles to breathe. Despite distant breath sounds, you hear end-expiratory rhonchi and a prolonged expiratory phase. An ECG shows peaked P waves in leads II, III, and aVF. Given this patient's history and physical examination, which of the following conditions does this patient most likely have?

a. Chronic bronchitis
b. Asthma
c. Emphysema
d. Congestive heart failure (CHF)
e. Pneumothorax

**54.** A 71-year-old woman presents to the ED after a reported mechanical fall 2 days ago. Her initial vitals include an HR of 55 beats per minute, a BP of 110/60 mm Hg, an RR of 14 breaths per minute, and an oxygen saturation of 96% on room air. The patient does not appear to be taking deep breaths. Her physical examination is significant for decreased breath sounds bilaterally and tenderness to palpation along the right side of her chest. After initial stabilization, which of the following is the diagnostic test of choice for this patient's condition?

a. Chest x-ray
b. Chest CT scan
c. ECG
d. Rib radiographs
e. Thoracentesis

**55.** A 29-year-old woman presents to the ED for hyperventilation. Her initial vitals include an RR of 28 breaths per minute with an oxygen saturation of 100% on room air. She is able to speak in full sentences and tells you that she cannot breathe and that her hands and feet are cramping up. She denies any trauma, past medical history, or illicit drug use. Chest auscultation reveals clear breath sounds bilaterally. A subsequent chest radiograph is normal. Upon reevaluation, the patient reports that she is breathing better. Her vitals include an RR of 12 breaths per minute with an oxygen saturation of 100% on room air. Which of the following conditions is most likely the etiology of this patient's symptoms?

a. Pneumothorax
b. Hemopneumothorax
c. Pleural effusion
d. Anxiety attack
e. Asthma exacerbation

**56.** A 42-year-old man presents to the ED via ambulance after activating EMS for dyspnea. He is currently on an oxygen face mask and was administered one nebulized treatment of a $\beta_2$-agonist by the paramedics. His initial vitals include an RR of 16 breaths per minute with an oxygen saturation of 96% on room air. The patient appears to be in mild distress with some intercostal retractions. Upon chest auscultation, there are minimal wheezes localized over bilateral lower lung fields. The patient's symptoms completely resolve after two more nebulizer treatments. Which of the following medications, in addition to a rescue $\beta_2$-agonist inhaler, should be prescribed for outpatient use?

a. Magnesium sulfate
b. *Epinephrine injection* (EpiPen)
c. Corticosteroids
d. Cromolyn sodium
e. Ipratropium

**57.** A 22-year-old woman is brought to the ED by paramedics who state that they found the patient hunched over on a park bench barely breathing. The patient is rousable only to painful stimuli. Her initial vitals include an HR of 78 beats per minute, a BP of 125/58 mm Hg, and a respiratory rate of 6 breaths per minute with an oxygen saturation of 94% on 2-L nasal cannula. Upon physical examination, the patient has clear breath sounds bilaterally and no signs of trauma. Her pupils are 2 mm bilaterally and reactive to light. Which of the following agents may be used to restore this patient's respirations?

a. Oxygen
b. Flumazenil
c. Anticholinergic inhaler treatment
d. $\beta_2$-Agonist nebulized treatment
e. Naloxone

**58.** A 43-year-old undomiciled man is brought to the ED after being found intoxicated on the street. He is currently rousable and expresses a request to be left alone. Initial vitals include an HR of 92 beats per minute, a BP of 125/80 mm Hg, and an RR of 14 breaths per minute with an oxygen saturation of 93% on room air. His rectal temperature is 101.2°F. A chest radiograph shows infiltrates involving the right lower lobe. Given this clinical presentation, what initial antibiotic coverage is most appropriate for this patient?

a. Gram-negative coverage only
b. Gram-positive coverage only
c. Broad-spectrum with anaerobic coverage
d. PCP coverage
e. Antifungal therapy

**59.** A 32-year-old man is brought into the ED by EMS with fever, shortness of breath, and stridor. The patient was treated yesterday in the ED for a viral syndrome. His BP is 90/50 mm Hg, HR is 110 beats per minute, temperature is 101.2°F, and his RR is 28 breaths per minute. A chest radiograph reveals a widened mediastinum. The patient is endotracheally intubated, given a 2-L bolus of normal saline, and started on antibiotics. His BP improves to 110/70 mm Hg and he is transferred to the intensive care unit (ICU). You see a friend that accompanied the patient to the hospital and ask him some questions. You find out that the patient is a drum maker and works with animal hides. What is the most likely organism that is responsible for the patient's presentation?

a. *Streptococcus pneumoniae*
b. *Corynebacterium diphtheriae*
c. *Coxiella burnetii*
d. *Haemophilus influenzae*
e. *Bacillus anthracis*

**60.** A 62-year-old man presents to the ED with gradual dyspnea over the last few weeks. He reports that he is a daily smoker and has not seen a physician in years. Upon physical examination, there are decreased breath sounds on the right as compared to the left. A chest radiograph indicates blunting of the right costophrenic angle with a fluid line. A thoracentesis is performed. Given this patient's history, which of the following most likely describes his effusion?

a. Transudative effusion
b. Exudative effusion
c. Transudative and exudative effusion
d. Lactate dehydrogenase < 200 units
e. Fluid-to-blood protein ratio < 0.5

**61.** A 40-year-old man with a history of untreated HIV for 8 years comes into the ED complaining of cough, fever, and malaise for 3 days. He is tachypneic and diaphoretic. Chest radiograph reveals bilateral infiltrates. Arterial blood gas (ABG) analysis is significant for a $PaO_2$ of 62 on room air. His chest radiograph is seen below. Which of the following is the most appropriate initial management?

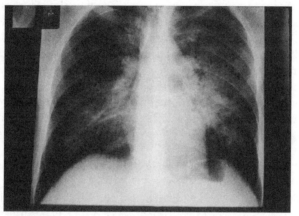

*(Reproduced, with permission, from Knoop KJ, Stack LB, Storrow AB. Atlas of Emergency Medicine. New York, NY: McGraw-Hill, 2002: 666.)*

a. Treat with corticosteroid prior to antibiotic therapy.
b. Treat immediately with IV trimethoprim/sulfamethoxazole (TMP/SMX).
c. Administer antibiotics after a rapid sputum Gram stain is obtained.
d. Treat with nebulizer.
e. Treat with racemic epinephrine.

# Shortness of Breath

## *Answers*

**41. The answer is d.** (*Harvey and Champe, pp 221-222.*) The patient has **angioedema**, a rare, but significant side effect of **angiotensin-converting enzyme (ACE-I) inhibitors**. This type of angioedema is usually limited to the **lips, tongue, and face**. If pharyngeal or laryngeal structures become involved, or there is significant tongue swelling, the patient may begin to **compromise their airway** and emergent intubation or surgical cricothyroidotomy needs to be performed. ACE-I–induced angioedema can occur after short- or long-term use of the medication. None of the other medications listed cause angioedema. The medication should be immediately discontinued.

**42. The answer is a.** (*Rosen, pp 1127-1136.*) The patient has a confirmed venous thrombosis and has symptoms consistent with a pulmonary thromboembolism. Data now show that almost every deep venous thrombosis (DVT) embolizes to some extent. The presence of a PE in this patient can be presumed by a confirmed DVT with pulmonary symptoms. All patients need to be on a monitor and should receive supplemental oxygen despite normal oxygen saturation. Oxygen acts as a pulmonary vasodilator. Heparin is the first-line therapy in this patient and should be administered promptly. Failure to achieve a therapeutic partial thromboplastin time (PTT) value within the first 24 hours leads to a 23% incidence of new embolism.

**(b)** A chest CT scan is not urgently needed since a DVT is already confirmed by duplex ultrasound and should not delay administration of anticoagulation. **(c)** Aspirin is not effective in preventing propagation of a DVT. The patient requires an anticoagulant, not an antiplatelet agent. **(d)** Although immobility can lead to increased thrombus, a patient with a diagnosed DVT should be monitored in bed while receiving anticoagulation. **(e)** Warfarin should never be started without concomitant administration of heparin. After the international normalized ratio (INR) is at a therapeutic level (2-3 IU), heparin can be stopped and warfarin can be taken alone. Warfarin initially causes a temporary hypercoagulable state because the anticoagulants, protein C and S (inhibited by warfarin), have shorter half-lives compared with the procoagulant vitamin K–dependent proteins that warfarin also inhibits.

**43. The answer is e.** *(Rosen, pp 939-943.)* A **spontaneous pneumothorax** typically presents with ipsilateral **pleuritic chest pain** and dyspnea while at rest. Physical findings tend to correlate with the degree of symptoms. Mild tachycardia, decreased breath sounds to auscultation, or hyperresonance to percussion are the most common findings. It typically occurs in healthy young men of taller than average stature without a precipitating factor. Mitral valve prolapse and Marfan syndrome are also associated with pneumothoraces. The most common condition associated with secondary spontaneous pneumothorax is chronic obstructive pulmonary disease (COPD). Although suggested by this patient's symptoms, the diagnosis of pneumothorax is generally made with a chest radiograph. The classic sign is the appearance of a thin, visceral, pleural line lying parallel to the chest wall, separated by a radiolucent band that is devoid of lung markings. If clinical suspicion is high with a negative initial chest x-ray, inspiratory and expiratory films, or a lateral decubitus film may be taken to evaluate for lung collapse.

An ECG **(a)** may be performed at a later time to investigate this patient's symptoms, but given the high likelihood of pneumothorax, a chest radiograph should be done first. A D-dimer **(b)** is a blood test used as a screening tool in patients who have a low pretest probability for a thromboembolism. A negative D-dimer can exclude the diagnosis of PE in patients with a low pretest probability. If the chest radiograph is unremarkable in this patient, sending a D-dimer may help in the workup of his dyspnea. A V/Q scan **(c)** also aides in the diagnosis of PE. Because spiral CT angiography has emerged as a test with high sensitivity and specificity, V/Q scan are being used less frequently. Its role is generally reserved for institutions that do not have access to spiral CT angiography and for individuals with a contraindication to spiral CT angiography (eg, contrast dye allergy, pregnancy). An upright abdominal x-ray **(d)** can assess for abdominal perforation, characteristically revealing air under the diaphragm.

**44. The answer is d.** *(Rosen, pp 1127-1136.)* In the history there are details that lead you to suspect **pulmonary embolus**: obesity, recent travel, progressive dyspnea despite inhaler treatment, and blood-streaked sputum. Objectively, her ECG shows right heart strain (large R waves and inverted

T waves in the precordial leads $V_1$-$V_3$), which is because of the heart beating against the high resistance of the pulmonary vasculature causing back flow, resulting in right ventricular enlargement. She is tachycardic, tachypneic, and hypoxic, cardinal signs of cardiovascular distress. Either dyspnea, pleuritic chest pain, or tachypnea is present in 95% of patients with a PE. The classic triad of dyspnea, pleuritic chest pain, and hemoptysis is uncommon and present in less than 25% of patients.

(a) *Mycoplasma pneumoniae* is the most common cause of atypical "walking" pneumonia. Most patients have constitutional symptoms, in addition to conjunctivitis, pharyngitis, or bullous myringitis. The hallmark of the disease is the disparity between the patient's clinically benign appearance and the extensive radiographic findings. (b) Q fever is caused by *C burnetii*. Infected individuals look ill, are diaphoretic, and febrile. (c) PCP is seen almost exclusively in patients who are immunocompromised, such as those with AIDS, malnourished, or on steroids. It is the most common opportunistic infection seen in HIV patients. Patients typically present with dyspnea, nonproductive cough, and fever. Chest radiograph may be normal in up to 20% to 30% of patients. The classic chest radiograph of PCP demonstrates bilateral diffuse interstitial infiltrates in the perihilar region and extending laterally in a "bat-wing" pattern. (e) The clinical hallmark of ARDS is severe hypoxemia unresponsive to increased concentrations of inspired oxygen. Many different conditions can precipitate ARDS; however, gram-negative sepsis is the most common.

**45. The answer is e.** (*Rosen, pp 888-903.*) This patient is suffering from an **acute asthma attack**. This is a reversible bronchospasm initiated by a variety of environmental factors that produce a narrowing and inflammation of the bronchial airways. The first-line treatment in order to open the airways includes a $\beta_2$-**agonist,** which acts to decrease bronchospasm of the smooth muscle.

Corticosteroids (a) are an effective measure for decreasing the late inflammatory changes involved in asthma. Magnesium sulfate (b) is also thought to act in a similar manner, but should be initiated in refractory cases of asthma. Epinephrine (c) decreases bronchospasm, but given its clinical side effects should only be administered in patients deemed to be in severe respiratory distress. Anticholinergics (d) are effective in patients with COPD, and are also administered in combination with a $\beta_2$-agonist to patients with an acute asthma exacerbation. However, it should never be given alone to treat asthma.

**46. The answer is e.** *(Rosen, pp 947-983.)* All patients with chest pain and shortness of breath should receive an **ECG**. It is a quick, noninvasive test that often provides substantive information. An ECG will show that this patient is having a large anterolateral wall myocardial infraction (MI) affecting much of her left ventricle, the reason for her heart murmur. An ECG must be performed in those crucial first moments so that the proper care can be delivered. This example reminds us of the importance of keeping the differential diagnosis broad in patients that present with respiratory distress. The other procedures may be done in a timely manner, but do not necessarily need to be performed as the next most critical step.

**47. The answer is c.** *(Rosen, pp 943-946.)* Pleural effusions are most easily detected on a **lateral decubitus film with the affected side down,** which in this case is the left side. Accumulations of 5 to 50 mL of fluid can be detected with this view.

Small effusions can be missed entirely on **(a)** supine views and are not generally apparent on PA views **(e)** and lateral views **(d)** until 200 mL or more of fluid are present.

**48. The answer is d.** *(Rosen, pp 761-762, 2033-2034.)* The **singed nares** seen in this patient should give you a clue to the possibility of severe **thermal burns.** Although there is minimal external involvement, damage from the heat may extend deep into the pulmonary system through inspiration. This results in a severe inflammatory reaction causing **pneumonitis.** Early intubation is critical.

Although you should always consider a foreign-body aspiration **(b)** in the differential diagnosis of respiratory distress, it is not consistent with the history of this individual. Reactive airway disease **(a)** typically presents with wheezing and pneumothorax **(e)** with decreased breath sounds. Decompression sickness **(c)** occurs when a scuba diver ascends too quickly and dissolved nitrogen bubbles reenter tissues and blood vessels.

**49. The answer is c.** *(Rosen, pp 1036-1053.)* **Pulmonary edema** can be divided into cardiogenic and noncardiogenic. Cardiogenic varieties are commonly seen in the ED and are usually a result of high hydrostatic pressures. It is seen in patients with MI or ischemia, cardiomyopathies, valvular heart disease, and hypertensive emergencies. **Nitroglycerin** acts to decrease the preload of the heart by venous dilation. This lowers the work of the heart so that it can function more effectively. A **loop diuretic** is used to induce diuresis and is also thought to act as a venous dilator. In conjunction with one another, these medications act to improve the overall functional capacity of the heart. If medical interventions are not stabilizing, preparation should be made for endotracheal intubation. Positive airway pressure devices (eg, BiPAP) may also be used as a temporizing measure for oxygen delivery.

(a) Morphine sulfate is a potent sedative and analgesic that also acts as a venous dilator. Its effects on preload and afterload are relatively minimal compared to nitroglycerin. It is also a respiratory depressant and should only be given in small quantities for patients with pulmonary edema. Aspirin (d) should be administered if there is suspicion of cardiac ischemia. If this patient had pneumonia then antibiotics (e) should have been administered. However, the chest radiograph and clinical presentation is consistent with acute pulmonary edema.

**50. The answer is e.** (*Rosen, pp 927-938.*) *Legionella pneumophila* is an intracellular organism that lives in aquatic environments. The organism may live in ordinary tap water and has probably been underdiagnosed in a number of community outbreaks. It is typically seen in the elderly and immunocompromised. Legionnaire disease is more common in the summer, especially in August. Patients often experience a prodrome of 1 to 2 days of mild headache and myalgias, followed by high fever, chills, and multiple rigors. Cough is present in 90% of cases. Other **pulmonary manifestations** include dyspnea, pleuritic chest pain, and hemoptysis. **GI symptoms** include nausea, vomiting, diarrhea, and anorexia. **Neurologic symptoms** include headache, altered mental status, and rarely, focal symptoms. **Urine antigen testing** is highly specific and sensitive and, if available, very rapid in making the diagnosis.

*Streptococcus pneumoniae* (a) is the most common etiology of community-acquired pneumonia among adults. It is found in the nasopharynx of almost half of the population and may manifest itself as a lobar pneumonia. *Haemophilus influenzae* (b) is common among patients with COPD, alcoholism, malnutrition, or malignancy. *Mycoplasma pneumoniae* (c) is another common cause of community-acquired pneumonia in patients under the age of 40. It presents as a mild, nonproductive cough with low-grade temperature and the typical chest x-ray appearing much worse than expected with diffuse infiltrates. Bullous myringitis may also be an associated symptom. *Chlamydophila pneumoniae* (d) is an intracellular parasite that is transmitted between humans by respiratory secretions or aerosols. It remains a relatively uncommon cause of pneumonia in the community.

**51. The answer is c.** (*Rosen, pp 927-938.*) **PCP** is a commonly seen opportunistic infection in the HIV/AIDS population. It typically presents with mild subjective symptoms of cough and general malaise. Objectively, patients are hypoxic and have a chest radiograph with a bilateral interstitial process. Risk factors include a **CD4 count less than 200.** Serum lactate dehydrogenase (LDH) is also considerably higher in AIDS patients with PCP. In fact, the greater the elevation in LDH, worse the prognosis. Despite the classic PCP radiograph demonstrating bilateral diffuse interstitial infiltrates, beginning in the perihilar region and extending into a "bat-wing" pattern, the chest radiograph may be normal in up to 30% of patients. In addition to Kaposi sarcoma involvement in the lungs, pulmonary infections, such as tuberculosis, cytomegalovirus, and fungal infections, should be considered.

Coccidioidomycosis (**a**) is caused by the fungus *C immitis*. The fungus is endemic in the southwestern United States. Conformation of the diagnosis is made through direct observation of the fungus in smear or culture, or through the detection of serum antibodies. The chest radiograph generally reveals mediastinal or hilar adenopathy, pleural effusions, nodules, cavitations, or infiltrates. *Mycobacterium tuberculosis* (**b**) is the causative organism of tuberculosis (TB). Patients can present with chronic cough, hemoptysis, and constitutional symptoms. Because TB can present in a clinically similar fashion as PCP in immunocompromised individuals, TB studies should also be performed on this patient. In classic reactivation TB, pulmonary lesions are located in the posterior segment of the right-upper lobe, apicoposterior segment of the left-upper lobe, and apical segments of the lower lobes. In the presence of HIV or other immunosuppressant disease, lesions are often atypical. Up to 20% of patients who are HIV positive with active disease have normal chest x-ray findings. Radiographic findings consistent with active primary TB are similar to those of lobar pneumonia with ipsilateral hilar adenopathy. *Mycoplasma pneumoniae* (**d**) is a common cause of community-acquired pneumonia in patients under the age of 40. Radiographic findings are variable, but abnormalities are usually more striking than the findings on physical examination. *Haemophilus influenzae* (**e**) is common among patients with COPD, alcoholism, malnutrition, or malignancy.

**52. The answer is c.** (*Rosen, pp 1511-1526.*) The patient is having an **anaphylactic reaction** to the shrimp she ate. Anaphylaxis refers to a severe systemic allergic reaction with variable features such as respiratory difficulty, cardiovascular collapse, pruritic skin rash, and abdominal cramping.

Anaphylaxis is a hypersensitivity reaction caused by an **IgE-mediated** reaction. Foods are the major cause in cases of anaphylaxis in which a source can be determined. Common foods that cause anaphylaxis include **nuts, shellfish,** and **eggs.** In the ED, attention is focused on reversing cardiovascular and respiratory disturbances. **Epinephrine** is the first drug of choice for patients with anaphylaxis. The route of administration is chosen by the severity of the patient's presentation. In a patient with severe upper airway obstruction or worsening hypotension, IV epinephrine should be administered. Patients with relatively stable vital signs can receive intramuscular epinephrine. Epinephrine should be used with caution in the elderly or any patient with coronary artery disease or dysrhythmias. However, in severe anaphylaxis, epinephrine can be life saving. Antihistamines, such as **diphenhydramine** and ranitidine, should be used in all cases. These drugs block the action of circulating histamines at target tissue receptors. Corticosteroids, such as **methylprednisolone,** have an onset of action approximately 4 to 6 hours after administration and, therefore are of limited value in the acute setting. However, since giving them early may blunt the biphasic reaction of anaphylaxis, therefore, it is advised to administer to patients in anaphylaxis.

Though aerosolized forms of albuterol **(d)** and epinephrine **(e)** are appropriate to give in the setting of anaphylaxis, they are adjunctive therapies and should never be given alone to treat anaphylaxis.

**53. The answer is c.** (*Rosen, pp 904-912.*) COPD is often referred to as a single disease but is in fact a triad of three distinct disease processes: emphysema, chronic bronchitis, and asthma. This clinical scenario paints a typical picture of **emphysema.** Individuals appear dyspneic, thin, and anxious. They generally have an increased anterior-posterior (AP) chest diameter and often use their accessory muscles to help with breathing. Lungs sounds are distant and associated with wheezes, rhonchi, and a prolonged expiratory phase. These individuals are often classified as "pink puffers" and use their pursed lips to push air that remains trapped in alveoli owing to the prolonged expiratory phase. Exacerbations should be treated with corticosteroids, anticholinergic inhalers, and intermittent $\beta_2$-agonists to decrease inflammation, decrease mucous production, and relax smooth muscle in an effort to open up the distal airways. Patients with COPD are at higher risk for developing bacterial bronchitis and pneumonia, therefore you should have a lower threshold to start them on antibiotics for atypical bacterial infections. COPD is generally caused by smoking but may also result from air pollution, occupational exposure, and genetic factors, such as $\alpha_1$-antitrypsin deficiency. Patients may require supplemental outpatient oxygen to function and perform basic activities of daily living.

Patients with chronic bronchitis (a) are considered "blue bloaters" given their mucous overproduction that causes hypoventilation. These patients generally have lowered oxygen saturation levels at baseline. They usually are stocky in build, have a productive cough, and have a normal AP chest diameter. Asthma (b) is characterized by airway hyperreactivity and inflammation. It is a reversible process whereas emphysema is not. This patient's signs and symptoms are not typical of CHF (d) or pneumothorax (e).

**54. The answer is d.** (*Rosen, pp 387-388.*) Given the history of trauma, a **rib fracture** is the most probable etiology of the patient's symptoms in this clinical scenario. Rib fractures usually occur at the **point of impact** or at the **posterior angle,** which is the weakest part of the rib. It is important to note that the true danger of rib fractures involves not the rib itself, but the risk of penetrating injury to underlying structures. A **rib series** is the most effective way to visualize these fractures. Treatment of patients with simple acute rib fractures includes pain relief so that respiratory splinting does not occur, which increases the rate of atelectasis and pneumonia. Chest binders should not be used as they promote hypoventilation. For multiple rib fractures, intercostal nerve blocks may be a more effective means of analgesia. Most rib fractures heal uneventfully within 3 to 6 weeks. The patient should be encouraged to take deep breaths to avoid developing pneumonia.

A chest radiograph (a) is valuable for investigating other associated injuries, but often obscures the ribs and fractures may remain hidden. A chest CT scan (b) is not indicated at this time and is only warranted with worsening symptoms or negative radiographs with a high clinical suspicion. An ECG (c) may be obtained to evaluate the general health of this patient but is not helpful in diagnosing a rib fracture. A thoracentesis (e), whether diagnostic or therapeutic, is indicated only in patients with pleural effusions.

**55. The answer is d.** (*Rosen, pp 1445-1451.*) The patient has normal vitals, a normal chest radiograph, and is stable. In fact, her symptoms self-resolve with time and without intervention. Only with this information can one be comfortable with making the diagnosis of an **anxiety attack** as the precipitant to the patient's symptoms. A history of a stressor may be helpful, but it is important to note that these symptoms are not under the voluntary control of the patient, and often patients may not even be able to identify a specific stressor. It is important to remember that the diagnosis of anxiety in the ED is a diagnosis of exclusion. Her extremity symptoms are typical of **carpal-pedal spasm** seen with tetany, a result of a transient decrease in calcium serum levels secondary to a respiratory alkalosis.

(a) A pneumothorax and hemopneumothorax (b) are generally seen with trauma and typically present with decreased breath sounds and abnormal oxygen saturation. A pleural effusion (c) has many etiologies and usually presents with decreased breath sounds at the point of effusion. Asthma (e) generally manifests itself with wheezing on examination.

**56. The answer is c.** *(Rosen, pp 896-901.)* **Corticosteroids** have been shown to improve asthma symptoms in subsequent days after an exacerbation and prevent acute recurrences in patients who are deemed suitable to be discharged from the ED. An acceptable dosage is 40 to 60 mg prednisone daily for 3 to 10 days after the initial event. Inhaled steroids may also be an alternative to prevent relapses in more intractable cases, and should be used daily with the guidance of the patient's primary care provider. Spacers are available to ensure adequate delivery of medications deep into the alveoli.

Cromolyn (d) acts as a mast cell stabilizer and is used primarily in the management of allergic rhinitis. Ipratropium (e) is an anticholinergic medication that is used in the management of COPD. Although it is usually administered in the acute care of asthma, it is not indicated for asthma maintenance. Adequate amounts of magnesium (a) should be obtained in the patient's diet. *Epinephrine injections* (EpiPens) (b) are only indicated for those patients who suffer severe allergic reactions and are not given on an outpatient basis in patients with asthma.

**57. The answer is e.** *(Rosen, pp 2047-2051.)* Attention to airway and breathing is of particular importance in **opioid intoxication,** as indicated by the patient's pinpoint pupils, because respiratory and central nervous system (CNS) depression are the most common life-threatening complications. **Naloxone** is a μ-opioid receptor-competitive antagonist and its rapid blockade of those receptors reverses the depressive effects of opioids.

Oxygen (a) and respiratory treatments (c and d) can aid in bringing saturations up, but will not treat the underlying cause. Flumazenil (b) is a benzodiazepine antagonist that works as a competitive inhibitor of the γ-aminobutyric acid (GABA) receptor.

**58. The answer is c.** *(Rosen, pp 933-934.)* **Aspiration pneumonia** occurs secondary to the inhalation of either oropharyngeal or gastric contents into the lower airways. Aspiration of gastric juices may cause a pulmonary inflammatory response. This type of mechanism of acquiring pneumonia is commonly seen in those with **swallowing difficulties** or a **relaxed lower esophageal sphincter** because of **alcohol**. Given these factors, this patient is in a high-risk category for aspiration pneumonia. The small degree of angulation of the right mainstem bronchus makes the right lung at higher risk. Most particles easily travel down this route, ending up in the **right middle or lower lobe** of the lung. **Antibiotic coverage** should be **broad**, covering for both **gram-positive and gram-negative organisms including anaerobes,** which are commonly present in the mouth. Given the severity, these patients may go on to develop ARDS, an inflammatory response to infection, and, subsequently, respiratory failure.

(a) Gram-negative organisms, such as *H influenzae, P aeruginosa, K pneumoniae,* and *E coli,* are the most frequent causes of nosocomial pneumonia. (b) Gram-positive organisms such as *S pneumoniae* and *Staphylococcus aureus* are most commonly associated with community-acquired pneumonia. (d) PCP is found in immunocompromised patients, such as those with AIDS, or those receiving immunosuppressants secondary to organ transplantation. They are also at risk for fungal pneumonias (e); however, treatment should not be initiated unless there is high clinical suspicion.

**59. The answer is e.** *(Rosen, pp 2498-2500.)* **Inhalation anthrax** is a rare, but life-threatening disease, with mortality rates exceeding 90%. It is caused by inhaling *B anthracis* spores into the lungs. Initially, the patient develops flu-like symptoms. Within 24 to 48 hours, the clinical course may abruptly deteriorate to septic shock, respiratory failure, and mediastinitis. Chest x-ray may reveal a widened mediastinum. Death usually results within 3 days. Anthrax is normally a disease of sheep, cattle, and horses. As there is no evidence for human-to-human transmission, disease in humans occurs when spores are inhaled. Working with untreated animal hides increases the risk for anthrax exposure.

Though *S pneumoniae* and *H influenzae* (a and d) can cause respiratory failure, it is unlikely to occur in a healthy 32-year-old man. (b) Diphtheria is a potentially life-threatening disease that is characterized by a gray-green pseudomembrane covering the tonsils and pharyngeal mucosa. *Coxiella burnetii* (c) is the organism that causes Q fever. It is similar to *B anthracis* in that sheep, cattle, and goats are the primary reservoirs. However, deterioration because of Q fever is not as rapid as that seen in anthrax.

**60. The answer is b.** *(Rosen, pp 943-946.)* Given this patient's long-standing history of **tobacco** use and having not seen a doctor for annual examinations, it is likely that the pleural effusion is **exudative** as a result of an underlying **malignancy.** Other causes of exudative effusions include the following: infection, connective tissue diseases, neoplasm, pulmonary emboli, uremia, pancreatitis, esophageal rupture—postsurgical, trauma, and drug induced. Pleural fluid analysis includes LDH, glucose, protein, amylase, cell count, Gram stain, culture, and cytology.

(**d and e**) Effusions that have an LDH greater than 200 units, fluid-to-blood LDH ratio greater than 0.6, and a fluid-to-blood protein ratio greater than 0.5 are classified as exudative. Levels less than these are classified as transudative. (**a**) Causes of transudative effusions include CHF, hypoalbuminemia, cirrhosis, myxedema, nephrotic syndrome, superior vena cava syndrome, and peritoneal dialysis. (**c**) An effusion cannot be both exudative and transudative.

**61. The answer is a.** *(Rosen, pp 933-936.)* In a patient with untreated **HIV** and bilateral **infiltrates** on chest x-ray, **PCP** must be considered, in addition to community-acquired pneumonia. Corticosteroids are shown to be beneficial as adjunctive therapy in patients with moderate to severe PCP. They (1) limit oxygen deterioration, (2) decrease mortality and respiratory failure, and (3) accelerate recovery. Therapy should be initiated to all children and adult patients with a $Po_2$ less than 70 mm Hg or an A-a gradient greater than 35 mm Hg. It is important to initiate steroid therapy prior to starting antibiotics to avoid worsening hypoxia that is secondary to the inflammatory reaction caused by dying organisms.

(**b**) Immediate treatment with IV TMP/SMX would be correct if the $Pao_2$ were greater than 70. (**c**) Delay of antibiotics is never appropriate in an ill patient with suspected pneumonia. Gram stain is unlikely to be useful in acutely identifying the organism in community-acquired pneumonia and silver stain is required to see pneumocystis. Nebulizer treatment (**d**) is ancillary and may provide relief of symptoms in a wheezing patient with pneumonia, but is not appropriate for initial management of this patient. Epinephrine (**e**) has no role in the acutely ill patient with PCP whose symptoms are less likely related to severe reactive airway disease.

# Abdominal and Pelvic Pain

## Questions

**62.** An 81-year-old diabetic woman with a history of atrial fibrillation is transferred to your emergency department (ED) from the local nursing home. The note from the facility states that the patient is complaining of abdominal pain, having already vomited once. Her vital signs in the ED are temperature 100.1°F, blood pressure (BP) 105/75 mm Hg, heart rate (HR) 95 beats per minute, and respiratory rate (RR) 18 breaths per minute. You examine the patient and focus on her abdomen. Considering that the patient has not stopped moaning in pain since arriving to the ED, you are surprised to find that her abdomen is soft on palpation. You decide to order an abdominal radiographic series. Which of the findings on plain abdominal film is strongly suggestive of mesenteric infarction?

a. Sentinel loop of bowel
b. No gas in the rectum
c. Presence of an ileus
d. Pneumatosis intestinalis
e. Air fluid levels

**63.** A husband and wife present to the ED with 1 day of subjective fever, vomiting, watery diarrhea, and abdominal cramps. They were at a restaurant a day before for dinner and both ate the seafood special, which consisted of raw shellfish. In the ED, they are both tachycardic with temperatures of 99.8°F and 99.6°F for him and her, respectively. Which of the following is responsible for the majority of acute episodes of diarrhea?

a. Parasites
b. Viruses
c. Enterotoxin-producing bacteria
d. Anaerobic bacteria
e. Invasive bacteria

**64.** A 49-year-old man presents to the ED with nausea, vomiting, and abdominal pain that began approximately 2 days ago. The patient states that he usually drinks a six pack of beer daily, but increased his drinking to 2 six packs daily over the last week because of pressures at work. He notes decreased appetite over the last 3 days and states he has not had anything to eat in 2 days. His BP is 125/75 mm Hg, HR is 105 beats per minute, and RR is 20 breaths per minute. You note generalized abdominal tenderness on examination. Laboratory results reveal the following:

White blood cells (WBC) 9000/μL
Hematocrit 48%
Platelets 210/μL
Aspartate transaminase (AST) 85 U/L
Alanine transaminase (ALT) 60 U/L

Alkaline phosphatase 75 U/L
Total bilirubin 0.5 mg/dL
Lipase 40 IU

Sodium 131 mEq/L
Potassium 3.5 mEq/L
Chloride 101 mEq/L
Bicarbonate 10 mEq/L
Blood urea nitrogen (BUN) 9 mg/dL
Creatinine 0.5 mg/dL
Glucose 190 mg/dL
Nitroprusside test weakly positive for ketones

Which of the following is the mainstay of therapy for patients with this condition?

a. Normal saline (NS) solution
b. Half normal saline (½ NS)
c. Glucose solution (D5W)
d. Solution containing both saline and glucose (D5/NS or D5 ½ NS)
e. The type of solution is irrelevant

**65.** As you palpate the right upper quadrant (RUQ) of a 38-year-old woman's abdomen, you notice that she stops her inspiration for a brief moment. During the history, the patient states that over the last 2 days she gets pain in her RUQ that radiates to her back shortly after eating. Her vitals include a temperature of 100.4°F, HR of 95 beats per minute, BP of 130/75 mm Hg, and RR of 16 breaths per minute. What is the initial diagnostic modality of choice for this disorder?

a. Plain film radiograph
b. Computed tomography (CT) scan
c. Magnetic resonance imaging (MRI)
d. Radioisotope cholescintigraphy (HIDA scan)
e. Ultrasonography

**66.** A 31-year-old man from Florida presents to the ED complaining of severe pain that starts in his left flank and radiates to his testicle. The pain lasts for about 1 hour and then improves. He had similar pain last week that resolved spontaneously. He noted some blood in his urine this morning. His BP is 145/75 mm Hg, HR is 90 beats per minute, temperature is 98.9°F, and his RR is 24 breaths per minute. His abdomen is soft and nontender. As you examine the patient, he vomits and has trouble lying still in his stretcher. Which of the following is the most appropriate next step in management?

a. Call surgery consult to evaluate the patient for appendicitis.
b. Order an abdominal CT.
c. Start intravenous (IV) fluids and administer an IV nonsteroidal anti-inflammatory drug (NSAID) and antiemetic.
d. Perform an ultrasound to evaluate for an abdominal aortic aneurysm (AAA).
e. Perform an ultrasound to evaluate for testicular torsion.

**67.** A 67-year-old man is brought to the ED by emergency medical service (EMS). His wife states that the patient was doing his usual chores around the house when all of a sudden he started complaining of severe abdominal pain. He has a past medical history of coronary artery disease and hypertension. His BP is 85/70 mm Hg, HR is 105 beats per minute, temperature is 98.9°F, and his RR is 18 breaths per minute. On physical examination, he is diaphoretic and in obvious pain. Upon palpating his abdomen, you feel a large pulsatile mass. An electrocardiogram (ECG) reveals sinus tachycardia. You place the patient on a monitor, administer oxygen, insert two large-bore IVs, and send his blood to the laboratory. His BP does not improve after a 1-L fluid bolus. Which of the following is the most appropriate next step in management?

a. Order a CT scan to evaluate his aorta.
b. Call the angiography suite and have them prepare the room for the patient.
c. Order a portable abdominal radiograph.
d. Call surgery and have them prepare the operating room (OR) for an exploratory laparotomy.
e. Call the cardiac catheterization laboratory to prepare for stent insertion.

**68.** A 57-year-old woman presents to the ED with a basin in her hand and actively vomiting. You insert an IV catheter, start IV fluids, and administer an antiemetic agent. The patient feels much better but also complains of severe crampy abdominal pain that comes in waves. You examine her abdomen and note that it is distended and that there is a small midline scar in the lower abdomen. Upon auscultation, you hear high-pitched noises that sound like "tinkles." Palpation elicits pain in all four quadrants but no rebound tenderness. She is guaiac negative. Which of the following is the most common cause of this patient's presentation?

a. Travel to Mexico
b. Ethanol abuse
c. Hysterectomy
d. Hernia
e. Constipation

**69.** An undomiciled 41-year-old man walks into the ED complaining of abdominal pain, nausea, and vomiting. He tells you that he has been drinking beer continuously over the previous 18 hours. On examination, his vitals are BP 150/75 mm Hg, HR 104 beats per minute, RR 16 breaths per minute, oxygen saturation 97% on room air, temperature of 99.1°F rectally, and finger stick glucose 81 mg/dL. The patient is alert and oriented, his pupils anicteric. You notice gynecomastia and spider angiomata. His abdomen is soft but tender in the RUQ. Laboratory tests reveal an AST of 212 U/L, ALT 170 U/L, alkaline phosphatase of 98 U/L, total bilirubin of 1.9 mg/dL, international normalized ratio (INR) of 1.3, WBC 12,000/μL. Urinalysis shows 1+ protein. Chest x-ray is unremarkable. Which of the following is the most appropriate next step in management?

a. Place a nasogastric tube in the patient's stomach to remove any remaining ethanol.
b. Order a HIDA scan to evaluate for acute cholecystitis.
c. Administer hepatitis B immune globulin.
d. Send viral hepatitis titers.
e. Provide supportive care by correcting any fluid and electrolyte imbalances.

**70.** A 48-year-old man with a past medical history of hepatitis C and cirrhosis presents to the ED complaining of acute-onset abdominal pain and chills. His BP is 118/75 mm Hg, HR is 105 beats per minute, RR is 16 breaths per minute, temperature is 101.2°F rectally, and oxygen saturation is 97% on room air. His abdomen is distended, and diffusely tender. You decide to perform a paracentesis and retrieve 1 L of cloudy fluid. Laboratory analysis of the fluid shows a neutrophil count of 550 cells/mm$^3$. Which of the following is the most appropriate choice of treatment?

a. Metronidazole
b. Vancomycin
c. Sulfamethoxazole/trimethoprim (SMX/TMP)
d. Neomycin and lactulose
e. Cefotaxime

**71.** A 24-year-old man woke up from sleep 1 hour ago with severe pain in his right testicle. He states that he is sexually active with multiple partners. On examination, the right scrotum is swollen, tender, and firm. You cannot elicit a cremasteric reflex. His BP is 145/75 mm Hg, HR is 103 beats per minute, RR is 14 breaths per minute, temperature is 98.9°F, and oxygen saturation is 99% on room air. Which of the following is the most appropriate next step in management?

a. Administer one dose of ceftriaxone and doxycycline for 10 days and have him follow-up with a urologist.
b. Swab his urethra, send a culture for gonorrhea and *Chlamydia*, and treat if positive.
c. Send a urinalysis and treat for a urinary tract infection (UTI) if positive.
d. Treat the patient for epididymitis and have him return if symptoms persist.
e. Order a statim (STAT) color Doppler ultrasound and urologic consultation.

**72.** A 28-year-old man presents to the ED complaining of constant vague, diffuse epigastric pain. He describes having a poor appetite and feeling nauseated ever since eating sushi last night. His BP is 125/75 mm Hg, HR is 96 beats per minute, temperature is 100.5°F, and his RR is 16 breaths per minute. On examination, his abdomen is soft and moderately tender in the right lower quadrant (RLQ). Laboratory results reveal a WBC of 12,000/µL. Urinalysis shows 1+ leukocyte esterase. The patient is convinced that this is food poisoning from the sushi and asks for some antacid. Which of the following is the most appropriate next step in management?

a. Order a plain radiograph to look for dilated bowel loops.
b. Administer 40 cc of Maalox and observe for 1 hour.
c. Send the patient for an abdominal ultrasound.
d. Order an abdominal CT scan.
e. Discharge the patient home with ciprofloxacin.

**73.** A 23-year-old woman presents to the ED in moderate pain in her left lower quadrant (LLQ). She states that the pain began suddenly and is associated with nausea and vomiting. She had a bout of diarrhea yesterday. This is the second time this month that she experienced pain in this location, however, never with this severity. Her BP is 120/75 mm Hg, HR is 101 beats per minute, temperature is 99.5°F, and RR is 18 breaths per minute. She has a tender LLQ on abdominal examination and a tender adnexa on pelvic examination. Which of the following is the most appropriate diagnostic test for the patient?

a. CT scan
b. MRI
c. X-ray
d. Doppler ultrasound
e. Laparoscopy

**74.** A 55-year-old man presents to the ED complaining of mild diffuse abdominal pain. He states that he underwent a routine colonoscopy yesterday and was told "everything is fine." The pain began upon waking up and is associated with some nausea. He denies fever, vomiting, diarrhea, and rectal bleeding. His BP is 143/71 mm Hg, HR is 87 beats per minute, temperature is 98.9°F, and RR is 16 breaths per minute. His abdomen is tense but only mildly tender. You order baseline laboratory tests. His chest radiograph is seen below. Which of the following is the most likely diagnosis?

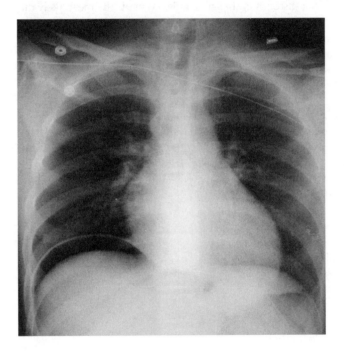

a. Ascending cholangitis
b. Acute pulmonary edema
c. Acute liver failure
d. Pancreatitis
e. Pneumoperitoneum

**75.** A 78-year-old woman is brought to the ED by EMS complaining of vomiting and abdominal pain that began during the night. EMS reports that her BP is 90/50 mm Hg, HR is 110 beats per minute, temperature is 101.2°F, and RR is 18 breaths per minute. After giving her a 500 mL bolus of NS, her BP is 115/70 mm Hg. During the examination, you notice that her face and chest appear jaundiced. Her lungs are clear to auscultation and you do not appreciate a murmur on cardiac examination. She winces when you palpate her RUQ. An ultrasound reveals dilation of the common bile duct and stones in the gallbladder. What is the most likely diagnosis?

a. Cholecystitis
b. Acute hepatitis
c. Cholangitis
d. Pancreatic cancer
e. Bowel obstruction

**76.** A 23-year-old woman presents to the ED complaining of lower abdominal pain and vaginal spotting for 2 days. Her menstrual cycle is irregular. She has a history of ovarian cysts and is sexually active but always uses condoms. Her BP is 115/75 mm Hg, HR is 75 beats per minute, temperature is 98.9°F, and RR is 16 breaths per minute. Which of the following tests should be obtained next?

a. *Chlamydia* antigen test.
b. β-Human chorionic gonadotropin (β-hCG).
c. Transvaginal ultrasound.
d. Abdominal radiograph.
e. Observe her abdominal pain, if it resolves discharge her with a diagnosis of menstruation.

**77.** A 71-year-old obese man is brought to the ED complaining of constant left mid quadrant (LMQ) abdominal pain with radiation into his back. His past medical history is significant for hypertension, peripheral vascular disease, peptic ulcer disease, kidney stones, and gallstones. He smokes a pack of cigarettes and consumes a pint of vodka daily. His BP is 145/80 mm Hg, HR is 90 beats per minute, temperature is 98.9°F, and RR is 16 breaths per minute. Abdominal examination is unremarkable. An ECG is read as sinus rhythm with an HR of 88 beats per minute. An abdominal radiograph reveals normal loops of bowel and curvilinear calcification of the aortic wall. Which of the following is the most likely diagnosis?

a. Biliary colic
b. Nephrolithiasis
c. Pancreatitis
d. Small bowel obstruction (SBO)
e. Abdominal aortic aneurysm

**78.** A 51-year-old man presents to the ED complaining of epigastric pain that radiates to his back. He states that he drinks six packs of beer daily. You suspect he has pancreatitis. His BP is 135/75 mm Hg, HR is 90 beats per minute, temperature is 100.1°F, and his RR is 17 breaths per minute. Laboratory results reveal WBC 13,000/µL, hematocrit 48%, platelets 110/µL, amylase 1150 U/L, lipase 1450 IU, lactate dehydrogenase (LDH) 150 U/L, sodium 135 mEq/L, potassium 3.5 mEq/L, chloride 105 mEq/L, bicarbonate 23 mEq/L, BUN 15 mg/dL, creatinine 1.1 mg/dL, and glucose 125 mg/dL. Which of the following laboratory values are most specific for pancreatitis?

a. Elevated amylase
b. Hyperglycemia
c. Elevated lipase
d. Elevated LDH
e. Leukocytosis

**79.** A 51-year-old man describes 1 week of gradually worsening scrotal pain and dysuria. He is sexually active with his wife. His temperature is 100.1°F, HR 81 beats per minute, BP 140/75 mm Hg, and oxygen saturation is 99% on room air. On physical examination, his scrotal skin is warm and erythematous. A cremasteric reflex is present. The posterior left testicle is swollen and tender to touch. Color Doppler ultrasonography demonstrates increased testicular blood flow. Urinalysis is positive for leukocyte esterase. What is the most likely diagnosis?

a. Epididymitis
b. Testicular torsion
c. UTI
d. Testicular tumor
e. Varicocele

**80.** A 22-year-old man presents to the ED complaining of dysuria for 3 days. He states that he has never had this feeling before. He is currently sexually active and uses a condom most of the time. He denies hematuria but notes a yellowish discharge from his urethra. His BP is 120/75 mm Hg, HR is 60 beats per minute, and temperature is 98.9°F. You send a clean catch urinalysis to the laboratory that returns positive for leukocyte esterase and 15 white blood cells per high power field (WBCs/hpf). Which of the following is the most appropriate next step in management?

a. Send a urethral swab for culture and administer 125 mg ceftriaxone intramuscularly and 1 g azithromycin orally.
b. Send urine for culture and administer SMX/TMP orally.
c. Discharge the patient with strict instructions to return if his symptoms worsen.
d. Order a CT scan to evaluate for a kidney stone.
e. Have him follow-up immediately with a urologist to evaluate for testicular cancer.

**81.** A 40-year-old woman presents to the ED complaining of fever and 1 day of increasingly severe pain in her RUQ. She denies nausea or vomiting and has no history of fatty food intolerance. The patient returned from a trip to Mexico 6 months ago. About 2 weeks ago she experienced intermittent diarrhea with blood-streaked mucus. Her BP is 130/80 mm Hg, HR is 107 beats per minute, temperature is 102°F, and RR is 17 breaths per minute. Physical examination reveals decreased breath sounds over the right lung base. Abdominal examination shows tenderness to percussion over the RUQ and normal active bowel sounds. There is no Murphy sign. Her WBC is 20,500/μL. Chest radiograph reveals a small right-pleural effusion. Which of the following is the most likely diagnosis?

a. Amebic abscess
b. Cholecystitis
c. Cryptosporidium
d. Enterobiasis
e. Pyogenic abscess

**82.** A 59-year-old woman presents to the ED complaining of worsening lower abdominal pain over the previous 3 days. She describes feeling constipated recently and some burning when she urinates. Her BP is 135/75 mm Hg, HR is 89 beats per minute, temperature is 101.2°F, and her RR is 18 breaths per minute. Her abdomen is mildly distended, tender in the LLQ, and positive for rebound tenderness. CT scan is consistent with diverticulitis with a 7-cm abscess. Which of the following is the most appropriate management for this condition?

a. Reserve the OR for emergent laparotomy.
b. Start treatment with ciprofloxacin and metronidazole and plan for CT-guided draining of the abscess.
c. Give an IV dose of ciprofloxacin and have the patient follow up with her primary physician.
d. Start treatment with ciprofloxacin and metronidazole and plan for an emergent barium enema.
e. Start treatment with ciprofloxacin and metronidazole and prepare for an emergent colonoscopy.

**83.** A 29-year-old man presents to the ED complaining of RLQ pain for 24 hours. He states that the pain first began as a dull feeling around his umbilicus and slowly migrated to his right side. He has no appetite, is nauseated, and vomited twice. His BP is 130/75 mm Hg, HR is 95 beats per minute, temperature is 100.9°F, and his RR is 16 breaths per minute. His WBC is 14,000/μL. As you palpate the LLQ of the patient's abdomen, he states that his RLQ is painful. What is the name of this sign?

a. Blumberg sign
b. Psoas sign
c. Obturator sign
d. Raynaud sign
e. Rovsing sign

**84.** A 60-year-old man is brought to the ED complaining of generalized crampy abdominal pain that occurs in waves. He has been vomiting intermittently over the last 6 hours. His BP is 150/75 mm Hg, HR is 90 beats per minute, temperature is 99.8°F, and his RR is 16 breaths per minute. On abdominal examination you notice an old midline scar across the length of his abdomen that he states was from surgery after a gunshot wound as a teenager. The abdomen is distended with hyperactive bowel sounds and mild tenderness without rebound. An abdominal plain film confirms your diagnosis. Which of the following is the most appropriate next step in management?

a. Begin fluid resuscitation, bowel decompression with a nasogastric tube, and request a surgical consult.
b. Begin fluid resuscitation, administer broad-spectrum antibiotics, and admit the patient to the medical service.
c. Begin fluid resuscitation, give the patient stool softener, and administer a rectal enema.
d. Begin fluid resuscitation, administer broad-spectrum antibiotics, and observe the patient for 24 hours.
e. Order an abdominal ultrasound, administer antiemetics, and provide pain relief.

**85.** A 25-year-old G3P1011 presents to the ED with a 6-hour history of worsening lower abdominal pain, mostly in the RLQ. She also noticed some vaginal spotting this morning. She is nauseated, but did not vomit. Her last menstrual period was 2 months ago, but her cycles are irregular. She is sexually active and has a history of pelvic inflammatory disease. Her BP is 120/75 mm Hg, HR is 95 beats per minute, temperature is 99.2°F, and RR is 16 breaths per minute. Her abdomen is tender in the RLQ. Pelvic examination reveals right adnexal tenderness. Her WBC count is slightly elevated and her β-hCG is positive. After establishing IV access, which of the following is the most appropriate next step in management?

a. Call the OR to prepare for laparoscopy.
b. Order an emergent CT scan of the abdomen.
c. Perform a transvaginal ultrasound.
d. Order a urinalysis.
e. Swab her cervix and treat for gonorrhea and *Chlamydia*.

**86.** A 59-year-old man presents to the ED complaining of vomiting and sharp abdominal pain in the epigastric area that began abruptly this afternoon. He describes feeling nauseated and has no appetite. Laboratory results reveal WBC 18,000/μL, hematocrit 48%, platelets 110/μL, AST 275 U/L, ALT 125 U/L, alkaline phosphatase 75 U/L, amylase 1150 U/L, lipase 1450 IU, LDH 400 U/L, sodium 135 mEq/L, potassium 3.5 mEq/L, chloride 110 mEq/L, bicarbonate 20 mEq/L, BUN 20 mg/dL, creatinine 1.5 mg/dL, and glucose 250 mg/dL. Which of the following laboratory results correlate with the poorest prognosis?

a. Amylase 950, lipase 1250, LDH 400
b. Lipase 1250, LDH 400, bicarbonate 20
c. Lipase 1250, creatinine 1.5, potassium 3.5
d. WBC 18,000, LDH 400, glucose 250
e. WBC 18,000, amylase 950, lipase 1250

**87.** A 19-year-old woman presents to the ED with 1 hour of acute-onset progressively worsening pain in her RLQ. She developed nausea shortly after the pain and vomited twice over the last hour. She had similar but less severe pain 2 weeks ago that resolved spontaneously. Her BP is 123/78 mm Hg, HR is 99 beats per minute, temperature is 99.1°F, and her RR is 16 breaths per minute. On physical examination, the patient appears uncomfortable, not moving on the gurney. Her abdomen is non-distended, diffusely tender, worst in the RLQ. Pelvic examination reveals a normal-sized uterus and moderate right-sided adnexal tenderness. Laboratory results reveal WBC 10,000/μL, hematocrit 38%, and a negative urinalysis and β-hCG. Pelvic ultrasound reveals an enlarged right ovary with decreased flow. Which of the following is the most appropriate management for this patient?

a. Admit to the gynecology service for observation.
b. Administer IV antibiotics and operate once inflammation resolves.
c. Attempt manual detorsion.
d. Order an abdominal CT.
e. Go for immediate laparoscopic surgery.

**88.** An 18-year-old woman presents to the ED complaining of acute onset of RLQ abdominal pain. She also describes the loss of appetite over the last 12 hours, but denies nausea and vomiting. Her BP is 124/77 mm Hg, HR is 110 beats per minute, temperature is 102.1°F, RR is 16 breaths per minute, and oxygen saturation is 100% on room air. Abdominal examination reveals lower abdominal tenderness bilaterally. On pelvic examination you elicit cervical motion tenderness and note cervical exudates. Her WBC is 20,500/μL and β-hCG is negative. Which of the following is the most appropriate next step in management?

a. Bring her to the OR for an appendectomy.
b. Begin antibiotic therapy.
c. Perform a culdocentesis.
d. Bring her to the OR for immediate laparoscopy.
e. Order an abdominal plain film.

**89.** A 73-year-old man is seen in the ED for abdominal pain, nausea, and vomiting. His symptoms have progressively worsened over the past 2 to 3 days. The pain is diffuse and comes in waves. He denies fever or chills, but has a history of constipation. He reports no flatus for 24 hours. Physical examination is notable for diffuse tenderness and voluntary guarding. There is no rebound tenderness. An abdominal radiograph is seen below. Which of the following is the most likely diagnosis?

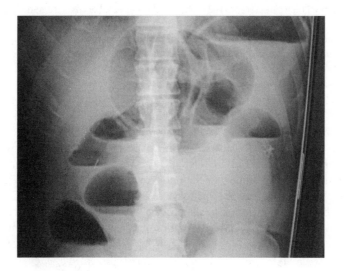

a. Constipation
b. SBO
c. Cholelithiasis
d. Large bowel obstruction
e. Inflammatory bowel disease

**90.** A 27-year-old man is seen in the ED for a leak around a surgical G-tube that was placed 2 weeks ago and has been used for enteral feeding for 1 week. Inspection reveals the tube is pulled out from the stoma, but is still in the cutaneous tissue. The abdomen is soft and nondistended and there are no signs of skin infection. Which of the following is the most appropriate next step in management?

a. Insert a Foley catheter into the tract and aspirate. If gastric contents are aspirated the tube can be used for feeding.
b. Insert a Foley catheter into the tract, instill water-soluble contrast, and obtain an abdominal radiograph prior to using for feeding.
c. Remove the tube and admit the patient for observation.
d. Remove the tube and immediately obtain a CT scan of the abdomen.
e. Return to the OR for closure of gastrotomy and placement of a new tube.

**91.** A 30-year-old man presents to the ED complaining of sudden onset of abdominal bloating and back pain lasting for 2 days. The pain woke him up from sleep 2 nights ago. It radiates from his back to his abdomen and down toward his scrotum. He is in severe pain and is vomiting. His temperature is 101.2°F and HR is 107 beats per minute. A CT scan reveals a 9-mm obstructing stone of the left ureter with hydronephrosis. Urinalysis is positive for 2+ blood, 2+ leukocytes, 2+ nitrites, 40 to 50 WBCs, and many bacteria. You administer pain medicine, antiemetics, and antibiotics. Which of the following is the most appropriate next step in management?

a. Admit for IV antibiotics and possible surgical removal of stone.
b. Observe in ED for another 6 hours to see if stone passes.
c. Discharge with antibiotics and pain medicine.
d. Discharge patient with instructions to consume large amounts of water.
e. Discharge patient with antibiotics, pain medicine, and instructions to drink large amounts of water and cranberry juice.

**92.** For which of the following patients is an abdominal CT scan contraindicated?

a. A 52-year-old man with abdominal pain after blunt trauma, negative focused assessment with sonography for trauma (FAST) examination, BP 125/78 mm Hg, and HR 109 beats per minute
b. A 22-year-old woman with RLQ pain, negative β-hCG, temperature 100.6°F
c. A 45-year-old man with abdominal pain, temperature 100.5°F, WBC 11,200/μL, BP 110/70 mm Hg, HR 110 beats per minute, and lipase 250 IU
d. A 70-year-old man with abdominal pain, an 11-cm pulsatile mass in the epigastrium, BP of 70/50 mm Hg, and HR of 110 beats per minute
e. A 65-year-old woman with right flank pain that radiates to her groin, microhematuria, BP 165/85 mm Hg, and HR 105 beats per minute

**93.** You are working in the ED on a Sunday afternoon when four people present with acute-onset vomiting and crampy abdominal pain. They were all at the same picnic and ate most of the same foods. The vomiting began approximately 4 hours into the picnic. They deny having any diarrhea. You believe they may have "food poisoning" so you place IV lines, administer IV fluids, and observe. Over the next few hours, the patients begin to improve, the vomiting stops, and their abdominal pain resolves. Which of the following is the most likely cause of their presentation?

a. Scombroid fish poisoning
b. Staphylococcal food poisoning
c. *Clostridium perfringens* food poisoning
d. *Campylobacter*
e. Salmonellosis

**94.** A 63-year-old man is brought to the ED by EMS complaining of severe abdominal pain that began suddenly 6 hours ago. His BP is 145/75 mm Hg and HR is 105 beats per minute and irregular. On examination, you note mild abdominal distention and diffuse abdominal tenderness without guarding. Stool is heme positive. Laboratory results reveal WBC 12,500/μL, hematocrit 48%, and lactate 4.2 U/L. ECG shows atrial fibrillation at a rate of 110. A CT scan is shown below. Which of the following is the most likely diagnosis?

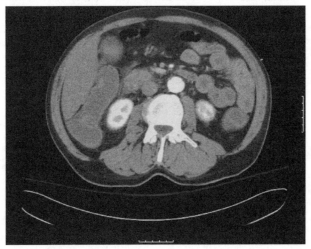

a. Abdominal aortic aneurysm
b. Mesenteric ischemia
c. Diverticulitis
d. SBO
e. Crohn disease

**95.** A 23-year-old woman presents to the ED with RLQ pain for the last 1 to 2 days. The pain is associated with nausea, vomiting, diarrhea, anorexia, and a fever of 100.9°F. She also reports dysuria. The patient returned 1 month ago from a trip to Mexico. She is sexually active with one partner but does not use contraception. She denies vaginal bleeding or discharge. Her last menstrual period was approximately 1 month ago. She has a history of pyelonephritis. Based on the principles of emergency medicine, what are the three priority considerations in the diagnosis of this patient?

a. Perihepatitis, gastroenteritis, cystitis
b. Ectopic pregnancy, appendicitis, pyelonephritis
c. Pelvic inflammatory disease (PID), gastroenteritis, cystitis
d. Ectopic pregnancy, PID, menstrual cramps
e. Gastroenteritis, amebic dysentery, menstrual cramps

**96.** A 24-year-old woman presents to the ED after being sexually assaulted. She is a college student with no past medical history. Her BP is 130/75 mm Hg, HR is 91 beats per minute, temperature is 98.6°F, and RR is 16 breaths per minute. On physical examination you observe vaginal trauma and scattered bruising and abrasions. Which of the following medications should be offered to the patient in this scenario?

a. Ceftriaxone, azithromycin, metronidazole, antiretrovirals, emergency contraception
b. Ceftriaxone, tetanus, metronidazole, antiretrovirals, emergency contraception
c. Ceftriaxone, azithromycin, tetanus, metronidazole, emergency contraception
d. Ceftriaxone, azithromycin, tetanus, antiretrovirals, emergency contraception
e. Ceftriaxone, azithromycin, tetanus, metronidazole, antiretrovirals, emergency contraception

**97.** A 22-year-old woman is brought to the ED by ambulance complaining of sudden onset of severe abdominal pain for 1 hour. The pain is in the RLQ and is not associated with nausea, vomiting, fever, or diarrhea. On the pelvic examination you palpate a tender right adnexal mass. The patient's last menstrual period was 6 weeks ago. Her BP is 95/65 mm Hg, HR is 124 beats per minute, temperature is 99.8°F, and RR is 20 breaths per minute. Which of the following are the most appropriate next steps in management?

a. Provide her oxygen via face mask and administer morphine sulfate.
b. Administer morphine sulfate, order an abdominal CT with contrast, and call an emergent surgery consult.
c. Send the patient's urine for analysis and order an abdominal CT.
d. Bolus 2 L NS, order a type and crossmatch and β-hCG, and call gynecology for possible surgery.
e. Provide oxygen via face mask, give morphine sulfate, and order a transvaginal ultrasound.

**98.** A 21-year-old woman presents to the ED complaining of diarrhea, abdominal cramps, fever, anorexia, and weight loss for 3 days. Her BP is 127/75 mm Hg, HR is 91 beats per minute, and temperature is 100.8°F. Her abdomen is soft and nontender without rebound or guarding. WBC is 9200/μL, β-hCG is negative, urinalysis is unremarkable, and stool is guaiac positive. She tells you that she has had this similar presentation four times over the past 2 months. Which of the following extraintestinal manifestations is associated with Crohn disease but not ulcerative colitis?

a. Ankylosing spondylitis
b. Erythema nodosum
c. Nephrolithiasis
d. Thromboembolic disease
e. Uveitis

**99.** A 23-year-old woman presents to the ED complaining of pain with urination. She has no other complaints. Her symptoms started 3 weeks ago. During this time, she has been to the clinic twice, with negative urine cultures each time. Her condition has not improved with antibiotic therapy with sulfonamides or quinolones. Physical examination is normal. Wet mount showed epithelial cells. Which of the following organisms is most likely responsible for the patient's symptoms?

a. *Staphylococcus aureus*
b. Herpes simplex virus
c. *Trichomonas vaginalis*
d. *Escherichia coli*
e. *Chlamydia trachomatis*

**100.** A 43-year-old man presents to the ED complaining of progressively worsening abdominal pain over the past 2 days. The pain is constant and radiates to his back. He also describes nausea and vomiting and states he usually drinks six pack of beer daily, but has not had a drink for 2 days. His BP is 144/75 mm Hg, HR is 101 beats per minute, temperature is 99.8°F, and RR is 14 breaths per minute. He is lying on his side with his knees flexed. Examination shows voluntary guarding and tenderness to palpation of his epigastrium. Laboratory results reveal WBC 10,500/μL, hematocrit 51%, platelets 225/μL, and lipase 620 IU. An abdominal radiograph reveals a nonspecific bowel gas pattern. There is no free air under the diaphragm. Which of the following is the most appropriate next step in management?

a. Observe in the ED.
b. Send home with antibiotic therapy.
c. Admit to the hospital for endoscopy.
d. Admit to the hospital for exploratory laparotomy.
e. Admit to the hospital for medical management and supportive care.

# Abdominal and Pelvic Pain

## Answers

**62. The answer is d.** (*Rosen, pp 1188-1192.*) There is a high suspicion that this patient has **mesenteric ischemia**, secondary to a **thromboembolism** from her **atrial fibrillation**. The typical patient with mesenteric ischemia may initially present with "pain that is out of proportion to the examination" (ie, although the patient is in pain, the abdomen is neither rigid, nor significantly tender on physical examination). Abdominal distention and peritoneal signs are late findings and signal the presence of bowel infarction. Plain abdominal radiographs are usually obtained early on in the workup. Although rare, the finding of **gas in either the bowel wall (pneumatosis intestinalis)** or in the portal venous system is strongly suggestive of intestinal infarct. This is a surgical emergency!

(**a, b, c, and e**) These are possible findings on radiography for patients with bowel infarction, although less sensitive and specific for infarction compared to pneumatosis intestinalis.

**63. The answer is b.** (*Rosen, pp 1200-1220.*) **Viral diarrheal** diseases are responsible for the majority of all acute episodes of diarrhea. *Rotavirus*, typically a disease of young children and **Norwalk virus** are the most frequent etiologic agents. In addition, enteric adenovirus is a common cause of gastroenteritis. Though dehydration is a common complication, these illnesses are usually self-limited, requiring only supportive care.

(**c, d, and e**) Bacterial causes of diarrheal disease comprise approximately 20% of all cases. (**a**) Parasitic causes are much more common outside of the United States.

**64. The answer is d.** (*Laoteppitaks, 2011.*) The patient's presentation is consistent with **alcoholic ketoacidosis (AKA)**. This is an acute metabolic acidosis that typically occurs in people who (1) chronically abuse alcohol and have a **recent history of binge drinking**, (2) have had little or **no recent food intake**, and (3) have had persistent vomiting. AKA is characterized by elevated serum ketone levels and a high anion gap ($\uparrow$AG = Na − [HCO3 + Cl] >12). A concomitant metabolic alkalosis is common, secondary to vomiting and volume depletion. AKA is the result of (1) starvation with glycogen depletion and counterregulatory hormone production; (2) a raised NADH/NAD+ ratio (related to the metabolism of ethanol); and (3) volume depletion, resulting in ketogenesis. The typical symptoms and physical findings relate to volume depletion and chronic alcohol abuse and include nausea, vomiting, abdominal pain, and/or hematemesis. The fruity odor of ketones may be present on the patient's breath. The patient's mental status may be impaired. Also associated with the presentation are dyspnea, tremulousness, and dizziness. Rarely do patients present with muscle pain, fever, diarrhea, syncope, seizure, or melena. In AKA, the β-hydroxybutyrate (β-OH)/acetyl acetate (AcAc) formation ratio is 5:1. The nitroprusside reaction (Acetest) may be negative or only weakly positive for serum ketones because nitroprusside reacts with AcAc, but not with β-OH. Therefore, ketosis may be more severe than would be inferred from a nitroprusside reaction alone.

Once the diagnosis of alcoholic ketoacidosis is established, the **mainstay of treatment is (b) hydration with 5% dextrose in normal saline ($D_5NS$ or ½ NS)**. With initial therapy, ketone formation shifts toward the production of AcAc so that measured ketone levels rise, although β-OH levels decrease. Carbohydrate and fluid replacement reverse the pathophysiologic derangements that lead to AKA by increasing serum insulin levels and suppressing the release of glucagon and other counterregulatory hormones. Dextrose stimulates the oxidation of NADH and aids in normalizing the NADH/NAD+ ratio.

As additional treatment, thiamine supplementation should be given as prophylaxis against Wernicke encephalopathy. In general, exogenous insulin is contraindicated in the treatment of AKA because it may cause life-threatening hypoglycemia in patients with depleted glycogen stores.

Fluids alone **(a, b, and c)** do not correct AKA as quickly as fluids and carbohydrates combined, thus making the type of solution quite relevant **(e)** to managing this patient indeed.

**65. The answer is e.** (*Rosen, pp 1168-1170.*) The patient's history and physical examination is consistent with **acute cholecystitis.** Because of the poor predictive value of the history, physical and laboratory findings in cholecystitis, the most important test for diagnosis is a strong clinical suspicion and **ultrasound imaging.** It is rapid and noninvasive. Ultrasound may show the presence of gallstones as small as 2 mm, gallbladder wall thickening and distention, and pericholecystic fluid.

(b) CT scanning may be useful when there are other intra-abdominal disorders in consideration. However, the sensitivity of a CT is less than that of ultrasound when diagnosing acute cholecystitis. (c) MRI usually has no role in the diagnosis of acute cholecystitis. (d) Radioisotope cholescintigraphy (HIDA scan) has a higher sensitivity and specificity than ultrasound making it the most accurate study for cholecystitis; however, it is reserved for cases where ultrasound is negative or equivocal. (a) Plain film radiographs demonstrate stones in the gallbladder only less than 25% of the time.

**66. The answer is c.** *(Rosen, pp 1307-1313.)* The patient's history of colicky flank pain that radiates to the groin and hematuria is consistent with a **ureteral stone.** Adequate **analgesia** is critical in treating a patient with a ureteral stone. Intravenous **ketorolac,** a nonsteroidal anti-inflammatory drug (NSAID), is frequently administered as a first-line analgesic, but morphine may be necessary for continued pain. In addition to their analgesia, NSAIDs decrease ureterospasm and renal capsular pressure in the obstructed kidney. Antiemetics, such as metoclopramide, help with the nausea and vomiting.

(a) Appendicitis is unlikely with a soft, nontender abdomen and no fever. An abdominal CT (b) will probably be necessary, but the patient's pain needs to be controlled first. An abdominal aortic aneurysm (d) can present with flank pain, however it is very rare in a 31-year-old man. Testicular torsion (e) should always be considered in a patient with groin pain. In this case, a stone is more consistent with the history.

**67. The answer is d.** *(Rosen, pp 1093-1102.)* The **classic triad** of a **ruptured abdominal aortic aneurysm (AAA)** is **pain, hypotension,** and a **pulsatile abdominal mass.** Sometimes patients have only one or two of the components and occasionally may have none. Most patients who are diagnosed with AAA are asymptomatic. However, rupture is often the first manifestation of an AAA. Most patients with a ruptured AAA experience pain in the abdomen, back, or flank. It is usually acute in onset and severe. Approximately 20% of the time, patients present to the ED with syncope. Patients with a ruptured AAA are unstable until their aorta is cross clamped in the OR. Therefore, any **hemodynamically unstable** patient with a diagnosed or strongly suspected AAA should be **taken immediately to the OR.**

(a) A CT scan is excellent for diagnosing an AAA in stable patients. (b) Angiography has no role in the emergent evaluation of a patient suspected of a ruptured AAA. (c) An abdominal radiograph can aid in the diagnosis of an AAA. However, when there is high clinical suspicion and the patient is hemodynamically unstable, the patient should be brought to the OR. (e) The patient is not complaining of chest pain and his ECG is not consistent with an acute coronary event. Therefore, cardiac catheterization is not required.

**68. The answer is c.** (*Rosen, pp 1184-1188.*) The patient presents with the clinical findings of **SBO:** vomiting, intermittent crampy abdominal pain, abdominal distention, hyperactive bowel sounds, and general tenderness. The most common cause of SBO in developed countries is **postoperative adhesions,** responsible for more than 50% of all SBO. There is a particularly high incidence of SBO after **gynecologic surgeries,** such as a **hysterectomy.** A common mnemonic for the causes of bowel obstruction is ABC: Adhesions, Bulges (hernia), and Cancer.

Hernias (d) are the second most common cause of obstruction. Traveling to Mexico (a) may give you diarrhea and abdominal pain from enteritis. Ethanol abuse (b) can lead to abdominal pain because of many causes, such as gastritis. Constipation (e) will not produce the hyperactive bowel sounds as seen in obstruction.

**69. The answer is e.** (*Rosen, pp 1159-1160.*) The patient's clinical presentation is consistent with **alcoholic hepatitis,** which is a potentially severe form of alcohol-induced liver disease. Most people remain subclinical, but the presentation ranges from nausea and vomiting to fulminant hepatitis and liver failure. Laboratory tests usually reveal moderate elevations of AST and ALT. Usually in alcoholic hepatitis, the **AST is greater than the ALT** (think "scotch" and "tonic" for AST > ALT). The patient exhibits stigmata of chronic alcohol disease seen by gynecomastia and spider angiomata. The management is principally **supportive,** with correction of any fluid or electrolyte imbalances, paying special attention to blood glucose (ethanol can suppress gluconeogenesis) and magnesium. Thiamine may also be deficient in chronic alcoholics.

Suctioning the patient's stomach with a nasogastric tube (a) is not indicated and should not be performed. A HIDA scan (b) is the most accurate test for establishing the diagnosis of cholecystitis. However, before an HIDA is performed, individuals with suspected cholecystitis should undergo ultrasound scanning. Unless this is a known needle stick or mucosal exposure, hepatitis immune globulin (c) is not acutely indicated. Viral hepatitis titers (d) can be drawn as an outpatient if suspicious for a viral infection.

**70. The answer is e.** *(Rosen, p 1162.)* Analysis of abdominal fluid and clinical presentation are consistent with **spontaneous bacterial peritonitis (SBP)**. It is recommended to start antibiotic treatment for SBP if the neutrophil count is greater than 250 cells/mm$^3$. Causative organisms include gram-negative enterococcus such as *E coli* and *Klebsiella*, as well as *Streptococcus* sp, and *Streptococcus pneumoniae*. Therefore, the most appropriate antibiotic for treatment is a **third-generation cephalosporin**, such as **cefotaxime**.

**71. The answer is e.** *(Rosen, pp 1314-1316.)* Testicular torsion is a **surgical** emergency. There are two peak periods in which torsion is likely to occur, the first year of life and at puberty. **Manual detorsion** can be attempted in most cases while arranging for definitive care. After appropriate analgesia, the anterior testicle should be twisted laterally, like opening a book. **Color Doppler ultrasound** is the best test of choice in most hospitals. Immediate evaluation and referral to a urologist is essential. **Prehn sign** (the physical lifting of the testicles relieves the pain of epididymitis but not pain caused by testicular torsion) is a medical diagnostic indicator that was once believed to help determine whether the presenting testicular pain is caused by acute epididymitis or from testicular torsion. Although elevation of the scrotum when differentiating epididymitis from testicular torsion is of clinical value, Prehn sign has been shown to be inferior to Doppler ultrasound to rule out testicular torsion.

To administer ceftriaxone and doxycycline (a) and swab his urethra (b) is the correct management for urethritis. A urinalysis (c) should be sent on most patients with scrotal pain but in this case the diagnosis of torsion takes precedence. Although epididymitis (d) and torsion have similar presentations, epididymitis usually has more of a gradual onset, reaching a peak over days. Epididymitis is the most common misdiagnosis of testicular torsion.

**72. The answer is d.** *(Rosen, pp 1193-1199.)* Appendicitis is the most common cause of the acute surgical abdomen. It can occur at any age but is most prevalent in the teens and twenties. It is classically described as starting with the vague onset of dull **periumbilical pain that migrates to**

**the RLQ.** It is associated with anorexia, nausea, and vomiting. A low-grade fever may develop. You should suspect appendicitis in any patient with RLQ pain. Approximately 90% of patients have a WBC greater than 10,000/mm$^3$ although, the WBC can be normal in appendicitis. Urinalysis can help differentiate urinary tract disease from acute appendicitis, although a mild pyuria may be seen in appendicitis if the appendix is irritating the ureter. **Abdominal CT with IV and oral or rectal contrast** is reported to have a sensitivity of up to 100% and specificity of 95%. CT findings of appendicitis include an enlarged appendix (> 6 mm), pericecal inflammation, and the presence of an appendicolith.

(a) Dilated loops of bowel are suggestive of bowel obstruction. (b) Many patients who ultimately are diagnosed with appendicitis initially believed they had food poisoning. If there is a low clinical suspicion for appendicitis and gastritis is more likely, than administering an antacid and observation is reasonable. However, any change in clinical examination should be attributed to a more significant process. (c) Abdominal ultrasound is commonly used initially in pregnant women and children with suspected appendicitis. Its sensitivity and specificity approaches 90%, but there may be inadequate studies as a result of body habitus or with a retrocecal appendix. (e) It would be inappropriate to discharge this patient home without first evaluating for appendicitis.

**73. The answer is d.** *(Rosen, pp 1325-1328.)* The patient's clinical picture is consistent with **ovarian torsion.** This phenomenon is most common in women in their mid-twenties. It is caused by the **ovary twisting on its stalk,** which leads to occlusion of venous draining from the ovary. This leads to ovarian edema, hemorrhage, and necrosis. Most occur in the presence of an enlarged ovary (ie, as a result of cyst, abscess, or tumor). Patients may give a history of similar pain that resolved spontaneously. The first choice to diagnose ovarian torsion is with **Doppler ultrasound** to demonstrate decreased or absent blood flow to the ovary. It can also identify an ovarian mass. If suspicion is high for ovarian torsion, the patient may immediately undergo laparoscopy, which is diagnostic and potentially therapeutic.

(a) CT scan may be necessary if the Doppler studies are equivocal. However, if torsion is suspected, the individual should undergo a laparoscopy, which is the definitive diagnostic procedure. (b) MRI and (c) x-ray have no role in the diagnosis of ovarian torsion. If there is high enough clinical suspicion, and diagnostic tests are equivocal, laparoscopy (e) can be used to visualize the ovaries in vivo.

**74. The answer is e.** *(Tintinalli, pp 606-613.)* Potential complications of colonoscopy include hemorrhage, perforation, retroperitoneal abscess, pneumoscrotum, pneumothorax, volvulus, and infection. **Perforation of the colon with pneumoperitoneum** is usually evident immediately, but can take several hours to manifest. Perforation is usually secondary to intrinsic disease of the colon (eg, diverticulitis) or to vigorous manipulation during colonoscopy. Most patients require immediate laparotomy. However, expectant management is appropriate in some patients with a late presentation (1-2 days later), or without signs of peritonitis. The radiograph in the figure demonstrates **air under the diaphragm,** which is pathognomonic for pneumoperitoneum.

Ascending cholangitis **(a)** and pancreatitis **(d)** may occur as a complication from endoscopic retrograde cholangiopancreatography (ERCP). **(b)** There is no evidence of pulmonary edema in this radiograph. **(c)** Liver failure with ascites does not cause pneumoperitoneum.

**75. The answer is c.** *(Rosen, p 1170.)* The patient's clinical picture is consistent with **cholangitis,** which is caused by an obstruction of the biliary tract leading to bacterial infection. Obstruction is commonly secondary to a stone, but may be because of malignancy or stricture. Cholangitis is a surgical emergency. The classic **triad** of physical findings described by **Charcot** is **RUQ pain, fever,** and **jaundice.** Sepsis is a common complication. Sonography may demonstrate intrahepatic or ductal dilation. The presence of stones in the gallbladder suggests obstruction as the etiology.

There is overlap in the clinical presentation with cholecystitis **(a),** however, the presence of jaundice and evidence of dilated common and intrahepatic ducts—which are not characteristic of cholecystitis—is helpful to distinguish it from cholangitis. Acute hepatitis **(b)** will not have the same sonographic findings seen in cholangitis. Pancreatic cancer **(d)** can present with jaundice, but it is usually painless. Bowel obstruction **(e)** generally presents with intermittent crampy abdominal pain, vomiting, and distention.

**76. The answer is b.** *(Rosen, pp 201-202, 2281-2285.)* β-**Human chronic gonadotropin (β-hCG)** should be obtained in all women of child-bearing age who present with abdominal pain or vaginal bleeding. Diagnostically, it is one of the most important tests in female patients. A positive pregnancy test in the setting of abdominal pain and vaginal bleeding demands that the physician rule out an ectopic pregnancy. Even though the patient states she always uses condoms during intercourse, there is still a small risk of pregnancy. (a) Women with lower abdominal pain and vaginal discharge may have cervicitis or pelvic inflammatory disease and require a *Chlamydia* antigen test. However, a pelvic examination should be performed first. (c) With a positive pregnancy test, transvaginal ultrasound is the next step in management. This is used to detect an intrauterine pregnancy. If no intrauterine pregnancy is detected, the suspicion for an ectopic pregnancy increases. (d) An abdominal radiograph may be obtained later in the workup, but is not currently indicated. (e) Observation is not an acceptable option in any patient with undifferentiated abdominal pain and vaginal bleeding. It is imperative that the clinician rule out an ectopic pregnancy in this individual.

**77. The answer is e.** *(Rosen, pp 1093-1102.)* The patient presents with multiple risk factors for an **AAA: age greater than 60, male gender, hypertension, cigarette smoking,** and **peripheral artery disease.** Classically, AAA presents with constant abdominal pain, often localizing to the left middle or lower quadrant with radiation to the back. Physical examination may reveal a **pulsatile abdominal mass.** Patients can present unstable if the aneurysm leaks or ruptures requiring emergent management in the OR. Evidence of an AAA is seen on plain radiograph approximately 66% to 75% of the time. The most common findings are curvilinear calcification of the aortic wall or a paravertebral soft tissue mass. Ultrasound and CT are the best diagnostic tools for the stable patient.

(a) Biliary colic occurs in the RUQ and usually lasts less than 6 hours. (b) The pain of a kidney stone is usually described as colicky in nature. Pain typically begins in the flank and radiates to the groin. (c) Pancreatitis typically presents with mid-epigastric pain that radiates to the back and is associated with nausea and vomiting. (d) SBO is diagnosed on radiography by evidence of dilated loops of bowel, air-fluid levels, and thickening of the bowel wall.

**78. The answer is c.** *(Rosen, pp 1176-1177.)* **Lipase is a pancreatic enzyme** that hydrolyzes triglycerides. In the presence of pancreatic inflammation it increases within 4 to 8 hours and peaks at 24 hours. At **five times the upper limits of normal,** lipase is **60% sensitive and 100% specific** for pancreatitis. The diagnosis is usually made with a lipase of two times the normal limit, thereby increasing its sensitivity.

(a) Elevations of amylase are approximately 70% specific for the diagnosis of pancreatitis. (b, d, and e) are all laboratory values that are used in the prognosis for pancreatitis, not for its diagnosis.

**79. The answer is a.** *(Rosen, pp 1316-1318.)* The patient has **epididymitis.** It is often difficult to distinguish epididymitis from testicular torsion and the clinician should always rule out torsion first if the diagnosis is in doubt. It is the most common misdiagnosis for testicular torsion. Epididymitis is generally a disease of adult men. The causative organism in men over 35 years is *E coli,* while *C trachomatis* and *Neisseria gonorrhoeae* predominate in men less than 35 years old. The older patient may have a history of gonococcal urethritis (GU) tract manipulation or a history of prostatitis. The onset is usually gradual and urinary tract symptoms may precede the pain.

Testicular torsion (b) should always be on the differential for a patient with scrotal pain. However, it is ruled out in this patient by the presence of blood flow on color Doppler. UTIs in men (c), in the absence of trauma or instrumentation, are rare. Scrotal pain is usually not present. Testicular tumors (d) are often mistakenly diagnosed as epididymitis. They usually occur in middle-aged men and have a higher prevalence in patients with cryptorchidism. Color Doppler can often distinguish a tumor from epididymitis. A varicocele (e) is a painless scrotal swelling that is caused by dilation and elongation of the veins of the pampiniform plexus. Varicocele is more common on the left side because the left spermatic vein drains into the left renal vein, whereas the right one drains into the inferior vena cava. Individuals may be asymptomatic or complain of a scrotal pain or heaviness. It is thought that varicoceles may decrease sperm production.

**80. The answer is a.** *(Rosen, pp 1289-1294.)* Dysuria in young men is almost always because of **urethritis,** which is commonly caused by a **sexually transmitted disease.** Urethritis is classically divided into gonococcal (GU) and nongonococcal (NGU) types. GU is caused by *N gonorrhoeae,* while the major pathogen in NGU is *C trachomatis.* Nearly all men with GU have purulent urethral discharge. NGU may be asymptomatic or with a yellow, mucopurulent discharge. It was demonstrated in multiple studies that the two pathogens coexist in men with urethritis up to 50% of the time. Therefore, antibiotics should be directed at eliminating both organisms. A third-generation cephalosporin or ciprofloxacin as a one-time dose is used to treat GU. Common antibiotics used to treat NGU include azithromycin as a single dose and doxycycline or erythromycin for 7 days. In addition, the patient should refer all of their sexual partners for evaluation and treatment. (**d and e**) There is no clinical suspicion for a kidney stone or testicular cancer.

(**b**) This choice might be correct if you suspect a patient has UTI. However, a young man with dysuria and urethral discharge needs to be treated for a sexually transmitted disease. (**c**) The patient should not be discharged prior to treatment and culture.

**81. The answer is a.** (*Rosen, pp 1164-1165.*) **Amebic abscesses** are common in countries with tropical and subtropical climates and areas with poor sanitation. **Entamoeba histolytica** causes an intestinal infection, and the liver is seeded via the portal system. The clinical presentation includes abdominal tenderness in the RUQ, leukocytosis, and fever. Diagnosis is supported by identifying a pathogenic protozoan in the stool. Management consists of supportive care and administering metronidazole. If medical therapy is unsuccessful, percutaneous catheter drainage is required.

(**b**) Cholecystitis will present with fever, leukocytosis, and pain. A Murphy sign is usually present. (**c**) Cryptosporidium is the most common cause of chronic diarrhea in individuals with AIDS. Patients present with profuse watery diarrhea, abdominal cramping, anorexia, nausea, and flatulence. Symptoms persist in the immunocompetent for approximately 1 to 3 weeks and are self-limited. Dehydration is common. There was a cryptosporidium outbreak in Milwaukee, Wisconsin in 1993 after a water purification plant was contaminated. More than 100 people died, among them mostly the elderly and immunocompromised. (**d**) Patients with enterobiasis or pinworms complain of itching in the anal region, particularly at night, as the adult worm lays eggs in the anus. (**e**) Pyogenic abscess is the most common type of liver abscess; however, the history of travel, and lack of primary source for the pyogenic abscess make it less likely a diagnosis. Underlying biliary disease with extrahepatic biliary obstruction leading to ascending cholangitis and abscess formation is the most common cause and is usually associated with choledocholithiasis, benign and malignant tumors, or postsurgical strictures.

**82. The answer is b.** (*Rosen, pp 1229-1232.*) Management for **complicated acute diverticulitis** involves **admission** and **antibiotic treatment**. Treatment is directed against both anaerobic and gram-negative bacteria. Intra-abdominal **abscess** formation secondary to diverticulitis requires prompt surgical consultation and should be **drained** using CT or ultrasound-guided percutaneous draining. Abscesses less than 5 cm in diameter may be treated with antibiotics alone.

The patient's vital signs are stable and there is no evidence for peritonitis, therefore she does not require an emergent laparotomy (**a**). The patient should not be discharged from the hospital (**c**). Because of the risk for bowel perforation, barium enema and colonoscopy are contraindicated (**d** and **e**); however, once the diverticulitis is controlled, the patient should undergo one of the procedures to look for other pathology and exclude complications, such as fistula formation.

**83. The answer is e.** *(Rosen, p 1194.)* **Rovsing sign** is the referred tenderness to the RLQ when the LLQ is palpated. It is seen with **acute appendicitis.**

Blumberg sign (**a**) is the occurrence of a sharp pain when the examiner presses his or her hand over McBurney point and then releases the hand pressure suddenly. This sign is indicative of peritoneal inflammation. The Psoas sign (**b**) is the increase of pain when the psoas muscle is stretched as the patient extends his or her hip. The Obturator sign (**c**) is the elicitation of pain as the hip is flexed and internally rotated. Raynaud sign (**d**) is a condition marked by symmetrical cyanosis of the extremities with persistent, uneven, mottled blue or red discoloration of the skin of the digits, wrists, and ankles, along with profuse sweating and coldness of the fingers and toes.

**84. The answer is a.** *(Rosen, pp 1184-1188.)* The patient's clinical picture is consistent with an **SBO. Fluid resuscitation** is important because of the inability of the distended bowel to absorb fluid and electrolytes at a normal rate. Compounded with vomiting, fluid loses can lead to hypovolemia and shock. **Nasogastric suction** provides enteral decompression by removing accumulated gas and fluid proximal to the obstruction. A **surgical consult** is necessary because definitive treatment may require taking the patient to the OR to relieve the obstruction. An old surgical adage states "Never let the sun set or rise on a bowel obstruction." Broad-spectrum antibiotics (**b and d**) are appropriate when surgery is planned or when there is suspicion for vascular compromise or bowel perforation.

Stool softener and enemas (**c**) have no role in acute intestinal obstructions caused by mechanical causes. Adult SBO are diagnosed with an abdominal plain film, or CT scan (**e**), not by ultrasound.

**85. The answer is c.** *(Rosen, pp 2281-2285.)* Any woman with abdominal pain, vaginal bleeding, and a positive pregnancy test needs to be ruled out for an **ectopic pregnancy.** Her vital signs are stable so that she can undergo a **transvaginal ultrasound.** This is used to document an intrauterine pregnancy and the health of the fetus. If no intrauterine pregnancy is observed, the suspicion for an ectopic pregnancy increases.

**(a)** Laparoscopy is an accurate diagnostic and therapeutic procedure that can be used in the patient with an unclear ultrasound and peritoneal signs on examination. **(b)** If an intrauterine pregnancy is documented and there is low suspicion for an ectopic pregnancy, yet the patient complains of severe RLQ pain, then the risks (eg, radiation exposure to the fetus) and benefits (eg, diagnosing appendicitis) of performing a CT scan must be discussed. **(d)** A urinalysis is part of the general workup, but is not emergently needed. **(e)** Any patient with a positive pregnancy test, abdominal pain, and vaginal bleeding needs to undergo an urgent evaluation for an ectopic pregnancy.

**86. The answer is d.** *(Rosen, pp 1176-1178.)* The patient's clinical picture is consistent with **acute pancreatitis.** Ranson developed criteria that help **predict mortality rates** in patients with pancreatitis. The presence of more than three criteria equals 1% mortality, while the presence of six or more criteria approaches 100% mortality. **Ranson criteria** at admission are age greater than 55, WBC greater than 16,000, glucose greater than 200, LDH greater than 350, and AST greater than 250. Within 48 hours of admission, hematocrit fall greater than 10%, BUN rise greater than 5, serum calcium less than 8, arterial $PO_2$ less than 60, base deficit greater than 4, and fluid sequestration greater than 6 L. The patient in the case fulfills four of Ranson criteria and has approximately 15% mortality risk. Note that lipase and amylase are not part of Ranson criteria despite being relevant in the diagnosis of acute pancreatitis.

**87. The answer is e.** *(Rosen, pp 1325-1328.)* The differential diagnosis in a woman with RLQ pain is expansive and includes GI pathology, such as appendicitis, inflammatory bowel disease, diverticulitis, and hernia. Gynecologic pathology includes ectopic pregnancy, tubo-ovarian abscess, ruptured corpus luteum cyst, and ovarian torsion. It is often difficult to initially distinguish between gastrointestinal (GI) and gynecologic (GYN) pathology and which diagnostic test, abdominal CT, or a pelvic ultrasound, is warranted. Often, the decision is based on the pelvic examination.

The patient in the question exhibits **adnexal tenderness** and therefore received a pelvic ultrasound that revealed a **unilateral enlarged ovary with decreased flow,** indicative of **ovarian torsion.** Ovarian torsion is a **gynecologic emergency** and conservative management has no place in the treatment decision of suspected torsion even if pain improves in the ED. Failure to surgically correct this entity may result in ischemia and subsequent necrosis of the involved ovary. Therefore, the mainstay of therapy is **laparoscopy** or **laparotomy.**

(a) Conservative management is not an option in suspected ovarian torsion. (b) Antibiotics and delayed surgery may be acceptable for a tubo-ovarian abscess. (c) Manual detorsion is not possible in the female patient. It can be attempted in the male patient. (d) If pelvic ultrasound was normal and there is suspicion for GI pathology, then abdominal CT is warranted.

**88. The answer is b.** *(Tintinalli, pp 716-720.)* **Pelvic inflammatory disease (PID)** comprises a spectrum of infections of the female upper reproductive tract. Although *N gonorrhoeae* and *C trachomatis* are thought to cause the majority of infections, new evidence points to greater rates of polymicrobial infections. Most cases of PID are thought to start with a sexually transmitted disease of the lower genital tract and ascend to the upper tract. Women typically present with lower abdominal pain and may have vaginal discharge, vaginal bleeding, dysuria, and fever. The examination usually reveals **lower abdominal tenderness** and **cervical motion tenderness** or **adnexal tenderness.** Many patients are treated as outpatients with antibiotics. Considerations for admission include those women who are pregnant, have failed outpatient therapy, are toxic appearing, have evidence for a tubo-ovarian abscess, or in whom a surgical emergency cannot be ruled out. Long-term outcomes are improved if antibiotics are begun immediately.

(a) The onset of appendicitis is more insidious than what is presented in this case. The initial symptoms are usually nausea or loss of appetite. Pain typically begins in the periumbilical area and migrates to the RLQ. Fever is usually not significant unless the appendix ruptures. (c) Culdocentesis is used to retrieve fluid in the cul-de-sac. The findings are limited and not specific to PID. (d) Laparoscopy is not indicated in an individual with cervicitis. It is useful to diagnose and manage ovarian torsion and other gynecologic pathology. (e) There is no role for a plain film in this patient. It would be useful if you suspected a bowel obstruction or free air.

**89. The answer is b.** *(Tintinalli, pp 581-583.)* The clinical scenario and radiograph are consistent with **SBO**. Patients usually present with **diffuse, crampy abdominal pain that** is often episodic in nature. Typically, the patient reports no recent bowel movements or flatus passage. The most common causes of SBO are **adhesions and hernias.** All patients with suspected SBO should have flat and upright abdominal radiographs performed. Flat-plate abdominal films can show distended loops of small bowel and the upright film can show multiple air-fluid levels in a stepladder appearance.

(**a**) Constipation is a diagnosis of exclusion, although fecal impaction is a common problem in debilitated elderly patients and may present with symptoms of colonic obstruction. (**c**) Cholelithiasis typically presents with RUQ pain and fever. Ultrasound is typically used to make the diagnosis of cholecystitis. (**d**) The most common causes of large bowel obstruction include neoplasm, diverticulitis, and sigmoid volvulus. The large bowel contains folds called haustra that do not cross the entire bowel width. In the above figure, we see **valvulae conniventes,** which are folds of the small bowel that cross the entire width of the bowel. (**e**) Neither the clinical scenario nor the plain film is consistent with inflammatory bowel disease. Most patients with inflammatory bowel disease are younger.

**90. The answer is b.** *(Tintinalli, pp 604-605.)* Although there are no studies stating how long it takes for a tract to mature, tracts that are 7 to 10 days old probably will remain open long enough to allow replacement. Insertion of a new tube should be performed with water-soluble lubricant. If resistance is met, the attempt should be aborted. After replacing the tube, 20- to 30-mL bolus of **water-soluble contrast** material should be instilled into the tube, and a supine **abdominal radiograph** should demonstrate rugae of the stomach. If there is any question of improper placement, immediate consultation should be obtained.

(**a**) Aspiration of gastric contents does not confirm proper placement of a G-tube. The intragastric location of a replaced tube should be confirmed by a contrast study before feedings. Many patients have received intraperitoneal feedings in the absence of such a confirmatory test. (**c**) If the tract is open, a tube should be replaced; otherwise observation would be appropriate until a new tube could be arranged. (**d**) A CT scan may be helpful to determine if the tube is out, but once it is, clinical signs would be sufficient to evaluate for intraperitoneal soilage. (**e**) Surgical G-tubes generally involve anchoring the stomach to the anterior abdominal wall.

Contamination is unlikely and the tube tract will be patent for a short time. There is no immediate indication for surgery.

**91. The answer is a.** *(Rosen, pp 1307-1313.)* An **obstructing stone with an overlying infection** is an impending **urologic emergency.** Bacteria in an obstructed collecting system can cause abscess formation, renal destruction, and severe systemic toxicity. The patient requires admission for IV antibiotics and removal and drainage of the stone. In addition to obstruction with infection, other indications for admission include persistent pain, persistent nausea and vomiting, urinary extravasation, and hypercalcemic crisis.

**(b)** Observation is not recommended. Stones smaller than 4 mm pass 90% of the time, stones 4 to 6 mm pass 50% of the time, and stones larger than 6 mm pass 10% of the time. The patient requires IV antibiotics and removal of the stone. **(c, d,** and **e)** The patient should not be discharged; rather, admission is required for an infected obstructing stone. Although it is important to keep the patient well hydrated, no evidence supports the notion that IV hydration increases likelihood of stone passage.

**92. The answer is d.** *(Tintinalli, CD e121.)* CT scanning has become an integral part of the ED evaluation of a patient. It is useful to differentiate abdominal pathologies when the history and physical examination are nonspecific, or in confirming a diagnosis suspected by the clinical presentation. Contrast materials for CT examinations in the ED are usually administered via oral and IV routes, which improves visualization of abdominal organs. **A patient must be relatively stable to undergo a CT scan.** The patient with abdominal pain and a BP of 70/50 mm Hg is not hemodynamically stable. His clinical presentation is consistent with a ruptured AAA. This is a surgical emergency and should be treated in the OR. Obtaining a CT scan first will delay definitive treatment and worsen the patient's hemorrhagic shock and ultimately decrease his chance of survival.

**(a)** This patient sustained blunt trauma and does not show evidence of an active bleed on the FAST examination. With stable vital signs, a CT scan is safe. **(b)** This patient may have appendicitis and requires a CT scan. If she was β-hCG positive, you would first perform a pelvic ultrasound to evaluate for an ectopic pregnancy. **(c)** Pancreatitis is high on the differential; a CT scan will help to evaluate his abdominal pain. **(e)** This patient most likely has a kidney stone, which is seen on abdominal CT scan.

**93. The answer is b.** (*Rosen, pp 1209-1214.*) **Staphylococcal food poisoning** is caused by an enterotoxin-forming strain of *Staphylococcus* organisms in the food before ingestion. Most **protein-rich foods** support the growth of staphylococci, particularly ham, eggs, custard, mayonnaise, and potato salad. The illness has an **abrupt onset**, beginning **1 to 6 hours** after ingestion of the contaminated food. Cramping and abdominal pain, with **violent and frequent retching and vomiting** are the predominant symptoms. Diarrhea is variable; it is usually mild, and occasionally absent. Although often aggressive in onset, staphylococcal food poisoning is **short lived** and usually **subsides in 6 to 8 hours,** rarely lasting more than 24 hours. The patient is often recovering when first seen by a physician. The **short incubation period** and **multiple cases** in people eating the same meal are highly suggestive of this disease.

(**a**) Scombroid fish poisoning results from the ingestion of heat-stable toxins produced by bacterial action on the dark meat of the fish (eg, tuna and mackerel). The symptoms occur abruptly within 20 to 30 minutes and resemble histamine intoxication, consisting of facial flushing, diarrhea, throbbing headache, palpitations, and abdominal cramps. Antihistamine therapy is usually curative. (**c**) *Clostridium perfringens* is probably the most common cause of acute food poisoning in the United States. Most cases occur in fairly large outbreaks and are caused by the ingestion of meat and poultry dishes. Symptoms usually appear within 6 to 12 hours but can occur up to 24 hours after ingestion of the contaminated food. Frequent, watery diarrhea and moderately severe abdominal cramping are the major symptoms. The illness is self-limited and rarely lasts for more than 24 hours. (**d**) *Campylobacter* is the most common bacterial cause of diarrhea in patients who seek medical attention. The incubation period is approximately 2 to 5 days. Onset of symptoms is usually rapid and consists of fever, crampy abdominal pain, and diarrhea. Constitutional symptoms are common. (**e**) Salmonellosis occurs most during the summer months and is acquired by the ingestion of contaminated food or drink. Poultry products, such as turkey, chicken, duck, and eggs constitute the most common sources. Family outbreaks and sporadic cases are more common than large epidemics. The typical patient presents with fever, colicky abdominal pain, and loose, watery diarrhea, occasionally with mucus and blood. Symptoms usually abate within 2 to 5 days and recovery is uneventful.

**94. The answer is b.** (*Rosen, pp 1188-1192.*) **Acute mesenteric ischemia** is caused by the lack of perfusion to the bowel. It primarily affects patients

**over the age of 50 years,** particularly those with significant cardiovascular or systemic disease. The etiology is either from arterial occlusion (eg, embolization from the heart); venous thrombosis that is associated with a hypercoagulable state; or nonocclusive, because of reduced cardiac output (eg, congestive heart failure [CHF], recent myocardial infraction [MI], hypovolemia). Most patients present with abdominal pain that is initially dull and diffuse. In this early state, patients frequently complain of severe pain, but have minimal tenderness on examination (ie, the characteristic "**pain out of proportion to examination**"). As infarction develops, abdominal distension and peritoneal signs develop. Sudden onset of pain suggests arterial vascular occlusion by emboli. This may occur with patients who present in **atrial fibrillation.** Insidious onset suggests venous thrombosis or nonocclusive infarction. Radiographs may reveal dilated loops of bowel, air in the bowel wall (**pneumatosis intestinalis**), and thickening of the bowel wall, as seen in the CT scan. Management involves fluid resuscitation, antibiotics, and surgical intervention.

(**a**) Classically, AAA present with constant abdominal pain, often localizing to the LMQ or LLQ, with radiation to the back. Physical examination may reveal a pulsatile abdominal mass. (**c**) Diverticulitis usually presents with LLQ abdominal pain and low-grade fever. (**d**) Patients with a SBO present with crampy abdominal pain and distention. Vomiting and obstipation are frequent symptoms. Distended loops of bowel and air-fluid levels are seen on radiographs. (**e**) Crohn disease may present with bloody diarrhea, abdominal pain, fevers, anorexia, and weight loss. There is a peak incidence between 15 and 22 years and 55 and 60 years.

**95. The answer is b.** (*Hamilton et al, p 6.*) The **emergency physician (EP)** approaches a problem by **considering the most serious disease** consistent with the patient complaint and working to exclude it. Thinking of the **worst** first is a reversal from the sequence of patient management in many other specialties. Once the EP rules out the life-threatening processes, more benign processes may be considered. This principle is particularly important when placed in the context of the patient population seen in the ED. Most of the patients are new to the EP; many are intoxicated or are brought to the ED by others. This leads to an array of fragmented histories, masked physical findings, and high emotional levels. In this setting, it is even more important for the EP to maintain a high level of suspicion for serious diseases.

All of the conditions listed as answer choices can be responsible for the patient's presentation. As discussed, it is important to first rule out the life-threatening processes. To address these processes, the patient requires a β-hCG to rule out an ectopic pregnancy; either an ultrasound or CT scan to evaluate for appendicitis; and a urinalysis to investigate pyelonephritis.

**96. The answer is e.** *(Riviello, 2005.)* When a sexual assault patient is evaluated in the ED, the EP not only has the standard responsibility to care for the patient's immediate physical and psychological health, but he/she must also consider how the encounter may affect the patient's life considerably once discharged from the ED. Once life-threatening injuries are addressed, EPs are responsible for collecting physical evidence necessary for prosecuting the assailant by conducting a sexual assault or "rape kit" with the patient's consent.

Most medications provided to sexually assaulted patients are provided as prophylaxis against sexually transmitted infections (STIs), pregnancy, and tetanus. Major STIs of concern are gonorrhea **(ceftriaxone)**, *Chlamydia* **(azithromycin or doxycycline)**, syphilis, and trichomoniasis **(metronidazole)** because of their relatively high incidence. The decision to provide **HIV postexposure prophylaxis (PEP)** after sexual assault must take into account the risks and benefits of treatment, the interval between exposure and treatment with antiretrovirals, and the likelihood of exposure to HIV. The average risk of HIV transmission per contact of unprotected receptive anal intercourse is approximately 1% to 5%. For unprotected insertive anal intercourse and receptive vaginal intercourse, the risk is approximately 0.1% to 1%. Some states mandate offering and providing HIV postexposure prophylaxis (PEP) to all sexually assaulted patients. The risk of pregnancy following sexual assault is approximately 5%. **Emergency contraception** is the use of hormone pills to prevent pregnancy. Hepatitis B vaccination should be administered to patients who never received the vaccine. If vaccination status is unclear, obtain hepatitis serology, and if not immune, proceed with vaccination. For patients who were previously fully vaccinated for hepatitis B, further therapy is not required. Tetanus is administered to patients who have sustained tetanus-prone injuries.

**97. The answer is d.** *(Rosen, pp 2281-2285.)* You should be concerned about a ruptured ectopic pregnancy in this patient. She missed her last menstrual period, has severe pain in the lower abdomen, and is hypotensive. This is a life-threatening condition that needs to be managed aggressively. The patient requires fluid resuscitation with 2 L NS. If her BP does not respond to the bolus, then blood should be administered. The patient will most likely be taken to the OR for a salpingectomy/oophorectomy. Risk factors for an ectopic pregnancy include history of pelvic inflammatory disease, prior ectopic pregnancy, pelvic surgery, and intrauterine device (IUD) use. **(a)** This will treat the pain but not its etiology. The patient is hypotensive and this needs to be addressed. **(b)** This is a plan for acute appendicitis, which is lower on the differential for this presentation than ectopic pregnancy. **(c)** This is a plan if you are suspecting a renal calculus, which would present with flank pain and microhematuria. **(e)** If the patient was stable then a pelvic ultrasound might be helpful in diagnosing an ectopic pregnancy.

**98. The answer is c.** *(Tintinalli, pp 536-539.)* **Crohn disease** is characterized by **chronic inflammation extending through all layers of the bowel wall**. Onset is generally between the ages of 15 and 40 years. Crohn disease should be suspected in any patient whose symptoms show a picture consistent with chronic inflammatory colitis. Extraintestinal manifestations are seen in 25% to 30% of patients. The incidence is similar for Crohn disease and ulcerative colitis. They include aphthous ulcers, erythema nodosum, iritis or episcleritis, arthritis, and gallstones. **Nephrolithiasis** is seen as a result of hyperoxaluria because of increased oxalate absorption in patients with ileal disease. Because ulcerative colitis affects only the large bowel, this extraintestinal manifestation is seen only in patients with Crohn disease.

**99. The answer is e.** *(Tintinalli, pp 630-637.)* *Chlamydia trachomatis* **urethritis** accounts for 5% to 20% of cases of dysuria, and its presence may be **suspected when urine cultures are sterile**. If clinical symptoms and urinalysis point to a UTI, urine cultures are sterile, and standard antibiotic regimens effective against most urinary pathogens fail, consider *Chlamydia* urethritis.

**(a)** Although group A streptococcus is a possible pathogen, it would be very rare and would be susceptible in most cases to the antibiotics that the patient has taken. **(b)** Initial episodes of herpes simplex virus can result in symptoms that mimic true dysuria secondary to sensitivity of lesions on the external genital surface or near the urethra. Generally, these episodes are accompanied by fever, chills, and systemic symptoms, in addition to extremely painful and tender lesions. Also, urinary frequency would not be common. **(c)** Although *T vaginalis* would not respond to the previous antibiotic therapy, trichomoniasis presents with a copious frothy vaginal discharge and would have been seen on wet mount preparation of the vaginal secretions. **(d)** *Escherichia coli* accounts for 70% to 90% of community-acquired UTIs in women. In a woman without recurrent UTIs, the antibiotics taken by this patient would be appropriate. In a patient with recurrent UTIs, it is more likely that the *E coli* would be resistant to standard antimicrobial regimens. This pathogen should have also been grown on the standard culture medium.

**100. The answer is e.** *(Tintinalli, pp 558-562.)* Abdominal pain that radiates to the back and is associated with nausea, vomiting, epigastric tenderness, and an elevated lipase in a patient with a history of ethanol abuse all point to a diagnosis of **alcoholic pancreatitis.** Although patients with mild pancreatitis, no evidence of systemic complications, and a low likelihood of biliary tract disease may be managed as outpatients, this patient requires admission for the potentially rapid progression of symptoms, severity of pain, and possible unreliability of the patient. The initial treatment for acute pancreatitis is **supportive: bowel rest, fluid resuscitation, and analgesia.** Ninety percent of patients recover without complications. Surgery is reserved for complications of alcoholic pancreatitis, such as pseudocysts, phlegmons, and abscesses.

**(a, b, and d)** As discussed above, this patient with pancreatitis requires admission to the hospital for medical management. An exploratory laparotomy is not indicated. **(c)** Endoscopy is used for patients with ulcerative disease. ERCP is also used in patients in whom the etiology of pancreatitis remains unclear after initial assessment.

# Trauma, Shock, and Resuscitation

## Questions

**101.** A 58-year-old woman is brought to the emergency department (ED) by emergency medical service (EMS) after slipping on a patch of ice while walking to work and hitting her head on the cement pavement. Bystanders acknowledged that the patient was unconscious for approximately 1 minute. On arrival, her vital signs are blood pressure (BP) 155/75 mm Hg, heart rate (HR) 89 beats per minute, respiratory rate (RR) 18 breaths per minute, and pulse oxygenation 98% on room air. She has a 5-cm laceration to the back of her head that is actively bleeding. You ask the patient what happened but she cannot remember. You inform her that she is in the hospital as a result of a fall. Over the next 10 minutes she asks you repeatedly what happened and where she is. You do not find any focal neurologic deficits. As you bring the patient to the CT scanner, she vomits once. CT results show a normal brain scan. Which of the following is the most likely diagnosis?

a. Cerebral concussion
b. Diffuse axonal injury
c. Cerebral contusion
d. Posttraumatic epilepsy
e. Trauma-induced Alzheimer disease

**102.** A 41-year-old man, the restrained driver in a high-speed motor vehicle collision, is brought to the ED by EMS. The patient is breathing without difficulty with bilateral and equal breaths sounds. He has strong pulses peripherally indicating a BP of at least 90 mm Hg. The HR is 121 beats per minute. His Glasgow coma scale (GCS) is 14. A secondary survey reveals chest wall bruising. You suspect a cardiac injury. Which of the following locations most commonly involve cardiac contusions?

a. Right atrium
b. Right ventricle
c. Left atrium
d. Left ventricle
e. Septum

**103.** A 25-year-old man is brought into the trauma resuscitation room after his motorcycle is struck by another vehicle. EMS reports that the patient was found 20 ft away from his motorcycle, which was badly damaged. His vital signs include a BP of 90/60 mm Hg, HR 115 beats per minute, RR 22 breaths per minute, and pulse oxygenation of 100% on facemask. Which of the following is the smallest amount of blood loss that produces a decrease in the systolic BP in adults?

a. Loss of 5% of blood volume
b. Loss of 10% of blood volume
c. Loss of 15% to 30% of blood volume
d. Loss of 30% to 40% of blood volume
e. Loss of greater than 40% of blood volume

**104.** You are notified by the EMS dispatcher that there is a multiple-car collision on the local highway with many injuries. He states that there are two people dead at the scene, one person is critically injured and hypotensive, and three people have significant injuries but with stable vital signs. Which of the following is the leading cause of death and disability in trauma victims?

a. Abdominal injury
b. Thoracic injury
c. Back injury
d. Cervical injury
e. Head injury

**105.** Paramedics bring a 17-year-old high school football player to the ED on a backboard and with a cervical collar. During a football game, the patient "speared" another player with his helmet and subsequently experienced severe neck pain. He denies paresthesias and is able to move all of his extremities. A cervical spine CT scan reveals multiple fractures of the first cervical vertebra. Which of the following best describes this fracture?

a. Odontoid fracture
b. Hangman's fracture
c. Jefferson fracture
d. Clay shoveler's fracture
e. Teardrop fracture

**106.** A 20-year-old man presents to the ED with multiple stab wounds to his chest. His BP is 85/50 mm Hg and HR is 123 beats per minute. Two large-bore IVs (intravenous) are established and running wide open. On examination, the patient is mumbling incomprehensibly, has good air entry on lung examination, and you notice jugular venous distension (JVD). As you are listening to his heart, the nurse calls out that the patient has lost his pulse and that she cannot get a BP reading. Which of the following is the most appropriate next step in management?

a. Atropine
b. Epinephrine
c. Bilateral chest tubes
d. ED thoracotomy
e. Pericardiocentesis

**107.** A 22-year-old man calls the ED from a local bar stating that he was punched in the face 10 minutes ago and is holding his front incisor tooth in his hand. He wants to know what the best way is to preserve the tooth. Which of the following is the most appropriate advice to give the caller?

a. Place the tooth in a napkin and bring it to the ED.
b. Place the tooth in a glass of water and bring it to the ED.
c. Place the tooth in a glass of beer and bring it to the ED.
d. Pour some water over the tooth and place it immediately back into the socket.
e. Place the tooth in a glass of milk and bring it to the ED.

**108.** A 19-year-old man is brought into the trauma room by EMS after a head-on cycling accident. The patient was not wearing a helmet. Upon presentation his BP is 125/75 mm Hg, HR is 105 beats per minute, RR is 19 breaths per minute, and oxygen saturation is 100% on mask. His eyes are closed but open to command. He can move his arms and legs on command. When you ask him questions, he is disoriented but able to converse. What is this patient's GCS score?

a. 11
b. 12
c. 13
d. 14
e. 15

**109.** An 18-year-old man presents to the ED after getting stabbed in his abdomen. His HR is 140 beats per minute and BP is 90/40 mm Hg. He is yelling that he is in pain. Two large-bore IVs are inserted into his antecubital fossa and fluids are running wide open. After 2 L of fluids, his BP does not improve. Which of the following is the most common organ injured in stab wounds?

a. Liver
b. Small bowel
c. Stomach
d. Colon
e. Spleen

**110.** A 61-year-old man presents to the ED with chest wall pain after a motor vehicle collision. He is speaking full sentences, breath sounds are equal bilaterally, and his extremities are well-perfused. His BP is 150/75 mm Hg, HR is 92 beats per minute, and oxygen saturation is 97% on room air. Chest radiography reveals fractures of the seventh and eighth ribs of the right anterolateral chest. He has no other identifiable injuries. Which of the following is the most appropriate treatment for this patient's rib fractures?

a. Apply adhesive tape on the chest wall perpendicular to the rib fractures.
b. Insert a chest tube into the right thorax.
c. Bring the patient to the OR for surgical fixation.
d. Analgesia and incentive spirometry.
e. Observation.

**111.** A 27-year-old man brought to the ED by paramedics after a motor vehicle collision. His RR is 45 breaths per minute, oxygen saturation is 89%, HR is 112 beats per minute, and BP is 115/75 mm Hg. You auscultate his chest and hear decreased breath sounds on the left. Which of the following is the most appropriate next step in management?

a. Order a stat chest radiograph.
b. Perform a pericardiocentesis.
c. Perform a diagnostic peritoneal lavage (DPL).
d. Perform an ED thoracotomy.
e. Perform a tube thoracostomy.

**112.** A 29-year-old man is brought to the ED by EMS after being stabbed in the left side of his back. His BP is 120/80 mm Hg, HR is 105 beats per minute, RR is 16 breaths per minute, and oxygen saturation is 98% on room air. On the secondary survey, you note motor weakness of his left lower extremity and the loss of pain sensation in the right lower extremity. Which of the following is the most likely diagnosis?

a. Spinal shock
b. Central cord syndrome
c. Anterior cord syndrome
d. Brown-Séquard syndrome
e. Cauda equina syndrome

**113.** A 33-year-old man, who was drinking heavily at a bar, presents to the ED after getting into a fight. A bystander tells paramedics that the patient was punched and kicked multiple times and sustained multiple blows to his head with a stool. In the ED, his BP is 150/75 mm Hg, HR is 90 beats per minute, RR is 13 breaths per minute, and oxygen saturation is 100% on non-rebreather. On examination, he opens his eyes to pain and his pupils are equal and reactive. There is a laceration on the right side of his head. He withdraws his arm to pain but otherwise does not move. You ask him questions, but he just moans. Which of the following is the most appropriate next step in management?

a. Prepare for intubation.
b. Suture repair of head laceration.
c. Administer mannitol.
d. Bilateral burr holes.
e. Neurosurgical intervention.

**114.** A 74-year-old man presents to the ED after being involved in a motor vehicle collision. He states he was wearing his seat belt in the driver's seat when a car hit him from behind. He thinks his chest hit the steering wheel and now complains of pain with breathing. His RR is 20 breaths per minute, oxygen saturation is 98% on room air, BP is 145/75 mm Hg, and HR is 90 beats per minute. On examination, you notice paradoxical respirations. Which of the following best describes a flail chest?

a. One rib with three fracture sites
b. Two adjacent ribs, each with two fracture sites
c. Three adjacent ribs, each with two fracture sites
d. One fractured right-sided rib and one fractured left-sided rib
e. Two fractured right-sided ribs and two fractured left-sided ribs

**115.** A 29-year-old man presents to the ED after being stabbed in his neck. The patient is speaking in full sentences. His breath sounds are equal bilaterally. His BP is 130/75 mm Hg, HR is 95 beats per minute, RR is 16 breaths per minute, and oxygen saturation is 99% on room air. The stab wound is located between the angle of the mandible and the cricoid cartilage and violates the platysma. There is blood oozing from the site although there is no expanding hematoma. Which of the following is the most appropriate next step in management?

a. Explore the wound and blind clamp any bleeding site.
b. Probe the wound looking for injured vessels.
c. Apply direct pressure and bring the patient immediately to the OR to explore the zone I injury.
d. Apply direct pressure and bring the patient immediately to the OR to explore the zone II injury.
e. Apply direct pressure and bring the patient immediately to the OR to explore the zone III injury.

**116.** A 45-year-old man is brought to the ED after a head-on motor vehicle collision. Paramedics at the scene tell you that the front end of the car is smashed. The patient's BP is 130/80 mm Hg, HR is 100 beats per minute, RR is 15 breaths per minute, and oxygen saturation is 98% on room air. Radiographs of the cervical spine reveal bilateral fractures of the C2 vertebra. The patient's neurologic examination is unremarkable. Which of the following best describes this fracture?

a. Colles fracture
b. Boxer's fracture
c. Jefferson fracture
d. Hangman's fracture
e. Clay shoveler's fracture

**117.** A 71-year-old man is found lying on the ground one story below the balcony of his apartment. Paramedics bring the patient into the ED. He is cool to touch with a core body temperature of 96°F. His HR is 119 beats per minute and BP is 90/70 mm Hg. His eyes are closed, but they open when you call his name. His limbs move to stimuli, and he answers your questions but is confused. On examination, you note clear fluid dripping from his left ear canal and an area of ecchymosis around the mastoid bone. Which of the following is the most likely diagnosis?

a. Le Fort fracture
b. Basilar skull fracture
c. Otitis interna
d. Otitis externa
e. Tripod fracture

**118.** A 34-year-old construction worker is brought to the ED by EMS after falling 30 ft from a scaffold. His vital signs are HR 124 beats per minute, BP 80/40 mm Hg, and oxygen saturation 93% on 100% oxygen. He has obvious head trauma with a scalp laceration overlying a skull fracture on his occiput. He does not speak when asked his name, his respirations are poor, and you hear gurgling with each attempted breath. Auscultation of the chest reveals diminished breath sounds on the right. There is no JVD or anterior chest wall crepitus. His pelvis is unstable with movement laterally to medially and you note blood at the urethral meatus. His right leg is grossly deformed at the knee and there is an obvious fracture of his left arm. Which of the following is the most appropriate next step in management?

a. Insert a 32F chest tube into the right thoracic cavity.
b. Perform a DPL to rule out intra-abdominal hemorrhage.
c. Create two Burr holes into the cranial vault to treat a potential epidural hematoma.
d. Immediately reduce the extremity injuries and place in a splint until the patient is stabilized.
e. Plan for endotracheal intubation of the airway with in-line stabilization of the cervical spine.

**119.** A 20-year-old man was found on the ground next to his car after it hit a tree on the side of the road. Bystanders state that the man got out of his car after the collision but collapsed within a few minutes. Paramedics subsequently found the man unconscious on the side of the road. In the ED, his BP is 175/90 mm Hg, HR is 65 beats per minute, temperature is 99.2°F, RR is 12 breaths per minute, and oxygen saturation is 97% on room air. Physical examination reveals a right-sided fixed and dilated pupil. A head CT is shown below. Which of the following is the most likely diagnosis?

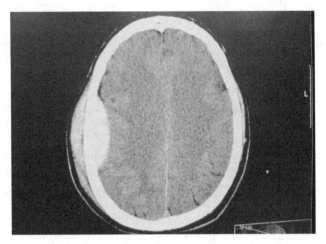

(Reproduced, with permission, from Knoop KJ, Stack LB, Storrow AB. Atlas of Emergency Medicine. New York, NY: McGraw-Hill, 2002: 162.)

a. Epidural hematoma
b. Subdural hematoma
c. Subarachnoid hemorrhage (SAH)
d. Intracerebral hematoma
e. Cerebral contusion

**120.** An 81-year-old woman presents to the ED after tripping over the sidewalk curb and landing on her chin causing a hyperextension of her neck. She was placed in a cervical collar by paramedics. On examination, she has no sensorimotor function of her upper extremities. She cannot wiggle her toes, has 1/5 motor function of her quadriceps, and only patchy lower extremity sensation. Rectal examination reveals decreased rectal tone. Which of the following is the most likely diagnosis?

a. Central cord syndrome
b. Anterior cord syndrome
c. Brown-Séquard syndrome
d. Transverse myelitis
e. Exacerbation of Parkinson disease

**121.** A 22-year-old man presents to the ED after being ejected from his vehicle following a high-speed motor vehicle collision. Upon arrival, his BP is 85/55 mm Hg and HR is 141 beats per minute. Two large-bore IVs are placed in the antecubital veins and lactated Ringer solution is being administered. After 3 L of crystalloid fluid, the patient's BP is 83/57 mm Hg. Which of the following statements is most appropriate regarding management of a hypotensive trauma patient who fails to respond to initial volume resuscitation?

a. It is important to wait for fully cross-matched blood prior to transfusion.
b. Whole blood should be used rather than packed red blood cells (RBCs).
c. Blood transfusion should begin after 4 L of crystalloid infusion.
d. Type O blood that is Rh-negative should be transfused.
e. Type O blood that is Rh-positive should be transfused.

**122.** A 24-year-old man is brought into the ED by paramedics after being run over by a car. His systolic BP is 90 mm Hg by palpation, HR is 121 beats per minute, RR is 28 breaths per minute, and oxygen saturation is 100% on non-rebreather. The airway is patent and breath sounds are equal bilaterally. You establish large-bore access and fluids are running wide open. Secondary survey reveals an unstable pelvis upon movement with lateral to medial force. Bedside focused abdominal sonography for trauma (FAST) is negative for intraperitoneal fluid. Which of the following is the most appropriate immediate next step in management?

a. Bilateral chest tubes
b. Application of external fixator
c. Application of pelvic binding apparatus
d. Venographic embolization
e. Angiographic embolization

**123.** A 32-year-old man is brought to the ED by paramedics after a diving accident. The lifeguard on duty accompanies the patient and states that he dove head first into the shallow end of the pool and did not resurface. On examination, the patient is speaking but cannot move his arms or legs and cannot feel pain below his clavicle. He is able to feel light touch and position of his four extremities. A cervical spine radiograph does not reveal a fracture. Which of the following is the most likely diagnosis?

a. Spinal cord injury without radiographic abnormality (SCIWORA)
b. Central cord syndrome
c. Anterior cord syndrome
d. Cauda equina syndrome
e. Brown-Séquard syndrome

**124.** A 22-year-old man is brought to the ED 20 minutes after a head-on motor vehicle collision in which he was the unrestrained driver. On arrival, he is alert and coherent but appears short of breath. His HR is 117 beats per minute, BP is 80/60 mm Hg, and oxygen saturation is 97% on a non-rebreather. Examination reveals bruising over the central portion of his chest. His neck veins are not distended. Breath sounds are present on the left but absent on the right. Following administration of 2 L of lactated Ringer solution, his systolic BP remains at 80 mm Hg. Which of the following is the most appropriate next step in management?

a. Sedate, paralyze, and intubate.
b. Perform a needle thoracostomy.
c. Perform a DPL.
d. Perform a FAST examination.
e. Perform a pericardiocentesis.

**125.** An 87-year-old man is brought to the ED on a long board and in a cervical collar after falling down a flight of steps. He denies losing consciousness. On arrival, his vital signs include an HR of 99 beats per minute, BP of 160/90 mm Hg, and RR of 16 breaths per minute. He is alert and speaking in full sentences. Breath sounds are equal bilaterally. Despite an obvious right arm fracture, his radial pulses are 2+ and symmetric. When examining his cervical spine, he denies tenderness to palpation and you do not feel any bony deformities. Which of the following is a true statement?

a. Epidural hematomas are very common in the elderly age population.
b. Cerebral atrophy in the elderly population provides protection against subdural hematomas.
c. Increased elasticity of their lungs allows elderly patients to recover from thoracic trauma more quickly than younger patients.
d. The most common cervical spine fracture in this age group is a wedge fracture of the sixth cervical vertebra.
e. Despite lack of cervical spine tenderness, imaging of his cervical spine is warranted.

**126.** A 45-year-old man is brought into the ED after a head-on motor vehicle collision. His BP is 85/45 mm Hg and HR is 130 beats per minute. He is speaking coherently. His breath sounds are equal bilaterally. After 2 L of fluid resuscitation, his BP is 80/40 mm Hg. A FAST examination reveals fluid in Morison pouch. Which of the following organs is most likely to be injured in blunt abdominal trauma?

a. Liver
b. Spleen
c. Kidney
d. Small bowel
e. Bladder

**127.** A 47-year-old man is brought into the ED after falling 20 ft from a ladder. His HR is 110 beats per minute, BP is 110/80 mm Hg, RR is 20 breaths per minute, and oxygen saturation is 100% on face mask. He is able to answer your questions without difficulty. His chest is clear with bilateral breath sounds, abdomen is nontender, pelvis is stable, and the FAST examination is negative. You note a large scrotal hematoma and blood at the urethral meatus. Which of the following is the most appropriate next step in management?

a. Scrotal ultrasound
b. Kidney-ureter-bladder (KUB) radiograph
c. IV pyelogram
d. Retrograde cystogram
e. Retrograde urethrogram

**128.** A 17-year-old man presents to the ED after getting hit in the right eye with a tennis ball during a tennis match. On arrival to the ED, you note periorbital swelling and ecchymosis. The patient's visual acuity is 20/20. When you are testing his extraocular muscles, you note that his right eye cannot look superiorly but his left eye can. He also describes pain in his right eye when attempting to look upward. Which of the following is the most likely diagnosis?

a. Zygomatic arch fracture
b. Orbital floor fracture
c. Retrobulbar hematoma
d. Ruptured globe
e. Mandible fracture with entrapment of the pterygoid

**129.** A 24-year-old man is brought to the ED after being shot once in the abdomen. On arrival, his BP is 100/60 mm Hg, HR is 115 beats per minute, and RR is 22 breaths per minute. His airway is patent and you hear breath sounds bilaterally. On abdominal examination, you note a single bullet entry wound approximately 1 cm to the right of the umbilicus. During the log roll, you see a single bullet exit wound approximately 3 cm to the right of the lumbar spine. His GCS score is 15. The patient's BP is now 85/65 mm Hg and HR is 125 beats per minute after 2 L of fluid. Which of the following is the most appropriate next step in management?

a. Probe the entry wound to see if it violates the peritoneum.
b. Perform a FAST examination.
c. Perform a DPL.
d. Take the patient directly to the CT scanner.
e. Take the patient directly to the OR.

**130.** A 55-year-old woman presents to the ED stating that her nose has been bleeding profusely for the last 3 hours. After 25 minutes of bilateral pressure on her nasal septum, there is still profuse bleeding. You place anterior nasal packing bilaterally, but bleeding still persists. The patient is starting to get anxious. Her BP is 110/70 mm Hg, HR is 80 beats per minute, RR is 18 breaths per minute, and oxygen saturation is 98%. Laboratory results reveal a white blood cell (WBC) count of 9000, hematocrit (HCT) 34%, platelets of 225,000, and international normalized ratio (INR) 1.1. Under direct visualization, you note the bleeding originating from the posterior aspect of her septum. Which of the following is the most appropriate management?

a. Place posterior nasal packing, start antibiotics, and admit the patient to a monitored hospital bed.
b. Place the patient supine and wait for spontaneous resolution of the bleeding.
c. Keep pressure on her nasal septum, and administer fresh frozen plasma (FFP) and platelets.
d. Place posterior nasal packing, and discharge the patient home with follow-up in 24 hours.
e. Apply silver nitrate to the nasal mucosa until the bleeding stops.

**131.** Paramedics bring a 44-year-old man to the ED. He was found in the middle of the street after being struck by a car. His systolic BP is 70 mm Hg; a diastolic BP cannot be obtained. The heart rate is 125 beats per minute, and oxygen saturation is 89% on room air. The patient's eyes are closed. You ask the patient his name and he doesn't respond. There is no response when you ask him to move his limbs. You notice that his left foot is severely deformed and there is a large laceration to his right arm. Which of the following is the most appropriate next step in management?

a. Prepare for emergent orotracheal intubation.
b. Begin aggressive fluid resuscitation and administer morphine for pain.
c. Apply a tourniquet just above his left foot and begin fluid resuscitation.
d. Apply pressure to the laceration, splint the left foot, and order a radiograph.
e. Administer packed RBCs and bring him to the CT scanner for a pan-scan.

**132.** A 17-year-old adolescent boy is found unconscious in a swimming pool. He is brought into the ED by paramedics already intubated. In the ED, the patient is unresponsive with spontaneous abdominal breathing at a rate of 16 breaths per minute, BP 80/50 mm Hg, and HR 49 beats per minute. In addition to hypoxemia, what condition must be considered earliest in the management of this patient?

a. Cervical spine injury
b. Electrolyte imbalance
c. Metabolic acidosis
d. Severe atelectasis
e. Toxic ingestion

**133.** A 22-year-old man is brought to the ED after sustaining a single gunshot wound (GSW) to his right thigh. On arrival, his HR is 105 beats per minute and BP is 115/75 mm Hg. You note a large hematoma of his medial thigh. The patient complains of numbness in his right foot. On extremity examination, the right foot is pale and you cannot palpate a distal pulse but can locate the dorsalis pedis by Doppler. In addition, the patient cannot move the foot. Which of the following is the most appropriate next step in management?

a. Angiography
b. Exploration and repair in the OR
c. Fasciotomy to treat compartment syndrome
d. Wound exploration
e. CT scan of the right extremity

**134.** A 67-year-old woman is brought to the ED after being struck by a cyclist while crossing the street. On arrival to the ED, her eyes remain closed to stimuli, she makes no verbal sounds, and withdraws only to painful stimuli. You assign her a GCS of 6. Her BP is 175/90 mm Hg and HR is 75 beats per minute. As you open her eye lids, you notice that her right pupil is 8 mm and nonreactive and her left is 4 mm and minimally reactive. Which of the following is the most common manifestation of increasing intracranial pressure (ICP) causing brain herniation?

a. Change in level of consciousness
b. Ipsilateral pupillary dilation
c. Contralateral pupillary dilation
d. Significantly elevated BP
e. Hemiparesis

**135.** A 34-year-old man is brought to the ED after being shot in the right side of his chest. The patient is awake and speaking. Breath sounds are diminished on the right. There is no bony crepitus or tracheal deviation. His BP is 95/65 mm Hg, HR is 121 beats per minute, and RR is 23 breaths per minute. Supine chest radiograph reveals a hazy appearance over the entire right lung field. You place a 36F chest tube into the right thoracic cavity and note 1200 cc of blood in the chest tube drainage system. Which of the following is an indication for thoracotomy?

a. 500 cc of initial chest tube drainage of blood
b. 1200 cc of initial chest tube drainage of blood
c. Persistent bleeding from the chest tube at a rate of 50 cc/h
d. Chest radiograph with greater than 50% lung field whiteout
e. Evidence of a pneumothorax (PTX)

**136.** A 32-year-old woman is brought to the ED by paramedics after being involved in a motor vehicle collision. The patient was the front-seat passenger of the car and was not wearing a seat belt. In the ED, the patient is speaking and complains of abdominal pain. Her breath sounds are equal bilaterally. You note a distended abdomen. A FAST examination is positive for fluid in the left upper quadrant (LUQ). Her BP is 90/70 mm Hg and HR is 120 beats per minute. You administer 2 L of crystalloid solution. Her repeat BP is 80/60 mm Hg. Which of the following is the most appropriate next step in management?

a. Administer a vasoconstrictor, such as epinephrine.
b. Administer another 2 L of crystalloid.
c. Administer type O, Rh-negative blood.
d. Bring patient to the CT scanner for an emergent scan.
e. Perform another FAST examination to see if the fluid is increasing.

**137.** A 27-year-old pregnant woman, in her third trimester, is brought to the ED after being involved in a low-speed motor vehicle collision. The patient was wearing a seat belt in the back seat of a car that was struck in the front by another car. Her BP is 120/70 mm Hg and HR is 107 beats per minute. Her airway is patent, breath sounds equal bilaterally, and skin is warm with 2+ pulses. FAST examination is negative for free fluid. Evaluation of the fetus reveals appropriate fetal HR and fetal movement. Repeat maternal BP is 120/75 mm Hg. Which of the following is the most appropriate next step in management?

a. Perform an immediate cesarean section in the OR.
b. Perform an immediate cesarean section in the ED.
c. CT scan of the abdomen and pelvis to rule out occult injury.
d. Discharge the patient if laboratory testing is normal.
e. Monitor the patient and fetus for a minimum of 4 hours.

**138.** A 61-year-old man presents to the ED with low back pain after slipping on an icy sidewalk yesterday. He states that the pain started on the left side of his lower back and now involves the right and radiates down both legs. He also noticed difficulty urinating since last night. On neurologic examination, he cannot plantar flex his feet. Rectal examination reveals diminished rectal tone. He has a medical history of chronic hypertension and underwent a "vessel surgery" many years earlier. Which of the following is the best diagnosis?

a. Abdominal aortic aneurysm (AAA)
b. Disk herniation
c. Spinal stenosis
d. Cauda equina syndrome
e. Osteomyelitis

**139.** Paramedics bring a 55-year-old woman to the ED after she was struck by a motor vehicle traveling at 30 miles/h. Her BP is 165/95 mm Hg, HR is 105 beats per minute, and RR is 20 breaths per minute. Upon arrival, she does not open her eyes, is verbal but not making any sense, and withdraws to painful stimuli. You assign her a GCS score of 8. As you prepare to intubate the patient, a colleague notices that her left pupil has become dilated compared to the right. Which of the following has the quickest effect to reduce ICP?

a. Cranial decompression
b. Dexamethasone
c. Furosemide
d. Hyperventilation
e. Mannitol

**140.** A car pulls up to your ED and drops off a 19-year-old man who was shot in the chest. The man tells you his name and complains of right-sided chest pain and difficulty breathing. On primary survey, his airway is patent and his oropharynx has no blood or displaced teeth. He is breathing at 32 beats per minute with retractions and an oxygen saturation of 88% on 15 L of oxygen. There is a bullet wound to his right mid-chest with another wound in his back. His trachea is deviated to the left. On auscultation, he has diminished breath sounds on the right side. Which of the following is the most appropriate next step in management?

a. Stat portable chest x-ray.
b. Intubation.
c. Perform ED thoracotomy.
d. Call the surgical service.
e. Needle decompression.

**141.** A 79-year-old woman with a history of coronary artery disease who underwent a coronary artery bypass graft (CABG) surgery 7 years ago is brought to the emergency department (ED) by her family for 2 days of worsening shortness of breath. For the past 2 days, she has not gotten out of bed and is confused. She does not have chest pain, fevers, or cough. Her temperature is 98.1°F, blood pressure (BP) is 85/50 mm Hg, heart rate (HR) is 125 beats per minute, and respiratory rate (RR) is 26 breaths per minute. On examination, she is unable to follow commands and is oriented only to name. The cardiovascular examination reveals tachycardia with no murmurs. Her lungs have rales bilaterally at the bases. The abdomen is soft, nontender, and nondistended. Lower extremities have 2+ edema to the knee bilaterally. Which of the following is the most likely diagnosis?

a. Hypovolemic shock
b. Neurogenic shock
c. Cardiogenic shock
d. Anaphylactic shock
e. Septic shock

**142.** A 32-year-old man with no past medical problems presents to the ED with palpitations. For the past 2 days he has been feeling weak and over the last 6 hours he has noticed that his heart is racing. He has no chest pain or shortness of breath. He has never felt this way before. His temperature is 98.9°F, BP is 140/82 mm Hg, HR is 180 beats per minute, and RR is 14 breaths per minute. His physical examination is normal. You obtain the following rhythm strip. What is your first-line treatment for this patient?

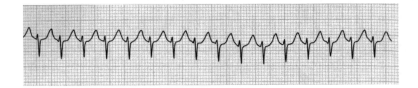

a. Synchronized cardioversion at 100 J
b. Adenosine 6-mg intravenous (IV) push
c. Adenosine 12-mg IV push
d. Valsalva maneuver
e. Verapamil 3-mg IV push

**143.** You are a passenger aboard an airplane and a 78-year-old woman is complaining of chest pain and difficulty breathing. You are the only medical professional available and volunteer to help. Fortunately, the aircraft is well-equipped with basic medical equipment, as well as with ACLS medications and a cardiac monitor. On examination, the passenger's BP is 75/40 mm Hg, HR is 180 beats per minute, and RR is 24 breaths per minute. On examination, the patient is in obvious distress but able to answer basic questions. Her heart is tachycardic, regular, and without murmurs, rubs, or gallops. Physical examination is remarkable for a bounding carotid pulse. You attach the cardiac monitor and see a regular rhythm at 180 beats per minute with wide QRS complexes and no obvious P waves. After asking the pilot to make an emergency landing, what do you do next?

a. Amiodarone IV
b. Synchronized cardioversion
c. Verapamil IV
d. Lidocaine IV
e. Procainamide IV

**144.** A 41-year-old man is brought into the ED by paramedics in cardio-pulmonary arrest. A friend states that the patient is a long-time user of IV heroin. You look at the monitor and see that the patient has pulseless electrical activity (PEA). Cardiopulmonary resuscitation is being performed and the patient is intubated. You decide to administer epinephrine to the patient but realize that he does not have IV access. Which of the following drugs is **ineffective** when administered through an endotracheal (ET) tube?

a. Atropine
b. Naloxone
c. Lidocaine
d. Epinephrine
e. Sodium bicarbonate

**145.** A 75-year-old man complaining of chest pain is brought into the ED by paramedics. He is barely able to speak to you because he is short of breath. The nurse immediately attaches him to the monitor, starts an IV, and gives him oxygen. His temperature is 98.9°F, BP is 70/40 mm Hg, HR is 140 beats per minute, RR is 28 breaths per minute, and oxygen saturation is 95% on room air. On examination, he is in mild distress. His heart is irregular and tachycardic. His lungs are clear to auscultation, with rales at the bases, bilaterally. An electrocardiogram (ECG) is shown below. What is your first-line treatment for this patient?

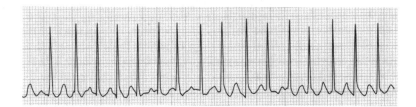

a. Heparin drip
b. Diltiazem 10-mg IV push
c. Metoprolol 5-mg IV push
d. Digoxin 0.5-mg IV
e. Synchronized cardioversion at 100 J

**146.** A 19-year-old man was struck by a motor vehicle while crossing the street. In the ED, he is awake, alert, and oriented but complaining of severe right leg pain. His temperature is 98.9°F, BP is 85/50 mm Hg, HR is 125 beats per minute, and RR is 24 breaths per minute. You confirm that his airway is patent, breath sounds are equal bilaterally, and his abdomen is soft and nontender. His right leg is shorter than his left leg, slightly angulated, and swollen in his anterior thigh area. There is no open wound. Which of the following is the most likely diagnosis?

a. Hypovolemic shock
b. Neurogenic shock
c. Cardiogenic shock
d. Anaphylactic shock
e. Septic shock

**147.** You are called to the bedside of a hypotensive patient with altered mental status. The nurse hands you an ECG which shows atrial flutter at 150 beats per minute with 2:1 arteriovenous (AV) block. You feel that the patient is unstable and elect to perform emergency cardioversion. You attach the monitor leads to the patient. What is the critical next step in electrical cardioversion?

a. Set the appropriate energy level.
b. Position conductor pads or paddles on patient.
c. Charge the defibrillator.
d. Turn on the synchronization mode.
e. Administer 25 μg of fentanyl IV.

**148.** Paramedics bring in a 54-year-old man who was found down in his apartment by his wife. He is successfully intubated in the field and paramedics are currently performing cardiopulmonary resuscitation (CPR). He is transferred to an ED gurney and quickly attached to the cardiac monitors. You ask the paramedics to hold CPR and assess the patient and the rhythm strip. The monitor shows sinus bradycardia, but no pulses are palpable. On examination you appreciate bilateral breath sounds with mechanical ventilation, a soft abdomen, no rashes, and a left arm AV graft. In addition to CPR with epinephrine and atropine every 3 to 5 minutes, which intervention should be performed next?

a. Administer 1 ampule of sodium bicarbonate.
b. Administer 1 ampule of calcium gluconate.
c. Administer 1 ampule of D50 (dextrose).
d. Place left-sided chest tube.
e. Perform pericardiocentesis.

**149.** A 72-year-old man is in the ED for the evaluation of generalized weakness over the previous 24 hours. He has a past medical history of coronary artery disease with a CABG performed 5 years ago, diabetes mellitus, and arthritis. The nurse places the patient on a cardiac monitor and begins to get his vital signs. While the nurse is obtaining the vital signs, she notices that the patient suddenly becomes unresponsive. You arrive at the bedside, look at the monitor, and see the following rhythm. Which of the following is the most appropriate next step in management?

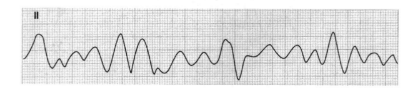

a. Wait 5 minutes to see if he awakens on his own.
b. Immediately defibrillate at 200 J (biphasic).
c. Perform synchronized cardioversion at 100 J.
d. Immediately intubate the patient.
e. Insert an IV line and administer amiodarone.

**150.** An 82-year-old nursing home patient presents to the ED in septic shock. Her BP is 75/40 mm Hg, HR is 117 beats per minute, temperature is 96.5°F, RR is 29 breaths per minute, and oxygen saturation is 87% on room air. As you perform laryngoscopy to intubate the patient, you easily visualize the vocal cords and subsequently pass the orotracheal tube through the vocal cords. You place the colorimetric end-tidal carbon dioxide device over the tube and get appropriate color change. There are equal, bilateral breath sounds on auscultation and you observe chest wall motion with ventilation. Which of the following is the most reliable method for verifying proper ET tube placement?

a. Chest radiograph
b. Visualization of the ET tube passing through the vocal cords
c. Observation of chest wall motion with ventilation
d. Hearing equal, bilateral breath sounds on auscultation
e. End-tidal carbon dioxide color change

**151.** A 25-year-old man fell off his surfboard and landed on rocks. He was pulled from the water by lifeguards and brought to the ED in full cervical and spinal immobilization. He is alert and oriented to person, place, and time. He is complaining of weakness in all of his extremities. His temperature is 98.4°F, BP is 85/50 mm Hg, HR is 60 beats per minute, RR is 20 breaths per minute, and oxygen saturation is 98% on room air. On examination, he has no external signs of head injury. His heart is bradycardic without murmurs. The lungs are clear to auscultation and the abdomen is soft and nontender. He has grossly normal peripheral sensation but no motor strength in all four extremities. Which of the following is the most likely diagnosis?

a. Hypovolemic shock
b. Neurogenic shock
c. Cardiogenic shock
d. Anaphylactic shock
e. Septic shock

**152.** A 48-year-old man is brought to the ED by paramedics for generalized weakness. His medical history is significant for a CABG last month. He has been unable to get out of bed for the past day because of dizziness when changing position. He denies chest pain, shortness of breath, or syncope. His temperature is 98.9°F, BP is 86/60 mm Hg, HR is 44 beats per minute, RR is 18 breaths per minute, and oxygen saturation is 98% on room air. There is a well-healing midline sternotomy incision. Cardiac examination reveals a III/VI systolic ejection murmur. There are minimal rales at his lung bases. He is immediately attached to the cardiac monitor. His rhythm strip is shown below. What is your initial treatment?

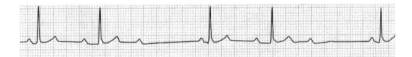

a. Observation on monitor
b. Transcutaneous pacing
c. Transvenous pacing
d. Atropine 0.5 mg IV
e. Epinephrine IV drip at 2 μg/minute

**153.** You are caring for a 54-year-old woman with a history of schizophrenia and coronary artery disease who presents to the ED for chest pain. Her vital signs are within normal limits and her ECG is normal sinus rhythm with nonspecific ST/T-wave changes. Her first troponin is sent to the laboratory and you are planning to admit her to the hospital for a complete acute coronary syndrome (ACS) evaluation. She receives aspirin and nitroglycerin and her chest pain resolves. A few minutes later, the nurse alerts you that the patient has become unconscious. You go to the bedside and find the patient awake and alert. You review the rhythm strip below. What is your next step in management?

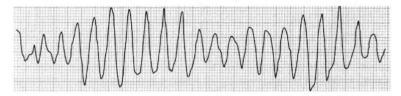

a. Observation of patient
b. Magnesium sulfate IV
c. Lidocaine IV
d. Transvenous pacemaker
e. Isoproterenol IV

**154.** A 19-year-old man is brought into the ED by paramedics with a stab wound to the right lower abdomen. The medics applied a pressure dressing and started an IV line en route to the hospital. On arrival, the patient has no complaints and wants to leave. His temperature is 98.4°F, BP is 130/95 mm Hg, HR is 111 beats per minute, RR is 20 breaths per minute, and oxygen saturation is 98% on room air. He is alert and oriented to person, place, and time. His abdomen is soft and nontender, with normal bowel sounds. He has a 2-cm stab wound with visible subcutaneous fat in his right lower quadrant (RLQ). You initiate the FAST examination. Which type of fluid should you start for his initial resuscitation?

a. 7% sodium chloride
b. 0.9% sodium chloride
c. 10% albumin
d. Type and cross-matched blood
e. Type-specific blood

**155.** An 82-year-old man with a history of COPD and hypertension presents with shortness of breath and fever. His medications include albuterol, ipratropium, prednisone, hydrochlorothiazide, and atenolol. His temperature is 102.1°F, BP is 70/40 mm Hg, HR is 110 beats per minute, RR is 24 breaths per minute, and oxygen saturation is 91% on room air. The patient is uncomfortable and mumbling incoherently. On chest examination, you appreciate rales on the left side of his chest. His heart is tachycardic, but regular with no murmurs, rubs, or gallops. His abdomen is soft and nontender. You believe this patient is in septic shock from pneumonia and start IV fluids, broad-spectrum antibiotics, and a dopamine drip. His BP remains at 75/50 mm Hg. Which of the following is the most appropriate next step in management?

a. D5 normal saline IV bolus
b. Phenylephrine IV drip
c. Fludrocortisone IV
d. Hydrocortisone IV
e. Epinephrine IV drip

**156.** A 64-year-old woman with a history of depression and hypertension was found down by her husband and brought in by the paramedics. Her husband says that she has recently been depressed and expressed thoughts of suicide. She usually takes fluoxetine for depression and atenolol for hypertension. On arrival, the patient is obtunded, but responds to pain and is maintaining her airway. Her temperature is 98.1°F, BP is 70/40 mm Hg, HR is 42 beats per minute, RR is 12 breaths per minute, and oxygen saturation is 94% on room air. On examination, her pupils are 3 mm and reactive bilaterally. Lungs are clear to auscultation. Heart is bradycardic, but regular, with no murmurs, rubs, or gallops. Extremities have no edema. An ECG shows first-degree AV block at 42 beats per minute, but no ST/T-wave changes. Blood sugar is 112 mg/dL. What is the most specific treatment for this patient's ingestion?

a. Fluid bolus
b. Atropine
c. Glucagon
d. Epinephrine
e. Cardiac pacing

**157.** A 19-year-old man suffers a single gunshot wound to the left chest and is brought in by his friends. He is complaining of chest pain. On examination, his temperature is 99°F, BP is 70/40 mm Hg, HR is 140 beats per minute, RR is 16 breaths per minute, and oxygen saturation is 96% on room air. He has distended neck veins, but his trachea is not deviated. Lungs are clear to auscultation bilaterally. Heart sounds are difficult to appreciate, but you feel a bounding, regular pulse. Abdomen is soft and nontender. Extremity examination is normal. Two large-bore IV lines are placed and the patient is given 2 L of normal saline. Chest radiograph shows a globular cardiac silhouette but a normal mediastinum and no pneumothorax. What is the definitive management of this patient?

a. Intubation
b. Tube thoracostomy
c. Pericardiocentesis
d. Thoracotomy
e. Blood transfusion

**158.** An 87-year-old woman with a history of dementia, arthritis, and hypertension presents to the ED for abdominal pain. Her caretaker reports that she is having mid-epigastric pain and had one episode of nonbloody, nonbilious vomiting prior to arrival. The patient is oriented to name only. Temperature is 99.8°F, HR is 110 beats per minute, BP is 80/44 mm Hg, RR is 16 breaths per minute, and oxygen saturation is 96% on room air. On examination, the abdomen is soft, nontender, with no masses, rebound or guarding. Stool is brown and guaiac negative. You place two IV lines and begin fluid resuscitation. You send her blood to the laboratory and order a radiograph of her chest that is shown below. Which of the following is the most appropriate next step in management?

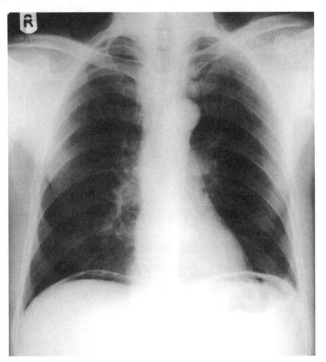

a. Start IV antibiotics.
b. Order a CT scan of her abdomen.
c. Call the surgery service.
d. Place a central venous line.
e. Discharge home with Maalox.

# Trauma, Shock, and Resuscitation

## Answers

**101. The answer is a.** (*Moore et al, pp 397-401.*) The patient sustained a **cerebral concussion**. This is caused by a head injury leading to a **brief loss of neurologic function**. These individuals are often amnestic to the event and frequently ask the same questions over and over again (perseverations). Headache with or without vomiting is generally present; however, there are no focal neurologic findings on examination. Loss of consciousness results from impairment of the reticular activating system (RAS). Patients show rapid clinical improvement. CT scan is normal.

Diffuse axonal injury (**b**) is caused by microscopic shearing of brain nerve fibers. Patients typically present unconscious and remain in a coma for a prolonged period of time. Although the CT scan does not show a mass lesion, patients have over a 33% mortality rate. The clinical features of a cerebral contusion (**c**) are similar to those of a concussion except that neurologic dysfunction is more profound and prolonged and focal deficits may be present if contusions occur in the sensorimotor area. These injuries occur when the brain impacts the skull. The lesion is typically seen on CT scan. Posttraumatic epilepsy (**d**) is associated with intracranial hematomas and depressed skull fractures. The seizures generally occur within the first week of the head injury. Some scientists believe that head trauma predisposes to Alzheimer disease (**e**); however, this would take years to develop.

**102. The answer is b.** (*Moore et al, pp 578-583.*) Blunt cardiac injuries usually result from high-speed vehicular collisions in which the chest wall strikes the steering wheel. Although they are all associated with potentially fatal complications, they should be viewed clinically as a continuous spectrum of myocardial damage: concussion (no permanent cell damage), contusion (permanent cell damage), infarction (cell death), tamponade (bleeding into the pericardium), and rupture (exsanguination). The mechanism of injury in a cardiac contusion involves a high-speed deceleration, which causes the heart to move forward, forcibly striking the sternum. In addition, the direct force of hitting an object (eg, the steering wheel) also can damage the heart. **The right ventricle** is **most commonly injured** because it is the most anterior aspect of the heart and is closest to the sternum.

**103. The answer is d.** (*Moore et al, pp 174-175, 219-223.*) Hypovolemia secondary to hemorrhage is the most common cause of shock in the trauma patient. The earliest signs of hemorrhagic shock are tachycardia and cutaneous vasoconstriction. The amount of blood loss present can be estimated based on the individual's initial clinical presentation. **Class I hemorrhage (a and b)** is characterized by 0% to 15% blood loss (0-750 mL). This stage exhibits minimal clinical signs and symptoms. The patient is normotensive with a slightly elevated HR (> 100). **Class II hemorrhage (c)** is characterized by 15% to 30% blood loss (750-1500 mL). This stage exhibits tachycardia (HR > 100) with a narrow pulse pressure, delayed capillary refill, mild anxiety, tachypnea, and a slight decrease in urine output. **Class III hemorrhage** is characterized by 30% to 40% blood loss (1500-2000 mL). This stage exhibits tachypnea, tachycardia (HR > 120), **decrease in systolic BP**, delayed capillary refill, decreased urine output, and a change in mental status. **Class IV hemorrhage (e)** is characterized by blood loss greater than 40% (> 2 L). This stage exhibits obvious shock, tachycardia (HR > 140), decreased systolic BP, extremely narrow pulse pressure, scant urine output, delayed capillary refill, confusion, and lethargy.

**104. The answer is e.** (*Moore et al, pp 26-32.*) Trauma is the leading cause of death between the ages of 1 and 44 years. Many of these injuries are treatable mainly because the patients are young and otherwise healthy. The primary role of the emergency physician is to assess, resuscitate, and stabilize the trauma patient by priority. There are three peak times for trauma deaths. The first, classified as **immediate death**, is the period with the greatest number of fatalities. This occurs within seconds to minutes of the injury and these patients generally die at the scene. The cause is most commonly because of massive **head injury**, followed by high cervical spine injury with spinal cord disruption, cardiac and great vessel rupture, and airway obstruction. The second peak period, classified as **early death**, occurs within minutes to a few hours of injury. This is the period called the "golden hour" where intervention is critical and significantly reduces the morbidity and mortality rate in these patients. Death in these patients is generally secondary to subdural and epidural hematomas. Other causes of death in this group include ruptured spleen, lacerated liver, hypovolemic shock, fracture of pelvis or multiple long bones, hemopneumothorax, tension pneumothorax, cardiac tamponade, and aortic dissection or rupture. The third peak period, classified as **delayed death**, occurs days to weeks following the initial injury. Death in these patients is usually a result of multisystem organ failure and sepsis.

**105. The answer is c.** *(Rosen, pp 337-350, 469.)* Spearing—hitting another player with the crown of the helmet—generates an axial loading force that is transmitted through the occipital condyles to the superior articular surfaces of the lateral masses of the first cervical vertebra (C1). This fracture is commonly referred to as a **Jefferson fracture**. It is considered an unstable fracture and is associated with C2 fractures 40% of the time. On plain radiograph, it is best seen on the open-mouth odontoid view as the lateral masses are shifted laterally. It is associated with diving accidents and in this scenario, "spearing" in a football game, which places an increased axial load to the cervical spine. Proper cervical spine precautions should remain in place throughout his management in the ED.

(a) Odontoid fractures occur when there is a fracture through the odontoid process of the C2 vertebra. (b) A hangman's fracture, or traumatic spondylolysis of C2, occurs when the cervicocranium is thrown into extreme hyperextension secondary to abrupt deceleration (eg, head-on, high-speed motor vehicle collisions). (d) Clay shoveler's fracture occurs secondary to cervical hyperextension or direct trauma to the posterior neck, resulting in an avulsion fracture of the spinous process (eg, assault with blunt object to back of neck). (e) A teardrop fracture occurs from severe hyperflexion of the cervical spine and is commonly seen after diving accidents. This injury disrupts all of the cervical ligaments, facet joints, and causes a triangular fracture of a portion of the vertebral body. It is associated with anterior cord syndrome.

**106. The answer is d.** *(Rosen, pp 403-406.)* The vignette describes a traumatic arrest after penetrating chest trauma. The most likely cause is **cardiac tamponade**, which occurs in approximately 2% of anterior penetrating chest traumas. Clinically, patients present with **hypotension, JVD,** and **muffled heart sounds**. These three signs are called **Beck triad**. In addition, tachycardia is often present. JVD may not be present if there is marked hypovolemia. The most effective method for relieving acute pericardial tamponade in the trauma setting is **thoracotomy** and incision of the pericardium with removal of blood from the pericardial sac. The indications to perform an ED thoracotomy generally include blunt or penetrating trauma patients who lose their vital signs in transport to or in the ED. Patients with penetrating wounds have a significantly better chance of surviving with thoracotomy; also patients with stab wounds are more likely to do better than GSWs.

(a and b) The role of advanced cardiac life support (ACLS) drugs in traumatic arrest is unclear. However, patients in traumatic arrest typically require surgical, rather than medical intervention. (c) Chest tube placement will not treat pericardial tamponade. If the patient had evidence of a tension PTX, chest tubes are the treatment of choice. (e) Pericardiocentesis may or may not be effective in acute traumatic tamponade because the pericardium is usually distended by clotted blood rather than by free blood. Pericardiocentesis is indicated for patients with suspected cardiac tamponade who have measurable vital signs that are stable.

**107. The answer is d.** (Rosen, pp 335-336, 854-856.) The patient has an **avulsed tooth**, which is a **dental emergency**. When a tooth is missing from a patient, the possibility of aspiration or entrapment in soft tissues should be considered. Avulsed permanent teeth require prompt intervention. The best environment for an avulsed tooth is its socket. **Replantation** is most successful if the tooth is **returned** to **its socket** within 30 minutes of the avulsion. A 1% chance of successful replantation is lost for every minute that the tooth is outside of its socket. The tooth should only be handled by the crown, so as not to disrupt the root. If the patient cannot replant the tooth, he or she should keep the tooth under his or her tongue or in the buccal pouch so that it is bathed in saliva. If that cannot be achieved, then the tooth can be placed in a cup of milk (e) or in saline. The best transport solution is **Hank solution**, which is a buffered chemical solution. However, it is typically unavailable in this setting.

(a) The worst situation is to transport the tooth in a dry medium. (b and c) Water and beer are less than ideal. Saliva, milk, or saline are better solutions.

**108. The answer is c.** (Rosen, pp 301-302, 307-308.) The GCS score, as seen below, may be used as a tool for classifying head injury and is an objective method for following a patient's neurologic status. The GCS assesses a person's **eye, verbal,** and **motor responsiveness.** Although the GCS was originally developed to assess head trauma at 6 hours postinjury, it is commonly used in the acute presentation. This patient received a score of 3 for eye opening to verbal command, 4 for disorientation, but conversant, and 6 for obeying verbal commands.

**A Glasgow Coma Scale**

| Eye opening | Spontaneous | 4 |
|---|---|---|
| | To verbal command | 3 |
| | To pain | 2 |
| | None | 1 |
| **Verbal responsiveness** | Oriented | 5 |
| | Confused | 4 |
| | Inappropriate words | 3 |
| | Incomprehensible sounds | 2 |
| | None | 1 |
| **Motor response** | Obeys | 6 |
| | Localized | 5 |
| | Withdraws (pain) | 4 |
| | Flexion (pain) | 3 |
| | Extension (pain) | 2 |
| | None | 1 |
| | **Total:** | _____ |

*(Reproduced, with permission, from Stone CK, Humphries RL, eds. The multiply injured patient. In: Current Diagnosis & Treatment: Emergency Medicine. 6th ed. New York, NY: McGraw-Hill, 2008: Figure 10-2.)*

**109. The answer is a.** *(Rosen, p 415.)* Since most people are right-handed and hold the offending instrument in their right hand, the LUQ is most commonly injured in stab wounds. However, the **liver** occupies the most space in the abdomen and therefore is the most common organ injured.

(b) The small bowel is the second most commonly injured organ in stab wounds and is the most common organ injured in projectile penetrating abdominal trauma (eg, GSW). The stomach, colon, and spleen (c, d, and e) are less commonly injured than the liver and small bowel in penetrating abdominal trauma.

**110. The answer is d.** *(Rosen, pp 387-388.)* **Simple rib fractures** are the most common form of significant chest injury. Ribs usually break at the point of impact or at the posterior angle, which is structurally the weakest area. The fourth through ninth ribs are most commonly involved. Rib fractures occur more commonly in adults than in children owing to the relative inelasticity of the adult chest wall compared to the more compliant chest wall of children. The presence of two or more rib fractures at any level is associated with a higher incidence of internal injuries. The treatment of patients with simple acute rib fractures includes **adequate pain relief** and **maintenance of pulmonary function**. Oral pain medications are usually sufficient for young and healthy patients. Older patients may require better analgesia with opioids, but care must be taken to avoid over sedation. Continuing daily activities and deep breathing are important to ensure ventilation and prevent atelectasis. If there is a question about the patient's ability to cough, breathe deeply, and maintain activity, particularly if two or more ribs are fractured, it is preferable to admit the patient to the hospital for aggressive pulmonary care.

(a) Attempts to relieve pain by immobilization or splinting should not be used. Although they may decrease pain, they also promote hypoventilation leading to atelectasis and pneumonia. (b) A chest tube is indicated only if a PTX or hemothorax is suspected. (c) Rib fractures heal spontaneously and do not require surgical fixation. (e) The main concern in treating rib fractures is preventing complications, such as atelectasis and pneumonia. Therefore, it is important that the patient have adequate analgesia.

**III. The answer is e.** *(Rosen, pp 393-396.)* A PTX can be divided into three classifications: simple, communicating, and tension. A PTX is considered simple when there is no communication with the atmosphere or any shift of the mediastinum or hemidiaphragm resulting from the accumulation of air within the pleural cavity. A communicating PTX is associated with a defect in the chest wall and is sometimes referred to as a "sucking chest wound." A tension PTX occurs when air enters the pleural cavity on inspiration, but cannot exit, which leads to compression of the vena cava and subsequent decreased cardiac output and hypotension. The progressive accumulation of air under pressure in the pleural cavity may lead to a shift of the mediastinum to the contralateral hemithorax.

Patients with a traumatic PTX typically present with shortness of breath, chest pain, and tachypnea. The physical examination may reveal decreased or absent breath sounds over the involved side, as well as subcutaneous emphysema. Any patient with respiratory symptoms in the setting of a PTX should be treated with a **tube thoracostomy (chest tube)**. The preferred site for insertion is the fourth or fifth intercostal space at the anterior or midaxillary line. The tube should be positioned posteriorly and toward the apex so that it can effectively remove both air and fluid.

(a) A chest radiograph may be helpful in diagnosing a PTX; however, the patient is unstable in the setting of blunt trauma and intervention should not wait for a chest radiograph. If the patient was stable, a chest radiograph could be used to confirm the presence of a PTX prior to chest tube insertion. (b) A pericardiocentesis is a procedure used to remove fluid from the pericardial sac, such as in the case of pericardial tamponade. It is more likely to occur after a penetrating trauma to the chest rather than a blunt trauma. (c) A DPL is used to diagnose fluid in the peritoneum. Although this may be necessary for this patient, it is important to follow the ABCs of resuscitation. In this patient, airway and breathing need to be addressed first. (d) ED thoracotomy is used in select circumstances, such as in blunt or penetrating trauma patients who lose their vital signs in transport to or in the ED.

**112. The answer is d.** *(Rosen, pp 354-356, 1390-1392.)* **Brown-Séquard syndrome** or **hemisection** of the spinal cord typically results from penetrating trauma, such as a gunshot or knife wound. Patients with this lesion have **ipsilateral motor paralysis** and **contralateral loss of pain** and **temperature** distal to the level of the injury. This syndrome has the best prognosis for recovery of all of the incomplete spinal cord lesions.

(a) Spinal shock is a clinical syndrome characterized by the bilateral loss of neurologic function and autonomic tone below the level of a spinal cord lesion. Patients typically exhibit flaccid paralysis with loss of sensory input, deep tendon reflexes, and urinary bladder tone. Also, they are usually bradycardic, hypotensive, and hypothermic. Spinal shock generally lasts less than 24 hours, but may last several days. (b) Central cord syndrome is often seen in patients with degenerative arthritis of the cervical vertebrae, whose necks are subjected to forced hyperextension (eg, a forward fall onto the face in an elderly person). Patients often have greater sensorimotor neurologic deficits in the upper extremities compared to the lower extremities. (c) Anterior cord syndrome results in variable degrees of motor paralysis and absent pain sensation below the level of the lesion. Its hallmark is preservation of vibratory sensation and proprioception because of an intact dorsal column. (e) Cauda equina injury causes peripheral nerve injury rather than direct spinal cord damage. Its presentation may

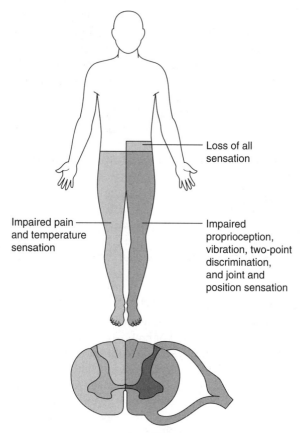

Loss of all
sensation

Impaired pain
and temperature
sensation

Impaired
proprioception,
vibration, two-point
discrimination,
and joint and
position sensation

*(Reproduced, with permission, from McPhee SJ, Lingappa VR, Ganong WF. Nervous system disorders. In: Lange Pathophysiology of Disease. 5th ed. New York, NY: McGraw-Hill, 2006: Figure 7-20.)*

include variable motor and sensory loss in the lower extremities, sciatica, bowel and bladder dysfunction, and saddle anesthesia.

**113. The answer is a.** *(Tintinalli, pp 1695-1698.)* Head injury severity is assessed on the mechanism of injury and on the initial neurologic examination. Although the GCS is currently used in multiple settings, it was initially developed for the clinical evaluation of hemodynamically stable, adequately oxygenated trauma patients with isolated head trauma. A score of 14 to 15 is associated with minor head injury, 9 to 13 indicates moderate, and **8 or less** is associated with **severe head injury.** His **GCS score is 8** (2 points for eye opening to pain, 2 points for mumbling speech, 4 points for withdrawing from pain). He is classified with a severe head injury. The overall mortality of severe head injury is almost 40%. It is recommended **to intubate** patients with a **GCS score of 8 or less** for airway protection. These patients are at risk for increased ICP and herniation, which can lead to rapid respiratory decline. All patients with severe traumatic brain injury require an emergent CT scan and should be admitted to the intensive care unit in a hospital with neurosurgical capabilities.

**(b)** Repairing his laceration is not a priority and can take place after diagnosing and stabilizing injuries that are more serious. If there is an active scalp bleed, staples can be rapidly placed to limit bleeding until definitive repair can take place. **(c)** Mannitol is an osmotic agent that is used to reduce ICP. It is administered if there are signs of impending or actual herniation (eg, fixed and dilated pupil). **(d)** Bilateral ED trephination (burr holes) is rarely, if ever, performed and is considered if definitive neurosurgical care is not available. **(e)** Although this individual may require neurosurgical intervention (eg, if there is any evidence of intracranial hemorrhage or declining neurologic status, indicating increased ICP), priority is given to his airway.

**114. The answer is c.** *(Rosen, pp 389-390.)* **Flail chest** results when **three or more adjacent ribs are fractured at two points**, allowing a freely moving segment of the chest wall to move in a **paradoxical motion.** It is one of the most commonly overlooked injuries resulting from blunt chest trauma. The paradoxical motion of the chest wall is the hallmark of this condition, with the flail segment paradoxically moving inward with inspiration and outward with expiration.

**115. The answer is d.** *(Rosen, pp 377-384.)* Owing to its lack of bony protection, the neck is especially vulnerable to severe, life-threatening injuries. Neck trauma is caused by three major mechanisms, including penetrating, blunt, and strangulation, which can affect the airway, digestive tract, vascular, and neurologic systems. The neck is divided into three zones, as seen in the picture below. Zone I extends superiorly from the sternal notch and clavicles to the cricoid cartilage. Injuries to this region can affect both neck and mediastinal structures. Zone II is the area between the cricoid

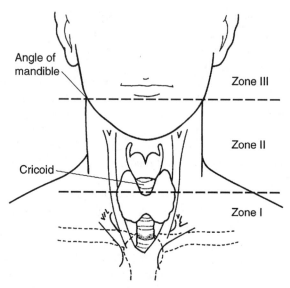

Angle of
mandible

Zone III

Zone II

Cricoid

Zone I

(Reproduced, with permission, from Doherty GM, Way LW. Current Surgical Diagnosis &
Treatment. New York, NY: McGraw-Hill, 2006: 210.)

cartilage and the angle of the mandible. Zone III extends from the angle
of the mandible to the base of the skull. Zones I and III injuries typically
pose a greater challenge to manage than zone II injuries because zones I
and III are much less exposed than zone II. **Generally, zone II injuries are
taken directly to the operating room for surgical exploration.** Injuries
in zones I and III may be taken to the operating room or managed conservatively using a combination of angiography, bronchoscopy, esophagoscopy,
and CT scanning.

Airway management is always given priority in trauma patients, particularly when neck structures are involved because of the potential for
rapid airway compromise. Active bleeding sites or wounds with blood
clots should not be probed because massive hemorrhage can occur. **Bleeding should be controlled by direct pressure.** Blind clamping should be
avoided because of the high concentration of neurovascular structures in
the neck.

**(a)** Blind clamping should be avoided because of the high concentration
of neurovascular structures in the neck. **(b)** Active bleeding sites or wounds

with blood clots should not be probed because massive hemorrhage can occur. **Bleeding should be controlled by direct pressure. (c and e)** The injury is in zone II of the neck.

**116. The answer is d.** *(Rosen, pp 337-350.)* The **hangman's fracture**, or **traumatic spondylolysis of C2**, occurs when the head is thrown into **extreme hyperextension** because of **abrupt deceleration**, resulting in bilateral fractures of the pedicles. The name "hangman's fracture" was derived from judicial hangings, where the knot of the noose was placed under the chin which caused extreme hyperextension of the head on the neck, resulting in a fracture at C2. However, many hangings resulted in death from strangulation rather than spinal cord damage. Today, the most common cause of a hangman's fracture is the result of head-on **automobile collisions**.

(a) Colles fracture is the most common wrist fracture seen in adults. It is a transverse fracture of the distal radial metaphysis, which is dorsally displaced and angulated. These fractures usually occur from a fall on an outstretched hand. (b) A boxer's fracture is a fracture of the neck of the fifth metacarpal. It is one of the most common fractures of the hand and usually occurs from a direct impact to the hand (eg, a punch with a closed fist). (c) A fracture of C1 is called a Jefferson fracture, which is typically produced by a vertical compression force. (e) Clay shoveler's fracture occurs secondary to cervical hyperextension or direct trauma to the posterior neck, resulting in an avulsion fracture of the spinous process.

**117. The answer is b.** *(Tintinalli, pp 1700-1701.)* The skull base comprises the floors of the anterior, middle, and posterior cranial fossae. Fractures in this region typically do not have localized symptoms. However, indirect signs of injury may include visible evidence of bleeding from the fracture into surrounding soft tissue. Ecchymosis around the mastoid bone is often described as **Battle sign** and periorbital ecchymosis is often described as "raccoon eyes." The most common **basilar skull fracture** involves the petrous portion of the temporal bone, the external auditory canal, and the tympanic membrane. It is commonly associated with a torn dura leading to **cerebrospinal fluid (CSF) otorrhea** or **rhinorrhea**. Other signs and symptoms of a basilar skull fracture include hemotympanum (eg, blood in the tympanic cavity of the middle ear), vertigo, decreased hearing or deafness, and seventh nerve palsy. Periorbital and mastoid ecchymosis develop gradually over hours after an injury and are often absent in the ED. If clear or pink fluid is seen from the nose or ear and a CSF leak is suspected, the fluid can be placed on filter paper and a "halo" or double ring may appear. This is a simple but nonsensitive test to confirm a CSF leak. Evidence of open communication, such as a CSF leak, mandates neurosurgical consultation and admission.

(a) Le Fort factures typically result from high-energy facial trauma and are classified according to their location. A **Le Fort I** involves a transverse fracture just above the teeth at the level of the nasal fossa, and allows movement of the alveolar ridge and hard palate. A **Le Fort II** is a pyramidal fracture with its apex just above the bridge of the nose and extending laterally and inferiorly through the infraorbital rims allowing movement of the maxilla, nose, and infraorbital rims. A **Le Fort III** represents complete craniofacial disruption and involves fractures of the zygoma, infraorbital rims, and maxilla. It is rare for these fractures to occur in isolation; they usually occur in combination. (c and d) Otitis interna and externa are inflammation of the inner ear and outer ear, respectively, and are not relevant in acute trauma. (e) Tripod fractures typically occur from blunt force applied to the lateral face causing fractures of zygomatic arch, the lateral orbital rim, the inferior orbital rim, and the anterior and lateral walls of the maxillary sinus. These fractures present clinically with asymmetrical facial flattening, edema, and ecchymosis.

**118. The answer is e.** (*Tintinalli, pp 1671-1675.*) Based on the principles of advanced trauma life support (ATLS), injured patients are assessed and treated in a fashion that establishes priorities based on their presenting vital signs, mental status, and injury mechanism. The approach to trauma care consists of a **primary survey**, rapid resuscitation, and a more thorough secondary survey followed by diagnostic testing. The goal of the primary survey is to quickly identify and treat immediately life-threatening injuries. The assessment of the ABCDEs **(airway, breathing, circulation, neurologic disability, exposure)** is a model that should be followed in all patients. Airway patency is first evaluated by listening for vocalizations, asking the patient to speak, and looking in the patient's mouth for signs of obstruction. Breathing is assessed by observing for symmetric rise and fall of the chest and listening for bilateral breath sounds over the anterior chest and axillae. The chest should be palpated for subcutaneous air and bony crepitus. Circulatory function is assessed by noting the patient's mental status, skin color and temperature, and pulses. The patient's neurologic status is assessed by noting level of consciousness and gross motor function. An initial GCS should be calculated in the ED. Last, the patient is completely undressed to evaluate for otherwise hidden bruises, lacerations, impaled foreign bodies, and open fractures. The secondary head-to-toe survey is undertaken only after the primary survey is complete, life-threatening injuries are addressed, and the patient is resuscitated and stabilized.

(a) This patient will require a chest tube for presumed hemo- or pneumothorax demonstrated by decreased breath sounds and oxygen saturation of 93%. However, the airway should first be secured. (b) A DPL or FAST examination is used to screen the abdomen for hemoperitoneum. However, airway and breathing take priority in this patient. (c) Bilateral ED trephination (burr holes) is rarely, if ever, performed and should only be considered in the case of severe neurologic impairment and definitive neurosurgical care is not available. (d) Extremity injuries are typically not life threatening and are assessed after the airway, breathing, and circulation are evaluated.

**119. The answer is a.** (*Tintinalli, pp 1700-1703.*) **Epidural hematomas** are the result of blood collecting in the potential space between the skull and the dura mater. Most epidural hematomas result from **blunt trauma** to the temporal or temporoparietal area with an associated skull fracture and middle **meningeal artery disruption**. The classic history of an epidural hematoma is a lucid period following immediate loss of consciousness after significant blunt head trauma. However, this clinical pattern occurs in a minority of cases. Most patients either never lose consciousness or never regain consciousness after the injury. On CT scan, epidural **hematomas appear lenticular or biconvex (football shaped)**, typically in the temporal region. The high-pressure arterial bleeding of an epidural hematoma can lead to herniation within hours after injury. Therefore, early recognition and evacuation are important to increase survival. Bilateral ED trephination (burr holes) is rarely, if ever, performed and should only be considered if definitive neurosurgical care is not available.

(b) Subdural hematomas appear as hyperdense, crescent-shaped lesions that cross suture lines. They result from a collection of blood below the dura and over the brain. To differentiate the CT finding from

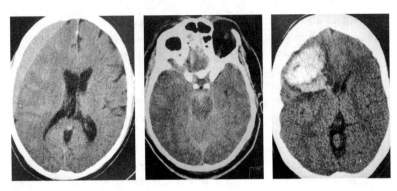

*(Courtesy of Adam J. Rosh MD.)*

an epidural hematoma, think about the high pressure created by the arterial tear of an epidural that causes the hematoma to expand inward. In contrast, the low-pressure venous bleed of a subdural hematoma layers along the calvarium. **(c)** Traumatic SAH is probably the most common CT abnormality in patients with moderate to severe traumatic brain injury. **(d and e)** Intracerebral hematomas and contusions occur secondary to traumatic tearing of intracerebral blood vessels. Contusions most commonly occur in the frontal, temporal, and occipital lobes. They may occur either at the site of the blunt trauma or on the opposite site of the brain, known as a contrecoup injury. Examples of each are seen above.

**120. The answer is a.** *(Rosen, pp 354-356, 1390-1392.)* **Central cord syndrome** is often seen in patients with degenerative arthritis of the cervical vertebrae, whose necks are subjected to **forced hyperextension**. Typically, it is seen in a forward fall onto the face in an elderly person. This causes the ligamentum flavum to buckle into the spinal cord, resulting in a contusion to the central portion of the cord. This injury affects the central gray matter and the most central portions of the pyramidal and spinothalamic tracts. Patients often have **greater neurologic deficits in the upper extremities, compared to the lower extremities,** since nerve fibers that innervate distal structures are located in the periphery of the spinal cord. In addition, patients with central cord syndrome usually have decreased rectal sphincter tone and patchy, unpredictable sensory deficits.

(b) Anterior cord syndrome results in variable degrees of motor paralysis, and loss of temperature and pain sensation below the level of

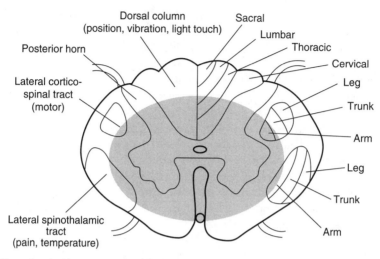

Dorsal column
(position, vibration, light touch)

Sacral

Lumbar

Thoracic

Cervical

Posterior horn

Lateral cortico-
spinal tract
(motor)

Leg

Trunk

Arm

Leg

Trunk

Lateral spinothalamic
tract
(pain, temperature)

Arm

*(Reproduced, with permission, from Schwartz DT. Emergency Radiology: Case Studies. New York, NY: McGraw-Hill, 2007: chap V-4, Figure 15.)*

the lesion. Its hallmark is preservation of vibratory sensation and proprioception because of an intact dorsal column. (c) Brown-Séquard syndrome results in ipsilateral loss of motor strength, vibratory sensation, and proprioception, and contralateral loss of pain and temperature sensation. (d) Transverse myelitis is an inflammatory process that produces complete motor and sensory loss below the level of the lesion. (e) Parkinson disease develops over years and does not result in paralysis.

**121. The answer is e.** *(Rosen, pp 39-40.)* The decision to begin blood transfusion in a trauma patient is based on the initial response to crystalloid volume resuscitation. **Blood products should be administered if vital signs transiently improve or remain unstable despite resuscitation with 2 to 3 L of crystalloid fluid.** However, if there is obvious major blood loss and the patient is unstable, blood transfusion should be started concomitantly with crystalloid administration. The main purpose in transfusing blood is to restore the oxygen-carrying capacity of the intravascular volume. Fully cross-matched blood is preferable (eg, type B, Rh-negative, antibody negative); however, this process may take more than 1 hour, which is inappropriate for the unstable trauma patient. Type-specific blood (eg, type A, Rh negative, unknown antibody) can be provided by most blood banks within 30 minutes. This blood is compatible with ABO and Rh blood types, but may be incompatible with other antibodies. If type-specific blood is unavailable, type O packed cells are indicated for patients who are unstable. Men should be administered type O, Rh-positive blood. To reduce sensitization and future complications, type O, Rh-negative blood is reserved for women of childbearing age.

(a) Fully cross-matched blood may take greater than 1 hour to prepare, which is inappropriate for an unstable patient. (b) Whole blood is rarely used by blood centers and was replaced by blood components, such as packed RBCs. Whole blood is not used because the extra plasma can contribute to transfusion associated circulatory overload, a potentially dangerous complication. (c) Blood transfusion should not be delayed in the unstable patient. As dictated in ATLS, if the individual does not respond to 2 to 3 L of crystalloid, blood transfusion should commence. (d) For life-threatening blood loss, type O, Rh-negative blood is reserved for women of childbearing age. This reduces complications of Rh incompatibility in future pregnancies. However, if type O, Rh-negative blood is unavailable, type O, Rh-positive blood should be administered to women.

**122. The answer is c.** (*Rosen, pp 605-616.*) This patient is hemodynamically unstable with a pelvic fracture. The retroperitoneum can accommodate up to 4 L of blood after severe pelvic trauma. A few options are useful in managing hemorrhage from an unstable pelvic fracture. However, the initial and simplest modality to use in a patient in shock from a pelvis fracture is placement of a **pelvic binding garment**. This device can be applied easily and rapidly and is typically effective in tamponading bleeding and stabilizing the pelvis.

(a) Bilateral chest tubes would be appropriate if there was evidence for a pneumo- or hemothorax. This patient has bilaterally equal breath sounds. (b) Although external fixation is an effective method to stabilize the pelvis, it may delay management of a trauma patient. Because a pelvic binding apparatus is quick and simple, it is preferred. (d) The source of retroperitoneal bleeding with pelvic fractures is typically the venous plexus or smaller veins. However, venography is not useful in managing these patients; even when venous bleeding is localized, embolization is ineffective because of the extensive anastomoses and valveless collateral flow. (e) In contrast, arteriography is a major diagnostic and therapeutic modality for the patient with severe pelvic hemorrhage from arterial sources. Angiography is indicated when hypovolemia persists in a patient with a major pelvic fracture, despite control of hemorrhage from other sources. Since angiography typically takes place in the angiography suite, patients should have a pelvic binding device applied, prior to being transferred to angiography.

**123. The answer is c.** (*Rosen, pp 354-356, 1390-1392.*) **Anterior cord syndrome** results from **cervical flexion injuries** (eg, diving in shallow water) that cause cord contusion or protrusion of a bony fragment or herniated intervertebral disk into the spinal canal. It may also occur from vascular pathology, such as laceration or thrombosis of the anterior spinal artery. The syndrome is characterized by different degrees of paralysis and loss of pain and temperature sensation below the level of injury. **Its hallmark is the preservation of the posterior columns, maintaining position, touch, and vibratory sensation.**

SCIWORA (**a**) is reserved for the pediatric population because the spinal cord is less elastic than the bony spine and ligaments. The diagnosis is associated with paresthesias and generalized weakness. This syndrome is coming under scrutiny since the advent of the magnetic resonance imaging (MRI) where spinal cord lesions are being identified in patients who otherwise had normal CT scans. Central cord syndrome (**b**) is often seen in patients with degenerative arthritis of the cervical vertebrae, whose necks are subjected to forced hyperextension. This is seen typically in a forward fall onto the face in an elderly person. Patients often have greater sensorimotor neurologic deficits in the upper extremities compared to the lower extremities. Cauda equina injury (**d**) causes peripheral nerve injury rather than direct spinal cord damage. Its presentation may include variable motor and sensory loss in the lower extremities, sciatica, bowel and bladder dysfunction, and saddle anesthesia. Brown-Séquard syndrome (**e**) results in ipsi-lateral loss of motor strength, vibratory sensation, and proprioception, and contralateral loss of pain and temperature sensation.

| Syndrome | Neurologic Deficits |
|---|---|
| Anterior cord | B/L paralysis below lesion, loss of pain and temperature, and preservation of proprioception and vibratory function |
| Central cord | Lower extremity paralysis > upper extremity paralysis, some loss of pain and temperature with upper > lower |
| Brown-Séquard | **Ipsilateral:** paresis, loss of proprioception, and vibratory sensation |
| | **Contralateral:** loss of pain and temperature |
| Cauda equina | Variable motor and sensory loss in lower extremities, bowel/bladder dysfunction, saddle anesthesia |

**124. The answer is b.** *(Tintinalli, pp 1753-1754.)* The treatment of a **tension** PTX involves immediate reduction in the intrapleural pressure on the affected side of the thoracic cavity. The simplest and quickest way to establish this is by inserting a 14-gauge catheter into the thoracic cavity in the second intercostal space in the midclavicular line. After this procedure, a chest tube should be inserted as definitive management. **Needle thoracostomy** is necessary when a patient's vital signs are unstable; otherwise, direct insertion of a chest tube is adequate for suspicion of a hemo- or pneumothorax. A tension PTX is a life-threatening emergency caused by air entering the pleural space that is not able to escape secondary to the creation of a one-way valve. This increased pressure causes the ipsilateral lung to collapse, shifting the mediastinum away from the injured lung, compromising vena caval blood return to the heart. The severely altered preload results in reduced stroke volume, increased cardiac output, and hypotension.

(**a**) Airway is the first component addressed in the ABCs; however, the patient is breathing on his own and does not require intubation. (**c and d**) If the BP does not elevate with insertion of a chest tube, the next area to focus on is an intra-abdominal injury, which can be assessed either by a DPL or FAST examination. (**e**) A pericardiocentesis is indicated in the stable trauma patient when there is suspicion for cardiac tamponade, which may present with tachycardia and Beck triad: hypotension, JVD, and muffled heart sounds.

**125. The answer is e.** *(Tintinalli, pp 1723-1726.)* The Canadian C-spine rule for radiography in alert and stable patients following blunt head or neck trauma identified **age greater than 65 years as a high risk factor for C-spine injury**, even among those with stable vital signs and a GCS score of 15. Therefore, C-spine imaging in all such elderly patients is warranted.

(**a**) It is thought that elderly patients experience a much lower incidence of epidural hematomas than the general population because of a relatively denser fibrous bond between the dura mater and the inner table of the skull in older individuals. (**b**) There is, however, a high incidence of subdural hematomas in elderly patients. As the brain mass decreases in size with age, there is greater stretching and tension of the bridging veins that pass from the brain to the dural sinuses. (**c**) In the elderly, diminished elasticity of the lungs can lead to a reduction in pulmonary compliance and in the ability to cough effectively, resulting in an increased risk for nosocomial gram-negative pneumonia. Geriatric patients are thus more susceptible to the development of hypoxia and respiratory infections following trauma.

(d) The most common cervical spine fractures in this age group are upper cervical, particularly fractures of the odontoid, not lower C6 fractures.

**126. The answer is b.** *(Tintinalli, pp 1765-1767.)* Blunt trauma is the most common mechanism of injury seen in the United States. The forces exerted on the abdomen put all of the organs at risk for injury. Motor vehicle collisions with another vehicle or with pedestrians are the major causes of blunt abdominal trauma. The **spleen** is the organ most often injured, and in approximately 66% of these cases, it is the only damaged intraperitoneal organ.

The liver (a) is the second most commonly injured intra-abdominal organ, third is the kidney (c), fourth is the small bowel (d), and fifth is the bladder (e).

**127. The answer is e.** *(Rosen, pp 437-440.)* **Urethral injuries** make up approximately 10% of genitourinary trauma. Anterior urethral injuries are most often attributed to falls with straddle injuries or a blunt force to the perineum. Approximately 95% of posterior urethral injuries are secondary to pelvic fractures. Signs and symptoms of urethral injury include perineal pain, inability to void, gross hematuria, blood at the urethral meatus, perineal or scrotal swelling or ecchymosis, and an absent, high-riding, or boggy prostate. A **retrograde urethrogram** is the study of choice when there is suspicion of a urethral injury. This procedure is performed by inserting an 8F urinary catheter 2 cm into the meatus and inflating the catheter balloon with 2-cc saline to create a seal. Then, 30 cc of radiopaque contrast is administered and a radiograph is obtained looking for extravasation of contrast from the urethra.

(a) A scrotal ultrasound may be necessary later on to evaluate for testicular injury, but it is not used to evaluate urethral injury. (b) A KUB is not useful to evaluate the urethra. Prior to CT scanning, it was commonly used to evaluate for kidney stones. (c) An IV pyelogram is an alternative to CT scanning for evaluating the kidney and ureter. (d) A retrograde cystogram is a useful study to evaluate the bladder for injury.

**128. The answer is b.** *(Rosen, pp 327-330.)* **Orbital floor fractures** typically occur when a blunt object with a radius of curvature less than 5 cm (eg, often a fist or ball smaller than a softball) strikes the orbit. The blunt force causes an increase in intraorbital pressure causing a fracture along the weakest part of the orbit, usually the inferior or sometimes medial wall. Patients usually complain of **pain that is greatest with upward**

eye movement. They may have **impaired ocular motility or diplopia** if the inferior rectus muscle becomes entrapped. They may also present **with infraorbital hypoesthesia** because of compression of the infraorbital nerve. Generally, the patient has normal visual acuity unless there is an associated ocular injury. A classic radiographic finding is the "teardrop sign," which represents herniated orbital fat and muscle in the roof of the maxillary sinus. There may also be an air-fluid level in the maxillary sinus as a result of bleeding into it. Patients usually do well and recover completely in mild to moderate fractures.

(**a**) Zygomatic arch fractures usually present with periauricular depression and point tenderness and may be complicated by trismus secondary to impingement of the coronoid process of the mandible on the arch during mouth opening. (**c**) A retrobulbar hematoma occurs secondary to blunt orbital trauma and typically causes exophthalmos. Patients usually present with periorbital edema, ecchymosis, a decrease in visual acuity, and an afferent papillary defect in the involved eye. (**d**) Open globe injuries typically result from penetrating trauma to the eye. Patients may present with leakage of aqueous humor, a teardrop-shaped pupil, or prolapse of choroid through the wound. (**e**) Patients with mandible fractures present with pain and decreased range of motion of the jaw, malocclusion or pain with teeth clenching, and inability to fully open the mouth.

**129. The answer is e.** (*Rosen, pp 428-430.*) An important concern with **anterior abdominal GSW** is to determine whether the missile traversed the peritoneal cavity. Patients with transabdominal GSWs nearly all have intra-abdominal injuries requiring surgery. Most of the time, this can be determined by approximating the trajectory. Therefore, a hole in both the anterior and posterior abdomen highly suggests a transabdominal trajectory. If there are a single or odd number of holes, a plain film may help estimate the trajectory. In cases of tangential or multiple GSWs, it may be impossible to determine trajectory with any certainty. In a patient with evidence of peritoneal penetration, a missile tract that clearly enters the abdominal cavity, or has a positive diagnostic study (eg, DPL, FAST, CT) in a tangential wound, he or she should undergo exploratory laparotomy. The standard algorithm for **penetrating abdominal trauma** recommends that any patient with **unstable** vital signs be taken directly to the OR to undergo an **exploratory laparotomy**. If their vital signs are stable, they should undergo further diagnostic studies, such as a FAST examination, DPL, or CT scan.

(a) In general, penetrating abdominal wounds should not be probed. This may worsen the injury and disrupt hemostasis, resulting in uncontrolled hemorrhage. Instead, gently separate the skin edges to see if the base of the wound can be visualized. (b, c, and d) In the setting of penetrating abdominal trauma, further diagnostic tests should only occur if the patient has stable vital signs. Otherwise, patients should go directly to the OR to undergo exploratory laparotomy.

**130. The answer is a.** *(Rosen, p 885.)* **Posterior epistaxis** is identified when posterior bleeding occurs with a properly placed anterior nasal packing. Posterior packing is mandated using either a commercially available balloon or a standard Foley catheter inserted into the posterior nares and inflated with water. Patients with posterior nasal packs should **be admitted to a monitored bed**. In addition to cardiac dysrhythmias, myocardial infarctions, cerebrovascular accidents, and aspiration have been reported in these patients. **Antibiotics** are often started to prevent sinusitis and toxic shock syndrome from obstruction of the nasal packing.

(b) Placing the patient supine increases risk of aspiration and has no benefit to stopping epistaxis. (c) If the patient had an elevated INR or was thrombocytopenic, then FFP and platelets should be administered. (d) Patients with posterior nasal packing require admission. (e) Silver nitrate is a therapy for anterior epistaxis. It has no role in posterior epistaxis.

**131. The answer is a.** *(Rosen, pp 247-249.)* Patients often present to the ED with life-threatening conditions that require rapid and simultaneous evaluation and treatment. The fundamentals of emergency medicine begin with the ABCs. **Airway assessment and management have priority over all other aspects of resuscitation in the critically ill or injured patient**. Moreover, airway management is not simply the passage of a tube through the trachea. It involves a series of actions ranging from repositioning a patient's head and neck, suctioning secretions in the posterior pharynx to supplying supplemental oxygen or performing an emergent cricothyrotomy. Whatever the intervention, it is important to know when and how to manage an airway. There are many reasons for definitive airway management with an orotracheal tube, the obvious being in patients who are not breathing. However, there are instances that require definitive management even when a patient is spontaneously breathing. Any patient who is at risk of losing the ability to protect their airway should be considered for intubation. This includes intoxicated patients, the poisoned patient, worsening hypoxia, those with evolving laryngeal edema or hematoma near the trachea, and patients with significant head injuries. Once the airway is addressed, it is appropriate to move onto the next critical component of the ABCs.

(b) The patient will certainly require volume resuscitation and pain control, but airway management takes priority. (c and d) It is important not to get distracted by other injuries in a critical patient who requires definitive airway management as first priority. (e) Although the patient will require a blood transfusion, the airway must be addressed first.

**132. The answer is a.** (*Rosen, pp 1929-1931.*) **Diving injuries** must always be suspected in near-drowning patients. This patient presents with abdominal breathing and spontaneous respirations. This pattern provides an important clue to a **cervical spine injury**. The diaphragm is innervated by the phrenic nerve that originates from the spinal cord at the C3-C4 level, whereas the intercostal muscles of the rib cage are supplied by nerves that originate in the thoracic spine. Therefore, abdominal breathing in the absence of thoracic breathing indicates an injury below C4. His bradycardia in the presence of **hypotension** is suspicious for **neurogenic hypotension**, which is caused by loss of vasomotor tone and **lack of reflex tachycardia** from the disruption of autonomic ganglia. However, this is a diagnosis of exclusion and should only be made once all other forms of shock are ruled out. It is important to maintain **C-spine immobilization** to prevent further progression of an injury.

(b) Electrolyte abnormalities are typically not a concern in near-drowning injuries. (c) Any patient with hypoxia and hypoperfusion generally also has a metabolic acidosis. Treating the underlying pathology will also treat the acidosis.

(d) All near-drowning cases (fresh or saltwater) involve the loss of surfactant and subsequent atelectasis with a high potential for hypoxia. (e) Although a toxic ingestion should always be considered, there are no specific indications for it in this patient.

**133. The answer is b.** (*Rosen, pp 456-463.*) Clinical manifestations of **penetrating arterial injury of the extremity** are generally divided into "hard signs" and "soft signs." Hard signs include pulsatile bleeding, expanding hematoma, palpable thrill or audible bruit, and evidence of distal ischemia (eg, pain, pallor, pulselessness, paralysis, paresthesia, poikilothermia). Soft signs include diminished ankle-brachial indices, asymmetrically absent or weak distal pulse, history of moderate hemorrhage or wound close to a major artery, and a peripheral nerve deficit. Emergent surgery is generally necessary when there are **hard signs** of vascular injury. Although the management of penetrating extremity injury is evolving, whenever there is **evidence of distal ischemia**, the patient should be taken to the OR **for exploration and repair.** When severe ischemia is present, the repair must be completed within 6 to 8 hours to prevent irreversible muscle ischemia and loss of limb function. In the presence of hard signs without evidence of ischemia, some surgeons may prefer to first perform angiography to better define the injury.

(a) Angiography is a frequently used modality in penetrating extremity trauma and is the study of choice with some injuries that present with **hard signs.** However, when there is evidence of limb ischemia, the patient should undergo exploration and repair immediately. (c) Fasciotomy is the treatment for compartment syndrome. Although compartment syndrome can occur with blunt and penetrating extremity trauma, it is more common in crush injuries or fractures with marked swelling. It may be required, but should be performed in conjunction with and after the establishment of arterial blood flow. (d) Local wound exploration is not recommended because it may disrupt hemostasis and cause a worsening of the hemorrhage. (e) CT scanning is not appropriate in the setting of limb ischemia.

**134. The answer is b.** (*Rosen, pp 300-301.*) Cerebral herniation occurs when increased ICP overwhelms the natural compensatory capacities of the central nervous system (CNS). Increased ICP may be the result of posttraumatic brain swelling, edema formation, traumatic mass lesion expansion, or any combination of the three. When increasing ICP cannot be controlled, the intracranial contents will shift and herniate through the cranial foramen. Herniation can occur within minutes or up to days after a traumatic brain injury. Once the signs of herniation are present, mortality approaches 100% without rapid reversal or temporizing measures. **Uncal herniation** is the most common clinically significant form of traumatic herniation and is often associated with traumatic extracranial bleeding. The classic signs and symptoms are caused by compression of the ipsilateral uncus of the temporal lobe. This causes **compression of cranial nerve III leading to anisocoria, ptosis, impaired extraocular movements, and a sluggish pupillary light reflex.** As herniation progresses, compression of the ipsilateral oculomotor nerve eventually causes ipsilateral pupillary dilation and nonreactivity.

(a) An altered level of consciousness is the hallmark of brain insult from any cause and results from an interruption of the RAS or a global event that affects both cortices. (c) Contralateral dilation is a late manifestation in brain herniation. (d) Progressive hypertension associated with bradycardia and diminished respiratory effort is described as Cushing reflex and is a late manifestation of herniation. (e) Contralateral hemiparesis develops as herniation progresses.

**135. The answer is b.** *(Rosen, p 396.)* A **hemothorax** is the accumulation of blood in the pleural space after blunt or penetrating chest trauma. It can lead to hypovolemic shock and can significantly reduce vital capacity if it is not recognized. It is associated with a PTX approximately 25% of the time. Hemorrhage from injured lung parenchyma is the most common cause of hemothorax, but this tends to be self-limiting unless there is a major laceration to the parenchyma. Specific vessels are less often the source of bleeding. A hemothorax is treated with **chest thoracostomy (chest tube)** that is generally placed in the fourth or fifth intercostal space at the anterior or midaxillary line, over the superior portion of the rib. The tube should be directed superior and **posterior** to allow it to drain blood from the dependent portions of the chest. In an isolated PTX, the tube is positioned anteriorly to allow it to suction air. Once the tube is inserted, it is important to closely monitor blood output. Indications for thoracotomy include

- Initial chest tube drainage of 1000 to 1500 cc of blood (**a and b**).
- 200 cc/h of persistent drainage (**c**).
- Patient remains hypotensive despite adequate blood replacement, and other sites of blood loss have been ruled out.
- Patient decompensates after initial response to resuscitation.
- Increasing hemothorax seen on chest x-ray studies.

**136. The answer is c.** *(Rosen, pp 40, 247-248.)* This question addresses the "C," **circulation**, in the ABCs. Initial fluid resuscitation usually begins with crystalloid fluids such as 0.9% normal saline or Ringer lactate. In general, if the patient remains hemodynamically unstable after 40 cc/kg of crystalloid administration (approximately 2-3 L), a **blood transfusion** should be started. Fully cross-matched blood is preferable; however, this is generally not available in the early resuscitation period. Therefore, **type-specific blood (type O, Rh-negative or type O, Rh-positive)** is a safe alternative and is usually ready within 5 to 15 minutes. Type O, Rh-negative blood is typically reserved for women in their childbearing years to prevent Rh sensitization. Type O, Rh-positive blood can be given to all men and women beyond their childbearing years. **(a)** The patient's underlying cause of hypotension is hypovolemia secondary to hemorrhage. Therefore, to treat her hypotension you should treat the underlying cause. She requires fluid resuscitation with blood and eventually may be taken to the OR to stop the bleeding. Epinephrine is used if the patient is in cardiopulmonary arrest and no longer has a pulse. However, the underlying cause, hypovolemia, must be corrected. **(b)** The best resuscitation fluid is blood. ATLS guidelines suggest starting resuscitation with crystalloid solution and adding blood if there is no response after a 40 cc/kg bolus of crystalloid fluid. **(d)** The patient is too unstable to be transferred for a CT scan. If the patient's BP normalizes, the trauma team may elect for a CT scan. If the patient remains hypotensive despite resuscitation, definitive measures need to take place, such as an exploratory laparotomy to stop the hemorrhage. **(e)** Once the FAST examination is positive, repeating it will not add valuable information. If the patient remains hypotensive, definitive management is a priority.

**137. The answer is e.** *(Rosen, pp 252-260.)* Trauma occurs in up to 7% of all pregnancies and is the leading cause of maternal death. It is important to **focus the primary examination on the patient and evaluate the fetus in the secondary examination**. The ABCs are followed in usual fashion. Once the patient is deemed stable, the fetus should be evaluated. Fetal evaluation focuses on the fetal HR and fetal movement. Minor trauma to the patient does not rule out injury to the fetus. Therefore, it is important to monitor the fetus. **Cardiotocographic (cardiofetal heartbeat, tocouterine contractions, graphy-measuring) observation of the viable fetus is recommended for a minimum of 4 hours** to detect any intrauterine pathology. The minimum should be extended to 24 hours if, at any time during the first 4 hours, there are more than three uterine contractions per hour, persistent uterine tenderness, a non-reassuring fetal monitor strip, vaginal bleeding, rupture of the membranes, or any serious maternal injury is present.

**(a)** Cesarean section in the OR may take place if the patient is stable, but the fetus is unstable and greater than 24 weeks' gestation. This decision should be made by the obstetrician. **(b)** Cesarean section in the ED, or perimortem cesarean section, is performed if uterine size exceeds the umbilicus, fetal heart tones are present, and maternal decompensation is acute. **(c)** Radiation from CT scanning in the setting of pregnancy is a concern. Shielding of the uterus in head and chest scans allows for an acceptable radiation exposure level. Abdominal and pelvic CT scanning incurs greater radiation exposure, and the risks and benefits of these studies should be discussed with the patient. Other diagnostic procedures can be used in the setting of blunt abdominal trauma, such as ultrasound, DPL, and MRI. **(d)** Minor trauma does not exempt the fetus from injury and direct impact is not necessary for fetoplacental pathology to occur. The mother with no obvious abdominal injury or even normal laboratory values still requires monitoring.

**138. The answer is d.** (*Rosen, pp 204-205, 592-595, 1391-1392.*) **Cauda equina syndrome** is an injury to the lumbar, sacral, and coccygeal nerve roots, causing peripheral nerve injury that can lead to permanent neurologic defects if not recognized and corrected rapidly. Because of the central location of the disk herniation, symptoms are often bilateral and involve **leg pain, saddle anesthesia, and impaired bowel and bladder function (retention or incontinence)**. On examination, patients may exhibit loss of rectal tone and display other motor and sensory losses in the lower extremities. Patients with suspected cauda equina syndrome require an urgent CT scan or MRI.

(**a**) AAA can present with low back pain and rarely a neurologic deficit if they get large enough and impinge a nerve root. AAA should always be considered in patients over 50 years with hypertension and low back pain. A bedside ultrasound can usually identify large abdominal aortic aneurysms. If there is still concern for an AAA, a CT scan can rule the diagnosis out. (**b**) Disk herniation can result in peripheral nerve root compression and irritation leading to sensory and motor deficits. Patients, however, should not exhibit altered bowel and bladder function, or have decreased rectal tone. If so, the condition is likely cauda equina syndrome and is a neurologic emergency. (**c**) Spinal stenosis is narrowing of the spinal canal, which may cause spinal cord compression that typically is worse with back extension and relieved with flexion. (**e**) Osteomyelitis is an infection of the bone that typically presents with fever.

**139. The answer is d.** (*Rosen, pp 304-306.*) **A unilateral dilated pupil** in the setting of head trauma is an **indicator of increased ICP**. If ICP is not lowered immediately, the patient has little chance of survival. Hyperventilation to produce an arterial $P_{CO_2}$ of 30 to 35 mm Hg will temporarily reduce ICP by promoting cerebral vasoconstriction and subsequent reduction in cerebral blood flow. The onset of action is within 30 seconds. In most patients, hyperventilation lowers the ICP by 25%. $PCO_2$ should not fall below 25 mm Hg because this may cause profound vasoconstriction and ischemia in normal and injured areas of the brain. **Hyperventilation is a temporary maneuver** and should only be used for a brief period of time during the acute resuscitation and only in patients demonstrating neurologic deterioration.

(a) ED cranial decompression (burr hole) should only be performed under extreme circumstances when all other attempts at reducing ICP have failed. (b) There is no evidence that steroids lower ICP and are not recommended in head trauma. (c) Furosemide has no role in acute traumatic brain injury. (e) Mannitol is the best osmotic agent to reduce ICP. Its onset is within 30 minutes and lasts up to 6 to 8 hours. Mannitol has the additional benefit of expanding volume, initially reducing hypotension, and improving the blood's oxygen-carrying capacity.

**140. The answer is e.** (*Tintinalli, p 1596.*) This patient has a tension pneumothorax. Secondary to the gunshot, air has entered the pleural space, secondary to the gunshot, and caused the right lung to collapse. This air cannot escape and pressure continues to increase, pushing the right lung into the mediastinum, causing the trachea to shift to the left. If this process is not corrected, venous return and cardiac output can be compromised and the patient will die. Classic symptoms of tension pneumothorax include dyspnea, tachypnea, tracheal deviation to the uninjured side, absent breath sounds on the injured side, and hypotension. Treatment of a tension pneumothorax is immediate needle decompression using a large 14- or 16-gauge IV catheter inserted into the pleural space (ie, second intercostals space in the midclavicular line). Air should come out of the catheter and the patient's clinical condition should improve. A tube thoracostomy should be performed after the needle decompression.

(a) Tension pneumothorax is a clinical diagnosis and, if suspected, should be treated immediately, without waiting for a chest x-ray. While intubation (b) is generally helpful for patients in respiratory distress, it can be dangerous in the setting of a tension pneumothorax. Positive-pressure ventilation worsens the tension pneumothorax leading to further cardiovascular compromise. This patient will likely require surgical management and the surgical team (d) should be called; however, needle decompression and tube thoracostomy are core emergency medicine skills and should be performed immediately by the emergency physician. ED thoracotomy

(c) is indicated in penetrating trauma patients who have witnessed loss of pulse in the field or in the ED.

**141. The answer is c.** (*Tintinalli, pp 385-389.*) This patient is in **cardiogenic shock** from **decreased cardiac output** producing inadequate tissue perfusion. Support for this diagnosis includes an older patient with a history of coronary artery disease and new mental status changes coupled with signs of volume overload. Common causes of cardiogenic shock include acute MI, pulmonary embolism, COPD exacerbation, and pneumonia. This patient should be stabilized with IV pressors since there is already pulmonary congestion evident on examination. A rapid workup including ECG, chest x-ray (CXR), laboratory tests, echocardiogram, and hemodynamic monitoring should help confirm the etiology and direct specific treatment of the underlying cause.

Hypovolemic shock (**a**) occurs when there is inadequate volume in the circulatory system, resulting in poor oxygen delivery to the tissues. Neurogenic shock (**b**) occurs after an acute spinal cord injury, which disrupts sympathetic innervation resulting in hypotension and bradycardia. Anaphylactic shock (**d**) is a severe systemic hypersensitivity reaction, resulting in hypotension and airway compromise. Septic shock (**e**) is a clinical syndrome of hypoperfusion and multiorgan dysfunction caused by infection.

**142. The answer is d.** (*Tintinalli, pp 136-143.*) This patient has **supraventricular tachycardia (SVT)**, a narrow complex, regular tachycardia. It is caused by a reentry or an ectopic pacemaker in areas of the heart above the bundle of His, usually the atria. Regular P waves will be present but may be difficult to discern owing to the very fast rate. The patient in this case has normal vital signs and examination, and is therefore stable. First-line treatment for a patient with stable SVT is **vagal maneuvers** to **slow conduction and prolong the refractory period in the AV node.** The Valsalva maneuver can be accomplished by asking the patient to bear down as if they are having a bowel movement and hold the strain for at least 10 seconds. Other vagal maneuvers include carotid sinus massage (after auscultating for carotid bruits) and facial immersion in cold water.

If vagal maneuvers fail, the next step is adenosine, a very short-acting AV nodal blocking medication. Initially, adenosine 6 mg (**b**) is rapidly pushed through the IV in a site as close to the heart as possible. Patients may experience a few seconds of discomfort, including chest pain and facial flushing on receiving the adenosine. If the patient remains in

SVT 2 minutes after receiving adenosine, a second dose of adenosine at 12 mg (c) is administered. If the second dose of adenosine fails and the patient remains stable, short-acting calcium channel blockers (eg, verapamil), (e) β-blockers, or digoxin can be administered. If at any time the patient is considered unstable (hypotension, pulmonary edema, severe chest pain, altered mental status, or other life-threatening concerns), synchronized cardioversion (a) should be performed immediately.

**143. The answer is b.** (*American Heart Association Guidelines, 2010; Tintinalli, pp 145-146.*) **Ventricular tachycardia (VT)** originates from ectopic ventricular pacemakers and is usually a regular rhythm with rate greater than 100 beats per minute and wide QRS complexes. Treatment of VT is primarily dependent on whether or not the patient is stable. Evidence of acute altered mental status, hypotension, continued chest pain, or other signs of shock are signs of instability. Unstable patients, such as the passenger on this airplane, should receive immediate **synchronized cardioversion**. It is critical that the cardioverter be placed in the synchronized mode, which permits a search for a large R wave and a corresponding shock around the incidence of such a wave. A shock administered outside of this constraint can induce ventricular fibrillation (VF).

Stable patients can be treated with antidysrhythmics. Amiodarone (a) 150 mg IV over 10 minutes is currently first-line treatment as recommended by the American Heart Association (AHA). Lidocaine (d) and procainamide (e) can also be administered. Verapamil (c) should not be used in VT as it may accelerate the HR and cause hypotension.

**144. The answer is e.** (*Roberts and Hedges, pp 443-450.*) **Endotracheal administration of drugs** is indicated whenever there is a need for emergent pharmacologic intervention in the absence of other access routes, such as IV or intraosseous. There are a limited number of emergency medications that can be administered safely and effectively via the endotracheal route. These include **naloxone, atropine, versed, epinephrine**, and **lidocaine**. This is remembered by the mnemonic **NAVEL**. Specific medications shown to be unsafe include sodium bicarbonate, isoproterenol, and bretylium. The endotracheal dosage of a medication should be at least equivalent to the IV route and is usually 2 to 2.5 times the IV dose administered. The patient in the scenario should receive epinephrine via the ET while IV access is established.

**145. The answer is e.** (*Tintinalli, pp 142-143.*) This ECG shows **atrial fibrillation with rapid ventricular response (RVR)**. Normally, one area of the atria depolarizes and causes uniform contraction of the atria. In atrial fibrillation, multiple areas of the atria continuously depolarize and contract, leading to multiple atrial impulses and an irregular ventricular response. Atrial fibrillation reduces the effectiveness of atrial contractions and may lead to or worsen heart failure in patients with left ventricular failure. Treatment of atrial fibrillation is dependent on whether or not the patient is stable or not. This patient is clinically **unstable**; the atrial fibrillation with RVR has pushed him into heart failure and he is hypotensive and tachypneic. Unstable patients like this should undergo **synchronized cardioversion**. Synchronized cardioversion is performed at 100 J and then at 200 J if the first attempt fails.

The focus of emergency management in stable patients with atrial fibrillation with RVR is ventricular rate control. Diltiazem **(b)** or verapamil are excellent choices for rate control. Metoprolol **(c)** or digoxin **(d)** may also be used, but may depress BP. Recall that patients in atrial fibrillation for longer than 48 hours are at risk for atrial thrombi. If these patients are cardioverted (electrically or chemically), they have a 1% to 2% risk of arterial embolism. Since it is often difficult to determine time of onset, ED patients are generally only cardioverted if they are unstable. Stable patients with atrial fibrillation should be anticoagulated with a loading dose of **(a)** heparin and oral warfarin for at least 1 month prior to elective cardioversion.

**146. The answer is a.** (*Tintinalli, pp 165-177.*) This patient is in **hypovolemic shock** secondary to blood loss from a **femoral fracture**. Hypovolemic shock occurs when there is inadequate volume in the circulatory system, resulting in poor oxygen delivery to the tissues. Hemorrhage, GI losses, burns, and environmental exposures can all be responsible for hypovolemic shock. In trauma, hemorrhage is the most common cause of hypovolemic shock. This patient fractured his femur, disrupting the nearby vascular supply, resulting in significant blood collection in the soft tissue.

This patient's hypovolemic shock can be treated with aggressive fluid and blood-product replacement. In the meantime, pain control and x-rays of the hip, femur, and knee should be performed. Once the femur fracture is confirmed, a Sager or Hare traction splint should be applied and orthopedics consulted. Other areas of life-threatening hemorrhage in trauma include the chest, abdomen, retroperitoneum, and pelvis. It is also important to keep in mind that significant blood loss could have occurred at the scene despite no obvious active bleeding in the ED.

Neurogenic shock **(b)** occurs after an acute spinal cord injury, which disrupts sympathetic innervation resulting in hypotension and bradycardia. Cardiogenic shock **(c)** is caused by decreased cardiac output producing inadequate tissue perfusion. Anaphylactic shock **(d)** is a severe systemic hypersensitivity reaction, resulting in hypotension and airway compromise. Septic shock **(e)** is a clinical syndrome of hypoperfusion and multiorgan dysfunction caused by infection.

**147. The answer is d.** (*Beinart, 2011.*) Low-energy cardioversion is very successful in converting atrial flutter to sinus rhythm. Remember, cardioversion is different than defibrillation. Cardioversion is performed on patients with organized cardiac electrical activity with pulses, whereas defibrillation is performed on patients without pulses (VF and VF without a pulse). Patients with heart beats who receive electrical energy during their heart's relative refractory period are at risk for VF. Therefore, cardioversion is a timed shock designed to avoid delivering a shock during the heart's relative refractory period. By activating **synchronization mode**, the machine will identify the patient's R waves and not deliver electrical energy during these times. The key step, when cardioverting, is to activate the synchronization mode and confirm the presence of sync markers on the R waves prior to delivering electrical energy.

**148. The answer is b.** (*American Heart Association Guidelines, 2010.*) This patient has cardiac electrical activity (sinus bradycardia) but no detectable pulses. He is therefore in a state of **pulseless electrical activity** (**PEA**), and management should be directed by the AHA PEA algorithm. Patients in PEA should be treated with CPR, epinephrine every 3 to 5 minutes, and atropine every 3 to 5 minutes (if PEA rate is < 60 per minute), but a search for an underlying etiology with targeted interventions should still be performed.

Common etiologies for PEA are shown in the following table along with their specific treatments. Many find the **H's** and **T's** in the table an easy way to remember the differential. Each etiology should be considered for every patient with PEA and causes that are more likely given a patient's history and physical should be treated first. This patient has an AV graft indicating that he has a history of renal disease. Since patients with end-stage renal disease are at risk for **hyperkalemia** and since hyperkalemia can cause PEA, **calcium gluconate** should be given first to stabilize the cardiac membranes.

| PEA Etiologies and Treatments | | | |
|---|---|---|---|
| **H's** | **Tx** | **T's** | **Tx** |
| Hypovolemia | IV fluids | Toxins | Antidotes |
| Hypoxia | Ventilation | Tamponade (cardiac) | Pericardiocentesis |
| Hydrogen ion (acidosis) | Sodium bicarbonate | Tension pneumothorax | Tube thoracostomy |
| Hypokalemia and Hypogly-cemia | KCl, calcium | Thrombosis (coronary and Hyperkalemia pulmonary) | Thrombolysis |
| Hypoglycemia | Dextrose | Trauma (hypovolemia and increased ICP) | IV fluids |
| Hypothermia | Warming | | |

If the patient does not improve with calcium, sodium bicarbonate (**a**) could be given to treat for metabolic acidosis and 50% dextrose (**c**) can be given for suspected hypoglycemia. Cardiac tamponade is a possible etiology in a patient with renal disease and pericardiocentesis (**e**) can be attempted if the patient is not improving with the aforementioned treatments. A bedside ultrasound may also be helpful to look for right ventricular collapse or other signs of tamponade. Pneumothorax is a less likely etiology in this particular patient. It is treated with a (**d**) chest tube.

**149. The answer is b.** (*Rosen, p 59.*) The rhythm is **VF**. Along with pulseless VT, these are **nonperfusing rhythms** that are treated identically because it is thought to be caused by the same mechanisms. The earlier a "shock" is administered in cardiac arrest, the more likely the patient will return to spontaneous circulation with a perfusing rhythm. If there is a delay to defibrillation (> 4 minutes), CPR should be administered for 60 to 90 seconds before defibrillation. If after defibrillation (200 J biphasic or 360 J monophasic) the patient's rhythm is still VF or pulseless VT, assisted ventilation and chest compressions should be started. Intubation should be performed and IV access obtained for the administration of epinephrine or vasopressin. If the rhythm is unchanged after administration of vasopressor therapy, another attempt at defibrillation at 360 J (or 200 J biphasic) with subsequent administration of an antidysrhythmic (eg, amiodarone) is recommended. Of note, monophasic defibrillation delivers a charge in only one direction. Biphasic defibrillation delivers a charge in one direction for half of the shock and in the electrically opposite direction for the second half. Biphasic defibrillation significantly decreases the energy necessary for successful defibrillation and decreases the risk of myocardial damage.

(a) There is no role for observation with VF. Successful return of a perfusing rhythm is most likely to result with immediate defibrillation. (c) Synchronized cardioversion is energy delivered to match the QRS complex. This reduces the chance that a shock will induce VF. Synchronization is used to treat tachydysrhythmias (eg, rapid atrial fibrillation) in hemodynamically unstable patients. It should not be used in VF or pulseless VT. (d) The most beneficial intervention for this patient is immediate defibrillation. If this fails, the patient's airway management (ABCs) will require him to be intubated. (e) Amiodarone, an antidysrhythmic, is used in patients with VF or pulseless VT after appropriate defibrillation and administration of vasopressor therapy.

**150. The answer is b.** *(Roberts and Hedges, p 72.)* The most serious complication of ET intubation is unrecognized esophageal intubation with resultant hypoxic brain injury. Esophageal placement is not always obvious. The best assurance that the tube is placed into the trachea is to **see it pass through the vocal cords**.

(a) The chest radiograph can be misleading and is essentially only useful to identify endobronchial intubation (ie, right main stem bronchus intubation). (c) Although the chest wall should expand with positive pressure and relax with expiration, this may not occur in patients with small tidal volumes or severe bronchospasm. (d) You may hear normal breath sounds if only the midline of the thorax is auscultated. (e) In cardiac arrest situations, low exhaled carbon dioxide levels are seen in both very-low-flow states and in esophageal intubation. In addition, colorimetric changes may be difficult to discern in reduced lighting situations, and secretions can interfere with color change.

**151. The answer is b.** *(Tintinalli, p 1722.)* This patient is in **neurogenic shock**. He suffered an acute cervical spine injury after his fall onto rocks and has **hypotension** and **bradycardia**. The pathophysiology behind neurogenic shock is still under investigation, but it's thought to be partially caused by **disrupted sympathetic outflow tracts** and **unopposed vagal tone**. Note that all other forms of shock attempt to compensate for hypotension with tachycardia. Neurogenic shock lacks sympathetic innervation; therefore bradycardia results. Given that this is a trauma patient, all other sources for hypotension must be ruled out. He should be treated with cervical spine immobilization and IV fluids. Pressors may be needed if hypotension does not respond to fluids or fluid overload becomes a concern.

Hypovolemic shock **(a)** occurs when there is inadequate volume in the circulatory system, resulting in poor oxygen delivery to the tissues. Cardiogenic shock **(c)** is caused by decreased cardiac output producing inadequate tissue perfusion. Anaphylactic shock **(d)** is a severe systemic hypersensitivity reaction, resulting in hypotension and airway compromise. Septic shock **(e)** is a clinical syndrome of hypoperfusion, hypotension, or multiorgan dysfunction caused by infection.

**152. The answer is d.** *(Tintinalli, pp 148-149.)* **Atropine** is the initial treatment of choice for patients in second-degree, Mobitz I AV block. The majority of patients respond to atropine without further treatment. Mobitz I is commonly seen with acute inferior MI, digoxin toxicity, myocarditis, and after cardiac surgery.

Observation alone **(a)** is appropriate for stable patients. However, this patient is hypotensive and needs more aggressive management. Transcutaneous (eg, electrical pads are placed externally, most commonly on the anterior chest wall) **(b)** or transvenous (eg, pacing wires are threaded into the right ventricle [RV] through a central vein) pacing **(c)** is an appropriate treatment and should be attempted if atropine is unsuccessful. Finally, if all else fails, epinephrine **(e)** or dopamine drips can be started. These treatments should be applied judiciously as the resulting increased HR may worsen patients with active ischemia as the etiology for their bradycardia. Furthermore, patients with acute inferior wall MI may have right ventricular failure and may be hypotensive because of decreased preload, not bradycardia. IV fluids would be the therapy of choice in patients with inferior MI.

**153. The answer is b.** *(Tintinalli, pp 145-147.)* This patient had a run of **torsade de pointes**, an atypical VT where the QRS axis swings from positive to negative within a single ECG lead. This dysrhythmia is frequently seen in patients with significant heart disease who have a prolonged QT interval. There are many possible causes of prolonged QT; however, common etiologies include drugs (eg, antidysrhythmics, psychotropics), electrolyte abnormalities, and coronary heart disease. This patient was likely on a phenothiazine for her schizophrenia leading to prolonged QT syndrome and an episode of torsade de pointes. Administration of **magnesium sulfate** has been shown to decrease runs of torsades. If the patient has a pulse but his or her vital signs are unstable, you should perform immediate cardioversion.

Observation alone (a), is not adequate. Conventional VT treatments such as lidocaine (c) are often ineffective. Procainamide can actually further prolong the QT interval. If magnesium is unsuccessful, the next strategy involves increasing the HR from 90 to 120 beats per minute, thereby reducing the QT interval and preventing recurrence of torsade de pointes. Increased HR is best achieved by placing a transvenous pacemaker (d); this technique is sometimes called overdrive pacing. During the time it takes for transvenous pacemaker placement, unstable patients can be started on isoproterenol (e), a β-adrenergic receptor agonist to medically increase the HR.

**154. The answer is b.** *(Tintinalli, pp 172-177.)* **Crystalloids** such as **normal saline (0.9% sodium chloride)** or **lactated Ringer** are the preferred resuscitation fluid in the United States. The patient is currently stable; however, he is tachycardic and has suffered an injury with the potential for significant morbidity. The FAST examination will help illustrate the extent of this patient's injury. In the meantime, the patient should be started on isotonic crystalloid solution. There is currently no convincing evidence that either solution—normal saline or Ringer lactate—is superior to the other.

Hypertonic saline (a) helps prevent the extravascular fluid shift seen with isotonic crystalloids but is volume limited owing to the risk of hypernatremia. Furthermore, clinical studies have not shown clear evidence of improved outcome using hypertonic saline. Colloid solutions (c) such as albumin, FFP, and dextran solutions have larger protein components and would therefore be expected to remain in the intravascular space. However, this is a theoretical benefit, as numerous studies have not shown improved outcome using colloid solutions. Blood (d and e) is the best resuscitation fluid. Cross-matched blood is preferred over type-specific blood, if time is available to perform the cross-match. In this case, the patient has only minimal tachycardia. He can receive crystalloid first with continuous monitoring while the diagnostic workup continues. Blood is indicated after 2 to 3 L of crystalloid infusion and only minimal improvement in vital signs or when the patient has obviously suffered significant blood loss.

**155. The answer is d.** *(Tintinalli, pp 1453-1456.)* This patient is in **septic shock** from pneumonia and also has **adrenal crisis**. Initial treatment with IV fluids, antibiotics, and dopamine is appropriate. Continued hypotension in a patient on maintenance steroid therapy should make you think of adrenal crisis. Exogenous glucocorticoids suppress hypothalamic release of corticotropin-releasing hormone (CRH) and subsequently anterior pituitary release of adrenocorticotropic hormone (ACTH). The adrenals subsequently atrophy from lack of stimulation. The patient is now faced with an acute stress from pneumonia and sepsis. His adrenals have atrophied and are unable to respond with increased cortisol secretion. Laboratory clues to adrenal crisis include hyponatremia and hyperkalemia caused by a lack of aldosterone. The treatment of adrenal crisis in the face of septic shock is **hydrocortisone.**

Mineralocorticoids, such as fludrocortisone (**c**), are not needed. Additional fluids (**a**) and pressors (**b and e**) are appropriate critical care management for sepsis and should be administered after glucocorticoids.

**156. The answer is c.** (*Tintinalli, pp 1264-1269.*) Toxic ingestions must always be considered, especially in suicidal patients. The patient regularly takes atenolol for hypertension and may have overdosed on this occasion. **β-Blocker toxicity** classically causes bradycardia and hypotension. Antidotes for β-blocker toxicity, such as **glucagon**, should be given to this patient immediately. Glucagon is thought to work through a separate receptor that is not blocked by β-adrenergic antagonists, ultimately enhancing inotropy and chronotropy. Patents who are hypotensive should receive intravenous fluids (normal saline) and be administered pressor agents, such as norepinephrine. Other medications that may be useful are phosphodiesterase inhibitors (eg, milrinone), which block cyclic adenosine monophosphate (cAMP) breakdown and maintain intracellular calcium levels. **High-dose insulin** is a promising treatment for β-blocker toxicity. Ultimately, the patient may require the other treatment options, but glucagon should be the first-line therapy.

You should administer an IV bolus of fluids (**a**), you may attempt to administer atropine (**b**), and place external cardiac pacers on the patient (**e**). However, because this is a β-blocker overdose, the administration of glucagon should treat the patient. (**d**) Epinephrine should be administered if the patient loses his pulse.

**157. The answer is d.** (*Tintinalli, pp 1758-1761.*) Patients with penetrating trauma to the chest with possible cardiac injury and signs of hemodynamic instability need immediate **operative thoracotomy.** This patient has signs of cardiac tamponade, a collection of blood surrounding the heart and interfering with the heart's ability to contract. He has Beck triad of hypotension, distended neck veins, and muffled heart sounds. His CXR also shows an enlarged heart. An echocardiogram would be helpful in confirming the diagnosis, but, since this patient is unstable and echocardiogram may not be readily available, the treatment is immediate thoracotomy in the operating room.

While pericardiocentesis (c) may help relieve tamponade, it is not the optimal procedure for traumatic tamponade. Pericardiocentesis may be difficult when clots fill the pericardium and may therefore give false-negative results. The procedure may also injure the heart and delay definitive treatment. Some clinicians perform bilateral tube thoracostomy (b) prior to thoracotomy to rule out a hemo- and pneumothorax. However, with equal breath sounds, midline trachea, and no evidence of pneumothorax or consolidation on radiograph, chest tubes are low yield in this patient. The patient is not in respiratory distress. Intubation (a) should be performed in the OR to prevent additional delays in definitive surgical care. IV fluids and blood transfusion (e) increase venous return to the heart and are excellent supportive measures prior to definitive thoracotomy.

**158. The answer is c.** (*Tintinalli, p 526.*) Abdominal pain in the elderly can be challenging for many reasons, including poor histories and deviation from classic presentations of diseases. However, abdominal pain in patients over 65 must be taken seriously since 25% to 44% require surgical intervention and more than 50% require admission to the hospital. This CXR reveals **free air under the right diaphragm**, likely from a perforated viscous. This is a **surgical emergency** and the surgical service should be contacted.

Antibiotics (a) and a central venous line (d) are appropriate and can be started after the surgical team has been notified. It is important to obtain large-bore IV access for this patient. If peripheral lines are not obtained, a central venous line should be inserted. A CT scan (b) is not necessary in this patient, especially with her low BP. She should be taken directly to the OR for an exploratory laparotomy. Although the patient has a benign abdominal examination, the caretakers report and her low BP is worrisome and sending the patient home (e) prior to a complete workup would be a mistake.

# Fever

## Questions

**159.** A 43-year-old man, who currently uses drugs intravenously (IV), presents to the emergency department (ED) with 2 weeks of fever, back pain, and progressive weakness in his legs bilaterally. He denies any history of trauma or prior surgery. His blood pressure (BP) is 130/75 mm Hg, heart rate (HR) is 106 beats per minute, temperature is 103°F, and respiratory rate (RR) is 16 breaths per minute. On physical examination, he has tenderness to palpation in the mid-lumbar spine, increased patellar reflexes, and decreased strength in the lower extremities bilaterally, with normal range of motion. Laboratory results reveal a white blood cell (WBC) count of 15,500/μL, hematocrit 40%, and platelets 225/μL. Urinalysis and spinal x-rays are unremarkable. Which of the following is the most likely diagnosis?

a. Fibromyalgia
b. Ankylosing spondylitis
c. Spinal epidural abscess
d. Vertebral compression fracture
e. Spinal metastatic lesion

**160.** An 81-year-old woman is brought to the ED by her children who state that the patient is acting more tired than usual, has had fever for the last 2 days, and is more confused. Ordinarily, the patient is high functioning: she is ambulatory, cooks for herself, and walks on a treadmill 30 minutes a day. Her vital signs are BP 85/60 mm Hg, HR 125, RR 20, temperature 101.3°F, and pulse oxygenation 97% on room air. On examination, the patient has dry mucous membranes but is otherwise unremarkable. She is oriented to person and place but states that the year is 1925. Her laboratory results show a WBC 14,300/μL, hematocrit 31%, and platelets 350/μL. Her electrolytes are within normal limits. Blood glucose is 92 mg/dL. A chest radiograph does not show any infiltrates. Urinalysis reveals 2+ protein, trace ketones, WBC > 100/hpf, red blood cell (RBC) 5 to 10/hpf, nitrite positive, and leukocyte esterase positive. After administering a 500-cc normal saline fluid bolus and broad-spectrum antibiotics through her peripheral IV line, the patient's BP is 82/60 mm Hg. You suspect that the patient is in septic shock due to an acute urinary tract infection. Which of the following is the next most appropriate course of action to manage this patient with early-goal-directed therapy (EGDT)?

a. Immediately start a norepinephrine infusion to increase the blood pressure given the low systolic blood pressure.

b. Prepare to transfuse uncrossed matched packed RBC to increase oxygen-carrying capacity given the low hematocrit.

c. Place a central venous line into the right internal jugular vein to measure central venous pressure (CVP).

d. Transport the patient to radiology for a stat CT scan of her head given the acute change in mental status.

e. Place a central venous line into the right internal jugular vein to measure mixed venous oxygen saturation (Svo$_2$).

**161.** A 23-year-old man presents to the ED with left lower abdominal pain and left testicular pain that started 1 to 2 weeks ago and has gradually worsened. He has some nausea and vomiting. His HR is 98 beats per minute, BP is 125/65 mm Hg, temperature is 100.9°F, and RR is 18 breaths per minute. Physical examination reveals a tender left testicle with a firm nodularity on the posterolateral aspect of the testicle. Pain is relieved slightly with elevation of the testicle and the cremasteric reflex in normal. You make the presumptive diagnosis of epididymitis. Which of the following is the next best step?

a. Prescribe pain medications and penicillin for coverage of syphilis, the most likely causative organism.
b. Recommend bed rest, ice, and scrotal elevation with prompt urology follow-up.
c. Give ceftriaxone 125 mg intramuscularly (IM), plus a one-time dose of azithromycin 1 g orally.
d. Give ceftriaxone 250 mg intramuscularly (IM), plus a 10-day course of oral doxycycline.
e. Confirm the diagnosis with transillumination of the testicle, and then consult urology for surgical drainage.

**162.** A 40-year-old man with insulin-dependent diabetes presents to the ED with complaints of 2 days of increasingly severe perineal pain and subjective fevers. His HR is 118 beats per minute, BP is 95/55 mm Hg, temperature is 103.4°F, and RR is 22 breaths per minute. The bedside sugar reading is "high." Physical examination demonstrates crepitus over the medial thigh and widespread erythema and purple discoloration with sharp demarcation over the scrotum. The scrotum is markedly tender, warm, and edematous. Which of the following is the most likely diagnosis?

a. Cutaneous candidiasis
b. Fournier syndrome
c. Phimosis
d. Paraphimosis
e. Testicular torsion

**163.** A 55-year-old man with a history of diabetes presents with complaints of developed left knee pain several days following a fall from standing height. The patient was brought to the ED by ambulance after being found on a park bench stating he was unable to walk because of the pain. On physical examination, there are no rashes or external signs of trauma. His left knee is warm, diffusely tender, and swollen with a large effusion. He has pain on passive range of motion and is refusing to walk. His BP is 150/85 mm Hg, HR is 105 beats per minute, temperature is 102.7°F, RR is 16 breaths per minute, and fingerstick glucose is 89 mg/dL. Which of the following is the most appropriate diagnostic test?

a. Knee radiographs
b. Magnetic resonance imaging (MRI)
c. Erythrocyte sedimentation rate (ESR) and C-reactive protein (CRP)
d. Arthrocentesis
e. Bone scan

**164.** A 35-year-old woman with systemic lupus erythematosus (SLE) is brought to the ED by her brother after he found her febrile and confused. Physical examination reveals fever, tachycardia, a waxing and waning mental status, petechiae over her oral mucosa, pallor, and mildly heme-positive stool. Her urinalysis is positive for blood, red cell casts, and proteinuria. Laboratory results reveal blood urea nitrogen (BUN) of 40 mg/dL and creatinine of 2 mg/dL. Her bilirubin is elevated (unconjugated > conjugated) and her international normalized ratio (INR) is 0.98. Her complete blood count reveals WBC 12,000/μL, hematocrit 29%, and platelet count 17,000/μL with schistocytes on the peripheral smear. Which of the following is the most appropriate next step in management?

a. Admit to the intensive care unit (ICU) for plasmapheresis and close monitoring for acute bleeds.
b. Admit to the ICU for platelet transfusion and monitoring for acute bleeds.
c. Admit to the ICU for corticosteroid infusion, transfusion of platelets, and prompt surgical consultation for emergent splenectomy.
d. Admit to the ICU for dialysis and close monitoring for acute bleeds.
e. Perform a noncontrast head computed tomography (CT) to screen for intracranial bleeding and mass effect followed by a lumbar puncture (LP) for analysis of cerebrospinal fluid (CSF). If negative, admit to telemetry for hemodynamic monitoring.

**165.** A 30-year-old woman presents to the ED with fever, headache, a "sunburn-like" rash, and confusion. A friend states that the patient has complained of nausea, vomiting, diarrhea, and a sore throat over the past few days. Her last menstrual period began 4 days ago. Vital signs are HR 110 beats per minute, BP 80/45 mm Hg, RR of 18 breaths per minute, and temperature of 103°F. On physical examination, you note an ill-appearing woman with a diffuse blanching erythroderma. Her neck is supple without signs of meningeal irritation. On pelvic examination, you remove a tampon. You note a fine desquamation of her skin, especially over the hands and feet, and hyperemia of her oropharyngeal, conjunctival, and vaginal mucous membranes. Laboratory results reveal a creatine phosphokinase (CPK) of 5000, WBC 15,000/μL, platelets of 90,000/μL, BUN 40 mg/dL, creatinine 2 mg/dL, and elevated liver enzymes. You suspect the diagnosis of toxic shock syndrome and initiate IV fluids. You target antibiotics at which of the following causative organism?

a. *Staphylococcus aureus*
b. *Rickettsia rickettsii*
c. *Streptococcus pyogenes*
d. *Neisseria meningitidis*
e. *Neisseria gonorrhoeae*

**166.** A 32-year-old diabetic man presents to the ED with a fever and 1 week of increasing right foot pain. He states he stepped on a nail while running barefoot 2 weeks ago but didn't think much of it at that time. On physical examination, his heel is mildly erythematous and diffusely tender to palpation, with overlying warmth and edema. There is a small amount of purulent drainage through the puncture hole in his heel. A plain radiograph of his foot demonstrates a slight lucency of the calcaneus. He has decreased range of motion, but you are able to passively dorsiflex and plantarflex his ankle without difficulty. His vital signs include a temperature of 101.4°F, HR of 98 beats per minute, BP of 130/75 mm Hg, and RR of 16 breaths per minute. Which of the following is the most common causative organism of this condition?

a. *Salmonella* sp
b. *Pseudomonas aeruginosa*
c. *Staphylococcus aureus*
d. Group B streptococci
e. *Pasteurella multocida*

**167.** A 75-year-old woman is transferred to your ED from the local nursing home for fever, cough, and increasing lethargy. Over the past 3 days, the nursing home staff noticed increasing yellow sputum and decreasing urine output from the patient. Her BP is 118/75 mm Hg, RR is 20 breaths per minute, HR is 105 beats per minute, temperature is 100.9°F, and pulse oxygenation is 94% on room air. On examination, auscultation of the lungs reveals bibasilar crackles. Laboratory results reveal WBC 14,500/μL, hematocrit 39%, platelets 250/μL, sodium 132 mEq/L, potassium 3.5 mEq/L, chloride 100 mEq/L, bicarbonate 18 mEq/L, BUN 27 mg/dL, creatinine 1.5 mg/dL, and glucose 85 mg/dL. Serum lactate is 4.7 mmol/dL. Chest radiography reveals bilateral lower lobe infiltrates. Based on this patient's presentation, which of the following is the most likely diagnosis?

a. Hospital-acquired pneumonia (HAP)
b. Community-acquired pneumonia (CAP)
c. Health care–associated pneumonia (HCAP)
d. Ventilator-associated pneumonia (VAP)
e. Atypical pneumonia

**168.** A 55-year-old man presents to the ED with fever, drooling, trismus, and a swollen neck. He reports a foul taste in his mouth caused by a tooth extraction 2 days ago. On physical examination, the patient appears anxious. He has bilateral submandibular swelling and elevation and protrusion of the tongue. He appears "bull-necked" with tense and markedly tender edema and brawny induration of the upper neck, and he is tender over the lower second and third molars. There is no cervical lymphadenopathy. These lungs are clear to auscultation with good air movement. His vital signs are HR 105 beats per minute, BP 140/85 mm Hg, RR 26 breaths per minute, and temperature 102°F. Which of the following is the most appropriate next step in management?

a. Obtain a sample for culture, administer a dose of IV antibiotics, and obtain a soft tissue radiograph of the neck.
b. Obtain a sample for culture, perform a broad incision and drainage at bedside, and administer a dose of IV antibiotics.
c. Administer a dose of IV antibiotics and obtain a CT scan of the soft tissues of the neck.
d. Administer a dose of IV antibiotics, obtain a CT scan of the soft tissues of the neck, and obtain an emergent ENT consult.
e. Secure his airway, administer a dose of IV antibiotics, and obtain an emergent ENT (ear, nose, and throat) consult.

**169.** A 67-year-old woman with a history of steroid-dependent COPD, non–insulin-dependent diabetes, and hypertension presents to the ED with complaints of a painful, red, swollen left lower leg. She states she noted a "bug bite" in that area 1 week ago and since then has had gradually increasing symptoms. On examination, you note a 12 cm × 10 cm sharply demarcated area of blanching erythema, warmth, and tenderness on the medial thigh with ascending erythema to the groin. You also note tender adenopathy in the left inguinal region. Her BP is 90/55 mm Hg, RR is 24 breaths per minute, HR is 105 beats per minute, temperature is 102.4°F, and pulse oxygenation is 98% on room air. Laboratory results reveal WBC 19,500/µL, hematocrit 39%, platelets 175/µL, sodium 132 mEq/L, potassium 3.5 mEq/L, chloride 100 mEq/L, bicarbonate 14 mEq/L, BUN 32 mg/dL, creatinine 1.7 mg/dL, and glucose 455 mg/dL. Serum lactate is 4.7 mmol/dL. Which of the following best describes her clinical state?

a. She has systemic inflammatory response syndrome (SIRS).
b. She has sepsis.
c. She has severe sepsis.
d. She is in septic shock.
e. She has multiple organ dysfunction syndrome (MODS).

**170.** An 84-year-old man presents to the ED with his family due to concerns that his condition is worsening despite being placed on levofloxacin for a urinary tract infection 5 days ago by his primary care physician. His is obtunded and unable to give any additional history. Physical examination does not reveal the source of infection. His BP is 84/45 mm Hg, HR is 135 beats per minute, temperature is 102.8°F, and his RR is 28 breaths per minute. Laboratory results reveal WBC 24,500/µL, hematocrit 19%, platelets 90/µL, sodium 132 mEq/L, potassium 7.5 mEq/L, chloride 100 mEq/L, bicarbonate 12 mEq/L, BUN 37 mg/dL, creatinine 6.5 mg/dL, and glucose 255 mg/dL. Serum lactate is 11.3 mmol/dL. Cardiac enzymes and troponin are mildly elevated, and he has hyperacute T-waves on electrocardiogram (ECG). His chest radiograph shows cardiomegaly with bilateral patchy opacities and pulmonary vascular congestion. Rapid urinalysis reveals 3+ WBCs and blood and nitrates. You secure his airway with intubation, initiate broad-spectrum antibiotics, IV fluids, and other supportive therapies, and emergently consult nephrology, cardiology, and pulmonology. Which of the following best describes his clinical state?

a. He has SIRS.
b. He has sepsis.
c. He has severe sepsis.
d. He is in septic shock.
e. He has MODS.

**171.** A 37-year-old man presents to the ED with complaints of 2 days of a sore throat and subjective fever at home. He denies cough or vomiting. His BP is 130/75 mm Hg, HR is 85 beats per minute, temperature is 101°F, and his RR is 14 breaths per minute. He has diffuse tonsillar swelling and bilateral exudates with bilaterally enlarged and tender lymph nodes of the neck. Which of the following is the next best step in management?

a. Administer penicillin and discharge the patient without further testing.
b. Perform a rapid antigen test. If it is negative, confirm with a throat culture, and administer penicillin if the results are positive.
c. Perform a rapid antigen test. If it is negative, administer penicillin and discharge the patient.
d. Perform a rapid antigen test. If it is positive, administer penicillin and discharge the patient.
e. Discharge the patient without treatment or further testing.

**172.** A 37-year-old man who just finished a full course of penicillin for pharyngitis presents to the ED requesting to be checked out again. He states he took the antibiotics exactly as prescribed and initially felt somewhat improved, but over the last 2 to 3 days has had increased pain and progressive difficulty swallowing. His BP is 130/65 mm Hg, HR is 95 beats per minute, temperature is 100.1°F, RR is 16 breaths per minute, and oxygen saturation is 99%. On examination, the patient is in no acute distress but has a fluctuant mass on the right side of his neck. You visualize a normal soft palate with swelling of the right tonsillar arch and deviation of the uvula to the left, but additional examination is limited because he is unable to open his mouth fully. Review of his records reveals a throat culture that was positive for *Streptococcus*. Which of the following is the most appropriate next step in management?

a. Attempt needle aspiration, treat him with a new course of antibiotics (either penicillin or clindamycin), and have him return in 24 hours.
b. Give him morphine for pain control, give him a dose of IV antibiotics, and observe him in the ED for 6 hours.
c. Admit him for incision and drainage in the OR under general anesthesia.
d. Switch his antibiotic to clindamycin and have him return in 24 hours.
e. Order a CT scan to visualize his neck, continue the penicillin, and have him return in 24 hours.

**173.** A 50-year-old man presents to the ED complaining of fever, headache, and neck pain for 24 hours. He states that 1 week ago he had rhinorrhea, nasal congestion, a sore throat, and occasional dry cough. He noted generalized weakness, myalgias, and malaise yesterday afternoon, and woke up today "feeling terrible." His BP is 145/75 mm Hg, HR is 102 beats per minute, temperature is 101.2°F, and his RR is 16 breaths per minute. On examination, he is awake, alert, and nontoxic appearing although he has discomfort in his neck with flexion. He has a nonfocal neurologic examination without increased deep tendon reflexes or opthalmoplegia. There are no rashes. Which of the following CSF results is most consistent with your clinical diagnosis of viral meningitis?

a. Identification of viral particles on Gram stain with an elevated CSF-to-serum glucose level
b. A mildly elevated total protein level with a decreased glucose level
c. A mildly elevated total protein level with a WBC count of fewer than 500 cells/mm$^3$
d. Increased turbidity with marked xanthochromia
e. A markedly elevated lymphocyte count, often exceeding 100,000 cells/mm$^3$ with a mildly elevated total protein level

**174.** A 32-year-old woman presents to the ED with 7 days of vaginal discharge and pelvic pain. She is sexually active and admits to several recent "one night stands." She denies trauma/injury and does not have any urinary or other abdominal complaints. Her HR is 85 beats per minute, BP is 135/90 mm Hg, RR is 18 breaths per minute, and temperature is 101.4°F. On bimanual examination, you note a copious, thin, white discharge with mild diffuse adnexal tenderness with significant cervical motion tenderness. There are no rashes, skin lesions, or adenopathy. Laboratory results are notable for a WBC of 18,000/µL. A urinalysis shows WBCs but is otherwise within normal limits. Which of the following is the most appropriate next step in management?

a. Prescribe her a 14-day course of levofloxacin (500 mg PO once per day) and urgent gynecology follow-up within 1 week.
b. Give her a dose of metronidazole (2 g PO) and prescribe her a 14-day course of cephalexin (500 mg) with urgent gynecology follow-up within 1 week.
c. Give her a one-time dose of oral metronidazole (2 g PO), azithromycin (1 g PO), and ceftriaxone (250 mg IM) with gynecology follow-up if she is not feeling better.
d. Give her a one-time dose azithromycin (1 g PO), and ceftriaxone (250 mg IM) with urgent gynecology follow-up within 1 week.
e. Give her a dose of ceftriaxone (250 mg IM), and prescribe her a 10-day course of doxycycline (100 mg PO BID) with urgent gynecology follow-up within 1 week.

**175.** A 45-year-old woman presents to the ED complaining of 3 days of fever and worsening throat pain and painful odynophagia without cough or coryza. She sits on a chair, leaning forward with her mouth slightly open. She is refusing to swallow and has a cup of saliva and a box of facial tissues at her side. Vitals are HR of 120 beats per minute, BP of 110/70 mm Hg, RR of 22 breaths per minute, oxygen saturation of 99% on room air, and temperature of 102.8°F. You note a slight wheezing noise coming from her anterior neck. Her voice is hoarse and she is able to open her mouth fully, making her examination quite difficult. From what you can visualize, her posterior oropharynx is moderately hyperemic, without exudates or tonsillar enlargement. A soft tissue lateral cervical radiograph shows marked edema of the prevertebral soft tissues and absence of the vallecular space. Which of the following is the most likely diagnosis?

a. Retropharyngeal abscess
b. Peritonsillar abscess
c. Epiglottitis
d. Pharyngitis
e. Laryngotracheitis

**176.** A 19-year-old woman presents with 4 days of bilateral lower abdominal pain right greater than left. She also complains of a fever, nausea, vomiting, and general malaise. Her last menstrual period was 5 days ago. Vitals are HR 98 beats per minute, BP 110/65 mm Hg, RR 18 breaths per minute, and temperature of 102.7°F. Pelvic examination demonstrates exquisite cervical motion tenderness and right adnexal tenderness. Laboratory reports are notable for a WBC 15,000/μL, an ESR of 95 mm/h, and a negative urine β-human chorionic gonadotropin (β-hCG). Transvaginal ultrasound demonstrates a right complex mass with cystic and solid components. Which of the following is the most appropriate next step in management?

a. Prescribe her a 14-day course of levofloxacin (500 mg PO once per day) and urgent gynecology follow-up within 1 week.
b. Give her a dose of metronidazole (2 g PO) and prescribe her a 14-day course of cephalexin (500 mg) with urgent gynecology follow-up within 1 week.
c. Give her a one-time dose of oral metronidazole (2 g PO), azithromycin (1 g PO), and ceftriaxone (250 mg IM) with gynecology follow-up if she is not feeling better.
d. Given her a one-time dose with emergent gynecology consultation for possible laparoscopic drainage.
e. Give her a dose of ceftriaxone (250 mg IM), and prescribe her a 10-day course of doxycycline (100 mg PO BID) with urgent gynecology follow-up within 1 week.

**177.** A 42-year-old IV drug user presents to the ED with fever, chills, pleuritic chest pain, myalgias, and general malaise. The patient's vitals include an HR of 110 beats per minute, BP of 110/65 mm Hg, RR of 18 breaths per minute, and temperature of 103.4°F. Physical examination is notable for retinal hemorrhages, petechiae on the conjunctivae and mucous membranes, a faint systolic ejection murmur, and splenomegaly. Which of the following is the most likely diagnosis?

a. Disseminated gonorrhea
b. Myocarditis
c. Pericarditis
d. Infectious mononucleosis
e. Endocarditis

**178.** A 51-year-old diabetic man complains of intense right-ear pain and discharge. On physical examination, his BP is 145/65 mm Hg, HR 91 beats per minute, and temperature 101°F. He withdraws when you retract the pinna of his ear. The external auditory canal is erythematous, edematous, and contains what looks like friable granulation tissue in the external auditory canal. The tympanic membrane is partially obstructed but appears to be erythematous, as well. You make the presumptive diagnosis of necrotizing (malignant) otitis externa. Which of the following statements regarding this condition is true?

a. It is an uncommon complication of otitis media in otherwise healthy patients.
b. The mainstay of treatment is outpatient with oral antibiotics.
c. Cranial nerve IX palsy is the most common complication.
d. *Pseudomonas aeruginosa* is the most common causative organism.
e. Hearing loss is the most common complication.

**179.** A 26-year-old woman presents to the ED with fever, malaise, and an evolving rash in the right axilla that she initially thought was from an insect bite that she received while hiking 1 week earlier. She complains of generalized fatigue, nausea, headache, and joint pain over the past several days. Her vitals are BP of 120/75 mm Hg, HR of 75 beats per minute, RR of 16 breaths per minute, and temperature of 101°F. On physical examination, she is awake and alert, with a nonfocal neurologic examination. Her neck is supple, but she is diffusely tender over the shoulder, knee, and hip joints bilaterally without any distinct effusions. Her abdomen is soft and nontender. She has a 9-cm erythematous annular plaque with partial central clearing and a bright red outer border and a target center under her right axilla. Which of the following is the next best step?

a. Treat empirically with broad-spectrum antibiotics and consult dermatology emergently for a biopsy of the rash.
b. Treat empirically for a cellulitis with cephalexin for 10 days and arrange follow-up with her primary care doctor.
c. Treat empirically for Lyme disease with doxycycline for 21 days and arrange follow-up with her primary-care doctor.
d. Treat empirically for an allergic dermatitis with prednisone, diphenhydramine, and famotidine for 3 days, and arrange follow-up with her primary care doctor.
e. Perform serologic testing for *Borrelia burgdorferi* to confirm the diagnosis of Lyme disease and arrange follow-up with her primary care doctor.

**180.** A 22-year-old man without medical complaints presents to the ED with a 3-day history of fever, malaise, and myalgias. He denies chest pain, shortness of breath, nausea or vomiting, abdominal pain, cough, sore throat, genitourinary symptoms, or respiratory tract complaints. On examination, the patient's BP is 100/60 mm Hg, HR is 110 beats per minute, RR is 20 breaths per minute, and temperature is 102°F. He appears awake, alert, and comfortable. His physical examination is normal. Which of the following is the most appropriate next step in management?

a. Discharge him with antipyretics and follow up with his primary care doctor in 1 or 2 days for a repeat examination.
b. Order a CBC, urinalysis, and chest x-ray. If normal, discharge him with antipyretics and follow up with his primary care doctor in 1 or 2 days for a repeat examination.
c. Order a CBC, urinalysis, chest x-ray, and two sets of blood cultures. If normal, discharge him with antipyretics and follow up with his primary care doctor in 1 or 2 days for a repeat examination.
d. Order a CBC, urinalysis, chest x-ray, two sets of blood cultures, and perform an LP. If normal, discharge him with antipyretics and follow up with his primary care doctor in 1 or 2 days for a repeat examination.
e. Order a CBC, urinalysis, chest x-ray, two sets of blood cultures, and perform an LP. Start empiric IV antibiotics and admit him for observation.

**181.** A 54-year-old man with a history of hepatitis C, alcohol abuse, and cirrhotic ascites presents with increasing abdominal girth and abdominal pain. He complains of increasing difficulty breathing, especially when lying down, caused by worsening ascites. On physical examination, the patient is cachectic and appears older than his stated age. He has a diffusely tender abdomen and tense ascites. The liver is palpable 4 cm below the costal margin. Vitals include a BP of 110/65 mm Hg, HR of 110 beats per minute, RR of 22 breaths per minute, and temperature of 102°F. Which of the following is the most common organism seen in spontaneous bacterial peritonitis?

a. *Pseudomonas aeruginosa*
b. *Enterococcus*
c. *Streptococcus pneumoniae*
d. Enterobacteriaceae
e. *Streptococcus viridans*

# Fever

## Answers

**159. The answer is c.** *(Rosen, pp 595, 1396.)* **Spinal abscesses** are most commonly found in **immunocompromised patients, IV drug users,** and the **elderly**. Signs and symptoms of epidural abscess usually develop over a week or two and include fever, localized pain, and progressive weakness. An elevated WBC count is also commonly seen. MRI is the most useful diagnostic test. *Staphylococcus aureus* is the most common causative organism, followed by gram-negative bacilli and tuberculosis bacillus.

Fibromyalgia (**a**) is a common cause of chronic back pain, but one would not expect the physical findings (weakness, hyperreflexia) or laboratory abnormalities. Inflammatory conditions, including ankylosing spondylitis (**b**), may cause back pain. The key findings in this disease include gradual onset of morning stiffness improved with exercise in a patient younger than 40 years. On physical examination, these patients may have limited back flexion, reduced chest expansion, and sacroiliac joint tenderness, all of which are nonspecific. Fever and weakness would not be expected. Back pain may result from vertebral compression fractures (**d**). These may be secondary to trauma or may be atraumatic in a patient with osteoporosis. Osteoporotic compression fractures usually involve patients older than 70 years or patients with acquired bone weakness (eg, prolonged steroid use). Metastatic lesions (**e**) invade the spinal bone marrow, leading to compression of the spinal cord. Most common primary tumors include breast, lung, thyroid, kidney, prostate (BLT with Kosher pickles), as well as lymphoma and multiple myeloma. Maintain a high level of suspicion for any cancer patient who develops back pain; these patients must be investigated for spinal metastases.

**160. The answer is c.** *(Pinsky, 2011.)* The treatment for sepsis has evolved considerably over the past 10 years with emphasis on the early recognition and aggressive therapy. This approach is known as **early-goal-directed therapy (EGDT)**. EGDT emphasizes early recognition of patients with potential sepsis in the ED, early broad-spectrum antibiotics, and a rapid crystalloid fluid bolus, followed by goal-directed therapy for those patients who remain hypotensive or severely ill after this initial therapy. EGDT is basically a three-step process, aimed at optimizing tissue perfusion:

- The first step involves titrating crystalloid fluid administration (up to 2 L) to achieve a CVP between 8 and 12 mm Hg. CVP is a surrogate for intravascular volume, as excess circulating blood volume is contained within the venous system.
- The second step, if the patient has not improved with fluid alone, is to administer vasopressors to attain a mean arterial pressure (MAP) > 65 mm Hg.
- The third step is to evaluate the central venous oxygen saturation (SvO$_2$). This is obtained from the central venous line, which, in turn, is a surrogate for peripheral tissue oxygenation and cardiac output. A central venous saturation of less than 70% is considered abnormal and indicative of suboptimal therapy. In this case, the hematocrit is checked and blood is transfused until a hematocrit > 30% is attained. Once this is attained and the central venous saturation is still low, dobutamine is initiated to increase cardiac output.

Vasopressor therapy (a) should not be started until the patient receives at least normal saline fluid boluses to achieve a CVP between 8 and 12 mm Hg or to maintain a MAP of at least 65 mm Hg. Packed RBCs (b) can be transfused if the SvO$_2$ is < 70% and the hematocrit is < 30%. However, this should not occur until after adequate fluid resuscitation. A CT scan (d) is not indicated at this time as the most reasonable explanation for the patient's change in mental status is the acute infection and hemodynamic changes and there is a great deal of risk involved in moving a hemodynamically unstable patient to the CT scanner (e) Although this patient should have central venous (subclavian or internal jugular) access, the evaluation of SvO$_2$ should occur after other resuscitative efforts have been maximized.

**161. The answer is d.** (*Tintinalli, pp 649-650.*) **Epididymitis** is an inflammation of the epididymis and has two distinct causes. In patients younger than 35 years, sexually transmitted diseases (STDs), such as gonorrhea and *Chlamydia*, are most common while urinary pathogens, such as *Escherichia coli* and *Klebsiella*, are most common in patients older than 40 years. Unlike testicular torsion, the onset of pain in epididymitis is usually gradual and the cremasteric reflex should be intact. Scrotal elevation may transiently relieve pain (positive Prehn sign). Treatment includes bed rest, scrotal elevation or support when ambulating, avoidance of heavy lifting, and antibiotics for infection. There is no approved one-time dose of antibiotics to treat epididymitis and patients must be treated for a total of 10 to 14 days.

This patient may require pain medications, (a) but coverage with appropriate antibiotics will help relieve symptoms. While penicillin is appropriate therapy for primary syphilis, it is not indicated to treat epididymitis. While scrotal elevation, ice, and rest (b) may be helpful, definitive treatment for epididymitis requires appropriate antibiotic coverage as described just previously. Although a lower dose of ceftriaxone and a one-time dose of azithromycin (c) are appropriate to treat urethritis, this is not adequate treatment of epididymitis. A hydrocele (e) is a fluid accumulation in a persistent tunica vaginalis owing to obstruction, which impedes lymphatic drainage of the testicle. On physical examination, transillumination may help confirm the diagnosis. Treatment includes reassurance, and possibly surgical follow-up for drainage.

**162. The answer is b.** (*Tintinalli, pp 647, 1020-1021.*) **Fournier syndrome** (also known as **Fournier gangrene**) is a **polymicrobial necrotizing fasciitis** of the **perineal subcutaneous tissue** that originates from the skin, urethra, or rectum. It is more common in male patients and usually begins as a simple abscess or benign infection that quickly spreads, especially in an immunocompromised patient. If not promptly diagnosed, it can lead to end-artery thrombosis in the subcutaneous tissue and widespread necrosis. Treatment includes aggressive fluid resuscitation; broad-spectrum antibiotics to cover gram-positive, gram-negative, and anaerobic bacteria; wide surgical debridement; and, possibly, hyperbaric oxygen therapy.

Cutaneous candidiasis (a) is common in diabetics with poorly controlled blood sugar and may be a presenting complaint in new-onset diabetes. However, this rash is nontoxic, without systemic signs and symptoms, and often limited to moist areas such as between skin folds. Phimosis (c) is the condition where the foreskin cannot be retracted from the glans penis and can lead to urinary retention. Paraphimosis (d) is the inability to reduce the proximal foreskin over the glans penis (the foreskin becomes "stuck" behind the glans penis). It may lead to decreased arterial flow and eventual gangrene. Testicular torsion (e) is the twisting of a testicle on its root that usually occurs during strenuous activity or following trauma but can occasionally occur during sleep. It is most common in infants and young adults.

**163. The answer is d.** (*Rosen, pp 1830-1835.*) This patient is exhibiting the common signs and symptoms of **septic arthritis**, an infection of a joint space, most commonly the knee, followed by the hip, shoulder, and wrist. Preexisting arthritis (osteoarthritis or rheumatoid arthritis), immunocompromised states (alcoholism, diabetes, or cancer), and risky sexual behavior are risk factors for the development of septic arthritis. Patients present with a warm, tender, erythematous, swollen joint and pain with passive range of motion. Fever and chills are common. Arthrocentesis is diagnostic with joint fluid demonstrating a WBC count > 50,000/μL with > 75% granulocytes. *Staphylococcus aureus* remains the predominant pathogen for all age groups. However, in young adults gonococcal septic arthritis is common and should also be included in the selection of antibiotic coverage. Patients with septic arthritis should receive a first dose of antibiotics in the ED prior to admission. If a coincident cellulitis is present over the involved joint, arthrocentesis may need to be delayed.

Plain radiographs (a) should be obtained to identify any underlying osteomyelitis or joint disease but are often nondiagnostic in acute septic arthritis. MRI (b) plays no role in the diagnosis of acute septic arthritis but may be useful in evaluating for chronic disease, osteomyelitis, and other musculoskeletal injuries involving the knee. The ESR and CRP (c) are often elevated in septic arthritis and can be trended to assess treatment success, but neither is specific or diagnostic. A bone scan (e) is useful in the detection of osteomyelitis that may not be immediately apparent on a plain radiograph, but is not sensitive in the diagnosis of septic arthritis.

**164. The answer is a.** (*Harrison, pp 720-722.*) This patient has **thrombotic thrombocytopenic purpura (TTP)**, caused by increased platelet destruction. In TTP, platelet-fibrin thrombi deposit in vessel and cause injury to RBCs and platelets, resulting in microangiopathy hemolytic anemia and thrombocytopenia. Patients tend to be females who are 10 to 45 years of age. Risk factors include pregnancy, autoimmune disorders (eg, SLE), infection, allogenic bone marrow transplantation, malignancy, and medications (such as quinine, clopidogrel, and ticlopidine). The **pentad** includes **Fever**, (microangiopathic hemolytic) **Anemia**, **Thrombocytopenia**, **Renal** (failure), and **Neurologic changes** (fluctuating symptoms with a waxing and waning mental status). Unfortunately, only 40% of patients presents with the classic pentad. Untreated, TTP carries a mortality rate up to 80%. Although steroids, splenectomy, anticoagulation, and exchange transfusion have been attempted, daily **plasmapheresis** until platelet count normalizes is the current initial treatment of choice. In addition, RBCs may be transfused in patients with symptomatic anemia. All patients with TTP should be admitted to an ICU for close monitoring of acute bleeds.

The initial therapy for TTP generally does not include platelet transfusion **(b)**, as this could worsen the condition and increase mortality. However, platelets should be administered in patients with a life-threatening bleed. Corticosteroids and splenectomy **(c)** are used in refractory cases but are not considered appropriate initial treatments. Fever and altered mental status may indicate meningitis, but this patient has other signs and symptoms consistent with TTP. A CT scan may be indicated to exclude intracranial bleeding but an LP **(d and e)** is unnecessary and could be dangerous given the very low platelet count. Additionally, this patient requires ICU monitoring.

**165. The answer is a.** (*Tintinalli, p 917, pp 999-1003, 1071-1072, p 1623.*) This patient suffers from **toxic shock syndrome (TSS)**, a toxin-mediated systemic inflammatory response that results in severe, rapidly progressive, life-threatening high fevers, diffuse macular erythroderma, profound hypotension, desquamation, and multisystem dysfunction (including vomiting or diarrhea, severe myalgias, mucous membrane hyperemia, renal or hepatic dysfunction, decreased platelets, and disorientation). TSS was initially recognized as a disease of young, healthy, menstruating women, in which tampon use increased the risk 33 times. With increased awareness and changes in tampon composition, cases of TSS have declined over the past 20 years. An **exotoxin** produced by *S aureus* is the presumed cause in menstrual-related TSS (MRTSS) and two endotoxins have been implicated in non–menstrual-related TSS (NMRTSS). TSS should be considered in any unexplained febrile illness associated with erythroderma, hypotension, and diffuse organ pathology. Patients with MRTSS usually present between the third and fifth day of menses. In severe cases, headache is the most common complaint. The rash is a diffuse, blanching erythroderma, often described as painless "sunburn" that fades within 3 days and is followed by desquamation, especially of the palms and soles. For severe cases, treatment includes aggressive IV fluid resuscitation, IV oxacillin or cefazolin, and hospital admission in a monitored setting.

Rocky Mountain spotted fever (RMSF) **(b)** is caused by *R rickettsii*, which is transmitted by ticks. The organism multiplies in endothelial cells lining small vessels, causing generalized vasculitis as well as headache, fever, confusion, rash, myalgias, and shock. The rash usually appears on days 2 to 3, initially on the wrists, ankles, palms, and soles, spreading rapidly to the extremities and trunk. Lesions begin as small, erythematous blanching macules that become maculopapular and petechial. The location and type of rash, along with the history distinguish RMSF from TSS. Serologic tests are confirmatory, but treatment with doxycycline or chloramphenicol should be started prior to confirmation. Streptococcal scarlet fever (c) is an acute febrile illness primarily affecting young children, caused by *S pyogenes* (group A streptococci [GAS]). The "sandpaper" rash of scarlet fever differs from the macular sunburn rash of TSS. The treatment is penicillin or macrolide in penicillin-allergic patients. While *S aureus* is the causative organism of TSS, a less common, but more aggressive, TSS-like syndrome, streptococcal TSS (STSS), has also been identified. The treatment is similar to that of TSS, with aggressive fluid management along with IV penicillin and clindamycin. These patients may progress to a necrotizing fasciitis or myositis, requiring surgical intervention. Meningococcemia (d) is an infectious vasculitis caused by disseminated *N meningitides*, a gram-negative diplococcus. Fever, headache, arthralgias, altered mental status, and abnormal vitals may also be found, along with neck stiffness. There is no indication of meningeal irritation in this patient. Furthermore, the rash of meningococcemia is distinctly different from that of TSS, involving petechial, hemorrhagic vesicles, macules, and papules with surrounding erythema, especially on the trunk and extremities. The treatment is IV ceftriaxone. Disseminated gonococcemia (e), usually seen in young, sexually active female patients, is caused by *N gonorrhoeae*. The rash of gonococcemia is pustular with an erythematous base, rather than petechial and hemorrhagic, as are the lesions of RMSF and meningococcemia. It can also be associated with fever and arthralgias. The treatment is IV ceftriaxone or oral ciprofloxacin.

**166. The answer is c.** *(Tintinalli, p 350.)* **Osteomyelitis** is an infection or inflammation of a bone with an incidence following plantar puncture wounds of 0.1% to 2%. Pain, swelling, fever, redness, and drainage may all occur, but pain is the presenting complaint in most cases. Risk factors include trauma, surgery, soft tissue infections, and being immunocompromised (eg, human immunodeficiency virus [HIV], diabetes, IV drug user, sickle-cell disease, alcoholism). Overall, *S aureus* is the leading cause of osteomyelitis, followed by various *Streptococcus* species. *Pseudomonas* is also implicated in specific subpopulations, as discussed in the following text. Definitive diagnosis is made by bone scan, which will demonstrate osteomyelitis within 72 hours of symptom onset. Radiographs may be normal early on but will demonstrate periosteal elevation within 10 days. ESR and CRP are often elevated, but normal or slightly elevated levels do not rule out the diagnosis and they are most valuable in following response to treatment, as levels should fall as the infection resolves. Blood cultures, which are positive in 50% of cases, should be used to guide antibiotic treatment. All patients with puncture wounds should receive tetanus prophylaxis.

Patients with sickle-cell disease and asplenism are at higher risk for *Salmonella* (a) osteomyelitis, although *S aureus* remains the most common cause. *Pseudomonas* (b) causes bone and joint infections primarily in three settings. First, patients receiving implanted prosthetic devices during orthopedic surgery are at higher risk for osteomyelitis from *Pseudomonas*. Puncture wounds to the foot also increase the risk of osteomyelitis from *Pseudomonas*. Second, *Pseudomonas* does not appear to grow on puncture objects but rather appears to grow on the footwear and may be inoculated into the wound. Third, IV drug users may develop hematogenous osteomyelitis, often in the spine, from *Pseudomonas* bacteria. (d) Overall, *Streptococcus* is the second most common cause of osteomyelitis; however, specific groups may be at increased risk. For example, in neonates group B *Streptococcus* is a common infecting bacterium of bone and joint infections, and in children aged 3 months to 14 years group A *Streptococcus* may be seen. *Pasteurella multocida* (e) is a common etiology of cellulitis following a cat bite.

**167. The answer is c.** (*Rosen, pp 1128-1141.*) **HCAP** is defined as the development of pneumonia in patients with recent (within 90 days) contact with the health care system, including hospitalization, outpatient dialysis, or residing in a nursing home or rehabilitation center. In comparison to CAP, HCAP tends to be caused by organisms with higher levels of resistance. Although specific treatments depend on local resistance patterns, hospital admission and initiation of broad-spectrum IV antibiotics that includes coverage for MRSA are generally recommended.

HCP (a) is defined as the development of a new pneumonia following at least 48 to 72 hours in the hospital. It is a common cause of nosocomial infection and the most common cause of death in ICUs. CAP (b) is defined as the development of pneumonia in any patient without specific health care contact. VAP (**d**) is defined as a new pneumonia that develops in a patient who has been on a ventilator for at least 48 hours. Atypical pneumonia (**e**) is caused by organisms such as *Mycoplasma pneumoniae*, viruses, or *Legionella*, and typically begins as a flu-like illness and lack of signs of consolidation on examination and radiography. Patients typically appear nontoxic and can be treated as outpatients.

**168. The answer is e.** (*Rosen, pp 977-978.*) **Ludwig angina (LA)** is a potentially life-threatening cellulitis of the connective tissue of the floor of the mouth and neck that **begins in the submandibular space** and is commonly caused by an infected or recently extracted tooth. Typically, it is a polymicrobial infection involving aerobic and anaerobic bacteria of the mouth, including streptococci, staphylococci, and bacteroides species. The most common physical findings are bilateral submandibular swelling and tongue protrusion or elevation. A tense edema and brawny induration of the neck above the hyoid may be present and is described as a "**bull neck.**" Marked tenderness to palpation of the neck and subcutaneous emphysema may be noted. Trismus and fever are often present but usually no palpable fluctuance or cervical lymphadenopathy. The involved teeth may be tender to palpation. Appropriate regimens include high-dose penicillin with metronidazole, or cefoxitin used alone. Clindamycin, ticarcillin-clavulanate, piperacillin-tazobactam, or ampicillin sulbactam may also be used. Oral antibiotics are not adequate.

Importantly, patients with LA should be considered to have an unstable airway regardless of the initial examination and should **never** be left alone because airway impairment can suddenly occur. Signs of impending airway compromise include stridor, tachypnea, dyspnea, drooling, and agitation. Patients should be left sitting upright to increase airway diameter and aid with airway protection. Of note, the upper airway may be severely distorted making endotracheal intubation difficult or impossible. Cricothyrotomy may also be difficult due to the swelling and increases the risk of spreading infection into the mediastinum. Therefore, fiberoptic nasotracheal intubation is preferred.

This is a clinical diagnosis, with soft tissue radiographs (**a**) and CT scans (**c and d**) of the neck confirm the diagnosis by demonstrating edema of the affected area, airway narrowing, and gas collections. However, radiographs *must* not delay treatment, compromise the patient's ability to protect their airway (such as by lying supine), or place the patient in an area where emergent airway management is difficult. Therefore, these studies should be delayed until the airway is stabilized. Prior to broad-spectrum antibiotics, incision and drainage (**b**) was the treatment of choice. Today, surgery is used only for those patients who fail to respond to antibiotic therapy or those with purulent collections. In these rare cases, surgery, including incision and drainage then excision of facial planes, would best be performed in an operating room (OR), not at the bedside. Additionally, cultures are often of little utility given the polymicrobial nature of the infection.

**169. The answer is b.** (*Tintinalli, pp 1014-1018.*) **Sepsis** represents the systemic inflammatory response, mediated by an inflammatory cascade triggered by an infection that overwhelms the body's regulatory systems. Initially, this leads to tachycardia, tachypnea, and fever, and may progress to shock, multiorgan failure, and death if not treated. Sepsis is a common cause of death in the United States with a mortality rate estimated between 20% and 50%. The initiation of early, aggressive therapy (known as EGDT) has been shown to improve outcomes of septic patients.

SIRS (**a**) is a systemic inflammatory response to a variety of clinical insults and can be defined according to various physiologic parameters, including elevated (or lowered) oral temperature, RR > 20, HR > 90, or elevated WBC count (or bandemia). Severe sepsis (**c**) is defined as sepsis with one or more

| SIRS | Sepsis | Severe Sepsis | Septic Shock |
|---|---|---|---|
| Two or more of the following criteria: | | | |
| HR > 90 | SIRS | Sepsis | Sepsis |
| Temperature > 100.4°F or < 96.8°F | + | + | + |
| | Suspected or proven infections | Acute organ dysfunction | Refractory hypotension |
| RR > 20, or $Pa_{CO_2}$ < 32 | | | |
| WBC >12,000 cells/mm³, or < 4000 cells/mm³, or > 10% band forms | | | |

signs of organ dysfunction, hypoperfusion, or hypotension such as metabolic acidosis, acute alteration in mental status, or respiratory distress syndrome. Septic Shock (**d**) is defined as severe sepsis with hypotension that is unresponsive to fluid resuscitation. These states are summarized in the following table. MODS (**e**) is defined as the dysfunction of more than one organ, requiring acute interventions to obtain homeostasis.

**170. The answer is e.** (*Rosen, pp 2211-2222.*) This patient has a urinary tract infection that appears to be resistant to treatment and is exhibiting signs of multiple organ system dysfunction seen by elevated cardiac enzymes and cardiomegaly (cardiac), an elevated BUN/creatinine, hyperkalemia (renal), and altered mental status (neurologic). He requires intubation, dialysis, and other acute interventions for this dysfunction.

SIRS (**a**) is defined according to various physiologic parameters, including elevated (or lowered) oral temperature, RR > 20, HR > 90, or elevated WBC count (or bandemia). Sepsis (**b**) is defined as SIRS that has a proven or suspected source of infection. Severe sepsis (**c**) is defined as sepsis with one or more signs of organ dysfunction, hypoperfusion, or hypotension such as metabolic acidosis, acute alteration in mental status, or respiratory distress syndrome. Septic shock (**d**) is defined as severe sepsis with hypotension that is unresponsive to fluid resuscitation.

**171. The answer is a.** (*Centor, 1981, pp 239-246.*) The patient has a **modified Centor** score of 4 (history of fever, tender adenopathy, no cough, exudates, age 15-45 years). The Centor criteria, seen below, are used for predicting streptococcal pharyngitis and whether or not to treat the patient with antibiotics. Because of his high score, it is likely that the patient has group A β-hemolytic streptococcal infection and that he should receive antibiotics. In addition, he should be treated symptomatically with fluids, topical anesthetics, and acetaminophen or ibuprofen.

Patients with a Centor criterion of 2 or 3 should have a rapid antigen test and a throat culture performed. If the rapid antigen test is negative, a confirmatory throat culture may be sent (**b**), but antibiotics (**c**) should not be initiated. If the rapid antigen test is positive, patients should be treated with an antibiotic (**d**). A patient with many predictive signs and symptoms should be treated with antibiotics rather than discharged (**e**).

| Centor Criteria | Points |
|---|---|
| Presence of tonsillar exudates | +1 |
| Tender anterior cervical adenopathy | +1 |
| Fever by history | +1 |
| Absence of cough | +1 |
| Age <15 years | +1 |
| Age >45 years | −1 |

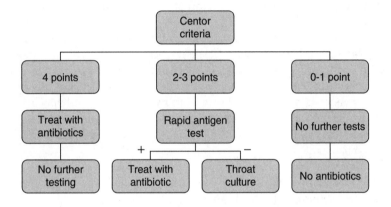

**172. The answer is a.** (*Rosen, pp 919-920.*) The patient's presentation is typical for a **peritonsillar abscess**. Signs and symptoms include a sore throat, muffled voice, trismus, fluctuant mass, deviation of the uvula, odynophagia, and drooling. Many of these patients have a history of being recently treated for strep throat. The abscess is **usually unilateral** and in the **superior pole of the tonsil**. Airway patency must be assessed because of the obstructing potential of an abscess. As with most abscesses, drainage—either through needle aspiration or incision and drainage—is the most important factor in treating these patients. However, antibiotics are useful adjunctive medications and should be prescribed.

The abscess will not resolve without an attempt at drainage. Antibiotics and pain control alone (**b**) are not sufficient. Incision and drainage of the abscess may be performed in the OR (c) if the abscess is large, complicated, or the patient's airway shows signs of compromise. However, this is not necessary in the patient described. Drainage of the abscess is the most important factor in treating these patients. Antibiotics alone (d) are not sufficient. A CT scan (e) may aid in the diagnosis of a peritonsillar abscess in patients with severe trismus, but should be ordered with caution given the potential for airway compromise. In this patient, it would be an unnecessary risk as he could be examined adequately.

**173. The answer is c.** *(Rosen, pp 920-921.)* **Viral meningitis** is an uncommon complication of viral infection and can follow seemingly mild respiratory, gastrointestinal, or urogenital infections. Viral meningitis is typically milder than bacterial meningitis and is **often self-limited** infection, though it may be associated with encephalitis (sometimes known as meningoencephalitis). Patients may often complain of preceding viral symptoms or have evidence of concurrent infection. Unfortunately, the physical findings in meningitis vary widely and many **patients will lack the classic findings** of meningeal irritation such as Kernig and Brudzinski signs. LP is necessary to confirm the diagnosis. Common CSF findings include **mildly elevated protein levels** and **WBC counts** with **normal glucose levels and polymorphonuclear neutrophil (PMN) and eosinophil counts**. There is no specific treatment for viral meningitis and treatment often is based on supportive care with antipyretics, pain medications, and fluids.

While specific viruses (such as West Nile virus and herpes simplex virus) can be identified in the CSF, they are not identified (a) by Gram stain. Additionally, patients with viral meningitis should have normal glucose levels (b) and, therefore, also have normal CSF-to-serum glucose level. Turbidity (d) refers to cloudiness due to leukocytosis at levels above 200 cells/mm$^3$ and should be only mild in cases of viral meningitis. Xanthochromia, a yellowish discoloration that results from RBC breakdown, raises the concern for subarachnoid hemorrhage. While the lymphocyte count may be mildly elevated (e), the WBC count is rarely elevated above 500 cells/mm$^3$.

**174. The answer is e.** *(Rosen, pp 1819-1820.)* The patient has **pelvic inflammatory disease (PID)**, due to an ascending vaginal or cervical infection. *Chlamydia trachomatis* and *N gonorrhoeae* are the most common causative organisms, but PID is often polymicrobial and numerous other organisms have been implicated. PID may be difficult to diagnose because it has a wide variety of presenting signs and symptoms, including lower abdominal or pelvic pain, vaginal discharge, abnormal vaginal or cervical bleeding, low-grade fevers, and nonspecific systemic symptoms (such as myalgias, malaise, and nausea). However, a hallmark of PID is the finding of significant **cervical motion tenderness** on bimanual pelvic examination. Current recommendations for the treatment of PID are varied and change frequently but generally require 10 days of total treatment. Most patients with PID can be safely discharged from the ED, but consideration for admission should be given to patients who appear toxic, are pregnant, have failed outpatient therapy, or have a concurrent intrauterine device (IUD) or tubo-ovarian abscess.

A 14-day course of levofloxacin (**a**) may be an appropriate treatment for pyelonephritis but is inappropriate antibiotic coverage for PID. A one-time dose of metronidazole (**b**) may treat trichomonas but is also inappropriate coverage for PID, even if combined with cephalexin. A one-time dose of the combination azithromycin and ceftriaxone (**d**) may be used to treat cervicitis but is not approved for the treatment of PID. When trichomonas cannot be excluded, metronidazole may be added (**c**) but is not approved for the treatment of PID.

**175. The answer is c.** (*Rosen, pp 1114-1117.*) **Epiglottitis** is a life-threatening inflammatory condition, usually infectious, of the epiglottis and the aryepiglottic and periglottic folds. Because most children are immunized against *Haemophilus influenzae* type B (Hib), **most cases of epiglottitis are now seen in adults**, with an average age of 46 years. Signs and symptoms include a prodromal period of 1 to 2 days consisting of constitutional symptoms, and then the patient exhibits high fever, dysphagia, odynophagia, drooling, inspiratory stridor, and dyspnea. The "**thumbprint sign**" (described in the question) is seen on lateral cervical radiograph that demonstrates a swollen epiglottis obliterating the vallecula.

Retropharyngeal abscess (**a**) can present with similar signs and symptoms as epiglottitis. Cervical lymphadenopathy is prominent and inflammation may be so severe that patients develop an inflammatory torticollis, causing the patient to rotate the head toward the affected side. Soft tissue cervical radiograph may demonstrate excess prevertebral swelling. Treatment is IV hydration and antibiotics, which should be started in the ED, and drainage in the OR. Peritonsillar abscess (**b**) presents with a unilaterally swollen and erythematous tonsil and uvula deviation toward the unaffected side. It is most common during the second and third decades of life. CT scan or ultrasound easily makes the diagnosis, but aspiration of purulent material is sufficient for diagnosis. Treatment is incision and drainage or needle aspiration, followed by high-dose penicillin or clindamycin. Pharyngitis (d) is an infection of the pharynx and tonsils that occur in adults, but has a peak incidence in children aged 4 to 7 years. The etiology is most often viral. *Streptococcus pyogenes* (group A β-hemolytic strep) is the most common cause of bacterial pharyngitis (5%-15%) in adults. Patients present with erythematous tonsils, tonsillar exudates, and enlarged and tender anterior cervical lymph nodes. Laryngotracheitis, or croup, (e) presents with stridor but lacks the other oropharyngeal findings and is generally seen in children aged 6 months to 3 years.

**176. The answer is d.** *(Rosen, pp 1569-1571.)* This patient has **a tubo-ovarian abscess (TOA)**, a common and potentially fatal complication of PID. While PID can usually be treated with outpatient antibiotics, patients with a TOA should be admitted for IV antibiotics, observation, and drainage if there is no response to medical management. Antibiotics should be directed at *Chlamydia trachomatis* and *N gonorrhoeae*, and may be curative in 60% to 80% of cases.

A 14-day course of levofloxacin (a) may be an appropriate treatment for pyelonephritis but is inappropriate antibiotic coverage for TOA. A one-time dose of metronidazole (b) may treat trichomonas but is inappropriate coverage for TOA, even if combined with cephalexin. A one-time dose of the combination metronidazole, azithromycin, and ceftriaxone (c) may be used to treat cervicitis and bacterial vaginosis but is not approved for the treatment of PID or TOA. When bacterial vaginosis cannot be excluded, metronidazole may be added (c) but is not approved for the treatment of PID.

**177. The answer is e.** *(Rosen, pp 1149-1152.)* Symptoms of **endocarditis** are nonspecific and vary widely, but the most common include fever (85%) and malaise (80%). In IV drug users, fever is present 98% of the time. Other symptoms include weakness, myalgias, dyspnea, chest pain, cough, headache, and anorexia. Neurologic signs and symptoms (eg, confusion, personality changes, decreased level of consciousness, and focal motor deficits) are seen in 30% to 40% of patients. Vasculitic lesions, including petechiae, splinter hemorrhages, tender fingertip nodules (Osler nodes), and nontender palmar plaques (Janeway lesions), are seen in 35% of patients. Splenomegaly, new heart murmur, and retinal hemorrhages may also be detected on physical examination. Risk factors for infective endocarditis include rheumatic or congenital heart disease, calcific degenerative valve disease, prosthetic heart valve, mitral valve prolapse, a history of IV drug use, or a history of endocarditis. Although any valve can be affected, IV drug use is the most common cause of right-sided endocarditis. The recurrence rate in these patients is 41%, significantly higher than the rate of < 20% in non-IV drug users.

Disseminated gonorrhea (a) often presents with the arthritis-dermatitis syndrome of fevers/chills, arthralgias, a rash, and tenosynovitis. One would not expect splenomegaly or vasculitic lesions. Myocarditis (b) is often infectious and results from inflammatory damage to the myocardium and presents with flu-like complaints, including fever, fatigue, and myalgias. Tachycardia out of proportion to the temperature or clinical picture may be present, but vasculitic lesions are not expected. Bacteria and enteroviruses, especially Coxsackie B virus and adenovirus, predominate as causative agents in the United States while Chagas disease is the leading cause, worldwide. Pericarditis (c) is caused by inflammation of the pericardial sac. The etiology is broad, including infection, trauma, metabolic diseases (eg, uremia), medications, systemic autoimmune diseases, and most often the cause is idiopathic. The diagnosis of infectious mononucleosis (d), a syndrome caused by the Epstein-Barr virus, is often made based on the triad of fever and chills, pharyngitis, and tender cervical lymphadenopathy.

**178. The answer is d.** (*Rosen, pp 1070-1071; Lee, 2010.*) **Necrotizing otitis externa (formerly known as malignant otitis externa)** is an uncommon complication of otitis externa that occurs primarily in adult **diabetics** and other **immunocompromised** individuals. It is primarily caused by a very aggressive *P aeruginosa* infection and is associated with a high mortality rate. The infection typically starts in the external ear canal and then progresses through the tissues into the bony junction of the external auditory meatus, base of the skull, and adjacent soft tissues. Thus, the condition is actually better described as an osteitis of the bone of the external auditory canal. It is distinguished by fever, intense ear pain, erythema, edema, and granulation tissue in the external canal. Cranial nerve palsies (CN VII, IX, X, and XI) and trismus can also occur. These patients require hospitalization and treatment with broad-spectrum, antipseudomonal IV antibiotics. Patients also require emergent ENT consultation for possible surgical debridement.

(a) Malignant otitis externa is rare in immunocompetent. Patients are usually diabetics, debilitated, or immunocompromised. (b) Owing to its high morbidity and mortality, this condition requires in-patient management with IV antibiotics. Although hearing loss (e) is a possibility, the most common cranial nerves involved is the facial nerve (cranial nerve VII), (c) but cranial nerves IX, X, and XI can also be involved.

**179. The answer is c.** *(Rosen, pp 2123-2128.)* **Lyme disease** is the most common vector-borne disease in the United States and is particularly prevalent in the northeast and upper midwest during late spring and early summer. It is caused by the spirochete *B burgdorferi* that is spread through the bite of the *Ixodes* tick. Lyme disease has three stages: early localized, early disseminated, and late. It typically begins with a **target rash** (known as **erythema migrans [EM]**) and associated flu-like symptoms. EM is the most characteristic clinical manifestation of Lyme disease and is recognized in 90% or more of patients. However, if untreated, neurologic, joint, or cardiac symptoms develop weeks to months later. These are followed by chronic arthritic and neurologic abnormalities weeks to years later. Recommended treatment for early Lyme disease includes doxycycline, amoxicillin (for children < 8 years or for pregnant or lactating women), or cefuroxime for a period of 3 weeks. The same drugs can be used for the second stage of disease, but their course of therapy needs to be longer. Neurologic disease requires long-term IV antibiotics.

Unfortunately, routine laboratory studies are nonspecific and nondiagnostic. This patient has early localized Lyme disease, and should be treated empirically based on the presence of the rash. Serologic testing may be positive weeks after inoculation, but a biopsy of the rash (a) would neither be necessary nor informative. Although the patient presents with an erythematous rash surrounding a purported bug bite, the classic appearance indicates erythema migrans and treatment for cellulitis (b) is inappropriate. It would also be inappropriate to mistake this for an urticarial rash and thus treat the patient for a cutaneous allergic reaction (d). Confirmatory serologic testing should be performed (e), but empiric treatment based on the presumptive diagnosis should not be delayed.

**180. The answer is a.** *(Rosen, pp 134-137.)* **Fever** is a very common presenting complaint to the emergency department and is associated with a high morbidity and mortality in pediatric and geriatric patients. In younger adults, however, fever is usually a benign disease or self-limited viral syndrome. Adult patients presenting with a fever should be assessed for the duration and magnitude of associated symptoms, recent travel, chronic illnesses, prior surgeries, and physical findings that suggest an infectious source. Stable, healthy patients without localizing signs and symptoms can be safely discharged with antipyretics. However, for **elderly** patients, the **immunocompromised**, and patients with **chronic illness, admission to the hospital** is usually warranted. Patients with unstable vital signs or life-threatening symptoms should be admitted to the ICU.

In this young, healthy adult man with stable vital signs and non-localizing signs and symptoms, additional evaluation (**b, c, d**) and initiation of antibiotics (**e**) is unnecessary.

**181. The answer is d.** (*Rosen, 1412-1413.*) **Spontaneous bacterial peritonitis (SBP)** is a common complication of cirrhotic ascites and should be suspected in all patients with a history of cirrhosis who present with fever, abdominal pain or tenderness, worsening ascites, or encephalopathy. **Paracentesis** should be performed to confirm the diagnosis. Ascitic fluid should be tested for glucose, total protein, lactate dehydrogenase (LDH), Gram stain, WBC count, and sent for culture. **Total WBC count > 1000/μL or neutrophil count > 250/μL is diagnostic for SBP.** Gram-negative Enterobacteriaceae (such as *E coli* and *Klebsiella*) account for up to 65% of all cases. Empiric treatment for suspected SBP includes third-generation cephalosporins, ticarcillin-clavulanic acid, piperacillin-tazobactam, or ampicillin-sulbactam.

(**a, b, c, and e**) Other causes of SBP include *S pneumoniae* and *S viridans* (15%), enterococci (6%-10%), and anaerobes (1%).

# Poisoning and Overdose

## Questions

**182.** After being fired from his job, a 35-year-old man attempts suicide by drinking from a bottle labeled "insecticide." Three hours later, emergency medical services (EMS) brings him into the emergency department (ED) and you notice that he is extremely diaphoretic, drooling, and vomiting. He is awake but confused. His vital signs include a blood pressure (BP) of 170/90 mm Hg, heart rate (HR) of 55 beats per minute, respiratory rate (RR) of 22 breaths per minute, temperature of 98.6°F, and oxygen saturation of 95% on room air. Physical examination demonstrates pinpoint pupils and crackles and wheezing on lung examination. What is the treatment to reverse this patient's poisoning?

a. Naloxone
b. N-acetylcysteine (NAC)
c. Atropine and pralidoxime (2-PAM)
d. Flumazenil
e. Physostigmine

**183.** A 19-year-old man is brought to the ED by EMS after he was found lying on the floor at a dance club. EMS states that the patient seemed unconscious at the dance club, but as soon as they transferred him onto the gurney, he became combative. Upon arrival in the ED, his BP is 120/65 mm Hg, HR is 75 beats per minute, temperature is 98.9°F, RR is 12 breaths per minute, and oxygen saturation is 98% on room air. On physical examination, his pupils are midsized, equal, and reactive to light. His skin is warm and dry. Lung, cardiac, and abdominal examinations are unremarkable. As you walk away from the bedside, you hear the monitor alarm signaling zero respirations and the oxygen saturation starts to drop. You perform a sternal rub and the patient sits up in bed and starts yelling at you. As you leave him for the second time, you hear the monitor alarm again signal zero respirations. You administer naloxone, but there is no change in his condition. Which of the following is most likely the substance ingested by this patient?

a. γ-Hydroxybutyrate (GHB)
b. Diazepam
c. Cocaine
d. Phencyclidine (PCP)
e. Heroin

**184.** A 43-year-old woman presents to the ED with a 3-week history of intermittent headache, nausea, and fatigue. She was seen at her private doctor's office 1 week ago along with her husband and children, who also have similar symptoms. They were diagnosed with a viral syndrome and told to increase their fluid intake. She states that the symptoms began approximately when it started to get cold outside. The symptoms are worse in the morning and improve while she is at work. Her BP is 123/75 mm Hg, HR is 83 beats per minute, temperature is 98.9°F, and oxygen saturation is 98% on room air. Physical examination is unremarkable. You suspect her first diagnosis was incorrect. Which of the following is the most appropriate next step to confirm your suspicion?

a. Order a mono spot test.
b. Perform a nasal pharyngeal swab to test for influenza.
c. Consult psychiatry to evaluate for malingering.
d. Order a carboxyhemoglobin (COHb) level.
e. Order a lead level.

**185.** An 18-year-old woman is brought to the ED by her mother. The patient is diaphoretic and vomiting. Her mom states that she thinks her daughter tried to commit suicide. The patient admits to ingesting a few handfuls of acetaminophen (Tylenol) approximately 3 hours ago. Her temperature is 99.1°F, BP is 105/70 mm Hg, HR is 92 beats per minute, RR is 17 breaths per minute, and oxygen saturation is 99% on room air. On examination, her head and neck are unremarkable. Cardiovascular and pulmonary examinations are within normal limits. She is mildly tender in her right upper quadrant, but there is no rebound or guarding. Bowel sounds are normoactive. She is alert and oriented and has no focal deficits on neurologic examination. You administer 50 g of activated charcoal. At this point, she appears well and has no complaints. Her serum acetaminophen (APAP) concentration 4 hours after the reported time of ingestion returns at 350 μg/mL. You plot the level on the nomogram seen below. Which of the following is the most appropriate next step in management?

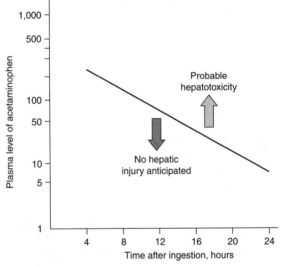

(Reproduced, with permission, from Brunton LL et al. Goodman and Gilman's The Pharmacological Basis Therapeutics. New York, NY: McGraw-Hill, 2006: 694.)

a. Discharge home with instructions to return if symptoms return.
b. Observe for 6 hours and, if the patient still has no complaints, discharge her home.
c. Repeat the acetaminophen level 4 hours after the patient arrived in the ED. Treat only if this level is above the line.
d. Admit to the psychiatry unit and keep on suicide watch while performing serial abdominal examinations.
e. Begin NAC and admit to the hospital.

**186.** A 47-year-old man is brought to the ED by EMS after being found wandering in the street mumbling. His BP is 150/75 mm Hg, HR is 110 beats per minute, temperature is 100.5°F, RR is 16 breaths per minute, oxygen saturation is 99% on room air, and fingerstick glucose is 98 mg/dL. On examination, the patient is confused with mumbling speech. His pupils are dilated and face is flushed. His mucous membranes and skin are dry. Which of the following toxic syndromes is this patient exhibiting?

a. Sympathomimetic syndrome
b. Anticholinergic syndrome
c. Cholinergic syndrome
d. Opioid syndrome
e. Ethanol syndrome

**187.** A 25-year-old man is carried into the ED by two of his friends who state that he is not breathing. The patient has a history of heroin abuse. His vital signs are BP 115/70 mm Hg, HR 99 beats per minute, temperature 98.9°F, RR 3 breaths per minute, and oxygen saturation 87% on room air. You notice fresh needle marks and miotic pupils. You begin bag-valve-mask ventilation and his oxygen saturation increases to 99%. Which of the following is the most appropriate next step in management?

a. Continue bag-valve-mask ventilation until he breathes on his own.
b. Perform endotracheal intubation of the patient.
c. Evaluate response to administration of naloxone.
d. Put the patient on supplemental oxygen.
e. Place a nasogastric tube and administer activated charcoal.

**188.** A 42-year-old man who is actively seizing is brought to the ED by EMS after a massive ingestion of an unknown substance. The man is known to have a history of acquired immunodeficiency syndrome (AIDS). An intravenous (IV) line is established and anticonvulsant therapy is administered. After high doses of diazepam, phenobarbital, and phenytoin, it is determined that the seizures are refractory to standard anticonvulsant therapy. Which of the following substances did this patient most likely ingest?

a. Cocaine
b. Diphenhydramine
c. Tricyclic antidepressant (TCA)
d. Haloperidol
e. Isoniazid (INH)

**189.** A 60-year-old woman with a history of diabetes is brought into the ED by EMS workers who state that the patient was found on a bus in a lethargic and diaphoretic condition. Her fingerstick glucose level at the scene was 35 mg/dL. EMS workers quickly administered dextrose through an IV line. The patient became alert and responsive, stating that she just took her normal medication. Her blood sugar went up to 110 mg/dL and she remained this way throughout her trip to the ED. However, in the ED you notice that the patient is again diaphoretic and is mumbling her speech. Her fingerstick glucose is now 47 mg/dL. You administer dextrose and she perks right up. Which of the following diabetes medications commonly causes hypoglycemia for which the patient is likely to require hospital admission?

a. Regular insulin
b. Metformin
c. Glyburide
d. Sitagliptin
e. Acarbose

**190.** A 23-year-old woman presents to the ED complaining of abdominal pain, nausea, and vomiting. She has a history of depression but is not currently taking any antidepressant medications. Upon further questioning, the patient states that she ingested a bottle of pills in her medicine cabinet approximately 3 hours ago. Her BP is 115/65 mm Hg, HR is 101 beats per minute, temperature is 100.1°F, RR is 29 breaths per minute, and oxygen saturation is 100% on room air. Physical examination is unremarkable except for mild diffuse abdominal tenderness. Laboratory results reveal a white blood cell (WBC) count of 10,300/$\mu$L, hematocrit 46%, platelets 275/$\mu$L, aspartate transaminase (AST) 70 U/L, alanine transaminase (ALT) 85 U/L, alkaline phosphatase 75 U/L, sodium 143 mEq/L, potassium 3.7 mEq/L, chloride 98 mEq/L, bicarbonate 8 mEq/L, blood urea nitrogen (BUN) 22 mg/dL, creatinine 0.9 mg/dL, and glucose 85 mg/dL. Arterial blood gas values on room air are pH 7.51, $P_{CO_2}$ 11 mm Hg, and $P_{O_2}$ 134 mm Hg. Which of the following substances did this patient most likely ingest?

a. Diphenhydramine
b. Ibuprofen
c. Acetaminophen
d. Aspirin
e. Pseudoephedrine

**191.** A 35-year-old agitated man presents to the ED in police custody. He denies any past medical history and takes no medication. He admits to using some drugs today. His BP is 195/90 mm Hg, HR is 121 beats per minute, temperature is 100.1°F, RR is 18 breaths per minute, and oxygen saturation is 99% on room air. On examination, he is diaphoretic, and has pupils that are 8 mm in diameter, along with 3+ patella reflexes bilaterally. Electrocardiogram (ECG) reveals sinus tachycardia with a rate of 123. Which of the following toxic syndromes is this patient exhibiting?

a. Anticholinergic
b. Cholinergic
c. Sympathomimetic
d. Opioid
e. Sedative hypnotic

**192.** A 31-year-old woman with a known psychiatric history presents to the ED after ingesting an unknown quantity of pills from her medication vial. In the ED, she complains of nausea, abdominal cramping, and feels unsteady on her feet. On physical examination, you observe that she is tachycardic and ataxic. Which of the following substances will *best* be treated by activated charcoal that could present like this?

a. Phenobarbital
b. Carbamazepine
c. Lye (sodium hydroxide)
d. Lithium
e. Acetaminophen

**193.** A 27-year-old man presents to the ED extremely agitated complaining of mild chest pain and dyspnea. He states that he was snorting cocaine all afternoon. You place him on a monitor and get his vital signs. His BP is 215/130 mm Hg, HR is 112 beats per minute, temperature is 100.1°F, RR is 17 breaths per minute, and oxygen saturation is 98% on room air. An ECG reveals sinus tachycardia at a rate of 116. Which of the following is the most appropriate medication to administer?

a. Haloperidol
b. Labetalol
c. Esmolol
d. Diltiazem
e. Diazepam

**194.** A 30-year-old man is brought to the ED by police officers. The patient is agitated, vomiting, and complaining of body aches. He states that he is withdrawing from his medication. His vital signs are BP 160/85 mm Hg, RR 20 breaths per minute, HR 107 beats per minute, and temperature 99.7°F. On examination he is diaphoretic, has rhinorrhea, piloerection, and hyperactive bowel sounds. Which of the following substances is this patient most likely withdrawing from?

a. Ethanol
b. Cocaine
c. Nicotine
d. Methadone
e. Clonidine

**195.** A 25-year-old man is brought into the ED by two police officers because of suspected drug use. The patient is extremely agitated and is fighting the police officers. It takes three hospital staff members and the two police officers to keep him on the stretcher. His vital signs are BP 150/80 mm Hg, HR 107 beats per minute, temperature 99.7°F, RR 18 breaths per minute, and oxygen saturation 99% on room air. Physical examination is unremarkable except for cool, diaphoretic skin, persistent vertical and horizontal nystagmus, and occasional myoclonic jerks. Which of the following is the most likely diagnosis?

a. Cocaine intoxication
b. Cocaine withdrawal
c. Anticholinergic toxidrome
d. PCP intoxication
e. Opiate withdrawal

**196.** An undomiciled 49-year-old man presents to the ED with altered mental status. His BP is 149/75 mm Hg, HR is 93 beats per minute, temperature is 97.5°F, RR is 18 breaths per minute, and $O_2$ saturation is 99% on room air. Physical examination reveals an unkempt man with the odor of "alcohol" on his breath. His head is atraumatic and pupils are 4 mm, equal, and reactive. The neck is supple. Cardiovascular, pulmonary, and abdominal examinations are unremarkable. There is no extremity edema and his pulses are 2+ and symmetric. Neurologically, he withdraws all four extremities to deep stimuli. ECG is sinus rhythm. Laboratory results reveal:

| | |
|---|---|
| Sodium 141 mEq/L | Arterial blood pH 7.26 |
| Potassium 3.5 mEq/L | Lactate 1.7 mEq/L |
| Chloride 101 mEq/L | Ethanol level undetectable |
| Bicarbonate 14 mEq/L | Measured serum osmolarity 352 mOsm/L |
| BUN 15 mg/dL | Calculated serum osmolarity 292 mOsm/kg |
| Creatinine 0.7 mg/dL | Urinalysis: no blood, ketones, or protein |
| Glucose 89 mg/dL | |

Which of the following statements best describes the laboratory findings?

a. Anion gap metabolic acidosis and osmol gap
b. Anion gap metabolic acidosis without osmol gap
c. Nonanion gap metabolic acidosis and osmol gap
d. Nonanion gap metabolic acidosis without osmol gap
e. Metabolic alkalosis with secondary acidosis

**197.** A 26-year-old woman with a history of depression is brought into the ED. She was found lying on the floor of her apartment next to an unlabeled empty pill bottle. Her HR is 117 beats per minute, BP is 95/65 mm Hg, RR is 14 breaths per minute, and oxygen saturation is 97% on 2-L nasal cannula. On examination, the patient appears obtunded, and her pupils are 3 mm and reactive. Her oropharynx is dry and there is no gag reflex to pharyngeal stimulation. Her neck is supple. The heart is tachycardic without murmurs, the lungs are clear to auscultation, and the abdomen is soft. There is normal rectal tone and brown stool that is heme negative. Her skin is cool and moist with no signs of needle tracks. Neurologically, she is unresponsive but withdraws all extremities to deep palpation. Fingerstick blood glucose is 85 mg/dL. Her ECG reveals sinus tachycardia at 119 with a QRS complex of 140 milliseconds and a terminal R wave in lead aVR. Which of the following is the most appropriate next step in management?

a. Orotracheal intubation, administer activated charcoal through orogastric tube, and IV naloxone

b. Orotracheal intubation, administer activated charcoal through orogastric tube, and IV sodium bicarbonate

c. Orotracheal intubation, administer activated charcoal through orogastric tube, and IV NAC

d. Orotracheal intubation, administer syrup of ipecac through orogastric tube, and IV sodium bicarbonate

e. Induce vomiting prior to intubation to lower the risk of aspiration then administer IV sodium bicarbonate

**198.** A 37-year-old woman is brought into the ED by her friend who states that the patient swallowed approximately 50 capsules of 325-mg acetaminophen (APAP) 6 hours ago in an attempted suicide. The patient states she feels nauseated and vomits while you take her history. Her BP is 100/75 mm Hg, HR is 97 beats per minute, temperature is 98.9°F, RR is 18 breaths per minute, and oxygen saturation is 99% on room air. Examination is unremarkable except for mild epigastric tenderness. Which of the following is the correct antidote for APAP overdose?

a. NAC

b. Physostigmine

c. Flumazenil

d. Naloxone

e. Digibind

**199.** A 31-year-old man is brought to the ED by EMS who state that the man was found lying on the floor of his garage. He is rousable in the ED, speaks with slurred speech, and vomits. His BP is 140/85 mm Hg, HR is 94 beats per minute, temperature is 98.8°F, RR is 17 breaths per minute, and oxygen saturation is 99% on room air. You place an IV line, draw blood, and start a liter of normal saline running through the line. Laboratory results reveal serum sodium 139 mEq/L, potassium 3.5 mEq/L, chloride 101 mEq/L, bicarbonate 14 mEq/L, BUN 15 mg/dL, creatinine 1 mg/dL, glucose 105 mg/dL, arterial blood pH 7.27, COHb 4%, and lactate 2.8 mEq/L. Urinalysis shows 1+ protein, trace ketones, WBC 4/hpf (high-power field), red blood cell (RBC) 2 to 3/hpf, and multiple envelope-shaped and needle-shaped crystals. Which of the following conditions would best explain his metabolic acidosis?

a. Ibuprofen toxicity
b. Ethylene glycol poisoning
c. Diabetic ketoacidosis (DKA)
d. Lactic acidosis
e. Isopropyl alcohol poisoning

**200.** A 35-year-old man who is employed as a forklift operator was found sitting outside a warehouse. He came stumbling out complaining of dizziness and headaches. Coworkers in an adjoining warehouse also complained of headache and nausea. After collapsing outside, he regained consciousness immediately but appeared confused. In the ED, his BP is 100/54 mm Hg, HR is 103 beats per minute, temperature is 100°F, pulse ox is 91% on room air, and RR is 23 breaths per minute. Physical examination is unremarkable. Laboratory results reveal WBC 10,500/μL, hematocrit 45%, platelets 110/μL, sodium 137 mEq/L, potassium 4 mEq/L, chloride 103 mEq/L, bicarbonate 21 mEq/L, BUN 8 mg/dL, creatinine 0.5 mg/dL, and glucose 89 mg/dL. Arterial blood gas results are pH 7.32, $P_{CO_2}$ 32 mm Hg, and $P_{O_2}$ 124 mm Hg. Which of the following is the most likely diagnosis?

a. Methemoglobinemia
b. Hypoglycemic syncope
c. Hydrocarbon poisoning
d. Opioid overdose
e. CO poisoning

**201.** A 51-year-old man presents to the ED complaining of nausea and abdominal pain after drinking some "bitter stuff." He is considered one of the "regulars" who is usually at triage with ethanol intoxication. His temperature is 97.9°F, BP is 130/65 mm Hg, HR is 90 beats per minute, RR is 16 breaths per minute, and oxygen saturation is 97% on room air. Physical examination is unremarkable, except for slurred speech and the smell of acetone on the patient's breath. Laboratory results reveal serum sodium 138 mEq/L, potassium 3.5 mEq/L, chloride 105 mEq/L, bicarbonate 23 mEq/L, BUN 10 mg/dL, creatinine 2.1 mg/dL, glucose 85 mg/dL, arterial blood pH 7.37, and lactate 1.4 mEq/L. Urinalysis shows moderate ketones. Which of the following is the most likely diagnosis?

a. DKA
b. Ethanol intoxication
c. Methanol intoxication
d. Isopropyl alcohol intoxication
e. Ethylene glycol intoxication

**202.** A 55-year-old man presents to the ED 6 hours after ingesting two bottles of his baby aspirin. He complains of nausea, vomiting, dizziness, and tinnitus. His temperature is 100.3°F, BP is 140/80 mm Hg, HR is 105 beats per minute, RR is 31 breaths per minute, and oxygen saturation is 99% on room air. Arterial blood gas on room air reveals a pH of 7.52, $P_{CO_2}$ 10 mm Hg, and $P_{O_2}$ 129 mm Hg. The blood salicylate level returns at 45 mg/dL. Which of the following is the most appropriate next step in management?

a. Administer activated charcoal, begin IV hydration, and administer sodium bicarbonate.
b. Administer activated charcoal, begin IV hydration, and intubate the patient for respiratory failure.
c. Administer activated charcoal, begin IV hydration, and administer NAC.
d. Arrange for immediate hemodialysis.
e. Gastric lavage, IV hydration, and repeat levels before beginning therapy.

**203.** A 40-year-old man with a known history of ethanol abuse states that 2 hours ago he ingested two bottles of extrastrength Tylenol. The patient has no medical complaints except for some nausea. At 4 hours postingestion, you send blood to the laboratory to measure the serum acetaminophen concentration. The level returns and falls above the treatment line when you plot it on the APAP nomogram. You administer activated charcoal and decide to start IV NAC. Which of the following is a known adverse effect of IV NAC administration?

a. Hepatic failure
b. Anaphylactoid reaction
c. Hypertensive crisis
d. Confusion
e. Change in urine color

**204.** A 19-year-old woman presents to the ED with abdominal pain, nausea, vomiting, diarrhea, and hematemesis after ingesting an unknown substance in a suicide attempt. Which of the following antidotes are correctly paired?

a. Organophosphate—Physostigmine
b. Iron overdose—Deferoxamine
c. Aspirin overdose—NAC
d. Acetaminophen overdose—Naloxone
e. Anticholinergic overdose—Fomepizole

**205.** A 34-year-old woman presents to the ED after ingesting an unknown quantity of her antidepressant pills. EMS workers found an empty bottle of amitriptyline on her apartment floor. She is awake but appears delirious. Her BP is 130/65 mm Hg, HR is 101 beats per minute, temperature is 99.1°F, RR is 16 breaths per minute, and oxygen saturation is 100% on room air. On examination, her pupils are 7 mm and reactive. Her face is flushed and mucous membranes are dry. Her lungs are clear and heart is without murmurs. The abdomen is soft, nontender, and with decreased bowel sounds. She is moving all four extremities. ECG reveals sinus rhythm at a rate of 99 and QRS just under 100 milliseconds. In a TCA overdose, which of the following is responsible for her mydriasis, dry mucous membranes, and delirium?

a. Sodium channel blockade
b. Muscarinic receptor blockade
c. Inhibition of serotonin and norepinephrine reuptake
d. Histamine receptor blockade
e. α-Receptor blockade

**206.** You receive notification from EMS that they are bringing in a 17-year-old adolescent boy who was found unconscious by a police officer. The police officer at the scene states that he snuck up on a group of kids that he thought were using drugs. Two of them got away and one just fell to the ground seconds after standing up. Lying on the ground next to the adolescent were plastic bags. The emergency medical technician (EMT) states that the patient was in ventricular fibrillation. He was shocked in the field and is now in a sinus rhythm. The EMT also administered IV dextrose, thiamine, and naloxone without any change in mental status. Which of the following substances was the patient most likely abusing?

a. Butane
b. Ethanol
c. Heroin
d. Cocaine
e. PCP

**207.** A 61-year-old man with a history of depression and hypertension is brought to the ED by EMS for altered mental status. The patient's wife states that he stopped taking his fluoxetine 1 month ago and now only takes metoprolol for his hypertension. The patient's BP is 75/40 mm Hg, HR is 39 beats per minute, RR is 14 breaths per minute, oxygen saturation is 99% on 100% oxygen, and fingerstick glucose is 61 mg/dL. The patient is awake and moaning, responding only to deep stimuli. His extremities are cool to the touch. You suspect an overdose of metoprolol. You endotracheally intubate the patient for airway control. Which of the following is the most appropriate next step in management?

a. Normal saline bolus, administer atropine, administer 1-g calcium gluconate bolus, then insert a transvenous cardiac pacer
b. Put the patient on pacer pads, then administer norepinephrine drip
c. Cardioversion with 200 J, then administer atropine
d. Normal saline bolus, atropine, norepinephrine
e. Normal saline bolus, atropine, glucagon

**208.** A 22-year-old woman presents to the ED by ambulance from a dance club. The paramedics report that the patient was agitated in the club and had a generalized seizure. Her BP is 165/100 mm Hg, HR is 119 beats per minute, temperature is 101.9°F, RR is 17 breaths per minute, oxygen saturation is 98% on room air, and fingerstick glucose is 92 mg/dL. On examination, the patient is hyperactive and appears to be hallucinating. Her pupils are dilated to 6 mm bilaterally and reactive. Her neck is supple. Examination of the heart is unremarkable except for tachycardia. Her lungs are clear and abdomen is soft and nontender. The patient moves all four extremities. Laboratory results are as follows:

Sodium 109 mEq/L          WBC 12,000/mm³
Potassium 3.5 mEq/L       Hct 49%
Chloride 83 mEq/L         Platelets 350/μL
Bicarbonate 20 mEq/L
BUN 10 mg/dL
Creatinine 1 mg/dL
Glucose 103 mg/dL

Which of the following substances did this patient most likely consume?

a. Cocaine
b. Heroin
c. 3,4-Methylenedioxymethamphetamine (MDMA)
d. Ketamine (special K)
e. PCP

**209.** An asymptomatic young adult was brought to the ED by a police officer after his home was raided. The patient swallowed five small packets of an unknown substance before being arrested. His BP is 125/75 mm Hg, HR is 85 beats per minute, temperature is 98.7°F, and RR is 16 breaths per minute. Physical examination is unremarkable. An abdominal radiograph confirms intraluminal small bowel densities. Which of the following is the most appropriate treatment?

a. Magnesium citrate
b. Gastric lavage
c. Activated charcoal and polyethylene glycol
d. Syrup of ipecac
e. NAC

**210.** A 33-year-old woman presents to the ED with a painful sprained ankle. She has a past medical history of depression for which she is taking phenelzine, a monoamine oxidase inhibitor. After you place an elastic wrap on her ankle, she asks you to prescribe her some pain medication. Which of the following medications is contraindicated in patients taking a monoamine oxidase inhibitor?

a. Ibuprofen
b. Acetaminophen
c. Meperidine
d. Oxycodone
e. Hydrocodone

**211.** A 27-year-old woman presents to the ED 6 hours after the onset of body aches, abdominal cramping, and diarrhea. She is currently visiting relatives and normally lives in another state. She regularly takes six to eight tablets daily of hydrocodone for chronic low-back pain, sumatriptan for migraines, and amitriptyline and paroxetine for bulimia nervosa. Her BP is 130/80 mm Hg, HR is 100 beats per minute, temperature is 98.6°F, RR is 16 breaths per minute, and oxygen saturation is 99% on room air. Examination shows diaphoresis, dilated pupils, and piloerection. Neurologically she is moving all four extremities and you do not note tremors. She is alert and cooperative but seems restless. She denies hallucinations or suicidal ideations. She becomes very angry when you ask her for the phone numbers of her regular physicians. Which of the following is the most likely explanation of her symptoms?

a. Anticholinergic overdose
b. TCA intoxication
c. Ethanol withdrawal
d. Serotonin syndrome
e. Opiate withdrawal

# Poisoning and Overdose

## Answers

**182. The answer is c.** *(Rosen, pp 2052-2059.)* The patient drank an **insecticide**. **The two most common classes of compounds are organophosphate compounds** (eg, Malathion) and carbamates (eg, Sevin). These compounds **inhibit acetylcholinesterase**, the enzyme responsible for the breakdown of acetylcholine. The patient is having a "cholinergic crisis." Overstimulation of muscarinic and nicotinic receptors leads to his symptoms, commonly remembered by the mnemonics **SLUDGE** (**s**alivation, **l**acrimation, **u**rination, **d**efecation, **g**astrointestinal [GI] upset, **e**mesis) or **DUMBBELS** (**d**efecation, **u**rination, **m**iosis, **b**ronchospasm, **b**ronchorrhea, **e**mesis, **l**acrimation, **s**alivation). The treatment for organophosphate toxicity is **atropine** and **pralidoxime (2-PAM)**. Atropine is an anticholinergic; therefore it competitively inhibits the excess acetylcholine, both peripherally and in the central nervous system (CNS). The dose of atropine is not limited to 3 mg as it is in advanced cardiac life support (ACLS) guidelines and should be dosed to dry secretions. Pralidoxime works to cause acetylcholinesterase to start working again, which causes acetylcholine levels to go down, reversing the toxicity.

(**a**) Naloxone is used to reverse opiate (eg, heroin) overdoses. (**b**) NAC is used in acetaminophen overdoses. (**d**) Flumazenil is a benzodiazepine antagonist but may lead to seizures. (**e**) Physostigmine is a reversible cholinesterase inhibitor. Its effect is to increase acetylcholine in the pre- and postsynaptic junctions. This will worsen the patient's condition by exacerbating the cholinergic syndrome.

**183. The answer is a.** *(Goldfrank et al, pp 1151-1153.)* **GHB** is a natural neurotransmitter that induces sleep. GHB has been sold as a muscle builder (sleep increases release of growth hormone), a diet aid, and a sleep aid. Patients with GHB overdose generally have a decreased level of consciousness. In contrast to other sedative/hypnotic overdoses, the level of consciousness tends to fluctuate quickly between agitation and depression. A distinctive feature of GHB intoxication is **respiratory depression with**

apnea, interrupted by periods of agitation and combativeness, especially following attempts at intubation.

(b) Diazepam, a benzodiazepine, also depresses mental and respiratory function but typically patients remain sedate. Any respiratory depression from diazepam will occur early in the ingestion. (c) Cocaine is a stimulant that increases HR, BP, and usually causes the pupils to dilate. (d) PCP intoxication may cause bizarre behavior, lethargy, agitation, confusion, or violence. Unlike GHB, this drug acts more as a stimulant than a depressant. (e) Heroin intoxication can cause respiratory depression. Patients usually present with miotic pupils and a decreased respiratory rate and depth.

**184. The answer is d.** (*Rosen, pp 2036-2038.*) The most useful diagnostic test obtainable in a suspected **CO poisoning** is a **COHb level**. Normal levels are less than 5% in nonsmokers as CO is a natural by-product of the metabolism of porphyrins. COHb levels may be slightly more elevated in smokers and those who live in large cities. CO poisoning should be suspected when multiple patients, usually in the same family, present with flu-like symptoms, and were exposed to products of combustion (eg, home heaters/generators). The level may not be elevated if they have not been exposed recently (< 12 hours). This most commonly occurs in colder, winter months. The mainstay of treatment is the delivery of oxygen. Hyperbaric oxygen is usually used for patients with COHb levels greater than 25%. The house in this question should be evaluated by the fire department or a heating and cooling specialist.

(a) Mono spot test can be helpful in detecting acute mononucleosis. Without pharyngitis, lymphadenopathy and given the duration of symptoms, this choice is not likely. (b) CO poisoning is often confused for a viral syndrome. Patients with influenza usually present to the ED with high fever. The duration of symptoms also makes this less likely. (c) Malingering is the intentional production of false or exaggerated symptoms motivated by external incentives. It is unlikely to happen in entire families. (e) Lead toxicity is mainly a disease of children resulting from ingestion of lead-based paints. Adults can be exposed to lead in a variety of occupational circumstances, such as welders, glassmakers, and scrap metal workers. There is no classic presentation of lead toxicity. Therefore, high suspicion and a thorough history are critical. The diagnosis is made by an elevated whole-blood lead level.

**185. The answer is e.** (*Rosen, pp 1948-1952.*) Acetaminophen is one of the most commonly used analgesic-antipyretic medications and causes more hospitalizations after overdose than by any other pharmaceutical agent. It also is the single most common drug that leads to death in overdose. In the case of a single acute ingestion, risk of hepatotoxicity is best established by plotting the acetaminophen concentration on the acetaminophen nomogram. Acetaminophen concentration must be measured between 4 and 24 hours after ingestion and then plotted on the nomogram. Patients with acetaminophen concentrations on or above the treatment line should be treated. This patient has a 4-hour serum acetaminophen concentration of 350 μg/mL. According to the nomogram, at 4 hours any concentration above 150 μg/mL (200 μg/mL outside of the United States) should be treated. Therefore, the **patient should be started on NAC** and **admitted to the hospital**. During her admission, she should be evaluated by a psychiatrist regarding her attempted suicide.

The patient is at risk for acetaminophen toxicity and meets criteria for treatment with NAC. Without treatment with NAC, she is at risk of developing liver failure and possible death. The patient is in first phase of an acetaminophen poisoning. This phase usually lasts 0.5 to 24 hours. Patients are usually asymptomatic or exhibit findings such as nausea, vomiting, anorexia, malaise, and diaphoresis.

In cases of chronic acetaminophen toxicity or with an unknown time of ingestion, the nomogram should not be used.

**186. The answer is b.** (*Rosen, pp 1943-1946.*) The term **toxidrome** refers to **a constellation of physical findings** that can provide important clues in a toxic ingestion. This is particularly useful in patients that cannot provide an adequate history. The **anticholinergic syndrome** typically presents with delirium, mumbling speech, tachycardia, elevated temperature, flushed face, dry mucous membranes and skin, dilated pupils, and hypoactive bowel sounds. The anticholinergic syndrome can be remembered by the phrase "blind as a bat (mydriasis), red as a beet (flushed skin), hot as a hare (hyperthermia secondary to lack of sweating), dry as a bone (dry mucous membranes), and mad as a hatter (mental status changes)."

(**a**) The sympathomimetic syndrome is usually seen after ingestion of cocaine, amphetamines, or decongestants. It typically presents with delirium, paranoia, tachycardia, hypertension, hyperpyrexia, diaphoresis, mydriasis, seizures, and hyperactive bowel sounds. Sympathomimetic and anticholinergic syndromes are frequently difficult to distinguish. The main difference is that sympathomimetics usually cause diaphoresis whereas anticholinergics cause dry skin. (**c**) The cholinergic syndrome is commonly remembered by the mnemonics SLUDGE or DUMBBELS. (**d and e**) Opioids and ethanol are part of the sedative-hypnotic syndrome. It typically presents with sedation, miosis, respiratory depression, hypotension, bradycardia, hypothermia, and decreased bowel sounds.

**187. The answer is c.** (*Goldfrank et al, pp 559-578.*) The patient presents to the ED with central nervous and respiratory depression and miotic pupils. Along with his history of heroin abuse and fresh needle marks, this is most likely a **heroin overdose**. Opioid toxicity is associated with the toxidrome of CNS depression, respiratory depression, and miosis. Attention is always first directed at **airway and breathing management** in emergency medicine. The first action for this patient is to provide oxygen via bag-valve-mask ventilation. Because his respiratory depression is most likely secondary to opioid overdose, an **opioid antagonist** should be administered. **Naloxone** is the antidote most frequently used to reverse opioid toxicity. The goal of naloxone therapy is not necessarily complete arousal; rather, it is to reinstitute adequate spontaneous respiration, while attempting to avoid inducing acute opioid withdrawal. The duration of action for naloxone is between 30 and 60 minutes. A patient like this may need more than one dose. If he does, consideration should be given to a naloxone drip.

(**a**) Theoretically, one can continue bag-valve-mask ventilation until the effects of the drug wear off; however, this is not practical. If the patient overdosed on a long-acting opioid, respiratory depression can last for more than 24 hours. (**b**) Similar to continued bag-valve-mask ventilation, the cause of this patient's respiratory depression is theoretically reversible with the administration of naloxone. If there is a delay to administration of naloxone or it is unsuccessful in restarting his respirations, the patient can be intubated. (**d**) His hypoxia is a result of central respiratory depression. As breathing is composed of both oxygenation and ventilation, administration of oxygen to this patient will mask his hypoventilation. In an otherwise healthy patient, hypoxia will only occur with hypoventilation and should not be addressed by supplemental oxygen without either end-tidal $CO_2$ monitoring or checking a blood gas. (**e**) Activated charcoal should not be administered in patients with CNS depression who are not intubated owing to the risk of emesis and aspiration.

**188. The answer is e.** (*Goldfrank et al, pp 205-206.*) An overdose of any of these agents can lead to seizures. However, **INH** is notorious for causing seizures that are refractory to standard therapy. Marked acidosis and respiratory compromise may also be present. Pyridoxine (vitamin $B_6$) is the treatment of choice for INH overdose. INH is used for the treatment of tuberculosis, which is seen with a greater incidence in patients with AIDS. The pathophysiology of these seizures is complex but related to decreased γ-aminobutyric acid (GABA) synthesis. There are many seizure-inducing substances that may be poorly responsive to benzodiazepines. Some of them include ipecac (a proemetic compound previously recommended for ingestions), camphor, false morel mushrooms (*Gyromitra* species), lindane (scabicide), theophylline (used for refractory chronic obstructive pulmonary disease [COPD]), and caffeine, All of the other substances listed as answer choices should respond to standard therapy with benzodiazepines.

**189. The answer is c.** *(Goldfrank et al, pp 714-723.)* **Glyburide** is a commonly prescribed **sulfonylurea**. Sulfonylureas are oral agents that stimulate the β cells of the pancreas to **secrete insulin**. Many of the sulfonylureas have relatively **long durations of action**. Glyburide can act up to 24 hours after ingestion. Hypoglycemia secondary to sulfonylureas generally **requires hospital admission** to monitor for **recurrent hypoglycemia**. **The antidote to this toxicity is octreotide. High serum glucose levels are what stimulate the pancreas to secrete insulin; therefore glucose boluses are likely to lead to large releases of insulin and a subsequent hypoglycemia.**

(a) Excess insulin is the most common cause of hypoglycemia in patients who present to the ED. Often, the hypoglycemia results from the unintentional overdose of short- or intermediate-acting insulin. After correcting the initial hypoglycemia, a meal and observation are usually enough for patients to be discharged. Very large injections of insulin, such as what can occur in suicide attempts, can lead to recurrent hypoglycemia, but this was not the scenario here. (b) Metformin, a biguanide, acts by increasing peripheral sensitivity to insulin and suppressing gluconeogenesis. Metformin should not produce hypoglycemia. (d) Sitagliptin is in the class of drugs known as dipeptidyl peptidase-4 inhibitors. It should not lead to hypoglycemia. (e) Acarbose is an α-glucosidase inhibitor that acts to decrease GI absorption of carbohydrates. It does not cause hypoglycemia.

**190. The answer is d.** *(Goldfrank et al, pp 508-517.)* The patient most likely ingested **aspirin**. Patients with an acute salicylate overdose may present with nausea, vomiting, tinnitus, fever, diaphoresis, and confusion. Salicylates are capable of producing several types of acid-base disturbances. Acute respiratory alkalosis, without hypoxia, is caused by salicylate stimulation of the respiratory center in the brainstem. The next stage of acid base disorders is a **mixed respiratory alkalosis and metabolic acidosis**. This is because of interference with the Krebs cycle, uncoupling oxidative-phosphorylation, and increased fatty acid metabolism as well as increasing amounts of exogenous acid. The next stage is a metabolic and respiratory acidosis.

The more acidotic the serum becomes, the more the equilibrium shifts toward the protonated form of the salicylate. The protonated form is more lipophilic, crosses the blood-brain barrier, and may lead to seizures. This shift may cause the serum levels to fall but heralds impending collapse. If the patient is hypoxic, salicylate-induced noncardiogenic pulmonary edema should be considered and is one of the indications for dialysis. If these patients need to be intubated, the vent settings must match or exceed the patient's minute ventilation.

(a) Diphenhydramine is a common decongestant that has antihistaminergic and anticholinergic properties. Overdoses may present as an anticholinergic toxidrome, including altered mental status, mydriasis, flushed skin, hyperthermia, and dry mucous membranes. The antihistaminergic properties may cause sedation. (b) Ibuprofen overdose includes GI symptoms (nausea, vomiting, and epigastric pain), mild CNS depression, renal failure and an elevated anion gap acidosis. Most of these effects are seen only in extremely high doses (> 100 mg/kg). (c) APAP overdose usually lacks clinical signs or symptoms in the first 24 hours. Patients may have nonspecific GI complaints. (e) Pseudoephedrine is a commonly used decongestant. An overdose may present with CNS stimulation, hypertension, tachycardia, and dysrhythmias.

**191. The answer is c.** *(Rosen, pp 1943-1944.)* The **sympathomimetic syndrome** usually is seen after acute abuse of cocaine, amphetamines, or decongestants. Patients are usually **hypertensive** and **tachycardic** and exhibit **mydriatic pupils**. In massive overdoses, cardiovascular collapse can result in shock and wide-complex dysrhythmias. CNS effects include seizures. Sympathomimetic syndrome is sometimes difficult to distinguish from anticholinergic syndrome. The difference is that patients usually present with dry mucous membranes with an anticholinergic overdose, whereas patients are **diaphoretic** with sympathomimetics.

(a) The anticholinergic syndrome typically presents with delirium, mumbling speech, tachycardia, elevated temperature, flushed face, dry mucous membranes and skin, dilated pupils, and hypoactive bowel sounds. **(b)** The cholinergic syndrome is commonly remembered by the mnemonics SLUDGE or DUMBBELS. **(d)** Opioids typically present with sedation, miosis, respiratory depression, hypotension, bradycardia, hypothermia, and decreased bowel sounds. **(e)** Sedative hypnotic toxidrome is characterized by a relatively normal set of vitals and a normal examination except for CNS depression.

**192. The answer is b.** (*Goldfrank et al, pp 90-100.*) A major change has occurred in the approach of GI decontamination over the past decade. Previous recommendations indicated that the stomach should be emptied by either syrup of ipecac or by gastric lavage. Ipecac is not recommended at all and gastric lavage is only recommended in patients who present early and symptomatic from an otherwise difficult-to-treat overdose. Activated charcoal alone has demonstrated similar or superior results and now is the recommended GI decontaminant. For certain compounds (carbamazepine, dapsone, theophylline, quinine, and phenobarbital), multiple doses of charcoal are recommended because of enterohepatic and enteroenteric recirculation. The complications of gastric emptying procedures, primarily aspiration, are largely avoided when only activated charcoal is used provided that the patient is awake enough to drink the charcoal. Repeated doses of sorbitol are not recommended. Most ingested drugs and chemicals are adsorbed to activated charcoal. The few agents that do not adsorb to charcoal include **ions** (eg, mineral acids and alkalis, lithium, borates, bromides), **hydrocarbons (HCs)**, **metals** (eg, iron), **alcohols** (eg, methanol, ethanol, and isopropanol) and **caustics (acids and bases)**.

The patient in question ingested **carbamazepine** that is used to treat her bipolar disorder. A carbamazepine level should be drawn and management-decided based on those results. Potential treatments include whole-bowel irrigation, multidose charcoal, dialysis, and charcoal hemoperfusion.

**193. The answer is e.** (*Goldfrank et al, pp 1095-1097; Rosen, pp 1997-1999.*) **Benzodiazepines (eg, diazepam)** should be used as the first-line agent for nearly all cocaine toxicities. Many effects of cocaine are thought to be mediated through CNS stimulation by the release or inhibiting the reuptake of catecholamines. The effects that acute cocaine intoxication has on the heart include coronary vasoconstriction with increasing myocardial oxygen demand. Benzodiazepines restore the CNS inhibitory tone on the peripheral nervous system. The use of β-adrenergic antagonists should be avoided with acute cocaine toxicity because of unopposed α-adrenergic receptor stimulation and coronary artery vasoconstriction. (a) Although haloperidol can be used for sedation, its anticholinergic and proseizure effects can limit cooling by impeding diaphoresis and may increase morbidity. (b and c) It is best to avoid β-adrenergic antagonists in the setting of cocaine intoxication. Their use leads to unopposed α-adrenergic stimulation that results in vasoconstriction. Although labetalol is an α- and β-adrenergic receptor blocker, it has substantially more β-adrenergic antagonism than α-adrenergic antagonist effects and is still not recommended as first-line treatment for this patient. (d) Calcium channel blockers are not recommended for the treatment of cocaine induced chest pain.

**194. The answer is d.** (*Rosen, pp 2048-2050.*) **Opioid withdrawal** initially presents with drug craving, yawning, rhinorrhea, and **piloerection**, and progresses to nausea, vomiting, diarrhea, hyperactive bowels, diaphoresis, myalgias, arthralgias, anxiety, fear, and mild tachycardia. **Methadone withdrawal** starts approximately 24 hours after the last dose and persists for 3 to 7 days. Heroin withdrawal begins about 6 hours after the last dose and usually fully manifests at 24 hours. Opioid withdrawal is not a life-threatening condition as long as adequate hydration and nutritional support are maintained. (a) Ethanol withdrawal is a life-threatening condition that develops 6 to 24 hours after the reduction of ethanol intake. It is characterized by autonomic hyperactivity, including nausea, anorexia, coarse tremor, tachycardia, hypertension, hyperreflexia, sleep disturbances, hallucinations, and seizure. To meet the definition of being in "DTs," the patient must be both delirious and tremulous. Treatment for this withdrawal state is benzodiazepines and very large doses may be required. (b) When cocaine use is stopped or when a binge ends, a crash follows almost immediately. This is accompanied by a strong craving for more cocaine, fatigue, lack of pleasure, anxiety, irritability, sleepiness, and sometimes agitation or extreme suspicion. Patients withdrawing from cocaine may be extremely difficult to wake up. (c) Nicotine withdrawal manifests largely as cigarette craving and subjective dysphoric symptoms. There are some symptoms of irritability and restlessness. (e) Discontinuation of clonidine leads to hypertension, headache, flushing, sweating, hallucinations, anxiety, and reflex tachycardia.

There is no piloerection in these patients and this is usually over within 24 hours.

**195. The answer is d.** (*Goldfrank et al, pp 1191-1198; Rosen, pp 2014-2016.*) **PCP intoxication** is characterized by a wide spectrum of findings. Behavior may be bizarre, agitated, confused, or violent. The hallmark of PCP toxicity is the **recurring delusion of superhuman strength and invulnerability** resulting from both the anesthetic and dissociative properties of the drug. Patients have broken police handcuffs, fracturing bones in doing so. The major cause of death or injury from PCP is behavioral toxicity leading to suicide and provoked homicide. Typical neurologic signs include **nystagmus** (horizontal, vertical, or rotary), ataxia, and altered gait. Pupils are usually midsized and reactive but can be mydriatic or miotic. Bizarre posturing, grimacing, and writhing may be seen. Management is conservative. To prevent self-injury, the patient must be safely restrained. Antipsychotics or benzodiazepines are frequently administered for chemical sedation. PCP intoxication usually ranges from 8 to 16 hours but can last longer in chronic users.

(**a**) Cocaine and amphetamines are sympathomimetics that can be confused with PCP intoxication. However, the hallmark to PCP intoxication that is not usually observed in sympathomimetic intoxication is the recurring delusion of superhuman strength and nystagmus. (**b**) When cocaine use is stopped or when a binge ends, a crash follows almost immediately. This is accompanied by a strong craving for more cocaine, fatigue, lack of pleasure, anxiety, irritability, sleepiness, and sometimes agitation or extreme suspicion. (**c**) While in the anticholinergic toxidrome, there may be an altered mental status and tachycardia, nystagmus is not classically associated with the anticholinergic toxidrome. Additionally, the skin would be dry. (**e**) Opioid withdrawal initially presents with drug craving, yawning, rhinorrhea, and piloerection, and progresses to nausea, vomiting, diarrhea, hyperactive bowel, diaphoresis, myalgias, arthralgias, anxiety, fear, and mild tachycardia.

**196. The answer is a.** (*Goldfrank et al, pp 1605-1612.*) An **anion gap** is the difference between unmeasured anions (eg, proteins, organic acids) and unmeasured cations (eg, potassium, calcium, magnesium). The anion gap can be calculated from the formula:

$$\text{Anion gap} = [Na^+] - [HCO_3^- + Cl^-]$$

The normal anion gap is approximately 6 to 10 mEq/L. The cause of increased anion gap is frequently remembered by the mnemonic **MUD PILES**:

| | |
|---|---|
| **M:** methanol, metformin | **P:** paraldehyde |
| **U:** uremia | **I:** iron, INH |
| **D:** DKA | **L:** lactate |
| | **E:** ethylene glycol, ethanol |
| | **S:** salicylate |

Our patient's anion gap is $(141) - (101 + 14) = 26$.

The **measured serum osmolarity** performed by the laboratory is measured by a depression in the freezing point or an elevation in the boiling point of the solution. If there is an increase in low-molecular-weight molecules, such as acetone, methanol, ethanol, mannitol, isopropyl alcohol, or ethylene glycol, the osmolarity increases more than what is calculated from the regular serum molecules.

The formula to calculate serum osmolarity is

$$Serum\ Osm\ (mOsm/kg) = 2[Na^+] + glucose/18 + BUN/1.8 + EtOH/4.6$$

The difference between the actual measured osmolarity and the calculated osmolarity is the **osmol gap (measure − calculated)**.

Our patient's osmol gap is $(352) - (292) = 60$. When the osmol gap is greater than 50 mOsm/L, it should be considered nearly diagnostic of **toxic alcohol** ingestion. However, a normal or even negative osmol gap does not exclude the presence of toxic alcohols.

The patient's clinical presentation of altered mental status, anion gap metabolic acidosis, and osmol gap is consistent with toxic alcohol ingestion. In this case, the ingested substance was methanol.

**197. The answer is b.** (*Goldfrank et al, pp 1049-1057; Rosen, pp 1964-1969.*) For young patients with altered mental status, toxic ingestion should be high on the differential. This clinical scenario is most consistent with toxic ingestion of a **TCA**. Treatment of all toxic ingestions should begin with assessment of airway, breathing, and circulation. As a result this patient's obtunded mental status and loss of gag reflex, **orotracheal intubation** is indicated for airway protection. Subsequently, **activated charcoal** can be administered but is not likely going to affect the outcome in this already very symptomatic patient. In an obtunded patient, it is important to first secure an airway prior to administering charcoal to prevent aspiration in the event of vomiting.

Acute cardiovascular toxicity is responsible for most of the mortalities from TCA overdose. The characteristic features are conduction delays, dysrhythmias, and hypotension. The sodium-blocking activity of TCAs leads to a widened QRS and rightward axis. It is believed that there is an increased chance of cardiac dysrhythmias if the QRS is greater than 100 milliseconds. It is recommended that you treat this condition with IV **sodium bicarbonate** until the QRS narrows to 100 milliseconds or the serum pH increases to 7.55. In addition, the patient is hypotensive and should receive a fluid bolus of normal saline and be placed in Trendelenburg position. If the hypotension does not resolve after these maneuvers and administration of bicarbonate, the patient should receive norepinephrine. TCA overdose may progress rapidly and while frequently difficult to predict, most fatalities occur before 4 to 6 hours of the onset of hypotension. It is common for a patient to present to the ED awake and alert and then develop life-threatening cardiovascular and CNS toxicity within a couple of hours.

(a) Narcan is the antidote for opioid toxicity; this patient requires sodium bicarbonate for a TCA overdose. Additionally, you should not give naloxone to an intubated patient. (c) NAC is the antidote for acetaminophen overdose. (d) Syrup of ipecac cannot be administered to a patient who is intubated and is not recommended generally. (e) Inducing vomiting is contraindicated given the potential for precipitous neurologic and hemodynamic deterioration.

**198. The answer is a.** (*Goldfrank et al, pp 500-507.*) **NAC** is the cornerstone of therapy for the potentially lethal acetaminophen overdose. NAC acts as a glutathione regenerator to reduce NAPQI (*N*-acetyl-*p*-benzoquinoneimine), the most toxic metabolite of acetaminophen. It can be administered orally or intravenously. NAC is most effective if administered within 8 hours of the ingestion; however, it may still be of benefit if given more than 24 hours after an acute acetaminophen overdose.

(b) Physostigmine is used for an anticholinergic overdose. (c) Flumazenil is a benzodiazepine antagonist used occasionally in a benzodiazepine overdose. Its use can precipitate benzodiazepine withdrawal and seizures in chronic benzodiazepine users. (d) Naloxone is a μ-receptor antagonist and is used in opioid overdoses. (e) Digibind is the antidote for digitalis glycoside poisoning.

**199. The answer is b.** (*Rosen, pp 2003-2007.*) **Ethylene glycol** is a colorless, odorless, slightly sweet-tasting liquid that is found in some antifreeze compounds. Ingestions of antifreeze are either accidental, suicidal, or in substitute of ethanol. Ethylene glycol is metabolized to glycolic acid, which results in a profound **anion gap metabolic acidosis** (Na) − ([Cl] + [HCO$_3$⁻]); (139 − [101 + 14]) = 24. Glycolic acid is subsequently metabolized to oxalic acid, which combines with calcium to form calcium oxalate crystals, which then precipitate in renal tubules, brain, and other tissues. The finding of **crystalluria** is considered the **hallmark of ethylene glycol ingestion**; however, its absence does not rule out the diagnosis. Another test that can be done in the ED involves examining freshly voided urine for fluorescence with a Wood lamp. Sodium fluorescein is added to most antifreeze products to aid in the detection of radiator leaks. This test may not be positive if the ingestion was not recent (< 4 hours). Ingestion of ethylene glycol is associated with neurologic, cardiopulmonary, and renal abnormalities.

(a) Ibuprofen can cause an elevated gap acidosis but would not give you crystalluria and should give you some GI symptoms or renal insufficiency in doses that would give you this degree of acidosis. (c) DKA can cause a metabolic acidosis. Patients usually have a history of diabetes, elevated blood glucose (> 200 mg/dL), and ketones in their urine. (d) Lactic acidosis can cause a metabolic acidosis. This patient's lactate is within normal limits. (e) Isopropyl alcohol (rubbing alcohol) is less toxic than methanol and ethylene glycol but more toxic than ethanol. Patients typically present with CNS depression. Isopropanol also causes a hemorrhagic gastritis. Unlike the other toxic alcohols, it is not usually associated with a high anion gap metabolic acidosis.

**200. The answer is e.** (*Goldfrank et al, pp 1658-1667.*) **CO poisoning** is the leading cause of poisoning morbidity and mortality in the United States. People are exposed to CO through fires, vehicle exhaust, home generators, and the metabolism of methylene chloride. Workers also become symptomatic from use of propane-powered equipment indoors, such as forklifts and ice skating resurfaces. Often, other people in the area have similar complaints. The earliest symptoms are nonspecific and readily confused with other illnesses such as viral syndromes. Mild symptoms include headache, nausea, and dizziness. Severe symptoms include chest pain, palpitations, and seizures. Diagnosis is made by detecting elevated CO in the blood. Normal levels range from 0% to 5%, while smokers may be as high as 10%. Treatment includes immediate oxygen therapy. Hyperbaric oxygen is the treatment of choice for patients with significant CO exposures.

(a) Methemoglobinemia occurs from exposures to nitrates, certain anesthetics, and various medications. Patients typically present cyanotic with a normal $PO_2$. They will typically be asymptomatic until levels are very high (> 25%). While patients with methemoglobinemia will have a low pulse ox, this patient does not have a source. (b) Hypoglycemia can cause syncope. However, this patient's blood glucose was normal. (c) Hydrocarbon poisoning (eg, kerosene, gasoline, nail polish remover) typically occurs from an intentional exposure. The pulmonary and CNS systems are most commonly affected. Certain hydrocarbons can lead to sudden death from oversensitization of the myocardium to catecholamines. This condition is sometimes called "sudden sniffing death." (d) Opioid overdose causes sedation and respiratory depression. In an otherwise healthy patient, this degree of hypoxia, if from an opioid, should have a respiratory acidosis.

**201. The answer is d.** (*Rosen, pp 2007-2009.*) **Isopropyl alcohol** is one of the **toxic alcohols** (ethylene glycol, methanol, and isopropyl alcohol). It is a clear, colorless liquid with a **bitter taste**. It is commonly used as a **rubbing alcohol** and as a solvent in haircare products, skin lotion, and home aerosols. Moreover, it is often ingested as an inexpensive and convenient substitute for ethanol. Clinically, GI and CNS complaints predominate. Its GI irritant properties cause patients to complain of abdominal pain, nausea, and vomiting. Pupillary size varies but miosis is commonly observed. Large ingestions can result in coma. Hypotension, although rare, signifies severe poisoning. Characteristically, metabolic acidosis, unlike the other **toxic alcohols**, is not present. This is because isopropyl alcohol is metabolized to **acetone**, a ketone, not an acid. It is also the cause for the presence of urinary ketones and the odor on the patient's breath. Isopropyl alcohol intoxication is often remembered by **ketosis without acidosis**. Another unique finding is the presence of "pseudo renal failure" or isolated false elevation of creatinine with a normal BUN. This results from interference of acetone and acetoacetate by the colorimetric method used to measure the creatinine level.

(a) If the patient had a history of diabetes with an elevated blood sugar and ketones present in the urine, DKA would be highly suspected. (b) Differentiating between ethanol and isopropyl alcohol ingestion can be very difficult. However, the patient's clinical presentation of drinking a bitter liquid, abdominal pain, nausea, vomiting, odor of acetone, and ketosis without acidosis is most consistent with isopropyl alcohol intoxication. (c and e) Methanol and ethylene glycol intoxications are typically associated with an anion gap metabolic acidosis.

**202. The answer is a.** *(Rosen, pp 1954-1956.)* The treatment of **salicy-late toxicity** has three objectives: (1) prevent further salicylate absorption, (2) correct fluid deficits and acid-base abnormalities, and (3) reduce tissue salicylate concentrations by increasing excretion. **Activated charcoal** should be administered as soon as possible to reduce salicylate absorption. Dehydration occurs early in salicylate intoxication and should be treated with **IV hydration**. **Sodium bicarbonate** alkalizes both the serum and, with some effort, the urine. Because salicylic acid is a weak acid, it is ionized in an alkaline environment and gets "trapped," limiting the amount that crosses the blood-brain barrier and increasing urinary excretion. **Serum alkalization** is done to keep the salicylic acid out of the brain and **urine alkalization** is done to keep the salicylate in the urine (prevent reabsorption in the distal tubule and collecting duct). Alkalization should be considered in patients with salicylate levels greater than 30 mg/dL. This is performed by administering IV sodium bicarbonate to maintain a serum pH between 7.45 and 7.55 and a urine pH greater than 7.5. Potassium supplementation is usually needed to achieve urinary alkalization.

(**b**) Endotracheal intubation may be necessary in respiratory failure; however, in a salicylate-poisoned patient, it is important to maintain or exceed the patient's minute ventilation. An alkaline serum is needed to keep salicylic acid ionized, which limits it from crossing the blood-brain barrier. It is difficult to maintain an appropriate level of hypocarbia and hyperventilation through assisted ventilation. (**c**) NAC is the antidote for APAP poisoning. It is important, however, to obtain an APAP and salicylate level in every overdose patient because they are common, deadly, and treatable. (**d**) Hemodialysis for aspirin overdose should be done in patients with severe salicylism associated with serum salicylate levels greater than 100 mg/dL; coma, renal, or liver failure; and pulmonary edema in levels less than 100 mg/dL with severe acid-base disturbances or the failure to respond to more conservative treatments such as activated charcoal and alkalization. (**e**) Gastric lavage is not recommended here. Gastric lavage should be done on intubated patients and that is something you want to avoid in salicylate toxicity. There is no need to repeat any levels before beginning therapy on this patient.

**203. The answer is b.** *(Rosen, pp 1948-1952.)* IV NAC has been responsible for **anaphylactoid reactions, including rash, bronchospasm, hypotension,** and **death**. These complications are dose and concentration dependent and are prevented by slow administration of dilute NAC. Some other side effects include GI disorders, tachycardia, and chest tightness. These are not seen with oral administration of NAC.

(a) NAC is used in the treatment of hepatic failure secondary to APAP overdose. (c and d) IV NAC is not known to cause these side effects. (e) Amitriptyline, indomethacin, doxorubicin, phenazopyridine, and rifampin are some medications known to cause urine to change color.

**204. The answer is b.** *(Rosen, pp 2019-2021.)* **Deferoxamine** is a specific chelator of **ferric iron (Fe$^{3+}$)**. It binds with iron to form a water-soluble compound, ferrioxamine, which can be excreted by the kidneys. Deferoxamine has a half-life of 1 hour, so continuous infusion is the preferred method of administration.

The patient's clinical presentation is consistent with **acute iron poisoning**. Initial presentation reflects the corrosive effects of iron on the gut and includes nausea, vomiting, diarrhea, and sometimes GI bleeding. Patients with severe overdose may present with shock or coma. In acute iron toxicity, there can be a brief quiescent period when the patient feels better.

Deferoxamine can cause hypotension; therefore correction of the patient's lost fluid from vomiting and diarrhea should be done quickly when deferoxamine is considered.

(a) The treatment for organophosphate toxicity is atropine and pralidoxime. Physostigmine is an antidote for the anticholinergic syndrome. (c) Aspirin overdose is treated with decontamination, alkalinization, and sometimes dialysis. NAC is the antidote for APAP overdose. (d) Flumazenil is a benzodiazepine antagonist but should not be given to adults without the understanding that any resulting seizures may be resistant to benzodiazepines and may require phenobarbital. Narcan is the antidote for opioid overdose. (e) Anticholinergic overdose can be treated with physostigmine. Fomepizole is the treatment for toxic alcohol ingestion (eg, ethylene glycol).

**205. The answer is b.** *(Goldfrank et al, pp 1049-1057; Rosen, pp 1964-1969.)* Overdose of **TCA** results in toxicity by a number of different mechanisms. The **anticholinergic properties** of TCAs result in the toxidrome "blind as a bat (mydriasis), red as a beet (flushed skin), hot as a hare (hyperthermia secondary to lack of sweating), dry as a bone (dry mucous membranes), mad as a hatter (mental status changes)." This toxidrome reflects the peripheral and central **muscarinic receptor blockade**. The cardinal signs of TCA overdose include ventricular dysrhythmias, hypotension, and decreased mental status.

(a) The most worrisome effect of TCAs is sodium channel blockade causing conduction delays and dysrhythmias as evidenced by QRS widening and wide-complex tachycardias. **Sodium bicarbonate** is a potentially lifesaving intervention in TCA overdose because an alkaline pH combined with a sodium load increases conductance through cardiac fast sodium channels and prevents ventricular dysrhythmias as evidenced by narrowing of the QRS complex on an ECG. The sodium channel blockade does not cause mydriasis, dry mucous membranes, and delirium. (c) Inhibition of serotonin and norepinephrine reuptake can cause hypertension and tachycardia acutely, and may contribute some to the mydriasis but should not affect the mucous membranes or delirium. (d) Histamine receptor blockade is associated with sedation. (e) α-Receptor blockade causes vasodilation, which causes a decrease in systemic vascular resistance. Hypotension, widened pulse pressure, and tachycardia result.

**206. The answer is a.** (*Rosen, pp 773, 2027-2030.*) **Hydrocarbons (HCs)** are a diverse group of organic compounds that contain hydrogen and carbon. Some common products containing HCs are household polishes, glues, paint remover, and industrial solvents. Acute HC toxicity usually affects three main target organs: the lungs, CNS, and heart. The lungs are most commonly affected by aspiration of ingested HCs. Pulmonary toxicity is associated with cough, crackles, bronchospasm, pulmonary edema, and pneumonitis on chest radiograph. Certain HCs (eg, toluene, benzene, gasoline, butane, chlorinated HCs) can have sedative/opioid-like effect and cause euphoria, disinhibition, confusion, and obtundation. HCs can also cause **sudden cardiac death**, particularly after sudden physical activity after intentional inhalation. It is thought that the HCs produce **myocardial sensitization** of endogenous and exogenous catecholamines, which precipitates ventricular dysrhythmias and myocardial dysfunction. One scenario is the solvent-abusing person. EMS workers often describe an individual who has used inhaled solvents, performed some type of physical activity, and then suddenly collapsed.

In the this scenario, the patient inhaling **butane** was approached by a police officer and tried to run away. This sudden exertion most likely led to a cardiac dysrhythmia. Paraphernalia is often found at the scene, including plastic bags used for "bagging" (pouring HCs in a bag, then deeply inhaling) or a HC-soaked cloth used for "huffing" (inhaling through a saturated cloth). Other paraphernalia includes gasoline containers, multiple butane lighters, and spray paint cans.

(b) Ethanol intoxication typically does not lead to ventricular fibrillation. (c) In patients with heroin overdose who become hypoxic, ventricular fibrillation is possible. However, in this scenario the patient's mental status did not change in response to naloxone, the reversal agent for opioids. (d) Cocaine intoxication may lead to ventricular fibrillation due to its cardiac affects; however, this scenario is more consistent with hydrocarbon abuse. (e) PCP generally does not lead to cardiac dysrhythmias.

**207. The answer is e.** (*Goldfrank et al, pp 896-906; Rosen, pp 1982-1985.*) β-Adrenergic receptor blockers (eg, Metoprolol) are commonly prescribed medications for hypertension. β-Adrenergic antagonist overdose is often benign, with about 33% of patients remaining asymptomatic. This is partially explained by the fact that β-adrenergic antagonism is often well tolerated in healthy persons who do not rely on sympathetic stimulation to maintain cardiac output. Conversely, those with cardiac abnormalities may rely on sympathetic stimulation to maintain HR or cardiac output. Selectivity and specificity are lost in overdose situations leading to systemic toxicity. The **hallmark of β-adrenergic receptor blocker toxicity is bradycardia with hypotension, cold extremities, and a low blood sugar.** Patients may also exhibit conduction and rhythm abnormalities. Onset of toxicity usually occurs within 4 hours of ingestion. If an adult remains asymptomatic after 6 hours, there is a low risk for subsequent morbidity unless a delayed-release preparation is involved.

Other drug classes that can cause bradycardia with hypotension include the central $\alpha_2$-agonists (eg, clonidine), calcium channel blockers (CCBs), and digoxin. β-Blockers usually have cooler extremities due to $\beta_2$-blockade in the periphery and unopposed $\alpha_1$-stimulation both of which lead to vasoconstriction. CCB patients have warm extremities because they lack the ability to vasoconstrict. Additionally, CCB patients are more likely to have elevated glucose measurements because calcium channels are needed for insulin release in the pancreas.

Management begins with addressing the ABCs. Airway and ventilation should be maintained with endotracheal intubation if necessary. The initial treatment of hypotension and bradycardia consists of **fluid resuscitation** and **atropine**. Whole-bowel irrigation should be considered in patients who have ingested sustained-release preparations. Patients with significant toxicity (HR < 40, BP < 80, congestive heart failure [CHF], altered mental status) should also receive **glucagon**, which does not rely on β-receptors for its actions and has both inotropic and chronotropic effects. It also helps counteract the hypoglycemia induced by β-blocker overdose. It is not unreasonable to think about transvenous and transcutaneous pacing early in these overdoses.

(a) This is an acceptable initial treatment for a calcium channel blocker, not a β-blocker. (b) While it might be reasonable to put the patient on pacer pads, atropine and glucagon are the first two lines of therapy for this patient. (c) Cardioversion is contraindicated in sinus rhythm. It is reserved for "shockable" rhythms such as ventricular fibrillation and pulseless ventricular tachycardia. (d) This selection may be attempted if the glucagon is ineffective and the patient continues to decompensate. Vasopressors such as norepinephrine are likely not going to help in severe β-blocker toxicity and may only serve to further decrease perfusion by increasing peripheral vascular resistance.

**208. The answer is c.** *(Goldfrank et al, pp 1078-1085.)* **MDMA** is currently one of the most widely abused **amphetamines** by college students and teenagers. It is commonly known as "ecstasy," "E," "XTC," and "M&M." MDMA is an entactogen, a substance capable of producing euphoria, inner peace, and a desire to socialize. Negative effects include ataxia, restlessness, confusion, poor concentration, and memory problems. MDMA, although classified as an amphetamine, is also a potent stimulus for the release of serotonin. MDMA can also cause significant **hyponatremia**. The increase in serotonin results in the excessive release of vasopressin (antidiuretic hormone [ADH]). Moreover, large free-water intake (increased thirst) combined with sodium loss from physical exertion (dancing) certainly contributes to the development of hyponatremia.

(a) Cocaine use can cause agitation and seizures but should not cause significant hyponatremia. (b) Heroin intoxication usually causes people to be more sedate rather than agitated. It should not cause seizures or hyponatremia. (d and e) Ketamine and PCP can cause agitation and hallucinations; however, significant hyponatremia is not usually present.

**209. The answer is c.** *(Goldfrank et al, pp 48-49, 1103-1106.)* Patients who swallow bags of drugs can be classified into two large categories. "**Body packers" are people who transport large amounts of drugs in very tightly wrapped packages.** This takes planning and is not done as the police are raiding. "Packers," if symptomatic, may need to go to the OR. Cocaine can lead to bowel perforation. Patients being arrested who swallow illicit drugs to conceal the evidence are referred to as "body stuffers." They commonly tend to ingest any and all the drugs they possess, potentially resulting in a polypharmaceutic overdose. Body stuffers are usually seen in the ED before symptoms have developed. **Activated charcoal** should be administered immediately and **whole-bowel irrigation** may be indicated. Sometimes there is radiographic evidence of the swallowed substances as seen in crack vials or staples on the packaging materials. Whole-bowel irrigation uses a **polyethylene glycol electrolyte solution (eg, GoLYTELY)**, which is not absorbed and flushes drugs or chemicals through the GI tract. This procedure seems to be most useful when radiopaque tablets or chemicals, swallowed packets of street drugs, or sustained-released drugs have been ingested.

(a) Magnesium citrate is a cathartic whose action begins 4 to 6 hours after ingestion. It is contraindicated in patients with renal failure. (b) Gastric lavage is not indicated for this patient. (d) Syrup of ipecac is also ineffective for the packets in the small bowel. (e) NAC is the antidote for acetaminophen toxicity.

**210. The answer is c.** (*Goldfrank et al, pp 1974-1976.*) Any patient taking a monoamine oxidase inhibitor (MAOI) is at risk for developing the **serotonin syndrome** if the individual congests a selective serotonin reuptake inhibitor (SSRI) or another drug that raises CNS serotonin levels. Some medications that can cause this interaction include indirect-acting and mixed-acting sympathomimetics (eg, cocaine, amphetamine), antidepressants (eg, TCA, SSRI), **meperidine (eg, Demerol)**, and dextromethorphan, which is found in many nonprescription antitussives. In contrast, morphine and its derivatives lack serotonin-potentiating effects. Serotonin syndrome is characterized by altered mental status, hyperthermia, neuromuscular dysfunction, and autonomic dysfunction. Symptoms may also include hyperreflexia, clonus (more in the lower extremities), shivering, trismus, akathisia, coma, and seizures.

(a, b, d, and e) Ibuprofen, acetaminophen, oxycodone, and hydrocodone are all safe to use in patients taking MAOIs.

**211. The answer is e.** (*Rosen, pp 2048-2050.*) Hydrocodone is an opioid used for pain relief. **Opioid withdrawal** occurs in tolerant individuals when opioid exposure is discontinued or an antagonist is administered. The effects of withdrawal are secondary to **increased sympathetic discharge**, which is responsible for the clinical signs and symptoms. Although these can be significant, they are typically not life threatening. Withdrawal is associated with CNS excitation, tachypnea, and mydriasis. Pulse and BP may be elevated. The patient may present with nausea, vomiting, diarrhea, abdominal cramps, myalgias, and insomnia. Examination often reveals **piloerection**, yawning, lacrimation, rhinorrhea, and diaphoresis. Neurologic manifestations include restlessness, agitation, and anxiety, but cognition and mental status are unaffected. Dysphoria and drug craving are usually prominent. This withdrawal state is uncomfortable but not life threatening.

(a and b) Amitriptyline is a TCA that has anticholinergic properties. Overdose of TCAs results in toxicity by a number of different mechanisms. The anticholinergic properties of TCAs results in the toxidrome "blind as a bat (mydriasis), red as a beet (flushed skin), hot as a hare (hyperthermia secondary to lack of sweating), dry as a bone (dry mucous membranes)." The cardinal signs of TCA overdose include ventricular dysrhythmias, hypotension, and decreased mental status. (c) Early alcohol withdrawal may occur 6 hours after cessation or decrease in alcohol consumption. It is characterized by autonomic hyperactivity: nausea, anorexia, coarse tremor, tachycardia, hyperreflexia, hypertension, fever, decreased seizure threshold, hallucinations, and delirium. (d) Serotonin syndrome occurs when a serotonin reuptake inhibitor is combined with another drug that potentiates serotonin. The opioid meperidine (Demerol), but not hydrocodone, is known to potentiate serotonin. It presents with abdominal pain, diarrhea, diaphoresis, hyperpyrexia, tachycardia, hypertension, myoclonus, irritability, agitation, seizures, and delirium. While sumatriptan is a medication that acts on serotonin receptors, they are not the receptors responsible for serotonin syndrome.

# Altered Mental Status

## Questions

**212.** A 69-year-old woman with a past medical history of hypertension, hypercholesterolemia, diabetes mellitus type 1, and alcohol abuse is brought to the emergency department (ED) by her daughter who states that her mom has been acting funny over the last hour. She states that the patient did not know where she was despite being in her own house. She also did not recognize her family and was speaking incomprehensibly. Her blood pressure (BP) is 150/80 mm Hg, heart rate (HR) is 90 beats per minute, temperature is 98.9°F, and her respiratory rate (RR) is 16 breaths per minute. On physical examination she is diaphoretic, agitated, and tremulous. Electrocardiogram (ECG) is sinus rhythm with normal ST segments and T waves. Which of the following is the most appropriate course of action for this patient?

a. Administer a benzodiazepine to treat her ethanol withdrawal.
b. Activate the stroke team and bring the patient directly to the computed tomographic (CT) scanner.
c. Get a stat fingerstick and administer dextrose if her blood sugar is low.
d. Request a psychiatric consult for probable sundowning.
e. Administer haloperidol for sedation.

**213.** A 74-year-old lethargic woman is brought to the ED by her family. Her daughter states that the patient has been progressively somnolent over the last week and could not be woken up today. The patient takes medications for diabetes, hypertension, hypothyroidism, and a recent ankle sprain, which is treated with a hydrocodone/acetaminophen combination. In the ED, the patient is profoundly lethargic, responsive only to pain, and has periorbital edema and delayed relaxation of the deep tendon reflexes. Her BP is 145/84 mm Hg, HR is 56 beats per minute, temperature is 94.8°F, and RR is 12 breaths per minute. Which of the following is the most likely diagnosis?

a. Hypoglycemia
b. Opioid overdose
c. Stroke
d. Myxedema coma
e. Depression

**214.** A 79-year-old man presents to the ED by paramedics with the chief complaint of agitation and confusion over the previous 12 hours. He has a past medical history of schizophrenia and is not taking any of his antipsychotics. His BP is 135/85 mm Hg, HR is 119 beats per minute, RR is 18 breaths per minute, oxygen saturation is 97% on room air, and fingerstick glucose is 135 mg/dL. Because of his agitation at triage, he was placed in wrist restraints. At this time, he is calm but confused. Examination reveals warm and clammy skin and 4-mm pupils that are equal and reactive. His cardiac examination reveals tachycardia and no murmurs. His lungs are clear to auscultation and his abdomen is soft and nontender. He is able to move all of his extremities. Which of the following is the most appropriate next step in management?

a. Administer haloperidol or lorazepam.
b. Consult psychiatry.
c. Order a CT scan of his head.
d. Send a urine toxicologic screen.
e. Obtain a rectal temperature.

**215.** A 25-year-old man is brought to the ED by emergency medical service (EMS) accompanied by his girlfriend who reports that the patient had a seizure 30 minutes ago and is still confused. The girlfriend reports that the patient is a known epileptic who has been doing well on his latest medication regimen. The exact seizure medications are unknown. On arrival to the ED, the patient develops continuous clonic movements of his upper and lower extremities. The patient's vital signs are BP of 162/85 mm Hg, HR of 110 beats per minute, and pulse oximetry of 91% on room air. Capillary glucose level is 95 mg/dL. Which of the following is the most appropriate next step in management?

a. Place the patient in a lateral decubitus position.
b. Administer lorazepam.
c. Administer phenytoin.
d. Perform rapid sequence intubation on the patient.
e. Look up the patient's medical records and administer his current antiepileptic regimen.

**216.** A 19-year-old college student presents to the ED complaining of headache, sore throat, myalgias, and rash that developed over the previous 12 hours. Her BP is 95/60 mm Hg, HR is 132 beats per minute, temperature is 103.9°F, RR is 19 breaths per minute, and oxygen saturation is 98% on room air. She is confused and oriented only to person. Physical examination is remarkable for pain with neck flexion, a petechial and purpuric rash on her extremities, and delayed capillary refill. Which of the following best describes the emergency physicians' priority in managing this patient?

a. Collect two sets of blood cultures prior to antibiotic administration.
b. Call the patient's parents and have them come immediately to the hospital.
c. Call her roommate to gather more information.
d. Begin fluid resuscitation, administer intravenous (IV) antibiotics, and perform a lumbar puncture (LP).
e. Administer acetaminophen to see if her headache and fever resolve.

**217.** A 21-year-old college student is brought to the ED by her roommate who states that the patient has been very sleepy today. She has a history of diabetes and has not refilled her medication in over a week. Her BP is 95/61 mm Hg, HR is 132 beats per minute, temperature is 99.7°F, and RR is 20 breaths per minute. Her fingerstick glucose is 530 mg/dL. Which of the following choices most closely matches what you would expect to find on her arterial blood gas with electrolytes and urinalysis?

a. pH 7.38, anion gap 5, normal urinalysis
b. pH 7.57, anion gap 21, presence of glucose and leukocytes in urine
c. pH 7.47, anion gap 12, presence of glucose and ketones in urine
d. pH 7.26, anion gap 12, presence of glucose and ketones in urine
e. pH 7.26, anion gap 21, presence of glucose and ketones in urine

**218.** A 65-year-old actively seizing woman is brought to the ED by EMS. She was found slumped over at the bus stop bench. EMS personnel state that when they found the woman, she was diaphoretic and her speech was garbled. En route to the hospital, she started to seize. As you wheel her to a room, the nurse gives you some of her vital signs that are a BP of 150/90 mm Hg, HR of 115 beats per minute, and oxygen saturation of 96%. Which of the following is the next best step in managing this patient?

a. Request a rectal temperature to rule out meningitis.
b. Call the CT technologist and tell them you are bringing over a seizing patient.
c. Ask for a stat ECG and administer an aspirin.
d. Check the patient's fingerstick blood glucose level.
e. Intubate the patient.

**219.** A 48-year-old man presents to the ED with ethanol intoxication. His BP is 150/70 mm Hg, HR is 95 beats per minute, temperature is 97.9°F, RR is 14 breaths per minute, and oxygen saturation is 93% on room air. The patient is somnolent and snoring loudly with occasional gasps for air. On examination, the patient's gag reflex is intact, his lungs are clear to auscultation, heart is without murmurs, and abdomen is soft and nontender. He is rousable to stimulation. A head CT is negative for intracranial injury. His ethanol level is 270 mg/dL. Which of the following actions is most appropriate to assist the patient with respirations?

a. Nasal airway
b. Oral airway
c. Bag-valve-mask ventilation
d. Laryngeal mask airway
e. Tracheoesophageal airway

**220.** A 52-year-old woman is brought to the ED by her husband for altered mental status for 1 day. The patient has hypertension and diabetes but has not been taking her medications for the last 5 days since she lost her insurance and could not afford her prescriptions. Her BP is 168/91 mm Hg, HR is 125 beats per minute, temperature is 99.8°F, and RR is 18 breaths per minute. Her fingerstick glucose is 900 mg/dL. There is glucose in her urine but no ketones. Which of the following is the most appropriate next step in management?

a. Administer IV fluids and insulin
b. Obtain head CT scan
c. Obtain ECG
d. Obtain chest radiograph and urine culture
e. Administer broad coverage antibiotics

**221.** A 45-year-old man is brought to the ED by his coworkers after collapsing to the floor while at work. A coworker states that the patient mistakenly took several tablets of his oral diabetic medications a few hours ago. The patient is unresponsive and diaphoretic. His BP is 142/78 mm Hg, HR is 115 beats per minute, temperature is 98.9°F, and RR is 12 breaths per minute. A bedside glucose reads 42 mg/dL. Which of the following is the most appropriate management of this patient?

a. Administer IV dextrose, obtain repeat fingerstick glucose every hour, and, if normal after 6 hours, discharge the patient home.
b. Administer IV dextrose and continue monitoring his blood sugar for at least 24 hours.
c. Administer IV fluids and insulin.
d. Administer IV fluids.
e. Administer activated charcoal and IV fluids.

**222.** A 59-year-old man is brought into the ED accompanied by his son who states that his father is acting irritable and occasionally confused. The son states that his father has a history of hepatitis from a transfusion he received many years ago. Over the past 5 years, his liver function slowly deteriorated. His vital signs include BP of 145/80 mm Hg, HR of 78 beats per minute, RR of 16 breaths per minute, oxygen saturation of 98%, and temperature of 98°F. Laboratory results are all within normal limits, except for an ammonia level that is significantly elevated. Which of the following is the best therapy?

a. Vancomycin and gentamycin
b. Lactulose and neomycin
c. Ampicillin and gentamycin
d. Levofloxacin
e. Ciprofloxacin

**223.** A 40-year-old man who is an employee of the hospital is brought to the ED actively seizing. A coworker states that the patient has a known seizure disorder and currently takes phenytoin for the disorder. He also tells you that the patient has been under stress recently and may not have taken his last few doses of medication. You call for the nurse to place a face mask with 100% oxygen and gain IV access. You then ask for a medication to be drawn up. Which is the most appropriate initial medication you should administer in this actively seizing patient?

a. Phenytoin
b. Diazepam
c. Phenobarbital
d. Valproic acid
e. Lithium

**224.** A 32-year-old gravida 1, para 1 who gave birth by normal vaginal delivery at 38 weeks' gestation 2 days ago presents to the ED complaining of bilateral hand swelling and severe headache that started 2 hours ago. Her BP is 187/110 mm Hg, HR is 85 beats per minute, temperature is 97.5°F, and RR is 15 breaths per minute. Urinalysis reveals 3+ protein. When you are examining the patient, she proceeds to have a generalized tonic-clonic seizure. Which of the following is the most appropriate next step in management?

a. Administer magnesium sulfate IV.
b. Administer labetalol to reduce her BP and morphine sulfate to address her headache.
c. Administer sumatriptan and place the patient into a dark quiet room.
d. Administer a loading dose of phenytoin, order a head CT scan, and call for a neurology consult.
e. Administer diazepam and normal saline IV.

**225.** An unconscious 51-year-old woman is brought to the ED by EMS. A friend states that the patient was complaining of feeling weak. She vomited and subsequently "blacked out" in the ambulance. The friend states that the patient has no medical problems and takes no medications. She also states that the patient smokes cigarettes and uses cocaine, and that they were snorting cocaine together prior to her blacking out. The patient's BP is 195/80 mm Hg, HR is 50 beats per minute, temperature is 98.6°F, and RR is 7 breaths per minute. What is the eponym associated with her vital signs?

a. Cushing syndrome
b. Cushing reflex
c. Cullen sign
d. Charcot triad
e. Chvostek sign

**226.** A 47-year-old man is brought to the ED by EMS after being persistently agitated at a business meeting. The patient's coworkers state that he has been working nonstop for a day and a half and that he always seemed like a healthy guy who frequented bars every night. EMS administered 25 g of dextrose and thiamine with no symptom improvement. In the ED, the patient is anxious, confused, tremulous, and diaphoretic. He denies any medical problems, medications, or drug ingestions. His BP is 182/92 mm Hg, HR is 139 beats per minute, temperature is 100.4°F, RR is 18 breaths per minute, and fingerstick glucose is 103 mg/dL. An ECG reveals sinus tachycardia. Which of the following is the next best step?

a. Administer acetaminophen.
b. Administer folate.
c. Administer diazepam.
d. Recheck fingerstick glucose.
e. Administer labetalol.

**227.** A 65-year-old man presents to the ED with a headache, drowsiness, and confusion. He has a history of long-standing hypertension. His BP is 230/120 mm Hg, pulse 87 beats per minute, RR 18 breaths per minutes, and oxygen saturation 97% on room air. On examination, you note papilledema. A head CT scan is performed and there is no evidence of ischemia or hemorrhage. Which of the following is the most appropriate method to lower his BP?

a. Administer propofol for rapid reduction in BP.
b. Administer mannitol for rapid reduction in BP and intracranial pressure (ICP).
c. Administer a high-dose diuretic to reduce preload.
d. Administer labetalol until his BP is 140/80 mm Hg.
e. Administer labetalol until his BP is 180/100 mm Hg.

**228.** A 74-year-old woman is brought to the ED by EMS for altered mental status. Her BP is 138/72 mm Hg, HR is 91 beats per minute, RR is 17 breaths per minute, and temperature is 100.9°F. A head CT is normal. LP results revealed the following:

> White blood cell (WBC) count 1020/mL with 90%
> polymorphonuclear cells
> Glucose 21 mg/dL
> Protein 225 g/L

Which of the following is the most likely diagnosis?

a. TB meningitis
b. Bacterial meningitis
c. Viral meningitis
d. Fungal meningitis
e. Encephalitis

**229.** A 67-year-old man presents to the ED for worsening confusion. His wife states that he received his first dose of chemotherapy for lung cancer 2 days ago. Over the last 24 hours, the patient became confused. His BP is 130/70 mm Hg, HR is 87 beats per minute, and temperature is 98.9°F. While in the ED, the patient seizes. You administer an antiepileptic and the seizure immediately stops. You compare his current electrolyte panel to one taken 2 days ago.

|  | Two Days Ago | Today |
|---|---|---|
| Sodium (mEq/L) | 139 | 113 |
| Potassium (mEq/L) | 4.1 | 3.9 |
| Chloride (mEq/L) | 105 | 98 |
| Bicarbonate (mEq/L) | 23 | 20 |
| Blood urea nitrogen (BUN) (mg/dL) | 13 | 17 |
| Creatinine (mg/dL) | 0.4 | 0.7 |
| Glucose (mg/dL) | 98 | 92 |

Which of the following is the most appropriate treatment?
a. 0.45% saline
b. 0.9% saline
c. 3% saline
d. 5% dextrose
e. 50% dextrose

**230.** A 31-year-old woman with a history of schizophrenia presents to the ED for altered mental status. A friend states that the patient is on multiple medications for her schizophrenia. Her BP is 150/80 mm Hg, HR 121 beats per minute, RR 20 breaths per minute, and temperature 104.5°F. On examination, the patient is diaphoretic with distinctive "lead-pipe" rigidity of her musculature. You believe the patient has neuroleptic malignant syndrome. After basic stabilizing measures, which of the following medications is most appropriate to administer?

a. Haloperidol
b. Droperidol
c. Dantrolene
d. Diphenhydramine
e. Acetaminophen

**231.** A 56-year-old man is brought in from the homeless shelter for strange, irrational behavior, and unsteady gait for 1 day. A worker at the shelter reports that the patient is a frequent abuser of alcohol. On examination, the patient is alert but oriented to name only and is unable to give full history. He does not appear clinically intoxicated. You note horizontal nystagmus and ataxia. What is the most likely diagnosis?

a. Wernicke encephalopathy
b. Korsakoff syndrome
c. Normal pressure hydrocephalus
d. Central vertigo
e. Alcohol withdrawal

**232.** An 18-year-old girl is brought to the ED from a party for agitation and attacking her boyfriend with a knife. Her boyfriend admits that she had several liquor shots and used intranasal cocaine at the party prior to becoming agitated, paranoid, and attacking him. Her BP is 145/80 mm Hg, HR is 126 beats per minute, temperature is 100.8°F, and RR is 20 breaths per minute. The patient is agitated, screaming, and resisting examination. What is the next best step in the management of this patient?

a. IV β-blocker
b. IV benzodiazepine
c. Acetaminophen
d. Lithium
e. Drug abuse specialist consult

**233.** A 78-year-old woman is transferred from a nursing home with altered mental status and fever. The nursing home reports that the patient was febrile to 102.3°F, disoriented, confused, and incontinent of urine. Her past medical history includes hypertension, a stroke with residual right-sided weakness, and nighttime agitation for which she was started on haloperidol 3 days ago. Her BP is 215/105 mm Hg, HR is 132 beats per minute, temperature is 102.8°F, and RR is 20 breaths per minute. On examination, the patient is oriented to name only, tremulous, diaphoretic, and has marked muscular rigidity and three out of five right upper- and lower-extremity strength. What is the most likely diagnosis?

a. Urinary tract infection
b. Malignant hyperthermia
c. Neuroleptic malignant syndrome
d. Recurrent stroke
e. Meningoencephalitis

**234.** A 54-year-old man is brought to the ED by his wife for bizarre behavior. The wife complains that her husband has not been acting like his usual self over the last several days. She states that he has not had any change in sleep, appetite, or activity level. She also recalls that her husband complained of morning headaches for the last 2 months. The patient is otherwise in good health and does not take any medications. His BP is 135/87 mm Hg, HR is 76 beats per minute, temperature is 98.9°F, and RR is 14 breaths per minute. His examination is otherwise unremarkable. Which of the following is the most likely diagnosis?

a. Migraine headache
b. Tension headache
c. Subarachnoid hemorrhage
d. Pseudotumor cerebri
e. Frontal lobe mass

**235.** A 27-year-old woman is brought to the ED by her husband after having a first-time seizure at home. She has no past medical history and had no complications while delivering her newborn vaginally 1 week prior to presentation. In the ED, her BP is 178/95 mm Hg, HR is 97 beats per minute, temperature is 99.1°F, and RR is 18 breaths per minute. On examination, she has mild edema of her hands and feet. The seizure stopped spontaneously, but the patient is postictal appearing and cannot answer your questions. Which of the following is the most appropriate diagnostic test?

a. Complete blood count
b. Head CT
c. LP
d. Urinalysis
e. ECG

**236.** A 46-year-old woman is brought to the ED by her husband for 1 day of worsening confusion. The patient has a history of systemic lupus erythematosus (SLE) and takes chronic oral steroids. She has not been feeling well for the last few days. Her BP is 167/92 mm Hg, HR is 95 beats per minute, temperature is 100.3°F, and RR is 16 breaths per minute. On examination, the patient is oriented to name and has diffuse petechiae on her torso and extremities. Laboratory results reveal hematocrit 23%, platelets 17,000/μL, BUN 38 mg/dL, and creatinine 1.9 mg/dL. Which of the following is the most likely diagnosis?

a. Henoch-Schönlein purpura (HSP)
b. Disseminated intravascular coagulopathy (DIC)
c. von Willebrand disease
d. Idiopathic thrombocytopenic purpura (ITP)
e. Thrombotic thrombocytopenic purpura (TTP)

**237.** A 63-year-old man presents to the ED complaining of headache, vomiting, and "not being able to think straight" for 1 day. The patient states that he has hypertension and diabetes but ran out of his medications in the last week. His BP is 245/138 mm Hg, HR is 90 beats per minute, temperature is 98.7°F, and his RR is 14 breaths per minute. Fingerstick glucose is 178 mg/dL. On examination, the patient appears slightly confused and oriented to name and place only. The neurologic examination is significant for papilledema. Which of the following is the most appropriate next step in management?

a. Nitroprusside IV
b. Magnesium sulfate IV
c. Metoprolol by mouth
d. Hydrochlorothiazide by mouth
e. Obtain head CT

**238.** A 26-year-old man with a long history of epilepsy is brought to the ED for a recent seizure. While in the ED, he is rhythmically moving his right leg and is unresponsive. Which of the following best describes this seizure pattern?

a. Petit mal seizure
b. Generalized tonic-clonic seizure
c. Partial seizure with secondary generalization
d. Simple partial seizure
e. Complex partial seizure

**239.** A 58-year-old woman is brought into the ED after a witnessed syncopal event. Upon arrival, the patient appears confused and agitated. Her vitals include HR of 89 beats per minute, BP of 145/70 mm Hg, RR of 16 breaths per minute, and oxygen saturation of 98% on room air. Within a few minutes, the patient is more alert and oriented. She denies any chest pain, headache, abdominal pain, or weakness preceding the event and is currently asymptomatic. She also states that she has not taken her antiepileptic medications in 2 days. The patient's examination is unremarkable including a nonfocal neurologic examination. Given this patient's history and evolving examination, what is the most likely etiology of this patient's syncopal event?

a. Cerebrovascular accident (CVA)
b. Transient ischemic attack (TIA)
c. Seizure
d. Aortic dissection
e. Pulmonary embolus

# Altered Mental Status

## Answers

**212. The answer is c.** (*Rosen, pp 1637-1639.*) The patient never received **fingerstick glucose** at triage. **Hypoglycemia** can mimic a CVA or seizure. Therefore, it is critical that all patients who present with altered mental status get fingerstick glucose. Glucose level should be considered a vital sign. Hypoglycemia is a common problem in patients with type 1 diabetes. The clinical presentation of hypoglycemia is caused by increased secretion of epinephrine, as well as central nervous system (CNS) dysfunction. Symptoms include diaphoresis, nervousness, tremor, tachycardia, hunger, and neurologic symptoms ranging from confusion and bizarre behavior to seizures and coma.

(a) Ethanol withdrawal can present in a similar fashion as hypoglycemia because both include symptoms of an adrenergic state (eg, tachycardia, hypertension, diaphoresis, agitation). Even if you suspect ethanol withdrawal, it is mandatory to check fingerstick glucose. (b) The stroke team should be activated in patients who present with signs and symptoms of a stroke that are not caused by hypoglycemia. Therefore, these patients need fingerstick glucose. (d) Sundowning refers to people who become increasingly confused at the end of the day and into the night. Sundowning isn't a disease but a symptom that often occurs in people with dementia, such as Alzheimer disease. It is more commonly observed on the hospital wards than in the ED. (e) Haloperidol is commonly used as a sedative for agitated patients. However, this patient is agitated because of an organic cause, hypoglycemia. By treating the underlying cause (administering glucose), the agitation will resolve.

**213. The answer is d.** (*Tintinalli, pp 1444-1447.*) **Myxedema coma** is a life-threatening **complication of hypothyroidism**. Mortality in myxedema coma approaches 20% to 50% even with appropriate management. The patient exhibits classic signs and symptoms of the disease: lethargy or coma, hypothermia, bradycardia, periorbital and nonpitting edema, and a delayed relaxation phase of deep tendon reflexes (areflexia in more severe cases). Myxedema coma can be triggered by sepsis, trauma, surgery, congestive heart failure, prolonged cold exposure, or use of sedatives or narcotics (as seen in this example). **(a)** It is critical that fingerstick glucose is checked. However, myxedema coma differs from the early stages of hypoglycemia in that myxedema coma results in the progressive slowing of all bodily functions; by contrast, in early hypoglycemia, the body is stimulated by the release of adrenergic hormones. **(b)** The classic findings in opioid toxicity include miotic pupils and respiratory depression. **(c)** Stroke should be on the differential in this case, but the patient's signs and symptoms are more consistent with an abnormal metabolic state than with purely neurovascular change. Depression **(e)** is an often forgotten diagnosis in the elderly and may present with a wide variety of signs and symptoms. Severe depression may appear as lethargy. It is unlikely, however, to have associated hypothermia and abnormal reflexes.

**214. The answer is e.** (*Roberts and Hedges, pp 16-20.*) Patients frequently present to the ED with agitation. It is important to discern what is causing their agitation; the range of etiologies is expansive, from ethanol intoxication to intracerebral bleeding. The approach to the emergency patient always begins with the **ABCs (airway, breathing, and circulation)**. In addition, the **vital signs** must be obtained early in a patient's assessment in order **to reveal potentially life-threatening conditions**. The patient in the vignette presents with agitation and tachycardia. Although it is tempting to attribute his agitation to his untreated schizophrenia, doing this without investigating medical causes of agitation can be disastrous. Finding out that the patient's temperature is 103.1°F, for instance, will lead you down a different clinical path than if his temperature is 98°F. This patient was ultimately diagnosed with meningitis.

**(a)** Administering a medication to control agitation or psychotic behavior is appropriate even when there are coexistent medical problems. Patients who are too agitated cannot be properly examined. However, it is critical to rule out potential life threats that may be causing the agitation. **(b)** A psychiatry consultation should be obtained once life-threatening conditions are excluded or in the case of the patient above, when he is stable and communicative as an inpatient. **(c and d)** A head CT and blood work will need to be obtained in this patient; however, all of the vital signs should be obtained first.

**215. The answer is a.** (*Tintinalli, pp 1153-1159.*) The initial approach to a seizing patient should involve protecting the patient from injury. Seizing patients should be immediately **placed in a lateral decubitus position to prevent aspiration of gastric contents**. Other initial measures are oxygen administration, pulse oxymetry, glucose level determination, and an IV line.

Benzodiazepines (eg, lorazepam) **(b)** are the first-line agents for an actively seizing patient. Benzodiazepines are sedative hypnotics which increase γ-aminobutyric acid (GABA) activity. Phenytoin **(c)** is a second-line anticonvulsant in a continuously seizing patient. It requires a loading dose and has to be administered slowly because rapid administration may cause hypotension and cardiac dysrhythmias. Rapid sequence intubation (RSI) **(d)** should not be performed at this time. The patient's pulse oximetry is 91% on room air and can be improved by supplemental oxygen and a nasopharyngeal airway if necessary. RSI should be done if the patient becomes apneic or his oxygen saturation drops despite oxygen supplementation. Patient's who are intubated and chemically paralyzed should be placed on continuous electroencephalogram (EEG) to monitor for underlying seizure activity. **(e)** Once the acute seizure is controlled, levels of the patient's anticonvulsant medications should be checked and supplemented if subtherapeutic.

**216. The answer is d.** (*Hamilton et al, p 5.*) The first question an emergency physician asks for each patient is whether a life-threatening process is causing the patient's complaint. Emergency medicine is primarily a complaint-oriented, rather than a disease-oriented specialty. Its emphasis rests on anticipating and recognizing a life-threatening process rather than seeking the diagnosis. The goal is to think about and plan to prevent the life-threatening things from happening or progressing in the patient. The patient in the vignette may have meningitis, a life-threatening condition, or a viral syndrome with dehydration. **The initial approach is stabilization and treatment or prevention of a life-threatening process.** This patient requires fluid resuscitation for her BP, altered mental status, and delayed capillary refill. Antibiotics should be started immediately and an LP performed once increased ICP is evaluated by funduscopic examination or CT scan. She should be placed in isolation. Her disposition is directed by her response to initial resuscitation and results of the LP.

**(a)** It is important to collect blood cultures; however, initial stabilization and treatment is priority. **(b)** The patient's parents should be contacted if the patient cannot do it herself, but treatment should proceed in the meantime. **(c)** Gathering more information is invaluable; however, this should be done after initial stabilization and treatment. **(e)** Observation in a patient with a life-threatening condition is not recommended.

**217. The answer is e.** *(Tintinalli, pp 1432-1438.)* This patient presents with an anion gap metabolic acidosis, glucosuria, and ketonuria, which is consistent with **diabetic ketoacidosis (DKA)**. DKA is an acute, life-threatening disorder occurring in patients with insulin insufficiency. It results in hyperglycemia, ketosis, and osmotic diuresis, and clinically presents with gastrointestinal (GI) distress, polyuria, fatigue, dehydration, mental confusion, lethargy, or coma. When the diagnosis of DKA is clinically suspected and hyperglycemia is confirmed by elevated fingerstick glucose, the results of a blood gas and urinalysis confirm the diagnosis. In DKA, the liver metabolizes free fatty acids into ketone bodies for alternative fuel in the setting of cellular glucose underutilization. The result is **ketonuria** and **anion gap metabolic acidosis (pH < 7.4 and HCO$_3^-$ < 24)**. **Glucosuria**, the result of hyperglycemia-related osmotic diuresis, is another manifestation of DKA.

The anion gap is calculated by subtracting Cl$^-$ and HCO$_3^-$ from Na$^+$.

$$\text{Anion gap (AG)} = [\text{Na}^+] - ([\text{Cl}^-] + [\text{HCO}_3^-])$$

A normal anion gap is 8 to 12 mEq/L. An elevated gap is a result of an increased concentration of unmeasured anions. In DKA, the elevated anion gap is caused by the production of ketones.

Other answers **(a, b, c, and d)** are incorrect choices in the DKA presentation.

**218. The answer is d.** *(Rosen, pp 1637-1639.)* In a patient who is **actively seizing**, it is essential to check the **blood glucose level**. **Hypoglycemia** is an easily **reversible** cause of seizure and is corrected with the administration of **dextrose**, not the usual anticonvulsants. Patients at both extremes of age are particularly susceptible to glucose stress during acute illness.

If the blood glucose level is normal, requesting a rectal temperature **(a)** is appropriate. However, this should be done concomitantly with addressing airway protection, gaining IV access, and administering an anticonvulsant. A CT scan **(b)** may be necessary in a seizure patient; however, this should occur once the patient is stabilized. An ECG and aspirin **(c)** are usually the initial management for patients with chest pain. In an actively seizing patient, nothing should be administered by mouth because there is an increased risk for aspiration and the patient may not have a gag reflex. Intubating (**e**) the patient may be necessary if the seizure cannot be medically controlled, the patient is hypoxic, or not protecting his or her airway. In the above patient, you'd expect the seizure to cease once glucose is administered. In addition, her oxygen saturation is 96%.

**219. The answer is a.** (*Tintinalli, pp 183-190.*) A **nasal airway** is made of a pliable material that allows it to be placed into the nostril of a somnolent patient with an **intact gag reflex**. The nasal airway is an excellent device that can be placed in a patient who may have decreased pharyngeal muscle tone and an obstructing soft palate and tongue. It allows air to bypass such obstructions. The patient in the vignette is intoxicated and appears to have episodes of transient obstruction.

(**b**) An oral airway is a rigid instrument that is used to prevent the base of the tongue from occluding the hypopharynx. It should be used to maintain the airway only in a patient with an absent gag reflex. (**c**) Bag-valve-mask ventilation is typically used to oxygenate a patient in preparation for a definitive airway, such as orotracheal intubation. (**d and e**) Laryngeal mask and tracheoesophageal and airways are devices typically used in the ED as rescue devices in failed intubation or in the prehospital setting when orotracheal intubation is not a viable option. These devices are designed to be placed in apneic, unconscious patients.

**220. The answer is a.** (*Tintinalli, pp 1440-1444.*) Profound hyperglycemia, absence of ketonuria, and diabetes medication noncompliance should raise your suspicion for **nonketotic hyperosmolar crisis (NKHC)** in this patient. This condition is a syndrome of hyperglycemia without ketoacidosis as small amounts of insulin protect against adipose tissue metabolism. This syndrome is more common in type 2 diabetics. Causes of NKHC are similar to those of DKA and include **diabetes medication noncompliance, infection, stroke, and myocardial infarction (MI)**. Patients are profoundly dehydrated because of osmotic diuresis. The mainstay of NKHC therapy consists of **replacing fluid losses**. Electrolyte deficiencies should be replaced and insulin administered. Fluid deficit in NKHC is significant and needs to be slowly corrected, as rapid correction may lead to cerebral edema. Insulin requirements in NKHC are usually less than in DKA.

Further diagnostic tests are important to obtain, depending on the patient's presentation and suspicion of an underlying etiology of NKHC. In this case, medication noncompliance is most likely. In other cases, head

CT for workup of intracranial pathology (**b**), ECG for evaluation of MI (**c**), or chest radiograph and urine culture for infectious etiology workup (**d**) might be necessary. Without an infectious etiology, broad coverage antibiotics (**e**) are not necessary in this patient.

**221. The answer is b.** *(Tintinalli, pp 1430-1432.)* This is a case of **hypoglycemia** caused by **oral hypoglycemic medication overdose**. Diabetic oral agents that cause hypoglycemia work by increasing pancreatic insulin secretion. This group includes sulfonylureas (glyburide, glipizide) and nonsulfonylurea secretagogues (repaglinide, nateglinide). Other common causes of hypoglycemia are insulin overdose, alcohol abuse (inhibition of gluconeogenesis), and sepsis. The presentation of a hypoglycemic patient generally involves signs and symptoms of CNS dysfunction owing to the release of counterregulatory hormones secondary to the unavailability of glucose. Symptoms include anxiety, diaphoresis, palpitations, and confusion. Don't be fooled by improved blood glucose levels after dextrose administration in overdose with oral hypoglycemic agents. **Hypoglycemia can last more than 24 hours because of long-lasting pancreatic effects** and will recur after dextrose infusion. Patients need to be observed in the hospital with frequent bedside glucose checks. They can be placed on a dextrose drip. Octreotide, an inhibitor of insulin release, can also be administered.

Choice (**a**) is inappropriate since hypoglycemia will recur after administration of a single bolus of dextrose. IV fluids and insulin (**c**) are treatments for hyperglycemia. IV fluid without dextrose (**d**) is not helpful in hypoglycemia management. Activated charcoal administration (**e**) is recommended within an hour after certain toxic ingestions or when there may be a coingestion of an unknown toxin.

**222. The answer is b.** *(Rosen, pp 1161-1162.)* The patient has **hepatic encephalopathy**, which is a clinical state of disordered cerebral function occurring secondary to acute or chronic liver disease. Laboratory tests may be normal in patients, but the **serum ammonia level is usually elevated**. **Lactulose** and **neomycin** represent the main therapeutic agents. Lactulose is a poorly absorbed sugar metabolized by colonic bacteria that traps ammonia and helps excrete it in the stool. Neomycin is a poorly absorbed aminoglycoside that is believed to act by reducing colonic bacteria responsible for producing ammonia. No other antibiotics (**a, c, d, and e**) are indicated in the management of hepatic encephalopathy.

**223. The answer is b.** (*Rosen, pp 2230-2234.*) Generally, the **first-line** pharmacologic treatment in an actively seizing patient is a parental **benzodiazepine**, such as diazepam (Valium), lorazepam (Ativan), or midazolam (Versed). Benzodiazepines are effective in terminating ictal activity in 75% to 90% of patients. Diazepam can be administered intravenously, intramuscularly, or down an endotracheal tube. Lorazepam and midazolam can be given intravenously or intramuscularly. All three have similar efficacy in terminating seizures.

Phenytoin (**a**) is a second-line agent that can be administered intravenously. Although the cause of the patient's seizure may be because of subtherapeutic levels of phenytoin, benzodiazepines are still the first-line therapy owing to their rapid onset. The onset of diazepam is 2 to 5 minutes while phenytoin is 10 to 30 minutes. In addition, phenytoin requires at least 20 minutes for administration because of its potential to cause hypotension and cardiac dysrhythmias. Phenobarbital (**c**) is a third-line agent. Its onset of action is 15 to 30 minutes. Valproic acid (**d**) is rarely used in the acute seizure setting. There is no role for lithium (**e**) in acute seizure management.

**224. The answer is a.** (*Rosen, pp 2287-2289.*) This patient has **postpartum eclampsia**, which needs to be managed with **magnesium sulfate** and admission to the obstetrical service. Preeclampsia is defined as new-onset hypertension (> 140/90 mm Hg) and proteinuria (1 g/L in random specimen or > 3 g/L over 24 hours). Some clinicians also use generalized edema as a requirement. Preeclampsia is most common in the third trimester. Eclampsia occurs with the development of seizures or coma in a patient with preeclampsia. A preeclamptic woman may worsen after delivery and develop late postpartum eclampsia, which usually occurs in the first 24 to 48 hours postpartum but may present several weeks after delivery. Management of eclamptic seizures in the ED involves administering magnesium sulfate, which is believed to act as a membrane stabilizer and vasodilator, reducing cerebral ischemia. Although magnesium sulfate is not a direct antihypertensive, the hypertension associated with eclampsia is often controlled adequately by treating the seizure.

(**b**) Treating the seizure will most likely also lower the patient's BP. Fewer than 10% of eclamptic patients require specific antihypertensive therapy. (**c**) This is the treatment for migraines, which this patient does not have. (**d and e**) This patient's seizure is secondary to eclampsia. The first-line treatment is with magnesium sulfate. If the seizure is not treated despite appropriate magnesium sulfate, a benzodiazepine can be administered and etiologies of seizure other than eclampsia should be sought.

**225. The answer is b.** *(Rosen, p 300.)* The patient has a triad of **hypertension, bradycardia,** and **respiratory depression,** which is called **Cushing reflex.** This is observed in one-third of patients with a potentially lethal **increase in ICP.** Increased ICP may result from traumatic brain injury or, as in this patient's case, from hemorrhagic stroke and subsequent brain edema. Tobacco and cocaine use are known risk factors for hemorrhagic stroke. Increasing ICP can result in cerebral herniation, which has a mortality rate close to 100%. For any chance of survival, it must be rapidly controlled by intubation, elevation of the head of the bed, hyperventilation, mannitol, and definitive neurosurgical intervention.

Cushing syndrome (a) describes the hyperadrenal state associated with increased production of cortisol, leading to hypertension, truncal obesity, abdominal striae, and hirsutism. Cullen sign (c) is purplish discoloration around the umbilicus that results from intraperitoneal hemorrhage. Charcot triad (d) constitutes fever, right upper quadrant (RUQ) pain, and jaundice, and is associated with cholangitis. Chvostek sign (e), associated with hypocalcemia, is twitching of the nose or lips with tapping of the facial nerve.

**226. The answer is c.** *(Tintinalli, pp 1967-1969.)* This patient presents with **alcohol withdrawal.** Signs and symptoms of this condition occur along a continuum ranging from simple shakes to delirium tremens (DTs) following a reduction or cessation of alcohol. Early symptoms usually appear 6 to 8 hours after cessation of drinking and involve tremulousness, anxiety, mild hypertension, and tachycardia. In more severe withdrawal, these symptoms worsen and paranoia, auditory, and visual hallucinations may develop proceeding to DTs with severe autonomic hyperactivity and profound altered mental status. DTs usually occur 3 to 5 days after alcohol cessation and carry 5% to 15% mortality even with supportive care. Additionally, alcohol withdrawal seizures may occur anywhere from 6 to 48 hours after cessation of alcohol. **Benzodiazepines** are the mainstay of therapy in alcohol withdrawal, as well as in sympathomimetic overdose and sedative-hypnotic withdrawal.

Acetaminophen (a) and labetalol (e) would treat the symptoms of low-grade fever and hypertension/tachycardia, respectively, without addressing the underlying etiology. Folate (b) should be given to all potentially undernourished patients, especially alcoholics, to prevent folate-deficient anemia. Dextrose was just administered by EMS without symptom improvement; however, fingerstick glucose (d) levels are important to check in all patients with altered mental status.

**227. The answer is e.** *(Rosen, pp 1079-1080.)* The patient has **hypertensive encephalopathy**, which is defined by a rapid rise in BP that is accompanied by **neurologic changes**. Patients typically present with a systolic BP greater than 220 mm Hg and diastolic BP greater than 110 mm Hg. Neurologic findings include severe headache, vomiting, drowsiness, confusion, seizure, blindness, focal neurologic deficits, or coma. Hypertensive emergency is a medical emergency. The goal of therapy is to stop and reverse the progression of end-organ dysfunction while maintaining organ perfusion and avoiding complications. Reduction in BP should be done rapidly but carefully. It is important to avoid dropping the pressure too low as this may lead to cerebral ischemia. The immediate goal is to reduce the mean arterial BP by 20% to 30% of pretreatment levels over the first hour of therapy. This can be accomplished by **labetalol**, a $\beta_1$-, $\beta_2$-, and $\alpha_1$-receptor blocker. Another useful medication is nitroprusside, which is a better choice if the patient's BP is being monitored through an intra-arterial line. Nitroprusside can cause a reflex tachycardia.

(a) Propofol is an excellent sedating agent that has a rapid onset of action and metabolizes quickly. It is also known to cause hypotension and apnea as side affects. However, it should not be used as an antihypertensive because of its unpredictable properties. (b) Mannitol is an osmotic agent that is used to lower ICP in patients with impending or actual brain herniation. It is not appropriate as an antihypertensive agent. (c) Diuretics are not useful to acutely lower BP but may be started as a maintenance antihypertensive. (d) Lowering the BP to 140/80 mm Hg can cause cerebral ischemia. The mean arterial pressure should only be lowered by 20% to 30% in the first hour.

**228. The answer is b.** *(Rosen, pp 2218-2225.)* The cerebrospinal fluid (CSF) analysis in bacterial meningitis typically shows an **elevated WBC count** with predominant **polymorphonuclear leukocytes. Protein is elevated and glucose is low**. A Gram stain may show bacteria. The most specific marker for the diagnosis is a positive culture. Tests that evaluate the presence of antigen in the CSF (eg, latex agglutination studies) are particularly useful in the diagnosis of partially treated bacterial meningitis.

(a) TB meningitis typically presents with less than 1000 WBC/μL with monocytic predominance. Symptoms are generally insidious in nature, typically not appearing until after a week has passed. (c) In viral meningitis, the CSF WBC count is made up of lymphocytes or monocytes, but early in the disease polys may predominate. CSF glucose is normal and protein is elevated in viral meningitis. A Gram stain will be negative and culture will show no growth. (d) Fungal meningitis is rare and generally presents in immunocompromised patients. LP usually reveals less than 500/μL WBCs. (e) Encephalitis is diagnosed by CSF culture or serology. CSF analysis that reveals blood is suspicious for herpes encephalitis.

| Test | Normal | Bacterial | Viral | Fungal | TB |
|------|--------|-----------|-------|--------|-----|
| Protein | < 50 | > 200 | < 200 | > 200 | > 200 |
| Glucose | > 40 | < 40 | > 40 | < 40 | < 40 |
| WBCs | < 5 | > 1000 | < 1000 | < 500 | < 1000 |
| Cell type | Monos | > 50% Polys | Monos | Monos | Monos |
| Gram stain | Neg | Pos | Neg | Neg | Pos (AFB) |

**229. The answer is c.** *(Tintinalli, pp 118-121.)* **Hyponatremia** is defined as a measured serum sodium less than 135 mEq/L. However, the development of symptoms secondary to hyponatremia is related more to the rate of change in the serum sodium than to the absolute value. Levels less than 120 mEq/L tend to cause symptoms regardless of the rate to reach this value. Symptoms can include confusion, lethargy, nausea, vomiting, anorexia, muscle cramps, and seizures. There are many causes of hyponatremia, including renal or GI losses, third-spacing, endocrine abnormalities, syndrome of inappropriate antidiuretic hormone (SIADH) release, cirrhosis, CHF, and nephrotic syndrome. Many medications cause SIADH, in addition to pulmonary and CNS disease. This patient, in particular, just started chemotherapy for lung cancer. The treatment for hyponatremia is guided by the cause of the process. However, if a patient is symptomatic (eg, seizing), **hypertonic saline (3%)** should be carefully administered to raise the serum sodium to 120 mEq/L. A known complication of hypertonic saline, when it is administered too fast and sodium levels rise rapidly, is the development of central pontine myelinosis.

(a and b) 0.45% and 0.9% do not provide adequate amounts of sodium to raise the serum level and can actually cause a drop in serum sodium in certain conditions. (d and e) Dextrose is the treatment of choice for hypoglycemic patients.

**230. The answer is c.** *(Tintinalli, pp 1209-1211.)* **Neuroleptic malignant syndrome (NMS)** is a rare but potentially fatal reaction commonly associated with the use of **antipsychotic drugs**. The classic triad for its clinical presentation includes **altered mental status, hyperthermia, and muscle rigidity**. The cornerstone of treatment is supportive care with rapid cooling, fluid and electrolyte repletion, and monitoring. **Dantrolene**, a nonspecific skeletal muscle relaxant, generally used in the treatment of malignant hyperthermia, is also effective for NMS. In addition, benzodiazepines are useful in the treatment of NMS. The offending agent should be discontinued.

**(a and b)** These are both antipsychotic medications that can worsen the symptoms of NMS and should not be administered. **(d)** Diphenhydramine, an anticholinergic, should be avoided as it is ineffective and may worsen the reaction by interfering with temperature regulation. **(e)** Acetaminophen, an antipyretic, may help in lowering the temperature. However, NMS is a centrally mediated process. External cooling is more effective.

**231. The answer is a.** *(Tintinalli, p 1144.)* This patient exhibits the classic triad of **Wernicke encephalopathy (WE): confusion, ataxia, and ophthalmoplegia**. WE is a result of **thiamine deficiency** leading to decreased glucose metabolism and neuronal destruction, primarily in the cerebellum, hypothalamus, vestibular system, and memory. It is typically found in **chronic alcoholics** caused by nutritional deficiency but can also occur in other malnutrition states, pregnancy, persistent vomiting, or dialysis. WE can mimic acute stroke symptoms and can lead to permanent nystagmus and ataxia. It carries 10% to 20% mortality if untreated.

Eye examination findings in WE include horizontal nystagmus, vertical gaze palsy, or cranial nerve VII palsy. Cerebellar destruction presents with ataxic, wide-based gait. WE is a clinical diagnosis. Thiamine deficiency can also lead to the development of high-output cardiac failure and Korsakoff syndrome. The treatment is parenteral thiamine supplementation.

Korsakoff syndrome **(b)** is another sign of thiamine deficiency and involves disorientation and confabulation. Normal-pressure hydrocephalus **(c)** presents with dementia, ataxic gait, and urinary incontinence. Head CT shows large ventricles. Central vertigo **(d)** is caused by lesions in the brainstem or cerebellum. It is associated with vertical or rotary nystagmus and nausea and vomiting. Alcohol withdrawal **(e)** typically presents with sympathetic and CNS overactivity.

**232. The answer is b.** (*Tintinalli, pp 1234-1238.*) The patient has **cocaine-induced autonomic and CNS hyperactivity** causing agitation, paranoia, and a hyperadrenergic state. More severe CNS manifestations of cocaine poisoning include hyperthermia, intracranial hemorrhage, seizures, spinal cord infarctions, and acute dystonic reactions. The CNS effects of cocaine are managed with **benzodiazepines**, which decrease sympathetic tone and prevent hyperthermia and seizures.

(a) β-Adrenergic receptor blockers decrease HR and BP. In this case, however, metoprolol administration does not address the underlying cause of the adrenergic hyperactivity. More importantly, β-adrenergic receptor blockade in cocaine poisoning leaves unopposed stimulated α-adrenergic receptors, thus worsening vasoconstriction. Therefore, β-receptor blocker use in cocaine poisoning is contraindicated. Acetaminophen (c) is not helpful in this situation. Fever or hyperthermia in cocaine poisoning is caused by hypothalamic stimulation, and not by inflammatory mediators. Hyperthermia should be treated with cooling methods, such as cool mist spray or ice-bath immersion. Lithium (d) is commonly used in the treatment of depressive and bipolar affective disorders. It has no role in the acute treatment of cocaine intoxication. Drug abuse specialists (e) should be consulted when the patient is medically cleared.

**233. The answer is c.** (*Tintinalli, pp 1209-1211.*) The patient presents with a rare but potentially life-threatening NMS. **Antipsychotic drugs (eg, haloperidol)** are the most common offending agents in the development of NMS, causing **central dopamine depletion**. The disorder is typically characterized by **hyperthermia, muscle rigidity, altered mental status**, and **autonomic instability**. Because NMS carries a high mortality, it is important to aggressively treat it with muscle relaxers, such as IV benzodiazepines, dantrolene, and dopamine agonists.

Urinary tract infection (a) in a debilitated or nursing home patient can easily lead to altered mental status and sepsis. The patient's muscular rigidity, however, does not fit this diagnosis. The presentation of malignant hyperthermia (b) is similar to NMS, also involving hyperthermia and muscle rigidity. It is caused by anesthetic agents, which this patient did not receive. Dantrolene is also used for muscle relaxation in malignant hyperthermia. Recurrent stroke (d) is unlikely in this presentation with hyperthermia and muscle rigidity. Right-sided motor findings on examination are residual deficits from the old stroke. Meningoencephalitis (e) is certainly high on the differential in this patient but is unlikely to cause generalized muscular rigidity. It typically presents with fever, headache, nuchal rigidity, altered mental status, and focal neurologic signs.

**234. The answer is e.** *(Tintinalli, p 1115.)* The most likely diagnosis in this patient is a **space-occupying lesion** in the **frontal lobe of the brain**. Brain tumors can present with **morning headaches associated with nausea and vomiting**. Neurologic examination is normal in most patients. Papilledema might provide an important clue of increased ICP and the presence of a brain mass. Frontal lobe tumors typically involve **personality changes** as seen in this patient.

Migraine headaches **(a)** are recurrent headaches that may be unilateral or bilateral. They occur with or without a prodrome. The aura of a migraine may consist of neurologic symptoms, such as dizziness, tinnitus, scotomas, photophobia, or visual scintillations. Persistent morning headaches and personality changes in this case are inconsistent with the diagnosis of tension headache **(b)**. Tension headache is described as bilateral pressure-like pain, not worsened with activity and associated with stress. Headaches in patients older than 50 years are unusual and should be taken seriously and well evaluated. Subarachnoid hemorrhage **(c)** typically presents with severe headache of acute onset, classically described as "the worst headache of my life," with associated nausea and vomiting. Pseudotumor cerebri **(d)** or benign intracranial hypertension is a disorder seen in young obese female patients complaining of chronic headaches.

**235. The answer is b.** *(Ross, p 2011.)* Eclampsia develops after the 20th week of gestation and is considered a complication of severe preeclampsia. The progression from severe preeclampsia to seizures and coma is thought to be a result of hypertensive encephalopathy, vasogenic edema-associated cortical ischemia, edema, or hemorrhage. Therefore, a head CT should be quickly obtained. Eclampsia is a clinical diagnosis with patients having seizures without evidence of CNS, metabolic, or any other seizure etiology. Most patients have systolic BP higher than 160 mm Hg or diastolic BP higher than 110 mm Hg and proteinuria; however, eclampsia can occur with minimally elevated BP—or elevated, relative to baseline—and without proteinuria. Evidence of end-organ damage prior to development of seizures is common. Symptoms include altered mental status, headache, visual disturbances, and abdominal pain; signs include hemolysis, impaired liver function with elevated liver enzyme levels, low platelets (HELLP [hemolysis, elevated liver enzymes, low platelets]), hemoconcentration, proteinuria, oliguria, pulmonary edema, generalized peripheral edema, microangiopathic hemolytic anemia, and fetal growth retardation. Eclampsia is most common during the antepartum period, yet 20% to 25% of cases occur during the postpartum period. Although postpartum eclampsia may occur as long after birth as 3 weeks postpartum, most cases (98%) occur on the first postpartum day. Eclampsia is not the cause of seizures that occur during the first trimester or well into the postpartum period. These seizures are suggestive of CNS pathology.

A complete blood count (a) and LP (c) are helpful if there is concern for an infectious etiology of the seizure, such as meningitis. In addition, if you are concerned for HELLP syndrome, a complete blood count is necessary. (d) A urinalysis is not required to make the diagnosis of eclampsia since proteinuria may or may not occur. A urinalysis can be used to rule out a urinary tract infection. An (e) ECG should be obtained to complete the patient's evaluation but can wait until after the head CT.

**236. The answer is e.** (*Tintinalli, pp 1490-1492.*) This patient presents with four of the five symptoms classically associated with **TTP**. These include **thrombocytopenia, hemolytic anemia, neurologic deficits, renal impairment, and fever**. TTP develops with fibrin-strand deposition in small vessels that attract platelets leading to platelet thrombi and thrombocytopenia. Passing RBCs get sheared in occluded vessels, resulting in microangiopathic hemolytic anemia. Renal and neurologic impairments occur because of the lodging of thrombi in respective circulations. Plasmapheresis decreases TTP mortality from 90% to 10%. Adjunct therapies include fresh frozen plasma infusion and steroids. It is important to realize that although patients may be severely thrombocytopenic, platelet infusion is contraindicated because it exacerbates the underlying cycle of thrombogenesis. Risk factors for TTP include pregnancy, autoimmune disorders, drugs, infection, and malignancy. Hemolytic-uremic syndrome (HUS) is a closely related entity usually seen in children. There is pronounced renal dysfunction without altered mentation.

HSP (a) is a small-vessel vasculitis mostly seen in children and associated with a preceding upper respiratory illness in about 50% of patients. It is characterized by purpura, usually lower extremities, abdominal pain, and hematuria. DIC (b) is a coagulopathic state triggered by major trauma, infection, malignancy, drugs, or pregnancy complications. The underlying process activates the coagulation cascade that leads to diffuse thrombosis and coagulopathy as platelets and coagulation factors are consumed.

Patients with DIC have profuse GI or puncture site bleeding, markedly prolonged PT/PTT times, thrombocytopenia, and elevated fibrin split products. DIC management involves treatment of the underlying disorder and replacement of depleted coagulation cascade components. von Wille-brand disease (**c**) is the most common bleeding disorder and involves deficiency or defect in von Willebrand factor, which normally aids in platelet adherence and carries factor VIII in plasma. von Willebrand disease presents clinically with GI bleeding, epis-taxis, easy bruising, and prolonged bleeding. ITP (**d**) is a disorder of antibody-mediated platelet destruction. It is acute in children, usually following a viral infection, and is chronic in adults who often require splenectomy for definitive treatment.

**237. The answer is a.** (*Tintinalli, pp 442-444.*) This patient presents with headache and altered mental status in the setting of severe hypertension leading to the diagnosis of **hypertensive encephalopathy**. A hypertensive emergency is defined by severe hypertension with evidence of organ dysfunction. The BP needs to be aggressively, but carefully, lowered to prevent cerebral bleeding and progression to coma and death. Patients can also present with seizures, focal neurologic deficits, visual acuity changes, or coma. Patients with hypertensive encephalopathy are managed with **short-acting titratable IV antihypertensive medications** such as IV **nitroprus-side** or labetalol. The BP should not be significantly lowered because it can result in brain hypoperfusion and infarction. Typically, the mean arterial pressure (MAP) is lowered by 20% to 25% in the first hour of treatment.

Magnesium sulfate (**b**) is used in the management of hypertension and seizures in eclampsia. It is not useful in other hypertensive emergency situations. Metoprolol (**c**) is a useful agent for hypertension but is not helpful in situations requiring rapid and precise BP control. Hydrochlorothiazide (**d**) is a good agent for chronic hypertension control. It does not offer rapid and precise BP control required in this case. Obtaining a head CT (**e**) should be considered in this patient since intracranial hemorrhage and brain tumor are in the differential diagnosis.

**238. The answer is e.** (*Tintinalli, p 1153.*) This is a **complex partial seizure**, also known as temporal seizure, although it does not necessarily originate in the temporal lobe. It is characterized by **focal electrical discharges** (partial seizure), such as clonic leg activity and **alteration of consciousness**.

Petit mal seizures (**a**), also known as absence seizures, involve sudden brief loss of consciousness without the loss of postural tone. Patients appear detached or withdrawn and do not respond to stimulation. The seizures might be frequent and classically occur in children. A generalized tonic-clonic seizure (b) involves both hemispheres and loss of consciousness (generalized component) and clonic activity of the extremities. Partial seizure with secondary generalization (c) starts with focal abnormal activity that spreads to involve bilateral cortex and mimics a generalized seizure. A simple partial seizure (d) is focal abnormal activity and intact consciousness.

**239. The answer is c.** (*Rosen, pp 142-148.*) The emergency medicine physician is often faced with differentiating whether the cause of a patient losing consciousness is a result of syncope or a **seizure**. The most likely etiology of this patient's symptoms is in the history that she gives. She tells you that she has **not taken her antiseizure medications** in 2 days. Also, given her evolving mental status and improvement in alertness, this patient most likely presented in a postictal state after she has seized. Without any focal deficit and further improvement in her mental status, one might be comfortable with this diagnosis. Serum testing of her antiepileptic drug levels must be performed to further investigate this suspicion. A CT of the head, ECG, and further investigation is warranted if these levels are normal and do not explain her loss of consciousness.

Other neurologic causes, such as a CVA (a) and TIA (b) should also be in the differential. Typical TIA symptoms include any neurologic symptom, which improves within 30 minutes. In this case, however, the patient's history and presentation most likely precludes this diagnosis. The possibility of her having a stroke is further diminished by her normal neurologic examination. This patient did not complain of any chest or abdominal symptoms (d and e), which place aortic dissection and pulmonary embolus further down on the differential list.

# Gastrointestinal Bleeding

## Questions

**240.** A 51-year-old man is brought to the emergency department (ED) by emergency medical services (EMS) with a blood pressure (BP) of 90/60 mm Hg, heart rate (HR) of 110 beats per minute, respiratory rate (RR) of 18 breaths per minute, and oxygen saturation of 97% on room air. The patient tells you that he has a history of bleeding ulcers. On examination, his abdomen is tender in the epigastric area. He is guaiac positive, with black stool. He has a bout of hematemesis and you notice that his BP is now 80/50 mm Hg, HR is 114 beats per minute, as he is slowly starting to drift off. Which of the following is the most appropriate next step in therapy?

a. Assess airway, establish two large-bore intravenous (IV) lines, cross-match for two units of blood, administer 1 to 2 L of normal saline, and schedule an emergent endoscopy.
b. Assess airway, establish two large-bore IVs, cross-match for 2 units of blood, and administer a proton pump inhibitor.
c. Place two large-bore IVs, cross-match for 2 units of blood, administer 1 to 2 L of normal saline, and schedule an emergent endoscopy.
d. Intubate the patient, establish two large-bore IVs, cross-match for 2 units of blood, administer 1 to 2 L of normal saline, and schedule an emergent endoscopy.
e. Intubate the patient, establish two large-bore IVs, cross-match for 2 units of blood, and administer a proton pump inhibitor.

**241.** A 45-year-old woman presents to the ED with 1 day of painful rectal bleeding. Review of systems is negative for weight loss, abdominal pain, nausea, and vomiting. On physical examination, you note an exquisitely tender swelling with engorgement and a bluish discoloration distal to the anal verge. Her vital signs are HR 105 beats per minute, BP 140/70 mm Hg, RR 18 breaths per minute, and temperature 99°F. Which of the following is the next best step in management?

a. Recommend warm sitz baths, topical analgesics, stool softeners, a high-fiber diet, and arrange for surgical follow-up.
b. Incision and drainage under local anesthesia or procedural sedation followed by packing and surgical follow-up.
c. Obtain a complete blood cell (CBC) count, clotting studies, type and cross, and arrange for emergent colonoscopy.
d. Excision under local anesthesia followed by sitz baths and analgesics.
e. Surgical consult for immediate operative management.

**242.** A 20-year-old man presents to the ED with fever and severe right lower quadrant (RLQ) pain for 1 day. Prior to this episode, he reports 2 months of crampy abdominal pain, generalized malaise, a 10-lb weight loss, and occasional bloody diarrhea. On examination, his HR is 115 beats per minute, BP is 125/70 mm Hg, RR is 18 breaths per minute, and temperature is 100.8°F. His only significant past medical history is recurrent perirectal abscesses. On physical examination, the patient appears uncomfortable and has a tender mass in the RLQ, without guarding or rebound. Rectal examination is positive for trace heme-positive stool. An abdominal computed tomographic (CT) scan reveals no periappendiceal fat stranding. There is inflammation of the distal ileum and several areas of the colon. There are no rectal inflammatory changes. Which of the following is the most likely diagnosis?

a. Crohn disease (CD)
b. Ulcerative colitis (UC)
c. Appendicitis
d. Pseudomembranous enterocolitis
e. Diverticulitis

**243.** A 62-year-old man with a history of hypertension presents to the ED with severe constant mid-epigastric pain for the past hour. Over the last several months, he has had intermittent pain shortly after eating, but never this severe. He states he now has generalized abdominal pain that began suddenly about 15 minutes ago. He has no history of trauma, has never had surgery, and takes no medications. His vitals include HR of 115 beats per minute lying supine, increasing to 135 when sitting up, BP of 170/105 mm Hg supine, falling to 145/85 mm Hg when sitting up. He appears pale. His abdomen is rigid and diffusely tender with guarding and rebound. Bowel sounds are absent and stool hemoccult is positive. The white blood cell (WBC) count is 8500/μL, hemoglobin 8.5 mg/dL, hematocrit 27%, and platelets 255/μL. Which of the following is the most likely diagnosis?

a. Boerhaave syndrome
b. Perforated gastric ulcer
c. Abdominal aortic aneurysm (AAA)
d. Inflammatory bowel disease (IBD)
e. Diverticulosis

**244.** A 60-year-old man with a history of alcohol abuse presents to the ED with hematemesis for 1 day. He denies abdominal or chest pain. On physical examination, his eyes appear reddened which he attributes to having drunken heavily the night before (he also reveals vomiting several times after this recent binge). Vital signs are HR 115 beats per minute, BP 130/85 mm Hg, RR 18 breaths per minute, and temperature 99.5°F. Chest radiograph is unremarkable. Laboratory results reveal a WBC 10,000/μL, hemoglobin 14 mg/dL, hematocrit 40%, and platelets 210/μL. Which diagnosis is endoscopic evaluation most likely to confirm?

a. Esophageal varices
b. Boerhaave syndrome
c. Curling ulcer
d. Perforated gastric ulcer
e. Mallory-Weiss tear

**245.** A 50-year-old man is brought to the ED by ambulance with significant hematemesis. In the ambulance, paramedics placed two large-bore IVs and began infusing normal saline. In the ED, his HR is 127 beats per minute, BP is 79/45 mm Hg, temperature is 97.9°F, RR is 24 breaths per minute, and oxygen saturation is 96%. On physical examination, his abdomen is nontender, but you note spider angiomata, palmar erythema, and gynecomastia. Laboratory results reveal WBC 9000/$\mu$L, hematocrit 28%, platelets 40/$\mu$L, aspartate transaminase (AST) 675 U/L, alanine transaminase (ALT) 325 U/L, alkaline phosphatase 95 U/L, total bilirubin 14.4 mg/dL, conjugated bilirubin 12.9 mg/dL, sodium 135 mEq/L, potassium 3.5 mEq/L, chloride 110 mEq/L, bicarbonate 26 mEq/L, blood urea nitrogen (BUN) 20 mg/dL, creatinine 1.1 mg/dL, and glucose 150 mg/dL. Which of the following is the most likely diagnosis?

a. Perforated gastric ulcer
b. Diverticulosis
c. Splenic laceration
d. Esophageal varices
e. Ruptured AAA

**246.** A 55-year-old man is brought to the ED by his family. They state that he has been vomiting large amounts of bright red blood. The patient is an alcoholic with cirrhotic liver disease and a history of portal hypertension and esophageal varices. His vitals on arrival are HR 110 beats per minute, BP 80/55 mm Hg, RR 22 breaths per minute, and temperature 99°F. The patient appears pale and is in moderate distress. Which of the following is an *inappropriate* option in the *initial* management of a hypotensive patient with a history of known esophageal varices presenting with hematemesis?

a. Sengstaken-Blakemore tube placement
b. Two large-bore IV lines and volume repletion with crystalloid solutions
c. Nasogastric (NG) lavage
d. IV octreotide
e. Gastrointestinal (GI) consult

**247.** A 70-year-old woman presents to the ED with dark stool for 3 weeks. She occasionally notes bright red blood mixed with the stool. Review of systems is positive for decreased appetite, constipation, and a 10-lb weight loss over 2 months. She denies abdominal pain, nausea, vomiting, and fever, but feels increased weakness and fatigue. She also describes a raspy cough with white sputum production over the previous 2 weeks. Examination reveals she is pale, with a supine BP of 115/60 mm Hg and HR of 90 beats per minute. Standing BP is 100/50 mm Hg, with a pulse of 105 beats per minute. Which of the following is the most likely diagnosis?

a. Hemorrhoids
b. Diverticulitis
c. Mallory-Weiss tear
d. Diverticulosis
e. Adenocarcinoma

**248.** A 76-year-old woman with a history of congestive heart failure, coronary artery disease, and an "irregular heart beat" is brought to the ED by her family. She has been complaining of increasing abdominal pain over the past several days. She denies nausea or vomiting and bowel movements remain unchanged. Vitals are HR of 114 beats per minute, BP 110/75 mm Hg, and temperature 98°F. On cardiac examination, her HR is irregularly irregular with no murmur detected. The abdomen is soft, nontender, and nondistended. The stool is heme-positive. This patient is at high risk for which of the following conditions?

a. Perforated gastric ulcer
b. Diverticulitis
c. Acute cholecystitis
d. Mesenteric ischemia
e. Sigmoid volvulus

**249.** A 70-year-old woman with a history of hypertension, congestive heart failure, and atrial fibrillation presents to the ED with several hours of acute onset diffuse abdominal pain. She denies any nausea or vomiting. The pain is constant, but she is unable to localize it. She was diagnosed with a renal artery thrombosis several years ago. Vital signs include HR of 95 beats per minute, BP of 110/70 mm Hg, and temperature of 98°F. Her abdomen is soft and mildly tender, despite her reported severe abdominal pain. Her WBC count is 12,000/µL, hematocrit 38%, platelets 250/µL, and lactate 8 mg/dL. The stool is traced heme-positive. You are concerned for acute mesenteric ischemia. What is the best way to diagnose this condition?

a. Serum lactate levels
b. Abdominal radiograph (supine and upright)
c. CT scan
d. Angiography
e. Barium contrast study

**250.** A 55-year-old man with hypertension and end-stage renal disease requiring hemodialysis presents with 2 days of painless hematochezia. He reports similar episodes of bleeding in the past, which were attributed to angiodysplasia. He denies abdominal pain, nausea, vomiting, diarrhea, and fever. His vitals include HR of 90 beats per minute, BP of 145/95 mm Hg, RR of 18 breaths per minute, and temperature of 98°F. His abdomen is soft and nontender and his stool is grossly positive for blood. Which of the following statements are true regarding angiodysplasia?

a. They are responsible for over 50% of acute lower GI bleeding.
b. They are more common in younger patients.
c. Angiography is the most sensitive method for identifying angiodysplasias.
d. They are less common in patients with end-stage renal disease.
e. The majority of angiodysplasias are located on the right side of the colon.

**251.** A 49-year-old man is brought to the ED by EMS stating that he vomited approximately three cups of blood over the last 2 hours. He also complains of epigastric pain. While examining the patient, he has another episode of hematemesis. You decide to place an NG tube. You insert the tube, confirm its placement, and attach it to suction. You retrieve 200 mL of coffee-ground blood. What is the most common etiology of an upper GI bleed?

a. Varices
b. Peptic ulcer
c. Gastric erosions
d. Mallory-Weiss tear
e. Esophagitis

**252.** A 68-year-old man presents to the ED 4 hours after an upper endoscopy was performed for 5 months of progressive dysphagia. During the procedure, a 1-cm ulcerated lesion was found and biopsied. Now, the patient complains of severe neck and chest pain. His vitals are as follows: BP 135/80 mm Hg, HR 123 beats per minute, RR 26 breaths per minute, and temperature 101°F. On physical examination, he appears diaphoretic and in moderate distress with crepitus in the neck and a crunching sound over the heart. You obtain an electrocardiogram (ECG), which is notable for sinus tachycardia. After obtaining a surgical consult, which of the following is the next best step in management?

a. Perform an immediate bronchoscopy.
b. Give aspirin 325 mg and obtain a cardiology consult for possible cardiac catheterization.
c. Repeat the endoscopy to evaluate the biopsy site.
d. Perform an immediate thoracotomy.
e. Order an immediate esophagram with water-soluble agent.

**253.** A 65-year-old man with a history of occasional painless rectal bleeding presents with 2 to 3 days of constant, dull RLQ pain. He also complains of fever, nausea, and decreased appetite. He had a colonoscopy 2 years ago that was significant for sigmoid and cecal diverticula but was otherwise normal. On physical examination he has RLQ tenderness with rebound and guarding. His vitals include HR of 95 beats per minute, BP of 130/85 mm Hg, and temperature of 101.3°F. The abdominal CT demonstrates the presence of sigmoid and cecal diverticula, inflammation of pericolic fat, thickening of the bowel wall, and a fluid-filled appendix. Which of the following is the most appropriate next step in management?

a. Discharge the patient with broad-spectrum oral antibiotics and surgical follow-up.
b. Begin IV hydration and broad-spectrum antibiotics, keep the patient npo (nothing by mouth), and admit the patient to the hospital.
c. Begin IV antibiotics and call a surgical consult for an emergent operative procedure.
d. Arrange for an emergent barium enema to confirm the diagnosis.
e. Begin sulfasalazine 3 to 4 g/d along with IV steroid therapy.

**254.** A 20-year-old man presents with several weeks of painful rectal bleeding. He denies fever, nausea, or vomiting. He is sexually active with women only and usually uses condoms. He denies any history of CD, UC, or malignancy. He states that the pain is most severe during and immediately after defecating. Bleeding is bright red and only enough to stain the toilet paper. Which of the following is the most common etiology of painful rectal bleeding?

a. External hemorrhoid
b. Anal fissure
c. Anorectal tumor
d. Internal hemorrhoid
e. Venereal proctitis

**255.** A 67-year-old woman with a history of hypertension and congestive heart failure presents with "burning" epigastric pain that began 2 hours after eating a meal. She states that she has had similar pain over the past several weeks, and has been taking antacids and a medication that her primary care physician had prescribed with moderate relief. The pain has occurred with increasing frequency and now awakens her from sleep. She states she came to the ED today because the pain was not relieved with her usual medications. She denies nausea, vomiting, diarrhea, or fever. She also denies hematemesis, black stool, or bright red blood per rectum. On physical examination, she is tender at the epigastrium, with an otherwise normal abdominal, pulmonary, and heart examination. Stool guaiac tests positive for occult blood. Which of the following is the most common serious complication of peptic ulcer disease?

a. GI hemorrhage
b. GI perforation
c. GI penetration
d. Gastric outlet obstruction
e. Pernicious anemia

**256.** A 78-year-old man with a history of atherosclerotic heart disease and congestive heart failure presents with increasing abdominal pain. The pain began suddenly a day ago and has progressively worsened since then. He denies nausea, vomiting, and diarrhea, but states that he had black tarry stool this morning. He denies any history of prior episodes of similar pain. Vitals are BP 120/65 mm Hg, HR 105 beats per minute, and temperature 99°F. The patient is at high risk for which of the following conditions?

a. Cholecystitis
b. Cecal volvulus
c. Mesenteric ischemia
d. Perforated peptic ulcer
e. Small bowel obstruction

# Gastrointestinal Bleeding

## Answers

**240. The answer is a.** (*Rosen, p 170.*) Emergency medicine always starts with an **assessment of the patient's airway**. For patients suspected of having a significant **GI bleed, two large-bore IV lines** need to be established rapidly. Treating an undifferentiated upper GI bleed is like treating a gunshot wound to the abdomen—you should expect the worst. Immediate volume resuscitation should begin with 1 to 2 L of normal saline. If there is no improvement in the BP of a hypotensive patient, blood should be administered. Sending a cross-match early is advisable because it can take up to an hour to retrieve. Use type O, Rh-negative (if female) or type O, Rh-positive (if male) if type-specific blood is not ready. It is crucial to remember that the initial hematocrit of the patient is a poor indicator of the severity of acute bleeding because it takes 24 to 72 hours to equilibrate.

**(b)** A proton pump inhibitor may be administered, but priority is to the airway, breathing, and circulation (ABCs) and this patient is hypotensive. **(c)** You must assess airway first. **(d and e)** The patient is maintaining his airway and does not need to be intubated emergently. However, if his BP worsens and he becomes altered or you anticipate his condition to worse, endotracheal intubation is appropriate.

**241. The answer is d.** (*Rosen, pp 1245-1247.*) Hemorrhoids are dilated venules of the hemorrhoidal plexuses. They are associated with constipation, straining, increased abdominal pressure, pregnancy, increased portal pressure, and a low-fiber diet. Hemorrhoids can be either internal or external. Those that arise above the dentate line are internal and painless. Those below the dentate line are external and painful. Individuals commonly present with thrombosed external hemorrhoids. On examination, there is a tender mass at the anal orifice that is typically bluish-purple in color. If pain is severe and the thrombosis is less than 48 hours, the physician should excise the thrombus under local anesthesia followed by a warm sitz baths. This patient is suffering from an acutely **thrombosed external**

**hemorrhoid**. If not excised, symptoms will most often resolve within several days when the hemorrhoid ulcerates and leaks the dark accumulated blood. Residual skin tags may persist. Excision provides both immediate- and long-term relief and prevents the formation of skin tags. (a) The symptoms of nonthrombosed external and nonprolapsing internal hemorrhoids can be improved by the **WASH** regimen. **Warm water**, via sitz baths or by directing a shower stream at the affected area for several minutes, reduces anal pressures; mild oral **analgesics** relieve pain; **stool softeners** ease the passage of stool to avoid straining; and a **high-fiber diet** produces stool that passes more easily. (b) **Incision** of a hemorrhoid (as opposed to **excision**) leads to incomplete clot evacuation, subsequent rebleeding, and swelling of lacerated vessels. (c) This patient has a thrombosed external hemorrhoid. The need for further evaluation of the rectal bleeding has not been established. (e) Hemorrhoids rarely require immediate operative management, unless there is evidence of thrombus formation with progression to gangrene.

**242. The answer is a.** *(Tintinalli, pp 536-540.)* **IBD** is a chronic inflammatory disease of the GI tract. There are two major types: CD and UC. **CD** can involve any part of the GI tract, from mouth to anus, and is characterized by segmental involvement. The distal ileum is involved in the majority of cases; therefore, acute presentations can mimic appendicitis. CD spares the rectum in 50% of cases. There is a bimodal age distribution, with the first peak occurring in patients 15 to 22 years of age and a second in patients 55 to 60 years of age. Definitive diagnosis is by upper GI series, air-contrast barium enema, and colonoscopy. Segmental involvement of the colon with rectal sparing is the most characteristic feature. Other findings on colonoscopy include involvement of all bowel wall layers, **skip lesions** (ie, interspersed normal and diseased bowel), **aphthous ulcers**, and **cobblestone** appearance from submucosal thickening interspersed with mucosal ulceration. Extraintestinal manifestations are seen in 25% to 30% of patients with CD.

(b) UC primarily involves the mucosa only with formation of crypt abscesses, epithelial necrosis, and mucosal ulceration. Rectal pain and bloody diarrhea are more common in UC than in CD. UC begins in the rectum, and fails to progress beyond this point in one-third of patients. Colonoscopy demonstrates inflammation of the mucosa only and continuous lesions of the GI tract. Although blood loss from sustained bleeding may be the most common complication, toxic megacolon must not be missed. (c) While appendicitis may be in the differential diagnosis, the acute on chronic nature of this disease and a normal-appearing appendix on abdominal CT rules it out. (d) Pseudomembranous enterocolitis is an inflammatory bowel disorder that results from toxin-producing *Clostridium difficile*, a spore-forming obligate anaerobic bacillus. The disease typically begins 7 to 10 days after the institution of antibiotic therapy, most often in hospitalized patients. However, incidence in the community is rising. (e) Diverticulitis is an acute inflammatory disease caused by bacterial proliferation within existing colonic diverticula. The most common presentation is pain, often in the left lower quadrant (LLQ). Abdominal CT demonstrates inflammation of pericolic fat, presence of diverticula, bowel wall thickening, or peridiverticular abscess.

**243. The answer is b.** (*Rosen, pp 165, 1145-1147.*) This patient had an untreated **gastric ulcer** that just **perforated**. The history of epigastric pain related to eating points to a gastric ulcer, whereas pain 2 to 3 hours after eating is more likely caused by a duodenal ulcer. The sudden onset of generalized abdominal pain associated with a rigid abdomen is concerning for a perforated viscus, in this case, a perforated gastric ulcer. This is a surgical emergency. An abdominal and upright chest radiograph can be performed quickly to look for **free air**, which will be seen **under the diaphragm** on the chest radiograph. This is useful for the majority of perforations, which are anterior, but may miss posterior perforations because the posterior duodenum is retroperitoneal. The treatment includes IV hydration, antibiotics, and immediate surgical correction.

(a) Boerhaave syndrome is a full-thickness tear of the left posterolateral aspect of the distal esophagus. It is typically associated with epigastric and retrosternal chest pain that often radiates to the back, neck, left chest, or shoulders. Although it may present similar to a perforated ulcer, in general the pain is more focused in the chest. (c) While the history of untreated hypertension is concerning for a ruptured AAA the history clearly points to previously undiagnosed peptic ulcer disease. (d) IBD is a chronic condition affecting the GI tract. The abdominal pain is usually crampy, while GI bleeding is generally associated with bloody diarrhea. (e) Diverticula are saclike herniations of colonic mucosa that occur at weak points in the bowel wall. They may bleed (diverticulosis) or become filled with fecal matter and lead to inflammation (diverticulitis). Diverticulosis is most commonly associated with substantial painless rectal bleeding but not with significant abdominal pain.

**244. The answer is e.** *(Rosen, pp 150-151, 1139-1140.)* A **Mallory-Weiss tear** usually follows a forceful bout of retching and vomiting and involves a 1- to 4-cm area of the mucosa or submucosa of the GI tract; 75% of cases occur in the stomach with the remainder near the gastroesophageal (GE) junction. Bleeding is usually mild and self-limited. However, 3% of deaths from upper GI bleeds result from Mallory-Weiss tears.

(a) Esophageal varices are dilated submucosal veins found in 50% of patients with cirrhosis of the liver. They usually develop as a result of portal hypertension. Up to 30% of patients with esophageal varices develop upper GI bleeds, and the bleeding is usually massive. Patients are often asymptomatic until the varices rupture and bleed. Although this patient is certainly predisposed to varices secondary to his ethanol abuse, his acute presentation of pain after vomiting is more consistent with a Mallory-Weiss tear. **(b)** Boerhaave syndrome involves a spontaneous full thickness perforation of the esophagus—80% involving the posterolateral aspect of the distal esophagus—that usually results from violent retching. Alcohol ingestion is a risk factor. Because the overlying pleura is torn, esophageal contents can spill into the mediastinum and thorax, leading to severe epigastric and retrosternal chest pain, with radiations to the back, neck, or shoulders. Characteristic findings on chest radiograph include a left pneumothorax, a left pleural effusion, mediastinal emphysema, and a widened mediastinum, all of which the individual in the question does not exhibit. Boerhaave syndrome represents a surgical emergency, with mortality approaching 50% if surgery is not performed within 24 hours. **(c)** A Curling ulcer is an ulcer or erosion caused by stress gastritis because of patients with severe burn injuries. The most common finding is painless GI bleeding. There is no evidence of severe burn injury in this patient. **(d)** A perforated gastric ulcer is a complication of chronic gastritis, which is usually associated with severe, acute abdominal pain. Perforations occur when an ulcer erodes through the wall and leaks air and digestive contents into the peritoneal cavity. Often, pain initially begins in the epigastrium but becomes generalized shortly thereafter. Patients usually lie still and avoid movement that might disturb the peritoneal cavity. An upright chest radiograph may demonstrate air under the diaphragm.

**245. The answer is d.** *(Tintinalli, pp 543-544, 566-572.)* **Esophageal varices** develop in patients with **chronic liver disease** in response to portal hypertension. Approximately 60% of patients with portal hypertension will develop varices. Of those who develop varices, 25% to 30%

will experience hemorrhage. Patients who develop varices from alcohol abuse have an even higher risk of bleeding, especially with ongoing alcohol consumption. This patient has evidence of chronic liver disease with thrombocytopenia and elevated bilirubin and liver enzymes. In alcoholic hepatitis, the AST is greater than the ALT by a factor of 2. Spider angiomata, palmar erythema, and gynecomastia further suggest underlying liver disease.

(a) A perforated gastric ulcer typically presents with severe sudden abdominal pain in a patient with a history of PUD. (b) Diverticulosis results from saclike herniations in the colonic mucosa (diverticula) that occur at weak points in the bowel wall, usually where arteries insert. Diverticulosis is most commonly associated with painless rectal bleeding. (c) Splenic laceration generally results from trauma. (e) The most common symptom with rupture of an AAA is sudden and severe abdominal pain. Back pain, also sudden and severe, is noted by half of patients. Incidence of AAA increases with age in both men and women and is typically associated with a history of hypertension.

**246. The answer is a.** (*McPhee et al, pp 540-638.*) Acute GI bleeding develops in fewer than one-third of patients with portal hypertension and varices. With upper GI bleeds, the initial step is assessment of the hemodynamic status. **Hypotension** with or without tachycardia identifies a **high-risk patient** with severe acute bleeding. This patient requires immediate treatment. If initial resuscitative efforts fail or if a patient remains hypotensive, more aggressive measures may be required, including consideration of Sengstaken-Blakemore tube is placed to physically tamponade the bleeding source, but this is not part of the initial management and has been associated with adverse reactions.

(b) In patients with significant bleeding, two 18-gauge or larger IV lines should be started prior to further diagnostic tests. Blood is sent for CBC, coagulation studies (prothrombin time [PT] with international normalized ratio [INR]), serum creatinine, liver enzymes, and cross-matching for 2 to 4 units or more of packed red blood cells (RBC). Patients with hemodynamic compromise should be resuscitated with crystalloid solutions and cross-matched blood. Cardiac monitoring and supplemental oxygen should also be instituted. (c) An NG tube should be placed in all patients with suspected upper GI bleeding. The aspiration of red blood or "coffee grounds" confirms an upper GI bleeding source, although 10% of patients with confirmed upper GI bleeding have nonbloody aspirates, especially when bleeding originates in the duodenum. An aspirate of bright red blood indicates active bleeding and is associated with the highest risk of bleeding and complications. Efforts to control bleeding by gastric lavage with large volumes of fluid are of no benefit and increase the risk of aspiration. (d) Octreotide reduces splanchnic blood flow and portal blood pressures and is effective in the initial control of bleeding related to portal hypertension. It should be administered promptly to all patients with active upper GI bleeding and evidence of liver disease or portal hypertension until the source of bleeding can be clarified by endoscopy. (e) A GI consult should be obtained in all cases of high-risk upper GI bleeds. Most patients with upper GI bleeding should undergo upper endoscopy after the patient is hemodynamically stable. High-risk patients or those with continued active bleeding require more urgent endoscopic evaluation to identify the source of bleeding, determine the risk of rebleeding, and provide hemostasis via sclerotherapy or rubber band ligation.

**247. The answer is e.** (*Rosen, pp 170-175, 1229-1232.*) The combination of lower GI bleed with weight loss and decreased appetite points toward carcinoma, most likely **adenocarcinoma of the colon**. The lack of esophageal, abdominal, or rectal pain makes the other choices unlikely, as does the lack of associated symptoms (nausea, vomiting, or fever). Anemia or rectal bleeding in an elderly person should be assumed to be malignancy until proven otherwise.

(a) Bleeding with defecation is the most common complaint with hemorrhoids, and unless the hemorrhoids are thrombosed, the bleeding is usually painless. Patients usually report bright red blood on the toilet paper or in the toilet bowl. Weight loss would not be expected, and only in rare circumstances is the blood loss substantial. (b) Diverticulitis occurs with inflammation of a diverticulum and is the most common complication of diverticulosis. Patients typically present with persistent abdominal pain. Initially, the pain may be vague and generalized, but it often becomes localized to the LLQ. Most patients can be managed medically with bowel rest, hydration, analgesics, and antibiotics. (c) A Mallory-Weiss tear is a partial tear of the esophagus that usually results from significant vomiting or retching. (d) Diverticulosis is the presence of diverticula with massive painless lower GI bleeding. It is one of the most common causes of massive GI bleeding in this population. In most instances, the bleeding stops spontaneously.

**248. The answer is d.** *(Rosen, pp 1188-1192.)* Patients with coronary artery disease, valvular heart disease, and arrhythmias, particularly **atrial fibrillation**, are at high risk for **mesenteric ischemia**. In addition, age greater than 50 years, congestive heart failure, recent myocardial infarction, critically ill patients with sepsis or hypotension, use of diuretics or vasoconstrictive medications, and hypercoagulable states place patients at higher risk. The most common cause of acute mesenteric ischemia is **arterial embolus**, which accounts for 50% of cases. The classic finding is "pain out of proportion to examination findings"; that is, a patient complains of severe pain but is not particularly tender on examination. A high degree of suspicion for mesenteric ischemia in an elderly patient with abdominal pain is warranted.

**(a)** Perforated gastric ulcer presents with acute onset of severe epigastric pain and bleeding, generally in someone with PUD. **(b)** Diverticulitis presents as LLQ pain that is usually described as dull and constant. **(c)** Acute cholecystitis occurs with an obstruction of the cystic duct with gallstones and is often accompanied by fever, chills, nausea, and a positive Murphy sign. It is the most common surgical emergency in elderly patients. **(e)** The classic triad for sigmoid volvulus includes abdominal pain, abdominal distention, and constipation. Nausea and vomiting are often present, and diagnosis can be made on plain radiograph in 80% of cases.

**249. The answer is d.** *(Rosen, pp 1190-1191.)* **Angiography** remains the "gold standard" in the diagnosis of **mesenteric ischemia**. Unlike any other diagnostic tools, it is capable of both **diagnosing and treating** the problem. It is capable of identifying all four types of acute mesenteric ischemia: (1) arterial embolus, (2) arterial thrombosis (3) venous thrombosis, and, under most circumstances, (4) nonocclusive mesenteric ischemia. Angiography should be obtained without delay when the diagnosis is suspected.

With the exception of angiography, the results of all other studies are most useful in ruling out other diagnoses or finding out baseline levels. Abdominal radiographs **(b)** should be performed on any patient with suspected mesenteric ischemia to rule out bowel obstruction or free air. However, in the early stages, plain radiographs are most often normal in patients with mesenteric ischemia and should not be used to rule out this entity. Positive findings include intraluminal gas or gas in the portal venous system, usually coincide with the development of necrotic bowel, and signify a grim prognosis. **(c)** Because of its availability, speed, and improved quality, CT is often used in the ED for assessing abdominal pain of unclear etiology in high-risk patients. CT may identify indirect signs of ischemia—including edema of the bowel wall or mesentery, abnormal gas patterns, intramural gas, and ascites. Occasionally, CT may accurately identify direct evidence of mesenteric venous thrombosis. As with abdominal radiographs, many patients may have normal or nonspecific findings on CT, so it cannot be used to rule out the diagnosis of mesenteric ischemia. While a few studies have found CT to be as sensitive as angiography, it is not currently the study of choice. (a) The sensitivity of serum lactate is high, nearly 100%, in the presence of mesenteric ischemia, but the specificity is low, ranging from 42% to 87%. Elevated serum lactate may best be used as a predictor of mortality. Some studies suggest that the presence of an unexplained acidosis should prompt a search for reversible causes of mesenteric ischemia. (e) Intraluminal barium contrast studies are contraindicated with suspected mesenteric ischemia because residual contrast material can limit visualization of the vasculature during diagnostic angiography.

**250. The answer is e.** *(Townsend et al, p 1216.)* **Angiodysplasias**, also known as **arteriovenous malformations**, are small ectatic blood vessels in the submucosa of the GI tract. More than half of angiodysplasias are located on the **right side of the colon**.

(a) Angiodysplasias are responsible for 3% to 20% of acute lower GI bleeds. (b) Although angiodysplasia accounts for the most common cause of lower GI bleeding in younger patients, its incidence overall increases with age over 50 years. (c) While angiography may identify angiodysplasias, colonoscopy remains the most sensitive diagnostic modality. On colonoscopy, angiodysplasias appear as red, flat lesions, measuring approximately 2 to 20 mm in diameter. (d) Angiodysplasias are associated with many medical problems, including end-stage renal disease, aortic stenosis, and von Willebrand disease, among others.

**251. The answer is b.** *(Rosen, pp 170-175.)* The most common cause of upper GI bleeds in adults is **peptic ulcer disease** accounting for approximately 45% of the cases. Hematemesis is the presentation in approximately 50% of patients with upper GI bleeds. The appearance of coffee-grounds in the stomach is caused by the conversion of hemoglobin to hematin or other pigments by hydrochloric acid in the stomach.

(a) Varices account for 10%, (c) erosions 23%, (d) Mallory-Weiss tear 7%, and (e) esophagitis 6%.

**252. The answer is e.** *(Rosen, pp 1139-1140.)* The patient most likely has an **esophageal perforation**, a serious, life-threatening **complication of endoscopy** that must be identified and treated quickly. Although sometimes reported as a result of forceful vomiting (eg, Boerhaave syndrome), the most common cause is iatrogenic. These usually occur as a complication of GI procedures, including upper endoscopy, dilation, sclerotherapy, and even NG tube placement or endotracheal intubation. The signs and symptoms may include chest pain near the rupture site, fever, respiratory distress, hoarseness, or dysphagia. Most patients have **mediastinal or cervical emphysema**, which may be noted by palpation or by a **crunching sound** heard during auscultation (**ie, Hamman sign**). An immediate esophagram with a water-soluble agent (eg, Gastrografin) is indicated.

(**a**) Bronchoscopy is used to evaluate a patient with suspected bronchial obstruction or endobronchial disease. It is not indicated in a case of suspected esophageal perforation. (**b**) The likelihood that this patient's chest pain is cardiac in origin is fairly small and the ECG demonstrates no ischemic changes. The diagnosis in a patient presenting with pain or fever following esophageal instrumentation should be considered esophageal perforation until proven otherwise. Also, if perforation is suspected, aspirin should be withheld. (**c**) Repeating the endoscopy may be useful, especially in cases of trauma; however, small perforations may be difficult or impossible to detect. An esophagram is better to evaluate for a suspected perforation. A chest radiograph and an upright abdominal radiograph are usually obtained first and may detect abnormalities in up to 90% of patients. These findings may include subcutaneous emphysema, pneumomediastinum, mediastinal widening, pleural effusion, or pulmonary infiltrate, but radiographic changes may not be present in the first few hours after the perforation. (**d**) Thoracotomy is the treatment for an esophageal perforation; however, an immediate esophagram with a water-soluble agent should be performed to confirm the diagnosis.

**253. The answer is b.** *(Tintinalli, pp 578-581.)* The diagnosis of **diverticulitis** is made by abdominal CT, which may demonstrate inflammation of pericolic fat, bowel wall thickening, the presence of diverticula, or peridiverticular abscess. The treatment of diverticulitis includes **IV hydration, bowel rest, and broad-spectrum antibiotics** to cover both aerobic and anaerobic bacteria. These typically include a combination of metronidazole and ciprofloxacin or levofloxacin. Well-appearing patients can be treated as outpatients with oral antibiotics and close follow-up, but patients with fever, signs of localized peritonitis or obstruction, and those who have failed outpatient therapy must be admitted to the hospital.

(a) This patient has systemic signs of infection (fever, rebound tenderness, guarding) and should be admitted for IV antibiotics and observation. If the patient manifests signs of bowel obstruction, an NG tube should also be placed. (c) The presentation of diverticulitis may be indistinguishable from acute appendicitis. This occurs when a patient has a redundant sigmoid lying on the right side of the abdomen or, as in this case, when a cecal diverticulum becomes inflamed. In this case, the abdominal CT demonstrates a normal fluid-filled appendix, effectively ruling out appendicitis. A prompt surgical consult should be obtained in the presence of intestinal obstruction, free perforation, abscess, or fistula formation. (d) The presence of diverticulitis is demonstrated on abdominal CT, which is more sensitive than a barium enema. Furthermore, both barium injected under high pressure and colonoscopy in the presence of acute diverticulitis carry the risk of perforation and are relatively contraindicated. (e) An exacerbation of CD, which may also present with RLQ pain and heme-positive stool, may be treated with sulfasalazine and steroid therapy, but neither is appropriate in the treatment of acute diverticulitis.

**254. The answer is b.** (*Tintinalli, pp 589-593.*) Pain and bleeding are common complaints associated with anorectal disorders. A good history and a thorough physical examination, including a digital rectal examination and anoscopy, should be performed whenever feasible. **Anal fissures (ie, fissures in ano)** result from linear tears of the anal canal at or just inferior to the dentate line and extend along the anal canal to the anal verge. This area has a rich supply of somatic sensory never fibers. Consequently, anal fissures are exquisitely painful and represent the **most common cause of painful rectal bleeding** in the first year of life and in adults. They are usually produced by the passage of a large, hard stool but may also occur with severe diarrhea.

(a) External hemorrhoids also arise from below the dentate line and are covered with well-innervated squamous epithelium making them painful. They often cause bleeding but not as common as anal fissures. (c) Early anorectal malignancies usually present with nonspecific symptoms, such as pruritus, pain, and bleeding mixed with stool, and represent less than 5% of all large bowel malignancies. (d) Internal hemorrhoids are detected by direct visualization using anoscopy. Uncomplicated internal hemorrhoids are painless because of lack of sensory innervation. Consequently, they present with **painless**, bright red bleeding with defecation. (**e**) Most venereal diseases involving the anorectal region present with pruritus, discharge, and mild to moderate pain or irritation, and may intermittently bleed.

**255. The answer is a.** (*Rosen, pp 1145-1147.*) The most serious complications of PUD include hemorrhage, perforation, penetration, and gastric outlet obstruction. **Hemorrhage**, which occurs in 15% of patients, is the **most common complication**.

(**b**) GI perforation occurs when an ulcer erodes through the stomach or bowel wall, and leaks air and digestive contents into the peritoneal cavity. It occurs in approximately 7% of patients and is the second most common serious complication of PUD. (**c**) GI penetration is similar to perforation, except the ulcer erodes into another organ, such as the liver or pancreas. (**d**) Gastric outlet obstruction, which occurs in 2% of patients, occurs because of edema and scarring near the gastric outlet. (**e**) Pernicious anemia results from an autoimmune disease in which the body develops antibodies to the acid-secreting cells in the gastric mucosa with ensuing loss of intrinsic factor, vitamin $B_{12}$ malabsorption, and the development of anemia. It is not a complication of PUD.

**256. The answer is c.** (*Tintinalli, pp 523, 546.*) The complaint of abdominal pain in the elderly patient should prompt the emergency physician to lower his or her threshold for considering more serious intra-abdominal conditions. Patients with a history of arrhythmias (especially atrial fibrillation), low cardiac output (such as congestive heart failure), or who take particular medications, such as digoxin, are at high risk for the elusive condition of **mesenteric ischemia.** A history of sudden onset abdominal pain with increasing severity, but with a benign physical examination should prompt consideration of this entity. Mesenteric ischemia is associated with a high mortality rate, and initial diagnosis is often incorrect. The diagnostic study of choice is angiography.

(**a**) Cholecystitis is the most common surgical emergency in elderly patients, but patients often localize pain to the RUQ. Ultrasonography is the initial diagnostic study of choice. (**b**) Sigmoid volvulus is two to three times more common than cecal volvulus among the elderly and presents with gradually increasing abdominal pain, along with nausea and vomiting. (**d**) Perforated peptic ulcer often presents with acute-onset epigastric pain followed by peritonitis and GI bleeding, and can be a similarly challenging condition to diagnose in elderly patients, who may lack dramatic pain or impressive peritoneal findings. The diagnostic study of choice is CT scan, although an upright chest or abdominal radiograph, which may show free air under the diaphragm, should be obtained immediately if the diagnosis is suspected. **(e)** Small bowel obstruction may also present with gradually increasing abdominal pain, nausea, and vomiting. It is not associated with the comorbid conditions listed, but rather with adhesions following abdominal surgery, incarcerated groin hernia, polyps, lymphomas, adenocarcinoma, abdominal abscess, and radiation therapy.

# Musculoskeletal Injuries

## Questions

**257.** While playing in his family's annual Thanksgiving Day touch-football game, a 41-year-old man fell onto his outstretched hand upon attempting to make the winning catch. He presents to the emergency department (ED) complaining of severe wrist pain. Which of the following carpal bones is most frequently injured in a fall on the outstretched hand (FOOSH)?

a. Triquetrum
b. Lunate
c. Capitate
d. Scaphoid
e. Pisiform

**258.** A 64-year-old man presents to the ED complaining of knee pain since yesterday. He denies trauma or similar presentation in the past. On examination, you note an erythematous, tender, and swollen knee. Radiographs do not reveal a fracture but do show calcium deposits. Arthrocentesis demonstrates 20,000/μL white blood cells (WBCs) with a predominance of neutrophils, a negative Gram stain, and rhomboid shaped crystals that are positively birefringent under polarized light. Which of the following is the most likely diagnosis?

a. Pseudogout
b. Gout
c. Septic joint
d. Rheumatoid arthritis
e. Osteoarthritis

**259.** A 22-year-old soccer player presents to the ED complaining of right knee pain and swelling. He states that earlier in the day he was in a soccer match and was running for the ball but stopped abruptly and tried to run in a new direction. Immediately thereafter, he felt intense pain in his knee with instant swelling. Which of the following is the most commonly injured major ligament of the knee?

a. Anterior cruciate ligament (ACL)
b. Posterior cruciate ligament (PCL)
c. Medial collateral ligament (MCL)
d. Lateral collateral ligament (LCL)
e. Patella ligament

**260.** A 45-year-old man is on his way to work and loses his footing while walking up a flight of steps. He feels excruciating pain at the back of his ankle and cannot ambulate. He arrives to the ED and states that he felt a snap in his leg during the injury. He has a past medical history of hypertension and hypercholesterolemia. He spends most of his free time in front of the television watching horror movies. On examination, you note swelling of the distal calf. Which of the following is likely to be positive in this individual?

a. Homan sign
b. Lachman test
c. McMurray test
d. Ballotable patella
e. Thompson test

**261.** A 24-year-old competitive ice skater is practicing for the Olympic trials when she falls during one of her jumps and lands on her outstretched hand. She is brought to the ED complaining of wrist pain. On examination, you note tenderness at the anatomic snuffbox and pain with axial loading of the thumb. You suspect she has a scaphoid fracture. In what part of a fractured scaphoid is the incidence of avascular necrosis highest?

a. Proximal scaphoid.
b. Waist (middle third) of the scaphoid.
c. Distal scaphoid.
d. Tubercle of the scaphoid.
e. The scaphoid is not at risk for avascular necrosis.

**262.** A 32-year-old male construction worker reports standing on scaffolding before it suddenly gave way beneath him. In an attempt to catch his fall, he spontaneously grabbed and hung on to an overhead beam for approximately 30 seconds. Two hours later in the ED, the patient presents with right shoulder pain and decreased range of motion. He denies any loss of consciousness or other sustained trauma. Vital signs are within normal limits, except for the patient's pain scale of 10/10. He is holding his right arm with the contralateral hand. On physical examination, the patient's shoulder appears swollen with no skin breakage. The upper extremity is without obvious deformity. The patient has palpable brachial, radial, and ulnar pulses with capillary refill that is less than 2 seconds. He can wiggle his fingers but cannot internally rotate his shoulder or raise his right arm above his head. Pinprick testing reveals paresthesias along the lateral deltoid of the affected arm. What is the most likely etiology of this patient's pain and paresthesias?

a. Acromioclavicular joint sprain
b. Posterior shoulder dislocation with axillary nerve impingement
c. Anterior shoulder dislocation with axillary nerve impingement
d. Anterior shoulder dislocation with median nerve impingement
e. Posterior shoulder dislocation with ulnar nerve impingement

**263.** A 22-year-old college volleyball player presents to the ED complaining of left shoulder pain that began while attempting a serve during a volleyball match. She states that this has happened to her before. On examination, the left shoulder looks "squared-off." She complains of severe pain when she tries to adduct or internally rotate the shoulder. A radiograph is seen below. What is the most common fracture associated with the patient's diagnosis?

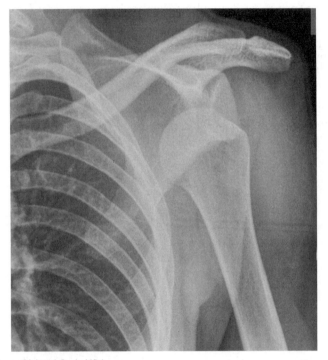

*(Courtesy of Adam J. Rosh, MD.)*

a. Bankart fracture
b. Hill-Sachs deformity
c. Clavicular fracture
d. Coronoid fracture
e. Scapular fracture

**264.** A 35-year-old man presents to the ED with right hand swelling, pain, and erythema that began 3 days ago. He denies any trauma, sick contacts, insect bites, or recent travel. The patient's vitals are significant for an oral temperature of 101°F. Upon physical examination, you note an area of erythema surrounding multiple punctate lacerations over the right third and fourth metacarpophalangeal (MCP) joints with localized tenderness. The patient is neurovascularly intact with limited flexion caused by the swelling and pain. Given the above presentation, what is the most appropriate disposition for this patient?

a. Suture and close follow-up with a hand surgeon
b. Suture and prescription for oral antibiotics
c. Wound irrigation and prescription for oral antibiotics
d. Wound irrigation and tetanus prophylaxis
e. Admission for intravenous (IV) antibiotics

**265.** A 23-year-old man presents to the ED complaining of finger pain. He states that while playing football, he went to catch a pass and the ball hit the tip of his finger and bent his finger backward. He thinks his finger is just "jammed." On examination, you notice that the distal phalanx is flexed and there is swelling and tenderness over the distal interphalangeal (DIP) joint, as seen below. In addition, he cannot extend his distal finger at the DIP joint. An x-ray does not reveal a fracture. Which of the following is the most appropriate way to manage this injury?

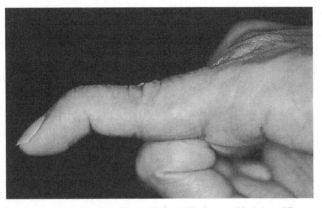

(Reproduced, with permission, from Knoop KJ, Stack LB, Storrow AB. Atlas of Emergency Medicine. New York, NY: McGraw-Hill, 2002: 305.)

a. Place a dorsal splint so that the proximal interphalangeal (PIP) and DIP joints are immobile; remove splint in 1 to 2 weeks.
b. Place a dorsal splint so that the PIP and DIP joints are immobile; remove splint in 1 week.
c. Buddy-tape the finger.
d. Place a dorsal splint to immobilize the DIP joint; remove splint in 1 to 2 weeks.
e. Place a dorsal splint to immobilize the DIP joint; remove splint in 6 to 8 weeks.

**266.** A 22-year-old college student presents to the ED with a painful, swollen finger. He states that he was playing with a roommate's dog and was bitten 3 days earlier. On physical examination, his heart rate (HR) is 70 beats per minute, blood pressure (BP) is 115/65 mm Hg, respiratory rate (RR) is 16 breaths per minute, and temperature is 101.6°F. Bilaterally, the radial pulses remain equal, and the hands and fingers are intact to sensation. His right second finger is held in flexion and is symmetrically swollen from the distal tip to the MCP joint. Both your attempt to extend the digit passively and palpate the flexor tendon sheath produce great pain. Based on these findings you make your diagnosis and notify the hand surgeon immediately. What name is given to the criteria used to make the diagnosis?

a. Finkelstein
b. Trousseau
c. Tinel
d. Kanavel
e. Phalen

**267.** A 41-year-old office worker presents to the ED with pain in her right wrist and fingers, which is associated with a tingling sensation. The pain occasionally awakens her from sleep and improves when the hand is shaken. She recalls falling on her wrist 2 years ago while she was ice-skating. Her symptoms are reproducible when her wrist is held in flexion for 60 seconds. Which of the following nerves is affected in patients with this syndrome?

a. Ulnar
b. Median
c. Axillary
d. Radial
e. Musculocutaneous

**268.** A 23-year-old man presents to the ED complaining of right hand pain. He states that he was mad at a friend and punched the wall in his bedroom. Immediately after he had punched the wall, he felt intense pain in his right hand. On physical examination, you note swelling and tenderness over the fifth metacarpal. When you ask him to make a fist, his fifth finger rotates to lie on top of his fourth finger. The radiograph is shown in below. What is the name of this type of fracture?

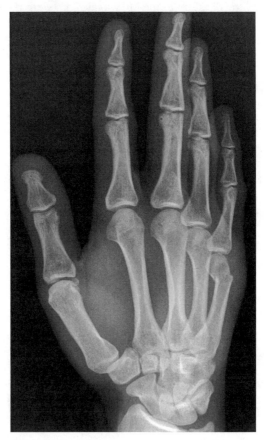

*(Courtesy of Adam J. Rosh, MD.)*

a. Colles fracture
b. Smith fracture
c. Scaphoid fracture
d. Galeazzi fracture
e. Boxer's fracture

**269.** A 43-year-old man presents to the ED after falling approximately 6 ft from the roof of his garage. The patient states that he landed on his feet but then fell to the ground. You assess his ABC (airway, breathing, and circulation), which are all normal. Vital signs are stable. Your secondary survey reveals a swollen and tender right heel. A radiograph reveals a fractured calcaneus. About 6 hours after the initial fall, the patient starts complaining of a constant burning in his right foot. You examine the foot and elicit pain with passive movement. There is decreased two-point discrimination. His dorsalis pedis pulse is 2+. Which of the following is the most appropriate next step in management?

a. Place ice on the foot and administer analgesia.
b. Order another radiograph to look for an occult fracture.
c. Elevate the leg and place an elastic bandage around the foot.
d. Order a duplex ultrasound for suspicion of a deep vein thrombosis (DVT).
e. Measure the intracompartmental pressure of the foot.

**270.** A 41-year-old man is brought into the ED after having a witnessed tonic-clonic seizure. He is alert and oriented, and states that he has not taken his seizure medication for the last week. His BP is 140/75 mm Hg, HR is 88 beats per minute, temperature is 99.7°F, and his RR is 16 breaths per minute. On examination you notice that his arm is internally rotated and adducted. He cannot externally rotate the arm and any movement of his shoulder elicits pain. Which of the following is the most likely diagnosis?

a. Humerus fracture
b. Clavicular fracture
c. Scapular fracture
d. Posterior shoulder dislocation
e. Anterior shoulder dislocation

**271.** A 24-year-old man presents to the ED complaining of right wrist pain that began after he had slipped, fallen, and landed on his outstretched hand. You examine the hand and wrist, and note no abnormalities except for snuffbox tenderness. A radiograph does not reveal a fracture. Which of the following is the most appropriate next step in management?

a. Place an ACE wrap around the hand and wrist until the pain resolves.
b. Immobilize the wrist in a thumb spica splint and have the patient follow up with an orthopedist for repeat radiographs in 10 to 14 days.
c. Continue to ice the wrist for 24 to 48 hours.
d. Order a CT scan to evaluate for an occult fracture.
e. Place the wrist and arm in a cast for 6 weeks.

**272.** A 29-year-old woman presents to the ED complaining of worsening left wrist pain for 1 month. She states that approximately 3 months ago she fell from a ladder and landed on her outstretched hand. She never went to the hospital and just dealt with the pain for a while. On examination, there is no deformity of the wrist. Neurovascular status is normal, but there is tenderness when you palpate the snuffbox. What is the most likely reason for this patient's wrist pain?

a. Fracture of the distal ulna
b. Acute fracture of the scaphoid
c. Avascular necrosis of the scaphoid
d. Hematoma of the radial artery
e. Fracture of the lunate

**273.** A 43-year-old warehouse worker is helping to stock large refrigerator boxes onto the forklift. One of the boxes starts to fall off the shelf and he tries to catch it before it falls. In doing so, his hand is hyperextended at the wrist and causes immediate pain. In the ED, you note limitation of the normal motion of the wrist with palpable fullness on the volar aspect. The patient also complains of tingling in the distribution of the median nerve. Which of the following injuries is most frequently associated with the development of acute carpal tunnel syndrome?

a. Lunate dislocation
b. Perilunate dislocation
c. Scapholunate dislocation
d. Capitate dislocation
e. Scaphoid fracture

**274.** A 22-year-old college football player presents to the ED with knee pain. He states that during the football game today, he received a direct blow to the lateral aspect of his knee. Radiograph of the knee is negative for fracture but shows an effusion. On examination, you confirm the hemarthrosis. As you examine his knee ligaments, you note joint instability with valgus stress in 30 degrees of flexion. The rest of your examination is unremarkable. With which of the following is this patient's injury most consistent?

a. Rupture of the LCL
b. Rupture of the MCL
c. Rupture of the ACL
d. Rupture of the PCL
e. Tear of the medial meniscus

**275.** A 31-year-old homebuilder is cutting a piece of wood when the table saw backfires and slices through the base of his left thumb. In the ED his BP is 135/70 mm Hg, HR 87, RR 18, and pulse oxygen is 99%. You stabilize the patient and call the vascular surgeon. In the meantime, what is the best method of preserving the amputated finger?

a. Irrigate it with 10% povidone-iodine solution to remove gross contamination, wrap it in sterile gauze moistened with normal saline, and place it between two ice packs.
b. Irrigate it with normal saline to remove gross contamination, wrap it in sterile gauze moistened with normal saline, and then place it on ice.
c. Irrigate it with normal saline to remove gross contamination, wrap it in sterile gauze moistened with normal saline, place it in a sterile watertight container, and store this container in ice water.
d. Place it in a container of 10% povidone-iodine solution and store this container in ice water.
e. Attempt to partially replant the part with 3-0 nylon sutures until the vascular surgeon arrives.

**276.** A 47-year-old man presents to the ED complaining of knee pain after slipping on ice on his way to work. On examination, you note significant swelling to his knee and palpate a large effusion. The patient has limited range of motion because of the swelling. You perform a palliative arthrocentesis and note blood and fat globules in the syringe. Which of the following findings is the presence of fat globules most suggestive of?

a. ACL tear
b. PCL tear
c. Medial meniscus tear
d. Fracture
e. Vascular injury

**277.** A 76-year-old woman is brought into the ED complaining of hip pain after a motor vehicle collision. She states that her knee slammed into the dashboard after her car struck another vehicle. On examination you note her right leg appears shortened, adducted, internally rotated, and flexed. She has no other injuries. The radiograph of her hip confirms your diagnosis of a hip dislocation. Which of the following statements regarding this type of injury is true?

a. The most common presentation of this injury is an abducted, externally rotated, and flexed lower extremity.
b. This type of injury accounts for 5% to 10% of all hip dislocations.
c. The injury is commonly caused by a direct force applied to a flexed knee.
d. The most common complication is injury to the femoral artery.
e. The femoral nerve is almost always injured in this type of dislocation.

**278.** A 33-year-old carpenter was working on a construction project to build a new house. When using a high-pressure paint gun, he inadvertently injected his left index finger. On arrival to the ED, he complains of intense hand pain. On examination, you note a 2-mm wound over the second proximal phalange. He has full range of motion and brisk capillary refill. Radiographs of the finger show soft tissue swelling, a small amount of subcutaneous air, but no fracture. His tetanus is up to date. Which of the following is the most appropriate disposition for this patient?

a. Place the hand in a radial gutter splint and have the patient follow up with an orthopedic surgeon in 1 week.
b. Discharge home with pain medication and have the patient return for repeat radiographs in 1 week.
c. Order a CT scan of the finger to confirm that there is no occult fracture before discharging the patient home.
d. Place the hand in a radial gutter splint, prescribe a 10-day course of antibiotics, and have the patient follow up with an orthopedic surgeon in 1 week.
e. Place the hand in a radial gutter splint, administer broad-spectrum antibiotics, and admit the orthopedic service for operative debridement.

**279.** A 29-year-old man is 10 ft up on a ladder, painting his barn ceiling when he loses his balance and falls off the ladder, landing on both of his feet and then falling to the ground. He is brought to the ED by emergency medical services (EMS). On examination there are no obvious deformities, but you note swelling, tenderness, and ecchymosis of the right hindfoot. He has full range of motion at the ankle, knee, and hip. There is mild tenderness over his lumbar spine. Hs neurovascular status is normal. Radiographs confirm the diagnosis. Which of the following statements regarding this type of injury is true?

a. This injury is the second most commonly fractured tarsal bone.
b. 10% are associated with compression fractures of the dorsolumbar spine.
c. 90% are bilateral.
d. The mechanism of injury is usually secondary to rotational force at the subtalar joint.
e. These fractures require operative repair to avoid gait defects.

**280.** A 39-year-old woman is brought to the ED by EMS on a backboard and cervical collar after being involved in a motor vehicle collision. The primary survey is unremarkable. However, the secondary survey reveals a deformity of the right arm involving the upper arm and elbow. Which of the following associations are paired *incorrectly*?

a. Olecranon fracture and ulnar nerve injury
b. Posterior elbow dislocation and ulnar and median nerve injury
c. Anterior elbow dislocation and brachial artery injury
d. Supracondylar fracture and brachial artery and median nerve injury
e. Humeral shaft fracture and axillary nerve injury

**281.** A 31-year-old man is riding his mountain bicycle down a steep hill when he hits a rock in the path and is thrown off the bicycle. In the ED, the individual complains only of left arm pain. Your primary survey is unremarkable. After administering medication for pain control, you send the patient for a radiograph of his arm. Which of the following injuries is consistent with this patient's radiograph as seen below?

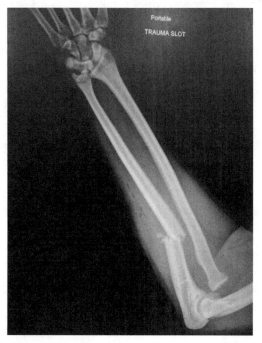

*(Courtesy of Adam J. Rosh, MD.)*

a. Monteggia fracture
b. Galeazzi fracture
c. Nightstick fracture
d. Colles fracture
e. Smith fracture

**282.** A 32-year-old dental hygienist presents to the ED with a painful lesion at the distal aspect of her right index finger. The individual states that she had a low-grade fever and malaise over the last week and subsequently developed pain and burning of the infected digit. Within the next week, she noted erythema, edema, and the development of small grouped vesicles on an erythematous base as depicted in the image below. Which of the following should be *avoided* when managing this condition?

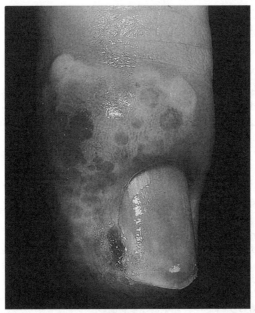

*(Reproduced, with permission, from Wolff K, Johnson RA, Suurmond R. Fitzpatrick's Color Atlas & Synopsis of Clinical Dermatology. 5th ed. New York, NY: McGraw-Hill; 2005: Figure 25-27.)*

a. Performing an incision and drainage to facilitate healing and avoid bacterial superinfection
b. Splinting the finger and recommending elevation and analgesics
c. Prescribing an antiviral agent, such as acyclovir
d. Applying a dry dressing over the lesions to prevent transmission
e. Prescribing an antibiotic if there is evidence of bacterial superinfection

**283.** A 43-year-old man presents to the ED complaining of right hand pain. The individual states that 3 days ago he accidentally punctured his index finger with a thumb tac. Subsequently, the finger became red and began to swell, and he had pain with movement of the finger. His tetanus status is up to date. You suspect the patient's diagnosis is tenosynovitis. Which of the following statements regarding Kanavel four cardinal signs of flexor tenosynovitis is correct?

a. The infected finger is held in slight flexion at rest.
b. Asymmetric swelling of the finger.
c. Tenderness along the extensor tendon sheath.
d. Painless with passive range of motion.
e. Purplish hue at the distal tip.

**284.** A 29-year-old figure skater lands incorrectly after a jump and injures her right ankle. She stands up on her own but has difficulty bearing weight so she calls EMS. She presents to the ED with swelling and tenderness of her lateral malleolus. You palpate a dorsalis pedis and posterior tibialis pulse. She is able to plantar and dorsiflex without difficulty. You are unsure if the patient requires an ankle radiograph because you think she only sustained a sprain. In addition to pain near the malleoli, which of the following is an indication for a radiograph according to the Ottawa ankle and foot rules?

a. Boney tenderness is present at the anterior edge of the distal 12 cm or at the tip of either malleolus.
b. The patient is able to bear weight for at least four steps immediately after the injury but not at the time of evaluation.
c. Boney tenderness is present at the navicular or at the base of the fifth metatarsal.
d. The Achilles reflex is diminished on the side of the injury.
e. An effusion is present on clinical examination.

# Musculoskeletal Injuries

## *Answers*

**257. The answer is d.** *(Tintinalli, pp 1813-1817.)* The **scaphoid** is the **most common carpal bone injured in a fall on the outstretched hand** (a **FOOSH** injury). On examination, patients exhibit tenderness at the anatomic snuffbox and pain referred to the anatomic snuffbox with longitudinal compression of the thumb. In the setting of a tender thumb, a thumb splint should be applied until films can be repeated after 1 week because initial films may not reveal the fracture. The application of the splint is especially important, because of the scaphoid's high risk for avascular necrosis.

(a) Triquetrum dorsal chip injury is the second most common carpal bone fracture and occurs with a FOOSH or direct blow to the dorsum of the hand. (b) Lunate fracture is the third most common carpal fracture. This injury is also at risk for avascular necrosis and any suspected injury should be placed in a thumb spica splint. (c) The capitate is the largest carpal bone and comprises 5% to 15% of all carpal fractures. (e) The pisiform is the only carpal bone with one articulation (the triquetrum). Anatomically it is important because the deep branch of the ulnar nerve and artery pass in close proximity to the radial surface of the bone. It is an uncommon fracture.

**258. The answer is a.** *(Simon and Sherman, pp 51-53.)* **Pseudogout** is the most common cause of acute **monoarticular arthritis** in the **elderly**. It affects women and men equally, primarily after their sixth decade of life. It is caused by the deposition of **calcium pyrophosphate crystals**. The knee is the most commonly involved joint, followed by the wrist and ankle. The synovial fluid **reveals rhomboid-shaped crystals** that are weakly **positive birefringent** under polarized light. Treatment is generally supportive with nonsteroidal anti-inflammatory drugs (NSAIDs).

Gout **(b)** occurs commonly in middle-aged men and elderly adults. Uric acid crystals usually deposit in the lower extremities, particularly the great toe (podagra). Evaluation of synovial fluid reveals needle-shaped crystals that exhibit negative birefringence under polarized light. Septic arthritis (c) is a medical emergency that most commonly affects the knee in adults. Joint fluid generally reveals greater than 50,000 WBC/mm$^3$ with mostly neutrophils. Rheumatoid arthritis (d) is an autoimmune disease that is characterized by a symmetric, progressive polyarthritis. Unlike osteoarthritis (e), rheumatoid arthritis has systemic manifestations.

**259. The answer is a.** (*Simon and Sherman, pp 458-468.*) The cruciate ligaments are the two internal bands extending from the tibia to the femur, one anteriorly and the other posteriorly. They control anteroposterior and rotary stability of the knee and prevent hyperextension. The **ACL is the most frequently injured ligament in the knee.** It has a rich blood supply that accounts for the high incidence of **hemarthrosis** when the ligament is injured. A history that includes a **pop** or **snap** at the time of injury (eg, during a sudden turn in direction while playing sports) suggests a rupture of the ACL until proven otherwise, particularly when associated with the rapid development of a knee effusion.

The PCL (b) is significantly stronger than the ACL and collateral ligaments. Therefore, injury to it is rare and is usually associated with severe knee injuries. (c and d) The MCL and LCL are often injured with excessive valgus (knee forced medially relative to leg) and varus (knee forced laterally relative to leg) forces, respectively. The patella ligament (e) runs from the patella to the tibial tuberosity and functions to help extend the leg at the knee. The ligament is commonly injured when an individual falls on a partially flexed knee.

**260. The answer is e.** (*Simon and Sherman, pp 546-547.*) The patient's diagnosis is an **Achilles tendon rupture**. The individual gives a history of a sudden excruciating pain and having heard or felt a **pop** or **snap**. This entity is most common in sedentary, middle-aged men or in athletes. The diagnosis can be made with the **Thompson test**. The patient is placed in the prone position. With normal function, squeezing the calf produces plantar flexion of the foot. With a complete tear of the Achilles tendon, plantar flexion will not occur. If doubt remains, magnetic resonance imaging (MRI) or ultrasound can be used to confirm the diagnosis. Treatment includes splinting the affected leg and discharging the patient with crutches. Orthopedic follow-up is required for repair.

Homan sign (a) is traditionally used to help diagnose a DVT. It is considered positive when passive dorsiflexion of the ankle elicits sharp pain in the calf. However, this sign is neither sensitive nor specific for

DVT. Lachman test **(b)** is used to detect an injury of the ACL of the knee. McMurray test **(c)** is used to detect an injury to the meniscus of the knee. A ballotable patella **(d)** signifies a significant knee effusion.

**261. The answer is a.** (*Simon and Sherman, pp 237-241.*) The blood supply to the scaphoid normally penetrates the cortex at the distal aspect of the bone. Therefore, there is **no direct blood supply to the proximal portion of the bone**, which predisposes this fragment to avascular necrosis and delayed union. The more proximal the fracture is in scaphoid injuries, the greater the likelihood of developing avascular necrosis.

All other scaphoid fractures **(a, b, and d)** increasing the risk for avascular necrosis, but proximal fractures are associated with the greatest risk. The scaphoid is prone **(e)** to avascular necrosis secondary to its limited blood supply.

**262. The answer is c.** (*Rosen, pp 579-585.*) This patient has **an anterior shoulder dislocation**. The glenohumeral joint is the most commonly dislocated joint in the body, mainly because of the lack of bony stability and its wide range of motion. Anterior dislocations account for 95% to 97% of cases and are most commonly seen in younger, athletic male patients and geriatric female patients. It usually happens by way of an indirect force that involves an abduction plus extension plus external rotation injury. Directly, it may occur due to a posterior blow that forces the humeral head out of the glenoid rim anteriorly. Radiographs obtained must include an axillary view to determine positioning of the humeral head. Patients usually present in severe pain, holding the affected arm with the contralateral hand in slight abduction. The lateral acromial process is prominent giving the shoulder a full or squared-off appearance. Patients typically cannot internally rotate their shoulder. **Axillary nerve injuries** can occur in up to 54% of anterior dislocations; however, these are neuropraxic in nature and tend to resolve on their own. Following the C5/C6 dermatome distribution, patients have a loss of sensation over the lateral aspect of the deltoid with decreased muscle contraction with abduction. After proper muscle relaxation with conscious sedation or intra-articular injection, closed reduction may be attempted using a variety of methods. After reduction, it is imperative to repeat a neurovascular examination and obtain confirmatory radiographs.

Acromioclavicular joint sprains **(a)** occur primarily in men and account for 25% of all dislocations. However, the mechanism of injury primarily involves a fall or direct blow to the adducted arm causing a downward and medial thrust to the scapula.

Posterior dislocations (**b and e**) are rare owing to the scapular angle on the thoracic ribs. They are seen, however, in convulsive seizures where the large internal rotator muscles overpower the weaker external rotators and cause the dislocation. Median nerve injuries (**d**) mainly involve weakness in the first three finger flexors. Ulnar nerve injuries (**e**) mainly involve weakness in the interossei muscles of the hand and paresthesias along the fifth digit.

**263. The answer is b.** (*Rosen, pp 579-582.*) The radiograph confirms an **anterior dislocation** of the left shoulder. Patient's typically present in severe pain with the dislocated arm held in slight abduction and external rotation by the opposite extremity. The patient leans away from the injured side and cannot adduct or internally rotate the shoulder without severe pain. Associated fractures may occur in up to 50% of anterior dislocations. The most common of these is a **compression fracture of the humeral head**, known as a **Hill-Sachs deformity**.

(**a**) Fracture of the anterior glenoid rim, or Bankart fracture, is also associated with anterior dislocations but is present in approximately 5% of cases. Choices (**c, d, and e**) are not commonly associated with anterior dislocations.

**264. The answer is e.** (*Rosen, pp 517, 740.*) This patient most likely sustained a **closed-fist injury**, which has high infection rates and evidence of poor wound healing. Wounds sustained by punches to the jaw and human bites, also known as "fight bites," are classically over the **metacarpal joints**. Penetration deep into the joint space and infection are common given the positioning of the hand during the injury, human oral flora, and delay in seeking treatment. Infected wounds are **polymicrobial** and specifically include **Eikenella corrodens**, a facultative anaerobic gram-negative rod harbored in human dental plaque. It acts synergistically with aerobic organisms to increase the morbidity of these injuries. The joint spaces must be examined under full range of motion to detect any tendon lacerations or presence of foreign bodies. Hand radiographs should also be obtained to examine for any bony involvement. **IV antibiotics** and **admission** are the appropriate disposition. The antibiotics of choice are **penicillin** and **second-generation cephalosporins** with broader coverage in the immunocompromised. The wounds should be left open with a sterile dressing, splinted in the position of function (hand-holding-glass position) and elevated. Human bites have resulted in the transmission of hepatitis B, hepatitis C, syphilis, and herpes. Although human immunodeficiency virus (HIV) is present in human saliva, it is in relatively small amounts and considered a low risk for transmission. Appropriate antivirals and testing should be considered in these patients.

(a and b) You should never suture these lacerations. (c and d) Wound irrigation and tetanus prophylaxis are warranted in conjunction with **IV antibiotics**.

**265. The answer is e.** *(Rosen, pp 512-513.)* The patient has a **mallet finger** or a **rupture of the extensor tendon** that inserts into the base of the distal phalanx. This type of injury occurs often from a sudden forceful flexion of an extended finger when an object, such as a football, strikes the tip of the finger. This is the common mechanism among athletes. Clinically, patients present with pain and swelling over the DIP joint, which is held in flexion of up to 40 degrees because of loss of the extensor mechanism. The most important aspect in managing these injuries is to **keep the DIP joint in continuous extension until healing occurs**. Therefore, a splint should be applied so that only the DIP is immobilized in extension for 6 to 8 weeks. The PIP and MCP joints should be mobile. Any disruption of the immobile DIP joint can result in improper healing.

**266. The answer is d.** *(Tintinalli, pp 1921-1922.)* **Kanavel criteria** for **flexor tenosynovitis** are known as **S.T.E.P.**: (1) **S**ymmetric swelling of the finger, (2) **T**enderness over the flexor tendon sheath, (3) **E**xtension (passive) of the digit is painful, and (4) **P**osture of the digit is flexed. A tenosynovitis is an infection of the flexor tendon sheath caused by penetrating trauma and dirty wounds (eg, a dog bite). Infection spreads along the tendon sheath; therefore, failure to diagnose and treat a flexor tenosynovitis may lead to loss of function of the affected digit and eventually the entire hand. It is, therefore, a surgical emergency. Treatment includes hand immobilization and elevation, immediate consultation with a hand surgeon, and IV antibiotics. Pain control and tetanus immunization should be provided, if not up to date.

(a) The Finkelstein test for DeQuervain tenosynovitis is positive when, with the thumb cupped in a closed fist, ulnar deviation reproduces pain along the extensor pollicis and abductor pollicis. (b) Trousseau sign for hypocalcemia is positive when a BP cuff inflated above the systolic BP for

3 minutes induces carpal spasm. **(c and e)** Compression of the median nerve may result in carpal tunnel syndrome, which presents with pain and paresthesias in the median nerve distribution. Tinel sign is positive when tapping over the median nerve at the wrist produces pain and paresthesia, while the Phalen test is positive when 1 minute of forced palmar flexion produces pain and paresthesia over the median nerve distribution.

**267. The answer is b.** (*Rosen, pp 538-539, 1406-1407.*) **Carpal tunnel syndrome** is a neuropathy of the **median nerve** that occurs due to compression of the nerve within the carpal tunnel of the wrist. Symptoms **include pares-thesias and pain** in the distribution of the median nerve; the volar thumb, second, third, and half of the fourth digit. Symptoms are usually worse after strenuous activities and at night. Pain improves with shaking of the hand or holding it in a dependent position. A sensitive test used to diagnose carpal tunnel is **Phalen test**. Have the patient hold the affected wrist in hyperflexion for 60 seconds. The test is positive if paresthesias or numbness develops in the median nerve distribution.

(**a**) The ulnar nerve's sensory distribution is over the fourth and fifth digits. (**d**) The radial nerve's sensory distribution is over the dorsal hand. (**c**) The axillary nerve's sensory distribution is over the proximal arm. (**e**) The musculocutaneous nerve's sensory distribution is over the lateral forearm.

**268. The answer is e.** (*Simon and Sherman, pp 192-194.*) A **boxer's fracture is a fracture of the neck of the fifth metacarpal**. It is one of the most common fractures of the hand and usually occurs from a direct impact to the hand (eg, a punch with a closed fist).

(**a**) Colles fracture is the most common wrist fracture seen in adults. It is a transverse fracture of the distal radial metaphysis, which is dorsally displaced and angulated. It usually occurs from a fall on an outstretched hand. (**b**) Smith fracture is a transverse fracture of the metaphysis of the distal radius, with associated volar displacement and angulation (opposite of a Colles). They typical occur secondary to a direct blow or fall onto the dorsum of the hand. (**c**) A scaphoid fracture is the most common fracture of the carpal bones. It is typically seen in young adults secondary to a FOOSH. (**d**) A Galeazzi fracture involves a fracture at the junction of the middle and distal thirds of the radius, with an associated dislocation of the distal radialulnar joint.

**269. The answer is e.** (*Simon and Sherman, pp 76-78.*) The patient is showing signs and symptoms of **compartment syndrome**. The syndrome occurs due to an increase in pressure within a confined osseofascial space that impedes neurovascular function. The end result is necrosis and damage to tissues. It can occur after crush injuries, circumferential burns, hemorrhage, edema, or any process that increases compartment pressure. Clinically, the patient complains of pain that is out of proportion to the injury. Physical examination may reveal swelling, sensory deficits, and pain with passive motion. **The presence of a pulse does not rule out compartment syndrome.** Late findings include pallor of the skin, diminished or absent pulses, and a cool extremity. The only way to diagnose compartment syndrome is to **measure intracompart-mental pressure with a Stryker device.** A pressure **greater than 30 mm Hg** is considered diagnostic and requires a **fasciotomy** to avoid tissue damage.

(a) Ice may decrease swelling but will not prevent compartment syndrome. There is also a risk of decreasing blood flow to the damaged tissue because of the vasoconstrictive effect of the ice. (b) There is no reason to suspect that an occult fracture is causing the pain. (c) Elevation to the level of the heart is recommended; however, all constrictive bandages should be removed. Elevation above the heart is not recommended. Again, this can limit blood flow to the damaged tissue. (d) A DVT should not cause this pain.

**270. The answer is d.** (*Rosen, pp 582-584.*) The patient's clinical presentation is consistent with a **posterior shoulder dislocation.** Posterior dislocations are rare and account for only 2% of all glenohumeral dislocations. Posterior dislocations are traditionally associated with **seizure patients, lightening injuries,** and **electrocutions.** However, the most common dislocation seen in postseizure patients is an anterior dislocation. Classically, the patient holds the dislocated arm across the chest in adduction and internal rotation. Abduction is limited and external rotation is blocked. Radiographs may reveal a **"light bulb" sign,** which is the light bulb appearance when the humeral head is profiled in internal rotation.

Although any type of injury can occur with a seizure (a, b, c, and e), the patient's clinical presentation is consistent with a posterior shoulder dislocation.

**271. The answer is b.** (*Rosen, pp 527-530.*) The **scaphoid** is the most commonly fractured carpal bone. It is typically seen in patients in their 20s to 30s after a FOOSH. Classically, physical examination reveals **tenderness in the anatomic snuffbox**, the space between the extensor pollicis longus and the extensor pollicis brevis. On radiography, however, up to 15% of scaphoid fractures are not detected. As the necrotic bone at the fracture site is resorbed, the fracture line often becomes apparent on radiographs at 10 to 14 days after injury. Therefore, patients with snuffbox tenderness and an initial radiograph should be splinted in **a thumb spica splint** and asked to return for **repeat radiographs in 10 to 14 days**.

(a) Placing an elastic wrap will not provide adequate immobilization and will lead to increased complications if a fracture is present. (c) Ice is recommended, but immobilization is also required. (d) Even a CT scan will not pick up the fracture immediately after injury. However, if there is snuffbox tenderness after 14 days and the radiograph remains negative, a CT scan is warranted. (e) This is unnecessary because it is not clear if the scaphoid is fractured.

**272. The answer is c.** *(Rosen, pp 527-530.)* **Avascular necrosis of the scaphoid** is seen in approximately 3% of scaphoid fractures. The typical presentation of a scaphoid fracture is a FOOSH. On examination patients **have snuffbox tenderness** or tenderness with axial loading of the thumb. Blood supply to the scaphoid is provided by a single artery that flows into the distal portion of the bone leaving the proximal portion vulnerable in the setting of a fracture. This increases the likelihood of complications, particularly avascular necrosis, in the setting of a poorly healed fracture.

(a) A fracture of the distal ulna would heal after 3 months. There is no tenderness over the ulna on examination. (b) This individual likely had an acute fracture of her scaphoid that she did not seek medical care for. The fracture did not heal properly subsequently leading to avascular necrosis. (d) A hematoma may have occurred at the time of injury from a venous bleed. However, it would not be present 3 months later. (e) Lunate fractures are rare but are also complicated by avascular necrosis. This patient has snuffbox tenderness, which is more likely because of a scaphoid injury.

**273. The answer is a.** *(Simon and Sherman, pp 257-259.)* The **median nerve** runs through the carpal tunnel between the flexor carpi radialis and the palmaris longus. It provides sensation to the palmar aspect of the radial three and one-half fingers as well as the dorsal aspect of the tips of the index and middle fingers and the radial half of the ring finger. Lunate dislocations are usually caused by hyperextension injuries. The **lunate**

is usually displaced volarly or dorsally. The **median nerve may be compressed** in the carpal tunnel by the lunate, and the patient may display signs of **acute carpal tunnel syndrome**.
(**b**) Perilunate dislocations are the most common wrist dislocation.
(**c**) Scapholunate dislocation is sometimes defined by the "Terry Thomas" or "Dave Letterman" sign, where there is a gap (>3 mm) in the space between the scaphoid and lunate (similar to a gap in the front teeth of these two people). (**d and e**) These dislocations are rare.

**274. The answer is b.** *(Simon and Sherman, pp 458-468.)* The most common mechanism of injury resulting in ligamentous injury is a **valgus stress** with an external rotary component on the flexed knee. This is common in skiing and football injuries. The **MCL** is commonly injured. On stability testing of the knee, patients with MCL tears usually **show instability with a valgus stress with the knee in 30 degrees of flexion.** Ligamentous tears are also associated with hemarthrosis.
(**a**) Rupture of the lateral collateral is caused by an unusual mechanism and may be seen when a skier fails to maintain a snowplow and the tips of his or her skis cross causing a varus stress. (**c**) Rupture of the ACL usually includes a history of a **pop** or **snap** and immediate development of a knee effusion. The Lachman test is used to identify ACL and PCL injuries. (**d**) PCL injuries occur when the tibia is forced posteriorly relative to the femur. (**e**) With meniscal injuries, patients typically complain that their knee locks in place or they hear a clicking sound. These injuries are usually caused by rotational force to a weight-bearing knee and are associated with effusions.

**275. The answer is c.** *(Rosen, pp 518-519.)* The best way to **preserve an amputated part** is to rinse it with normal saline to remove gross contamination, wrap it in sterile gauze moistened with saline or lactated ringers, and place it in a sterile, watertight container. Then store this container in ice water.
(**a and d**) Povidone-iodine is a strong antiseptic solution that is used commonly in the hospital setting, particularly in the operating room to create a sterile field. However, it is thought to be injurious to fibroblasts and may limit wound healing. (**b**) The amputated part should not be placed directly on ice or in ice water because this may also damage the tissue. (**e**) Replantation of the thumb should be performed by a vascular surgeon in the operating room. There is an increased risk of tissue death the longer the severed part is not properly stored.

**276. The answer is d.** (*Tintinalli, pp 1856-1864.*) Frequently, there is a **fracture** to account for the presence of fat within the joint because the fat has entered from the bone marrow cavity. The presence of fat globules may be seen in the joint aspirate and even on the radiograph of the knee showing a joint effusion with a fat-fluid level.

(**a and b**) Cruciate ligament tears are associated with early hemarthrosis. (**c**) Meniscal tears are associated with effusions that develop gradually over 6 to 24 hours postinjury. (**e**) Vascular injuries of the knee occur with fractures and dislocations and are a medical emergency.

**277. The answer is c.** (*Simon and Sherman, pp 415-419.*) The patient sustained a **posterior hip dislocation**. The most common mechanism for this to occur is during a motor vehicle collision in which a **direct force is applied to the flexed knee** (eg, the patient's knee hits the dashboard at high velocity). The limb appears shortened, adducted, internally rotated, and flexed. Because of the strong forces needed to cause such an injury, hip dislocations rarely occur in isolation. Life-threatening injuries should always be addressed first, prior to treating hip dislocations. Nonetheless, early reduction is required because the likelihood of **avascular necrosis** of the femoral head increases in direct proportion to a delay in reduction. Early complications of posterior dislocations include **sciatic nerve injury**. Late complications include avascular necrosis of the femoral head, as mentioned above.

(**a**) This is the most common presentation of an anterior hip dislocation. (**b**) Posterior hip dislocations account for approximately 80% of hip dislocations. (**d**) The most common complication is avascular necrosis. (**e**) The sciatic nerve is at risk for injury.

**278. The answer is e.** (*Simon and Sherman, p 203.*) The patient sustained a **high-pressure injection injury** of his finger—this is a surgical emergency. These injuries may involve **extensive tissue loss** and are associated with a **high infection rate**. Most of these injuries involve grease, paint, or other industrial toxins. Paint generates a large, early inflammatory response, resulting in a high percentage of amputations. Within several hours after the digit has been injected, the extremity becomes painful and swollen. Initially, there may be anesthesia and even vascular insufficiency of the extremity. In the late stages, marked breakdown of the skin occurs, resulting in ulcers and draining sinuses. If the material injected into the extremity is radiopaque, it is possible to determine its degree of spread.

Management involves **splinting** and **elevating** the extremity, administration of **antibiotics, tetanus prophylaxis** updated as indicated, **analgesia,** and immediate **orthopedic consultation.**

**279. The answer is b.** *(Simon and Sherman, pp 520-525.)* This individual sustained a **calcaneal fracture** of the right foot.

The calcaneus is the most commonly fractured tarsal bone **(a)**; the talus is the second most commonly injured tarsal bone. A calcaneal fracture is usually caused by a **compression injury (d)**, such as a fall from a height with the patient landing on his or her feet. The examination reveals swelling, tenderness, and ecchymosis of the hindfoot and the inability to bear weight on the fracture. Ten percent are bilateral **(c)** and 10% are associated with **compression fractures of the dorsolumbar spine.** Therefore, it is important to examine the patient's entire spine. Treatment varies depending on the extent of injury. In general, nondisplaced or minor extra-articular fractures only require supportive care with immobilization in a posterior splint and follow-up with an orthopedic surgeon **(e).** The management of intra-articular or displaced calcaneal fractures remains controversial regarding nonoperative versus immediate surgical reduction.

**280. The answer is e.** *(Simon and Sherman, pp 284-302, 311-314.)* **Humeral shaft fractures** most commonly occur from a direct blow to the mid-upper arm. The fracture usually involves the middle third of the humeral shaft. The most common associated injury is damage to the **radial nerve** that causes wrist drop and loss of sensation in the first dorsal web space. Ulnar and median nerve injuries may also occur but are much less common.

Olecranon fractures **(a)** are associated with injury to the ulnar nerve. Individuals may experience paresthesias and numbness in the ulnar nerve distribution or weakness of the interossei muscles. Posterior elbow dislocations **(b)** are associated with injuries to the ulnar and median nerves. Anterior elbow dislocations **(c)**, although uncommon, have a much higher incidence of vascular injuries than posterior dislocations. It is important to evaluate for a brachial artery injury. Supracondylar fractures **(d)**, common in young individuals, are associated with injuries to the brachial artery and median nerve as the distal humeral fragment is displaced posteriorly, thus placing the sharp fracture fragments anteriorly.

**281. The answer is a.** *(Simon and Sherman, pp 269-274.)* **Monteggia fractures** are of the **proximal one-third of the ulnar shaft** combined with a **radial head dislocation**. This injury commonly occurs from either a direct blow to the posterior aspect of the ulna or a FOOSH with the forearm in forced pronation. This fracture is associated with an injury to the radial nerve. It is important to always look for an associated fracture or dislocation when one is noted in a forearm bone.

A Galeazzi fracture (**b**) is a fracture of the distal radial shaft associated with a distal radioulnar dislocation at the distal radioulnar joint (DRUJ). This fracture is often confused with Monteggia fracture. A way to remember the difference is to recall that Monteggia ends in an "a" and in this fracture, the ulna (also ends in "a") is fractured. A Nightstick fracture (**c**) is an isolated fracture of the shaft of the ulna. This injury can occur after a direct blow to the ulna and usually occurs when an individual raises his or her forearm up to protect their face from a blow. A Colles fracture (**d**) is a transverse fracture of the metaphysis of the distal radius with dorsal displacement of the distal fragment. The median nerve is at risk for injury. A Smith fracture (**e**) is a transverse fracture of the distal radial metaphysis with volar displacement of the distal fragment. As in a Colles fracture, the median nerve is at risk for injury.

**282. The answer is a.** (*Omori, 2010.*) The patient has a **herpetic whitlow**, a viral infection of the distal finger. It is caused by the herpes simplex virus type I or II. This condition typically occurs in health care providers with exposure to oral secretions and in patients with coexistent herpes infections. It generally presents with a prodrome period of fever and malaise. Subsequently, there is localized burning, itching, and pain that precede the development of the classic clear herpetic vesicles. Typically, only one finger is involved. The diagnosis is usually made clinically, but, if doubt remains or if the presentation is atypical, it can be confirmed with a Tzanck smear or viral culture. When managing this condition, it is important to note that **surgical drainage is contraindicated**. It can result in secondary infection and delayed healing.

All of the other answer choices (**b, c, d, and e**) are acceptable management options.

**283. The answer is a.** (*Simon and Sherman, pp 226-227.*) **Flexor tenosynovitis** typically results from a puncture wound. The causative agents are usually *Staphylococcus aureus* or *Streptococcus*.

The diagnosis is based on the presence of **Kanavel four cardinal signs** of flexor tendon synovitis. These include the finger held in slight flexion at rest, **(b)** symmetric swelling or sausage digit of the finger, **(c)** tenderness along the flexor tendon sheath, and **(d)** pain with passive range of motion of the finger. Answer choice **(e)** is not one of Kanavel signs.

**284. The answer is c.** *(Young, 2011.)* The **Ottawa rules** are a prospectively validated clinical decision tree for radiograph ordering in adults. By following these rules, emergency physicians can eliminate up to 30% of radiographs that are routinely ordered without missing clinically significant fractures. Radiographs are required only if there is bony pain in the malleolar or midfoot area and if any one of the following conditions applies: Bony tenderness at the navicular bone or at the base of the fifth metatarsal; **(a)** bony tenderness is present at the posterior edge of the distal 6 cm or at the tip of either malleolus; and **(b)** the patient is unable to bear weight for at least four steps immediately after the injury and at the time of evaluation. A diminished Achilles reflex **(d)** or effusions **(e)** are not part of the Ottawa criteria.

# Headache, Weakness, and Dizziness

## Questions

**285.** A 21-year-old college student is brought by her roommate to the emergency department (ED). The roommate states that earlier in the day the patient complained of a severe headache, stiff neck, and photophobia. On their way to the ED, the roommate states that the patient was confused. Her vital signs are blood pressure (BP) 110/80 mm Hg, heart rate (HR) 110 beats per minutes, respiration rate (RR) 16 breaths per minute, and temperature 102°F. What is the next step in the management of this patient?

a. Start empiric antibiotics, noncontrast head computed tomography (CT) before performing lumbar puncture (LP).
b. Order a noncontrast head CT and start antibiotics once the results are back.
c. Give 1 g of acetaminophen, start fluid hydration, and perform an LP.
d. Perform an LP and start antibiotics once the results are back.
e. Order a noncontrast head CT, perform an LP, then start antibiotics.

**286.** A 29-year-old woman presents to the ED complaining of a generalized headache over the last 2 months. She has seen many doctors for it but has yet to get a correct diagnosis. She describes the headache as moderate in intensity and worse with eye movement. Occasionally, it awakes her from sleep and is worse when tying her shoes. She is scared because her vision gets blurry for a few minutes every day. Her only medication is acetaminophen and an oral contraceptive. Her BP is 140/75 mm Hg, HR is 75 beats per minute, temperature is 98.9°F, and RR is 16 breaths per minute. On physical examination you appreciate papilledema. Which of the following is the most appropriate next step in management?

a. Consult neurosurgery.
b. Administer 2 g of ceftriaxone then perform an LP rule out meningitis.
c. Order a magnetic resonance imaging (MRI) to look for a carotid artery dissection.
d. Diagnose a migraine headache and prescribe her a triptan.
e. Perform a CT scan, and if negative perform, an LP specifically to measure the opening pressure.

**287.** A 67-year-old woman presents to the ED complaining of a 2-day history of general malaise, subjective fevers, chills, diffuse headache, and right-sided jaw pain. She also notes diminished vision in her right eye. Her symptoms are minimally relieved with acetaminophen. She denies any sick contacts. The patient's vitals include an oral temperature of 100.6°F, HR is 95 beats per minute, BP is 130/75 mm Hg, and RR is 16 breaths per minute with oxygen saturation of 99% on room air. She is tender on the right side of her scalp. You initiate empirical treatment. Which of the following tests will confirm your diagnosis?

a. Influenza A/B assay
b. Rapid strep test
c. Erythrocyte sedimentation rate (ESR)
d. Complete blood count (CBC)
e. Temporal artery biopsy

**288.** A 25-year-old stockbroker presents to the ED complaining of 6 weeks of daily headaches. Her headaches are band-like in distribution and are not associated with nausea, vomiting, visual phenomena, or neurologic symptoms. Normally they respond to acetaminophen, but they have increased in frequency in the past week as she stopped taking a medication that had been prescribed to prevent them. What type of primary headache syndrome is the patient likely experiencing?

a. Migraine headaches
b. Cluster-type headaches
c. Trigeminal neuralgia
d. Postherpetic neuralgia
e. Tension headache

**289.** A 22-year-old woman presents to the ED complaining of headache. She states that while at home, she experienced a headache that was associated with blurry vision in both eyes with a shimmering line in her vision. She subsequently lost her vision and felt uncoordinated, followed by increased pain at the base of her skull. Upon arrival in the ED, her vision returned to normal. A head CT scan and an LP are both negative. She now complains of a persistent, severe, pulsatile headache. She has had two similar episodes in the past year with the headache refractory to over-the-counter medications. Which of the following is likely to relieve her symptoms?

a. Diazepam
b. High-flow oxygen
c. Sumatriptan
d. Acetaminophen
e. LP with removal of 15-cc cerebrospinal fluid (CSF)

**290.** A 25-year-old man presents to the ED complaining of headache for 2 days. He describes the pain as pulsatile and occipital. The patient had an LP 3 days back and was diagnosed with viral meningitis after 4 days of symptoms. Noncontrast head CT at that time was normal. He improved shortly thereafter with defervescence of his fever and resolution of his constitutional and nuchal symptoms. He states that his new headache is different than his previous in that it is exacerbated by standing or sitting upright and is relieved by sitting down and is not associated with photophobia or neck stiffness. The headache is not relieved by over-the-counter pain medications. He is afebrile and nontoxic appearing. Which of the following is definitive therapy for this patient's headache?

a. A 1-L bolus of intravenous (IV) normal saline
b. Treatment with standard pharmacologic agents for migraine
c. Treatment with meclizine
d. Consultation with anesthesia for a blood patch
e. Repeat LP to improve symptoms

**291.** A 27-year-old woman with known idiopathic intracranial hypertension (IIH) presents to the ED complaining of a bifrontotemporal headache several times a day for 6 weeks after running out of her medications. She complains of occasional pulsatile tinnitus but no visual disturbances. Funduscopic examination reveals no papilledema and normal venous pulsations. Which of the following factors determines the need for urgent treatment in patients with IIH?

a. The presence of papilledema on funduscopic examination
b. A history of pulsatile tinnitus
c. Presence of an empty sella on CT scan
d. Complaint of visual loss or visual disturbances
e. A history of concomitant minocycline use

**292.** A 57-year-old man with a past medical history of hypertension and migraines presents to the ED complaining of a headache that started 2 days ago. He states the headache began suddenly with peak intensity while he was defecating. The pain is continuous particularly in the occipital region and is associated with mild nuchal rigidity and mild photophobia. He denies having a recent fever. A noncontrast head CT is obtained and is normal. Which of the following is the most appropriate next step in management?

a. Metoclopramide for nausea relief and ketorolac (Toradol) for pain control
b. LP
c. Empiric treatment for meningitis with IV antibiotics
d. IV mannitol to lower intracranial pressure (ICP)
e. Angiography to evaluate for an aneurysm

**293.** A 27-year-old woman presents to the ED complaining of headache lasting approximately 1 hour in duration that is unrelieved by aspirin and acetaminophen. She states the headache was not preceded by any visual phenomena, is left sided, pulsatile, and has occurred nearly monthly coinciding with her menstrual period for the past 6 months. She also complains of nausea and sensitivity to sound and light. Which of the following is the most appropriate therapy for this patient at the time of presentation?

a. IV morphine sulfate
b. Another trial of aspirin and acetaminophen
c. Sumatriptan (Imitrex)
d. Topiramate (Topamax)
e. Hydromorphone and acetaminophen

**294.** A 55-year-old woman presents to the ED complaining of 1 day of a left-sided headache that is associated with scalp and ear pain. She describes the pain as gradual in onset, dull, and constant. She describes a week of constitutional symptoms before the onset of her headache syndrome, including joint pain, tenderness of the muscles of her lower extremities, and fatigue. She is afebrile with no nuchal symptoms, photophobia, or phonophobia. Physical examination reveals a tender scalp and a thickened, painful temporal artery. Which of the following is the most appropriate next step in management?

a. Initiate corticosteroid therapy.
b. LP to rule out subarachnoid hemorrhage (SAH).
c. Injection of lidocaine at the base of the occiput.
d. Initiate antibiotic therapy.
e. Send an ESR.

**295.** A 28-year-old male military recruit presents to the ED complaining of headache, fever, and neck stiffness. His temperature is 102.2°F and he refuses to move his neck. He is somewhat lethargic appearing and winces when the lights are turned on in the examining room. He has a nonfocal neurologic examination and you proceed with LP. Which of the following is the most specific finding for suspected bacterial meningitis?

a. The presence of phonophobia, photophobia, and neck stiffness
b. Fever higher than 102.2°F
c. Elevated polymorphonuclear white blood cell (WBC) count on CSF analysis
d. Elevated protein on CSF analysis
e. Increased glucose on CSF analysis

**296.** As a senior resident in the ED, an intern calls you over to see a patient he treated for a migraine headache. The patient is a 21-year-old woman with a history of poorly controlled migraines. The patient was using a number of migraine medications at home and several were administered intravenously. When you approach the patient, you note her tongue is protruding and her head is tilted to the left. She is grimacing. The intern is concerned that the patient is having an acute stroke and would like to obtain a head CT scan. You advise the intern that the symptoms are likely the result of a medication side effect. Which of the following medications is likely to have caused the patient's symptoms?

a. Morphine sulfate
b. Acetaminophen
c. Metoclopramide
d. Caffeine
e. Sumatriptan

**297.** A 63-year-old man who lives in a homeless shelter presents to the ED complaining of headache with photophobia for 6 hours. Upon arrival to the ED, the triage nurse places him in an isolation room. The triage note states that the patient was alert and conversant during the nursing interview. You enter the isolation room and attempt to speak to the patient, but he is lethargic and combative. You note that his temperature is 103°F. He is unwilling to move his neck and winces when you attempt to check his pupillary reflexes with a penlight. The nurse informs you that laboratory analyses are delayed this evening because of staffing issues. Which of the following is the most appropriate next step in management?

a. Diagnostic LP
b. Initiation of IV antibiotic therapy
c. A loading dose of IV corticosteroids
d. Aggressive antipyretic therapy
e. Sedation of the patient and noncontrast head CT

**298.** A 22-year-old woman with known IIH who is scheduled for a ventriculoperitoneal shunt in 2 weeks presents to the ED complaining of severe headache. She states the headache is similar to the normal headaches associated with her condition except that it is refractor to her regular medications, including triptans and opiates. Her neurologist increased her dose of acetazolamide, but this also did not help. Her noncontrast head CT is unchanged from previous and she does not have papilledema. Which of the following is likely to provide prompt relief?

a. IV corticosteroids
b. Infusion of mannitol
c. LP with removal of 15 cc of CSF
d. IV metoclopramide
e. Nonsteroidal anti-inflammatory drugs (NSAIDs)

**299.** A 55-year-old woman with a past medical history of diabetes presents to the ED with fevers, headache, vision complaints, and right-sided weakness. She was treated for otitis media 2 weeks ago with amoxicillin as an outpatient. You obtain the CT scan seen below. What is the most likely diagnosis?

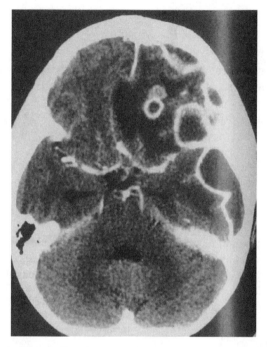

*(Reproduced, with permission, from Schwartz DT, Reisdorff EJ.* Emergency Radiology. *New York, NY: McGraw-Hill, 2000: 430.)*

a. Central nervous system (CNS) toxoplasmosis
b. Subdural hygroma
c. Glioblastoma multiforme
d. Brain abscess
e. SAH

**300.** A 35-year-old woman presents to the ED for the second time. She is complaining of fever, neck stiffness, and photophobia. She was seen in your ED 2 days ago for the same symptoms. At that time, she had a normal neurologic examination, was otherwise well-appearing, and underwent diagnostic LP. The results of her CSF analysis were as follows:

| | |
|---|---|
| Glucose | 82 mg/dL |
| Protein | 60 mg/dL |
| WBC | 150/L (98% lymphocytes) |
| Gram stain | No organisms seen |

The patient was sent home after a period of observation with presumed viral meningitis. She was told to return if her symptoms were not better in 48 hours. Since then, her fever increased (100.4°F-102.2°F). What is the next most appropriate step in management?

a. Administration of acyclovir
b. Aggressive antipyretic therapy and observation
c. CT scan of the sinuses
d. CT of the head and, if no contraindication, repeat LP
e. Viral cultures and polymerase chain reaction (PCR) from previously obtained CSF

**301.** A 68-year-old man presents to the ED complaining of a daily headache for almost a month. He describes the headache as being dull, difficult to localize, most intense in the morning, and abating in the early afternoon. He also noticed progressive weakness of his right upper and lower extremity. Which of the following headache syndromes are the signs and symptoms most consistent with?

a. Headache caused by a mass lesion
b. Cluster headache
c. Tension-type headache
d. Headache from intracranial hypertension
e. Waking or morning migraine

**302.** A 75-year-old man presents to the ED with a depressed level of consciousness. His wife is at the bedside and states he was stacking heavy boxes when he complained of a sudden intense headache. He subsequently sat down on the couch and progressively lost consciousness. She states that he had a headache the previous week that was also sudden but not as intense. He had gone to visit his primary care physician who sent him to have a CT scan of the brain, which was normal. Over the course of the past week, he complained of intermittent pulsating headaches for which he took sumatriptan. In the ED, you intubate the patient and obtain the noncontrast head CT seen below. The scan is most consistent with which diagnosis?

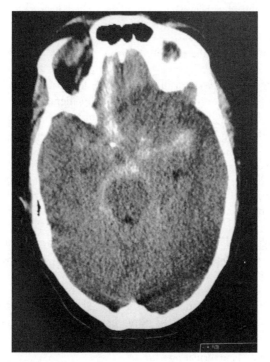

*(Courtesy of Adam J Rosh, MD.)*

a. Meningoencephalitis
b. SAH
c. Normal-pressure hydrocephalus
d. Epidural hematoma
e. Subdural hematoma (SDH)

**303.** A 43-year-old homeless man presents to the ED with fever and nuchal rigidity. His mental status is depressed, but his neurologic examination is otherwise nonfocal. Noncontrast head CT is normal. You obtain an LP for diagnostic purposes and initiate empiric antibiotic treatment for bacterial meningitis. The result of the CSF analysis is complete after 1 hour. The protein and glucose are within normal range, but the WBC count consists of 220 mononuclear cells. The Gram stain is negative. The patient was recently purified protein derivative (PPD) negative and had a normal chest x-ray. In addition to the treatment already initiated, what is the next most appropriate step in this patient's management?

a. Empiric treatment with isoniazid
b. Empiric treatment with antiviral medications for herpes virus
c. Empiric treatment with antifungals
d. Antibiotic coverage for *Bartonella* sp
e. Addition of steroids to the antibiotic regimen

**304.** During a busy day working in the ED, five patients come in all of whom you believe require an LP to evaluate for meningitis. From the following list of patients, which one can you forgo a CT scan and proceed directly to an LP?

a. A 65-year-old man with fever and headache
b. A 49-year-old woman with acquired immunodeficiency syndrome (AIDS)
c. A 74-year-old man with new right lower-extremity motor weakness
d. A 19-year-old man with a fever who is lethargic and disoriented
e. A 51-year-old woman who is febrile and complains of neck stiffness

**305.** A 53-year-old man presents to your ED stating he has had an excruciating right-sided headache since leaving the movie theater. He states that the headache is unilateral, severe, and associated with nausea and vomiting. His vision is blurry and notes seeing halos around objects. He denies trauma or a history of headaches in the past. Physical examination reveals right conjunctival injection and a pupil that reacts only marginally. Which examination is likely to yield the correct diagnosis?

a. Measurement of intraocular pressure
b. Funduscopic examination
c. Fluorescein examination
d. LP with cell count
e. Visual acuity testing

**306.** A 78-year-old man presents to triage of your ED complaining of gradual onset of headache over the course of the day. The headache is present almost every day and wonders if it is related to the unusually cold temperatures this winter. He describes the headache as bounding and constant. You notice that his face is very ruddy in appearance. He is afebrile but looks rather lethargic and somewhat short of breath. He is afebrile and saturating 100% on pulse oximetry. One of your coworkers informs you that the patient's wife is in another part of the emergency room with a similar presentation. Two more ambulances arrive, one with a patient complaining of a similar headache and another with a patient who is obtunded. All live in the same building. What is the next most appropriate step in the management of these patients?

a. Place the patient in respiratory isolation for presumed *Neisseria meningitidis* infection.
b. Draw a blood gas and send it for cooximetry.
c. Start antibiotic therapy and perform an LP.
d. Treatment for migraine with triptans or IV antiemetics.
e. Transfer of all three patients to the nearest hyperbaric facility.

**307.** A 35-year-old man presents to the ED complaining of a headache over the previous 4 weeks. He was assaulted with a bat 4 weeks ago and was admitted to the hospital for observation in the setting of a small traumatic SDH. Repeat noncontrast CT scan of the head 2 weeks ago was normal with resolution of the hematoma. He states he has headaches several times each day. They last from 5 minutes to several hours. They are sometimes band-like; other times they are localized to the site where he was struck. They can be pulsating or constant and are associated with sensitivity to sound. A head CT scan today is normal. Which of the following is the most likely diagnosis?

a. Postconcussive syndrome
b. Posttraumatic hydrocephalus
c. Subdural hygroma
d. Cluster headache
e. Posttraumatic stress disorder

**308.** A 35-year-old woman presents to the ED complaining of headache and blurry vision. She has had daily headaches for 3 months associated with blurry vision. She is afebrile, not losing weight, and has a normal neurologic examination, including fundoscopy. You ask when her last menstrual period was and she states she has not menstruated for 5 months and is not taking oral contraceptive pills. She also complains of galactorrhea. Noncontrast head CT is normal. An LP is performed and reveals a normal opening pressure. Which of the following is the most appropriate next step in managing the patient's headaches?

a. Repeat head CT with administration of IV contrast
b. Initiation of therapy with bromocriptine
c. Evaluation of CSF for xanthochromia and RBCs
d. Treatment of her headache with analgesia and an MRI
e. Repeat LP with removal of 15-mL CSF for therapeutic benefit

**309.** A 37-year-old woman with a history of migraines presents to the ED complaining of crampy lower abdominal pain for 3 days. Workup reveals an intrauterine pregnancy and early prenatal care is arranged with obstetrics as an outpatient. You are concerned because her headaches are controlled with a significant number of medications. She uses medications for both abortive therapy and for prophylaxis. Which of the following classes of medications do you advise she discontinue while pregnant?

a. Anticonvulsants
b. β-Blockers
c. Triptans
d. Acetaminophen
e. Antiemetics

**310.** A 78-year-old man presents to the ED complaining of left arm weakness that started 10 minutes ago in the clinic. The patient states that he has a history of hypertension and diabetes but has never had similar symptoms in the past. He is feeling well otherwise. His BP is 157/85 mm Hg, HR is 87 beats per minute, temperature is 98.8°F, and RR is 14 breaths per minute. His neurologic examination is unremarkable and the patient embarrassingly states that his left arm is no longer weak. Which of the following is the most likely diagnosis?

a. Thrombotic stroke
b. Conversion disorder
c. Migraine with focal neurologic deficit
d. Transient ischemic attack (TIA)
e. Todd paralysis

**311.** A 56-year-old man presents to the ED complaining of intermittent light-headedness and nausea throughout the day. He believes it started after eating leftover shrimp salad in the morning. On further questioning, he reports that during the light-headedness episodes the room is spinning around him and the episodes are triggered by turning his head to the right. He denies hearing loss, tinnitus, or other associated symptoms. His BP is 137/85 mm Hg, HR is 67 beats per minute, temperature is 98.5°F, and RR is 14 breaths per minute. The patient reproduces the symptoms by turning his head to the right. Which of the following is the most likely diagnosis?

a. Benign positional vertigo (BPV)
b. Food poisoning
c. Meniere disease
d. Labyrinthitis
e. TIA

**312.** A 29-year-old woman presents to the ED complaining of double vision for 3 days. She states that she has been feeling very tired lately, particularly at the end of the day, when even her eyelids feel heavy. She feels better in the morning and after lunch when she is able to rest for an hour. Her BP is 132/75 mm Hg, HR is 70 beats per minute, temperature is 98.4°F, and RR is 12 breaths per minute. On examination, you find ptosis and proximal muscle weakness. What is the most appropriate diagnostic test to perform?

a. Edrophonium test
b. Serologic testing for antibodies to acetylcholine receptors
c. Head CT scan
d. Electrolyte panel
e. Lumbar puncture

## Questions 313 and 314

**313.** A 40-year-old woman is brought to the ED by the paramedics complaining of bilateral foot weakness and numbness that started a few hours ago and is progressively worsening. She denies similar episodes in the past. On the review of systems, she describes having abdominal cramps with nausea, vomiting, and diarrhea 2 weeks ago that resolved after 2 to 3 days. Her BP is 124/67 mm Hg, HR is 68 beats per minute, temperature is 98.8°F, and RR is 12 breaths per minute. On examination, you elicit 2/5 strength, decreased sensation, and loss of deep tendon reflexes in the lower extremities below the hips. Which of the following is the most likely diagnosis?

a. Hypokalemic periodic paralysis
b. Guillain-Barré syndrome
c. Peripheral vascular disease
d. Tetanus
e. Brain abscess

**314.** What life-threatening complication is associated with this disease process described in the previous question?

a. Permanent paralysis
b. Thrombocytopenia
c. Respiratory failure
d. Need for surgery
e. Kidney failure

**315.** A 58-year-old man presents to the ED complaining of generalized weakness for the last 2 days. He states that a few days ago he had abdominal cramps, vomiting, and diarrhea when his whole family got sick after a picnic. These symptoms resolved a day and a half ago, but he has not been eating well and now feels weak all over. The patient has a history of hypertension for which he takes hydrochlorothiazide (HCTZ), which was recently increased. His BP is 144/87 mm Hg, HR is 89 beats per minute, temperature is 98.7°F, and RR is 12 breaths per minute. The physical examination reveals hyporeflexia. His electrocardiogram (ECG) is shown below. Which of the following is the most likely diagnosis?

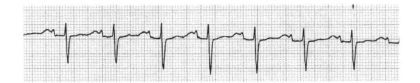

a. Hypernatremia
b. Hyponatremia
c. Hyperkalemia
d. Hypokalemia
e. Hypercalcemia

**316.** A 69-year-old man is brought to the ED by his son. His son, who states that his father developed left arm and leg weakness this afternoon and now has difficulty walking. The patient states that he has a history of heart palpitations and recently stopped taking his blood-thinning medicine because it was giving him an upset stomach. His BP is 165/90 mm Hg, HR is 97 beats per minute, temperature is 98.9°F, and RR is 16 breaths per minute. You suspect the patient is having a stroke and rush him to the CT scanner. The result of the head CT is seen below. What percentage of all stroke patients will have this type of stroke?

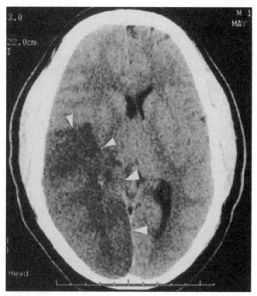

*(Reproduced, with permission, from Brunicardi CF et al. Schwartz's Principles of Surgery. New York, NY: McGraw-Hill, 2005: 1616.)*

a. 20%
b. 40%
c. 60%
d. 80%
e. 95%

## Questions 317 and 318

**317.** A 35-year-old woman presents to the ED complaining of left arm weakness and right facial pain for 1 day. She denies any past medical history but on the review of systems remembers having pain and decreased vision in her left eye approximately 4 months ago that has since resolved. She attributed it to being stressed and tired and did not see a physician at the time. Her BP is 126/75 mm Hg, HR is 76 beats per minute, temperature is 98.8°F, and RR is 12 breaths per minute. The physical examination is unremarkable except for 4/5 strength in the left upper extremity. Which of the following is the most likely diagnosis?

a. Myasthenia gravis
b. Multiple sclerosis (MS)
c. Vertebrobasilar artery occlusion
d. Encephalitis
e. Guillain-Barré syndrome

**318.** Which of the following is the best test to confirm your diagnosis in the previous question?

a. Edrophonium test
b. Angiogram of the carotid arteries
c. LP and CSF analysis
d. Head CT
e. MRI

**319.** A 58-year-old woman is brought to the ED by paramedics complaining of worsening left arm and leg weakness. She reports a history of hypertension, diabetes, and smoking. She denies any past surgeries. Her BP is 165/83 mm Hg, HR is 110 beats per minute, temperature is 98.4°F, RR is 18 breaths per minute, pulse oxymetry is 98% on room air, and capillary glucose is 147 mg/dL. On examination, the patient's speech is slurred and you notice a left-sided facial droop. Her left arm and leg strength is 2/5 and there is decreased sensation. The patient's head CT is normal. It has been 130 minutes since the onset of symptoms. Which of the following is the most appropriate next step in management?

a. Observation since she is out of the thrombolytic window.
b. Administer nitroprusside to lower her BP; then give thrombolytics.
c. Administer heparin only since she is out of the thrombolytic window.
d. Administer thrombolytic therapy.
e. Administer aspirin only since she is out of the thrombolytic window.

**320.** A 37-year-old woman presents to urgent care complaining of general weakness and blurry vision over the last month. She states that she feels great in the morning, but by dinner she has trouble cooking and complains of double vision. Her husband notices that her eyelids sometimes look droopy in the evening. On physical examination, her cranial nerves are intact, pupils are equal and reactive, extraocular muscles are intact; however, you notice slight ptosis. What is the most likely diagnosis of this patient?

a. Botulism
b. Lambert-Eaton myasthenic syndrome
c. Ophthalmoplegia of the third cranial nerve
d. Guillain-Barré syndrome
e. Myasthenia gravis

**321.** A 63-year-old woman accompanied by her husband is brought to the ED by EMS with worsening right arm weakness that started 90 minutes ago at the opera. Her husband states that she has a history of hypertension and long smoking. She has no surgical history. The husband states that his wife was fine when going to the opera. The patient's BP is 215/118 mm Hg, HR is 97 beats per minute, temperature is 99.3°F, and RR is 14 breaths per minute. On examination, the patient is anxious, mildly aphasic, has 2/5 strength, and diminished sensation in the right upper extremity. An emergent head CT scan is normal. It has been 2 hours since the onset of symptoms. Which of the following is the most appropriate next step in management?

a. Administer labetalol.
b. Administer fibrinolytic therapy.
c. Administer aspirin before fibrinolytic therapy to reduce platelet aggregation.
d. Administer phenytoin before fibrinolytic therapy as seizure prophylaxis.
e. Administer mannitol to reduce intracranial pressure before fibrinolytic therapy.

**322.** A 46-year-old woman presents to the ED with her husband complaining of flu-like symptoms, headache, vomiting, and dyspnea. She states that she never had similar symptoms in the past and that her husband is getting sick with similar symptoms as well but refuses to see a doctor. She reports feeling well yesterday and even helped her husband set up a home generator in their garage. Her BP is 142/85 mm Hg, HR is 97 beats per minute, temperature is 100.6°F, and RR is 20 breaths per minute. On examination the patient is slow to respond to questions. Which of the following is the most appropriate diagnostic test?

a. Send blood to check the WBC count.
b. Order a head CT scan.
c. Send blood to check the carboxyhemoglobin level.
d. Perform an LP.
e. No testing is necessary at this point.

**323.** An 82-year-old right-handed woman is brought to the ED by her daughter stating that her mother has not been able to walk after waking up from a nap 30 minutes ago. The patient has a history of hypertension and diabetes. Her BP is 179/76 mm Hg, HR is 91 beats per minute, temperature is 98.9°F, and RR is 14 breaths per minute. On examination, you elicit neurologic deficits and emergently bring her to the CT scanner. The radiologist tells you there is an abnormality in the left parietal lobe and a likely middle cerebral artery stroke. Which of the following motor deficits are you likely to find in this patient?

a. Right sensorimotor deficit in arm greater than leg and aphasia
b. Left sensorimotor deficit in arm greater than leg and aphasia
c. Right sensorimotor deficit in leg greater than arm, slowed response to questions, and impaired judgment
d. Right motor deficit and left facial droop
e. Right leg hemiplegia only

**324.** A 67-year-old man is brought to the ED by his wife who states that her husband's face looks different and that he has been nauseated, vomiting, and unsteady on his feet since yesterday. The patient also states that he has been having blurry vision and difficulty swallowing, in addition to feeling like the room is tilting from side to side. The patient attributes this to eating leftover salmon last night. The patient's past medical history is notable for obesity and hypertension. His BP is 187/89 mm Hg, HR is 86 beats per minute, temperature is 99.3°F, and RR is 13 breaths per minute. On examination, you find a right facial droop, diplopia, vertical nystagmus, and severe ataxia. Which of the following is the most likely diagnosis?

a. Lacunar infarct
b. BPV
c. Labyrinthitis
d. Posterior cerebral artery occlusion
e. Vertebrobasilar artery occlusion

**325.** A 45-year-old man presents to the ED complaining of recurrent episodes of light-headedness and nausea overnight. He describes the episodes as a room swaying from side to side when he lies on his left side. He reports mild headache now and denies tinnitus, hearing loss, fevers, or vomiting. He has no medical problems and takes no medications except for occasional acetaminophen. His BP is 123/65 mm Hg, HR is 69 beats per minute, temperature is 98.5°F, and RR is 12 breaths per minute. The patient is asymptomatic now and the examination is unremarkable. Which of the following is the most appropriate diagnostic test?

a. Dix-Hallpike maneuver
b. Caloric stimulation testing
c. Orthostatic vital signs
d. Head CT scan
e. ECG

**326.** A 23-year-old woman presents to the ED complaining of dizziness and weakness for 2 days. She complains that she does not have energy to perform her duties at work and even gets short of breath going up the stairs to her third-floor apartment. She denies shortness of breath at rest, fever, nausea, vomiting, diarrhea, chest pain, headache, recent travel, or other associated symptoms. She does not have any medical problems and takes no medications. On further questioning, she reports that she is on day 9 of her menstrual period, which has been heavy. Her periods are regular and last about 10 days. Her BP is 122/75 mm Hg, HR is 108 beats per minute, temperature is 98.7°F, and RR is 12 breaths per minute. Physical examination is unremarkable except for pale conjunctiva and mild tachycardia. Which of the following is the most appropriate initial diagnostic test?

a. Basic metabolic panel
b. Complete blood count
c. ECG
d. Chest x-ray
e. Chest CT with contrast

**327.** A 57-year-old man presents to the ED with generalized weakness and pain, abdominal discomfort, and nausea for 2 days. On the review of systems, he also admits to recent polydipsia, polyuria, and a 10-lb weight loss. His medical history includes hypertension for which he takes no medications. He has a 20-pack-year smoking history. The vital signs are remarkable for mild tachycardia and hypertension. Laboratory results reveal a serum sodium 131 mEq/L, potassium 3.5 mEq/L, chloride 101 mEq/L, bicarbonate 22 mEq/L, blood urea nitrogen (BUN) 15 mg/dL, creatinine 1.1 mg/dL, glucose 125 mg/dL, and serum calcium level of 12.6 mEq/L. Which of the following is the most appropriate next step in management?

a. Administer calcitonin.
b. Start 0.9% normal saline intravenous (IV) bolus.
c. Administer furosemide.
d. Obtain chest radiograph.
e. Obtain ECG.

## Questions 328 and 329

**328.** A 46-year-old woman presents to the ED with left-sided arm and leg weakness for half an hour. She has no medical problems except for chronic neck pain after a motor vehicle collision 5 years ago. On examination she has right eye miosis, partial ptosis, and 3/5 strength in her left upper and lower extremities. Which of the following is consistent with the patient's ocular findings?

a. Oculomotor nerve palsy
b. Bell palsy
c. Horner syndrome
d. Kehr sign
e. Nikolsky sign

**329.** On further questioning, the patient mentioned in the previous question states that earlier in the day she saw a chiropractor for her neck pain. After the session she developed severe right-sided neck pain. About an hour later she noticed difficulty using her left side of her body. Which of the following is the most likely diagnosis?

a. Internal carotid artery (ICA) dissection
b. Cavernous sinus syndrome
c. MS
d. Transverse myelitis
e. Spinous process fracture of a cervical vertebra

**330.** A 64-year-old man presents to the ED complaining of an episode of vertigo he experienced while exercising in the gym today. He states that he has been having similar episodes with exercise for a week. His routine consists of running on a treadmill, lifting weights, and doing leg presses. The vertigo usually occurs mid-routine when he is lifting weights and resolves with cessation of exercise. He also noticed unusual left arm pain during these episodes. He has hypertension for which he takes antihypertensive medication and had a myocardial infarction 6 years ago. He decreased his smoking from one pack per day to five cigarettes per day over the last 6 years. His BP in the right arm is 148/80 mm Hg and in the left arm it is 129/74 mm Hg. Which of the following is the most likely diagnosis?

a. Superior vena cava syndrome
b. Aortic dissection
c. Subclavian steal syndrome
d. Angina pectoris
e. Vestibular neuronitis

**331.** A 36-year-old woman presents to the ED complaining of worsening weakness over the past few weeks. She states that initially she attributed it to being overworked, but for the last few days she has been having unusual difficulty getting out of chair or walking the steps to her fourth-floor apartment. She has no prior medical history and takes no medications. Her vital signs are unremarkable. On examination, she has 5/5 strength in her bilateral upper and lower extremities distally but 3/5 strength proximally. Sensory examination and reflexes are normal. You also notice a red confluent macular rash on her eyelids. Which of the following is the most likely diagnosis?

a. Myasthenia gravis
b. MS
c. Dermatomyositis
d. Rhabdomyolysis
e. Disseminated gonococcal infection

**332.** A 32-year-old woman presents to the ED complaining of sudden onset of left facial weakness that began half an hour ago that was noticed by her coworker. She denies having medical problems or taking medications. On the review of systems, she admits to subjective fevers, fatigue, and arthralgias for the last week, which she attributed to the flu. She also reports having a rash on the back of her thigh a month ago, around the time she was hiking in Rhode Island. On examination she has left facial paralysis. Which of the following is the most likely diagnosis?

a. Bell palsy
b. Lyme disease
c. Ramsay Hunt syndrome
d. Brain tumor
e. Rocky Mountain spotted fever (RMSF)

**333.** A 24-year-old woman presents to the ED complaining of dizziness and numbness and tingling in her fingertips with decreased range of motion. Her initial vitals include an HR of 100 beats per minute, an RR of 30 breaths per minute, and an oxygen saturation of 100% on room air. The patient denies any other symptoms. Upon physical examination, the patient appears anxious, tachypneic with a clawed appearance to both hands that are difficult to range. An arterial blood gas is drawn that shows a pH of 7.55 with a decreased carbon dioxide level and normal bicarbonate level. Which of the following underlying metabolic disturbances is responsible for this patient's symptoms?

a. Metabolic acidosis
b. Metabolic alkalosis
c. Respiratory acidosis
d. Respiratory alkalosis
e. Hyperthyroidism

# Headache, Weakness, and Dizziness

## Answers

**285. The answer is a.** *(Rosen, pp 2218-2222.)* This patient presents with symptoms consistent with **meningitis**. **Antibiotics** are administered **empirically** as diagnostic workup proceeds. The best choice in this patient is **ceftriaxone**, which has good CNS penetration. In order to avoid transtentorial herniation in this patient with a **neurologic deficit (confusion)**, a **noncontrast head CT** should be performed **before LP**. It is controversial whether or not a head CT needs to be performed before all LPs. However, if there is papilledema or a neurologic deficit, head CT is mandatory.

**(b)** It is not prudent to wait for results from a head CT. This will only delay treatment of a potentially fatal disease. **(c)** Although this patient can benefit from acetaminophen and hydration, starting antibiotics empirically is more important. In addition, this patient requires a head CT before LP. **(d and e)** As previously stated, antibiotics should be started early in management and not be delayed while waiting for results.

**286. The answer is e.** *(Rosen, pp 1363-1364.)* The patient most likely has **IIH (pseudotumor cerebri)**, a neurologic disease seen primarily in **young obese women** of **childbearing age**. Clinically, patients complain of a generalized headache of gradual onset and moderate severity. It may worsen with eye movements or with the Valsalva maneuver. Visual complaints are common and may occur several times a day and can become permanent in 10% of patients. Patients typically have papilledema and visual field defects on physical examination. Diagnosis is made by a normal neuroimaging scan (eg, head CT scan) and an elevated intracerebral pressure ($>200$ mm $H_2O$) measured by the opening pressure from an LP. This is also therapeutic.

This patient does not require immediate surgery **(a)** but may require a ventricular shunt in the future if she exhibits impending vision loss. Neurosurgery consultation can wait until after the diagnosis is made. Two grams of ceftriaxone **(b)** is therapy for meningitis, which this patient does not have. She is afebrile with no other constitutional symptoms. A carotid artery dissection (c) presents classically with the triad of unilateral headache, ipsilateral partial Horner syndrome, and contralateral hemispheric findings, such as aphasia, visual disturbances, or hemiparesis. This patient does not exhibit any of these findings. Migraines (d) tend to be unilateral and pulsating and associated with nausea, vomiting, photophobia, phonophobia, blurred vision, and light-headedness. Patients should not exhibit papilledema.

**287. The answer is e.** (Rosen, pp 1504.) This patient's clinical picture is consistent with **temporal arteritis (TA)**. Patients are usually **middle-aged women** (age > 50) who present with malaise, fevers, and headache. A complete physical examination would have revealed temporal artery tenderness to palpation. This patient also complains of symptoms consistent with **polymyalgia rheumatica**, a general achiness that may become confused with influenza. Temporal or giant-cell arteritis is a granulomatous inflammation that involves the large- and medium-sized arteries of the body, commonly the carotid artery and its branches. Symptoms are produced as a result of ischemia to the organs fed by the branches of the artery. Visual loss in one eye, transient diplopia and jaw claudication are common symptoms when the branches of the internal and external carotid are affected. A **temporal artery biopsy** is the **diagnostic test of choice and will confirm the diagnosis. However, it is important to note that TA is segmental in nature and false negatives do occur.** Treatment up until the time of biopsy should include high-dose **glucocorticoids**, namely prednisone or methylprednisolone. This does not alter biopsy results and may prevent progression of the disease. Hospitalization is warranted in patients with severe debilitation or impending visual loss and may require high-dose steroids.

(a) Symptoms of influenza closely mimic those of polymyalgia rheumatica, were it not for the specific eye/jaw symptoms. (b) Patients with streptococcal pharyngitis may present with profound general malaise; however, they are typically more febrile and have a history of sick contacts and dry cough. Tonsillar exudates and anterior cervical adenopathy might be evident upon physical examination. (c) An ESR between 50 and 100 mm/h is a good initial test to further the suspicion of TA; however, it is not the diagnostic test of choice. An elevated C-reactive protein may also be present. (d) A CBC may indicate anemia, which results from the arterial inflammation that furthers the breakdown of red blood cells (RBCs). However, this and an elevated WBC count are nonspecific findings.

**288. The answer is e.** (*Aminoff et al, Ch 2 Headache and facial pain.*) Tension headaches often occur **daily**, and classically cause bilateral occipital pain that is described as a **band tightening** around the head. In general, people experience a constant, dull pain that is nonthrobbing and without the ancillary features associated with migraines (visual phenomena, aura, neurologic complaints, nausea, vomiting). There is often secondary contraction of the neck and scalp musculature. First-line treatment includes NSAIDs and acetaminophen. If the headaches occur frequently enough to cause dysfunction in daily activities, patients may benefit from preventive therapy, such as amitriptyline, desipramine, or propranolol.

Migraine headaches (**a**) classically begin with visual phenomena or another aura and are pulsatile, unilateral, associated with nausea, vomiting, photophobia, and phonophobia. They may also have associated neurologic phenomena. Cluster headaches (**b**) are more common in men and are unilateral, boring, and may be associated with neurologic phenomena or autonomic activation. They are short lived and generally recur daily at the same time for days or weeks before the patient has remission of their symptoms. Trigeminal neuralgia (**c**) is thought to result from microvascular compression of the trigeminal nerve roots. It presents as shooting facial pain, in the distribution of the fifth cranial nerve, particularly the second and third nerve roots. In fewer than 5% of cases, it involves the first division of the trigeminal nerve and patients will present complaining of headache. Treatment includes carbamazepine or other antiepileptic drugs. Postherpetic neuralgia (**d**) is pain that continues after an eruption of herpes zoster. It is often described as a burning or stabbing pain that is constant in the dermatome originally affected by the zoster outbreak. In 50% of patients it subsides after 6 months. In some patients it lasts for years. Treatment is with gabapentin, phenytoin, or amitriptyline.

**289. The answer is c.** (*Tintinalli, p 1152.*) The patient is experiencing a **migraine** variant known as a **basilar migraine**. Its onset is similar to other migraines in that it can begin with scotomata or aura. The visual symptoms are often bilateral and followed by a brief period of cortical blindness. Symptoms related to the basilar circulation then predominate, including incoordination, dysarthria, vertigo, and numbness and tingling in the arms or legs. These symptoms generally last 10 to 30 minutes then resolve. Occasionally, transient coma or quadriplegia can develop but persist for only several hours. The resulting headache is occipital and pulsating. The symptoms may mimic a vertebrobasilar ischemic event. Treatment with first-line agents for migraine is recommended. Threshold should be low to seek neurologic consultation unless the diagnosis is certain.

Diazepam (a) is useful for treating cervical muscle spasm and torticollis. At high doses, it has the principal side effect of respiratory depression. It is unlikely to relieve the pain associated with a migraine although it may be useful for associated scalp and trapezius spasm. High-flow oxygen (b) is beneficial to migraine patients but is not the mainstay of treatment. Other adjuncts to pharmacotherapy include decreasing ambient light and noise and putting a cool cloth over the forehead. Acetaminophen (d) is a useful first-line treatment with NSAIDs for migraine and tension-type headaches. They represent a safer first-line treatment to triptans, which are contraindicated in patients with dysrhythmias, poorly controlled hypertension, or coronary artery disease. Therapeutic removal of CSF (e) is indicated in cases of IIH.

**290. The answer is d.** (*Rosen, pp 1364-1365.*) The patient has a **post-LP headache**. The headache is thought to be caused by the removal of CSF during LP with a continued leakage of CSF. It is exquisitely **sensitive to position** and many patients will experience complete relief of pain after being placed in Trendelenburg position. A **blood patch** is placed by injecting an aliquot of the patient's blood in a sterile fashion just external to the dura mater at the same interspace where the LP occurred. The majority of patients have relief of symptoms with this procedure. Prevention of the post-LP headache includes using a 22-gauge or smaller needle, removing as little fluid as possible, and facing the bevel up when the patient is in the lateral position.

Administering IV fluids (a) is thought to increase intravascular volume and CSF production, thereby reducing symptoms. It should be administered to this individual; however, it is not definitive treatment. Standard migraine treatments (b) are often ineffective in treating the post-LP headache. The headache often responds well to caffeine-based therapy. Meclizine (c) is a medication used to treat peripheral vertigo and is ineffective in the treatment of the post-LP headache. Repeat LP (e) is unlikely to yield new diagnostic information and is likely to exacerbate the headache. Headaches that improve after dural puncture are those typically associated with IIH. There are case reports of spontaneous SDH post-LP caused by relative descent of the brain in the setting of decreased CSF with stretch on bridging veins. If this is a diagnostic consideration, a head CT scan should be obtained.

**291. The answer is d.** *(Goldman, pp 1448-1449.)* IIH formerly **pseudotumor cerebri**, requires urgent treatment when there is a history of visual phenomena, particularly transient vision loss. Agents used to lower ICP in this setting include carbonic anhydrase inhibitors (ie, acetazolamide) and loop diuretics (ie, furosemide). Transient visual loss, pain, or blurring occurs frequently and can be permanent in up to 10% of patients. Treatment of the headache itself often employs the same agents used to treat migraines: ergots, antiemetics, and occasionally steroids. The headache is often refractory and difficult to manage. The condition is associated with obesity and weight loss is sometimes helpful.

Papilledema **(a)** in the setting of intermittent frontotemporal headaches and an otherwise normal neurologic examination is consistent with IIH. Its presence does not rule in or out other intracranial pathology. It is not by itself a risk factor in patients with IIH for neurologic deterioration. A history of pulsatile tinnitus **(b)** is often associated with IIH, but its prognostic significance is unclear. An empty sella **(c)** is frequently seen on CT scan of IIH patients. It is likely caused by herniation of arachnoid CSF into the sellar space and is sometimes reversible with lowering of CSF pressure. Another finding to look for on CT scan is an occluded venous sinus, which indicates a secondary cause of elevated ICP. Minocycline, oral contraceptive pills, vitamin A, and anabolic steroids **(e)** have been associated with the development of IIH.

**292. The answer is b**. *(Rosen, pp 1360-1361; Manno, pp 347-366.)* The patient presents with a clinical history that is consistent with a **SAH**. Brain CT without contrast is the procedure of choice for diagnosing SAH and should be done in any individual with a new onset of a severe or persistent headache. It has a sensitivity of 95% for detecting SAH. If the CT is negative, an LP should be performed because some patients with SAH have a normal CT scan. A yellow supernatant liquid (xanthochromia), obtained by centrifuging a bloody CSF sample, can help distinguish SAH from a traumatic tap. If the diagnosis is still in question, an angiography may be required.

Administration of metoclopramide and ketorolac **(a)** is useful in managing pain as a result of a migraine syndrome. Because of their antiplatelet activity, ketorolac (Toradol) and other NSAIDs are contraindicated in patients who may be actively bleeding. Treatment of meningitis **(c)** with IV antibiotics should not be delayed if the diagnosis is suspected. However, the patient's clinical history is inconsistent with this diagnosis (he is afebrile and without constitutional symptoms) and LP is readily available. Infusion of IV mannitol **(d)** lowers ICP acutely via osmotic diuresis. It is indicated in patients displaying symptoms of increased ICP or when impending herniation is suspected. Angiography **(e)** is the gold standard for diagnosis of a cerebral aneurysm, but LP should be performed to confirm the presence of intracranial bleeding before contrast-based imaging.

**293. The answer is c.** *(Tintinalli, pp 1379-1381.)* The headache described is a **menstrual migraine**, a common **variant of the migraine headache syndrome**. Appropriate abortive therapies (this headache is just starting) are diverse and include IV ergot, triptans, and antiemetics. Sumatriptan (Imitrex) is a triptan that acts by blocking the 5-hydroxytryptamine (5-HT, serotonin) 1D receptor. It also has less associated nausea and vomiting than ergots. It may have a higher incidence of minor side effects (flushing, injection site reaction) and a higher relapse rate than ergots. Contraindications to triptans or ergots include pregnancy, hypertension, coronary artery disease, or use of either class of agent within the last 24 hours.

Opioid analgesics **(a and e)** are reserved for failed abortive therapy or when there are contraindications to readily available abortive drugs. Opioids decrease the pain associated with headache syndromes but fail to interrupt the neurochemical dysfunction. Frequent use of opioids for primary headache syndromes is associated with poor outcomes. **(b)** NSAIDs and acetaminophen are appropriate first-line therapy for patients with minor migraine symptoms. If a patient has tried these in the past and they have been ineffective, there is little utility in trying again. **(d)** Topiramate (Topamax) is an antiepileptic drug that is used for migraine prevention in patients with frequent and difficult-to-control headache syndromes.

**294. The answer is a.** *(Goldman and Ausiello, pp 2059-2062.)* In a case of suspected TA, **initiation of corticosteroid therapy is indicated emergently** to prevent irreversible complications. **Loss of vision** is known to occur and prompt initiation of corticosteroid therapy decreases this possibility. TA, also referred to as giant-cell arteritis, is a granulomatous inflammation of the proximal great vessels and its carotid bifurcations. It has an overlapping clinical syndrome with **polymyalgia rheumatica**.

The description of this headache syndrome is inconsistent with a SAH **(b)**, which classically presents with sudden onset of pain and is associated with nausea, photophobia, and nuchal rigidity. It is rarely preceded by constitutional symptoms. Injection of lidocaine at the base of the occiput is an effective treatment for cervical neuralgia (**c**) but has no place in the treatment or diagnosis of TA. (**d**) The patient's clinical history is inconsistent with meningitis. ESR (**e**) is normally elevated to the 50 to 100 range, but a mildly elevated sedimentation rate does not rule out the diagnosis. Laboratory analysis is helpful in diagnosing TA, but waiting for serum analysis inappropriately delays treatment. The confirmatory diagnostic test of choice is a temporal artery biopsy.

**295. The answer is c.** *(Rosen, pp 1418-1425.)* The normal number of **WBCs** in the CSF is 5 or fewer with 1 or less **polymorphonuclear neutrophils (PMN)**. Numbers greater than these should be taken as evidence for CNS infection. In cases of **acute bacterial meningitis**, cell counts of 1000/µL to 20,000/µL WBCs are observed, often with neutrophil predominance. In cases of aseptic (viral) meningitis, cell counts are generally lower with lymphocyte predominance. Initial treatment with antibiotics before LP is unlikely to affect the cell count. After 6 hours the culture is less likely to return positive. It should be noted that a subset of patients with bacterial meningitis may present with lymphocytic predominance. Therefore, lymphocytic predominance does not rule out bacterial meningitis and antibiotics should be given.

The classic clinical presentation of bacterial meningitis includes photophobia, headache, fever, and nuchal rigidity. None of these symptoms are specific (**a**) and an LP must be obtained. The classic clinical presentation is altered in states of immunocompromised (human immunodeficiency virus [HIV], corticosteroid use), so clinical suspicion should be higher in these patients. Fevers (**b**) are generally thought to be high in bacterial meningitis, but there is no number that is specific for its diagnosis. CSF protein level (**d**) generally ranges from 15 to 45 mg/dL. Levels greater than 150 mg/dL are often seen in acute bacterial meningitis but can result from many other conditions, including CNS abscesses, encephalitis, and fungal infections. Fungal infections often have CSF proteins that are markedly elevated, often greater than 1000 mg/dL. Glucose levels are generally depressed (**e**) in cases of bacterial meningitis.

**296. The answer is c.** *(Rosen, pp 1048, 1208-1209, 1953-1954.)* **Dystonic reactions** may occur with the use of dopamine-blocking agents. Medications classically associated with dystonic reactions are typical antipsychotics (eg, haloperidol) but can also occur with the antiemetics used to treat migraines. They are generally not life threatening and respond almost immediately to administration of diphenhydramine (Benadryl) given intravenously or intramuscularly or benzodiazepines. Common dystonic reactions include oculogyric crises (eyes deviating in different directions), torticollis, tongue protrusion, facial grimacing, and difficulty speaking.

Morphine sulfate (a) has the principal side effect of respiratory depression. This effect and the drug's analgesic properties are reversed by naloxone. Localized reactions including erythema, swelling, and pruritus are common after intramuscular or subcutaneous injection. Anaphylaxis has been described but is rare. Acetaminophen (b) has the principal side effect of hepatotoxicity. In patients using it chronically without following dose-based guidelines, liver damage is possible. (d) Caffeine is a methylxanthine. Side effects include palpitations, anxiety, tremulousness, and dry mouth. Sumatriptan (e) has side effects related to the cardiovascular system. They include hypertension and coronary artery vasospasm. Several cases of myocardial infarctions have been observed after its use.

**297. The answer is b.** *(Tintinalli, pp 1172-1175.)* The clinical presentation is consistent with **meningitis**. The patient's mental status has declined between initial nursing assessment and the physician's interview. Delay in antibiotic therapy in order to first confirm the diagnosis with CSF analysis may lead to increased mortality.

LP (a) performed even several hours after initiation of antibiotic therapy is often still culture positive for the causative organism. Administration of IV corticosteroids before antibiotic administration (c) has been shown in some studies to reduce the mortality of patients with bacterial meningitis. Their use in the ED for undifferentiated cases of meningitis has not been sufficiently studied. Antipyretics (d) are used to reduce fever but will not stop the primary pathologic process. Noncontrast head CT (e) should be obtained before LP when question of mass effect or increased ICP might lead to herniation from CSF removal. Antibiotic therapy should not be delayed in cases of suspected meningitis for neuroimaging.

**298. The answer is c.** *(Rosen, pp 1363-1364.)* IIH is an idiopathic elevation of ICP. In the setting of a normal CT, the diagnosis is made by LP with an elevated opening pressure often between 250 and 450 mm $H_2O$. Patients often experience complete relief of their symptoms with **LP** and return of their ICP to levels less than 200 mm $H_2O$.

Corticosteroids (a) are controversial in the management of headache in IIH, but many neurologists use them routinely. Mannitol (b) is an osmotic diuretic that is used to acutely lower ICP, often in the setting of trauma to prevent impending herniation. Its use is not recommended in the setting of IIH. It should not be confused with acetazolamide, a carbonic anhydrase inhibitor that works as a diuretic and is part of maintenance treatment for IIH. Metoclopramide (**d**) is normally used as an antiemetic but is also highly effective in the treatment of migraines. Ketorolac and other NSAIDs (**e**) are the mainstays of treatment for many headache syndromes, including tension headaches, migraines, cluster headaches, and others. Their use should be avoided when there is suspicion that the patient has an intracranial bleed because they have antiplatelet effects and can exacerbate bleeding.

**299. The answer is d.** (*Goldman and Ausiello, pp 2271-2273; Tintinalli, pp 1177-1178.*) **Brain abscesses** are uncommon and their incidence has decreased over the past several years as a result of better antibiotic treatment of the remote infections that cause them. Today, the majority of brain abscesses in developed countries are the result of contiguous spread from otitis media, mastoiditis, paranasal sinusitis, or meningitis. They can also occur after trauma, classically after a basilar skull fracture. Presentation is often nonspecific, with almost half present with headache alone. Focal weakness, fevers, and nausea are other common presenting complaints. Antibiotic choice should be guided by suspected source and ability to penetrate the CNS. In general, MRI is more sensitive at detecting CNS infection than CT. With contrast CT, the walls of the abscess enhance and there is a central necrotic area of lower density. On this CT with IV contrast, there are multiple ring-enhancing lesions with surrounding edema in the left frontal lobe. The large extra-axial collections with enhancing margins represent emphysemas. There is also midline shift secondary to mass effect of the abscesses.

(**a**) CNS toxoplasmosis is uncommon in the developed world outside the setting of advanced HIV or other immunocompromised states. Patients often present with altered mental status, neurologic deficits, or seizures. On contrast enhanced CT, there are often multiple, small, ring-enhancing lesions. (**b**) Subdural hygromas are fluid-filled subdural pockets containing xanthochromic fluid. They are often the result of trauma and present with signs and symptoms of increased ICP or with neurologic deficits. They are thought to result from tears in the arachnoid with fluid accumulation. (**c**) Glioblastoma multiforme is the most common and most aggressive of the primary brain tumors. On CT scans, glioblastomas usually appear as irregularly shaped hypodense lesions with a peripheral ringlike zone of contrast enhancement and a penumbra of cerebral edema. **(e)** Spontaneous SAHs present as severe headaches associated with nausea, vomiting, nuchal rigidity, and can have neurologic deficits associated with them. It appears on noncontrast CT as hyperdense fluid that may fill the cisterns and subarachnoid space.

**300. The answer is d.** (*Tintinalli, pp 1174-1176.*) Patients with CSF analysis consistent with viral meningitis can be managed as outpatients with close follow-up. These patients must be reliable for follow-up, not immunocompromised and otherwise well appearing. They should be told to return for reevaluation if their symptoms do not improve within 48 hours. If they have not improved, **reevaluation** including **neuroimaging**, **repeat LP**, and treatment with antibiotics is indicated.

Administration of acyclovir **(a)** is indicated in patients with presumed meningoencephalitis caused by herpes virus. Antipyretic therapy **(b)** is indicated for patient comfort, but repeat diagnostic evaluation is essential. Sinus pain **(c)** can often present as a frontal, pulsating headache. Patients may be febrile and can seed the CSF from direct extension of sinusitis. Nevertheless, meningitis must still be ruled out and treated, even if there is CT confirmation of sinus opacification. Analyzing CSF already in the laboratory **(e)** from a previous LP is not recommended.

**301. The answer is a.** (*Tintinalli, p 1115.*) Headaches caused by a **mass lesion** are classically described as **worse in the morning**, associated with **nausea and vomiting**, and **worse with position**. Rarely do patients present with focal neurologic symptoms. When they do, imaging is a necessary adjunct before leaving the ED. If a mass lesion is part of the differential diagnosis, LP should be deferred until neuroimaging has been performed because of the risk of herniation.

Cluster headaches **(b)** are rare, generally occur in male patients, last less than 2 hours, and present as unilateral eye or temporal pain. There is often unilateral tearing, swelling, or nasal congestion. In contrast to the migraine patient, patients with cluster headaches are typically restless. Cluster headaches respond to ergots, triptans, and often high-flow oxygen. Tension-type **(c)** headaches are bilateral, not pulsating, not worsened by exertion, and should not be associated with nausea or vomiting. They generally respond to NSAIDs or acetaminophen. Headaches associated with intracranial hypertension **(d)** are exacerbated by changes in position (eg, squatting), are often frontotemporal, and may be associated with disturbances of gait and incontinence. They are difficult to control. Migraines (**e**) are generally unilateral, pulsating, associated with phonophobia or photophobia, nausea, and vomiting. They are slow in onset and generally last 4 to 72 hours. There is considerable heterogeneity in their presentation. Most patients who are chronic migraineurs can describe their headache syndrome and are able to differentiate between their normal migraine and another headache. Change in the character, intensity, location, or duration of a migraine should prompt suspicion of another cause.

**302. The answer is b.** (*Tintinalli, pp 1118-1121.*) The CT depicts subarachnoid arachnoid blood. This patient may have had a sentinel bleed, a small SAH, the previous week. Noncontrast CT misses a small percentage of SAH and therefore, in cases of high suspicion, an LP must be obtained to exclude the diagnosis.

Irritation of the meninges or inflammation of the brain (**a**) may not appear at all on noncontrast CT of the brain. If contrast is used, meningeal or cerebral enhancement may be apparent, but diagnosis of these conditions is not based on imaging. High clinical suspicion must be present for either condition and LP is used to confirm the diagnosis. Hydrocephalus (**c**) appears as dilated ventricles on CT scan. If all of the ventricles are patent and dilated, it is termed *communicating hydrocephalus*. If part of the ventricular system is collapsed and the others dilated, an obstructive cause of hydrocephalus is present. Epidural hematomas (**d**) are the result of brisk arterial bleeds into the space between the dura and the calvarium. They are classically caused by trauma and are associated with a "lucid period" during which level of consciousness is normal before neurologic deterioration. On noncontrast CT, they appear as hyperdense intracranial collections of blood that are bilenticular in shape. SDHs (**e**) are intracranial blood collections that result from tearing of the bridging veins between the dura and the brain. Risk factors for SDH include advanced age and chronic alcohol use. Both conditions are associated with decreased brain volume and provide stretch on these delicate veins. On noncontrast CT, SDHs appear as crescent-shaped collections of hyperdense blood.

**303. The answer is b.** (*Tintinalli, pp 1175-1176.*) The CSF analysis in this patient is consistent with a **viral or atypical cause of meningitis**. Although patients may have a mononuclear predominance and still have bacterial meningitis, viral causes should be considered. CSF should be sent for PCR analysis and empiric treatment initiated for **herpes encephalitis**. The mortality of meningoencephalitis caused by herpes simplex virus (HSV) is exceptionally high if untreated.

Tuberculosis (TB) meningitis **(a)** should be considered in this undomiciled patient. Other risk factors for TB include immunocompromise and living in an endemic region. However, the patient is recently PPD and chest x-ray negative, making this possibility less likely. In an immunocompromised patient, PPD may be less reliable so a CSF acid fast stain and mycobacterial culture should still be sent. Fungal causes **(c)** of CNS pathology are also a diagnostic consideration but are less likely than viral causes. In this patient, fungal cultures are recommended in addition to CSF cryptococcal antigen. *Bartonella* sp **(d)** and other rare causes of meningitis are not considered until other first- and second-tier analyses are conducted. When given simultaneously with (or before) the first dose of antibiotic, steroids **(e)** reduce the incidence of sensorineural hearing loss associated with bacterial meningitis in children. It also decreases the risk of an unfavorable outcome in adults with bacterial meningitis.

**304. The answer is e.** *(Hasbun, p 1727.)* Indications for brain CT scanning before LP include: patients older than 60 years, patients who are immunocompromised, patients with known CNS lesions, patients who presented with a seizure or who had a seizure within 1 week of presentation, patients with abnormal level of consciousness, patients with focal findings on neurologic examination, and patients with papilledema seen on physical examination with clinical suspicion of elevated ICP. All of the patients in this scenario presented fit one of these contraindications except for the 51-year-old woman with fever and neck stiffness.

**305. The answer is a.** *(Tintinalli, pp 1543-1544.)* The patient presents with **acute angle closure glaucoma** that results from obstruction of aqueous outflow of the anterior chamber of the eye with a resulting **rise in intraocular pressure**. It is the result of a shallow anterior chamber or a chamber distorted by the development of a cataract. Classically, it occurs when a patient leaves a prolonged dimly lit situation. When the iris becomes mid-dilated, it maximally obstructs the trabecular meshwork occluding aqueous humor flow. Intraocular pressures may rise from normal (10-21 mm Hg) to levels as high as 50 to 100. **Visual acuity is usually decreased** in the affected eye as a result of corneal edema. Treatment is aimed at lowering intraocular pressure with acetazolamide, ophthalmic β-blockers, prostaglandin analogues, and pilocarpine to induce miosis. Ophthalmologic consultation and follow-up are indicated. Patients may present complaining of headache, nausea, and vomiting but will often endorse that the symptoms began with acute eye pain. Funduscopic examination (**b**) is occasionally abnormal in acute glaucoma, but associated papilledema rarely develops acutely. Corneal examination with fluorescein (**c**) is used to diagnose corneal abrasions or other corneal pathology (ie, ulcers, keratitis, foreign body, corneal rupture). The cornea may appear normal or "steamy" in the setting of acute glaucoma as the edges accumulate edema from the increase pressure of the anterior chamber. The cornea should not take up fluorescein. LP (**d**) is used to diagnose intracranial pathology. The acute unilateral pain of glaucoma may make the clinician consider a SAH, but glaucoma should always be considered. A change in visual acuity (**e**) is nonspecific and should not be diagnostic for glaucoma.

**306. The answer is b.** (*Rosen, pp 2036-2038.*) The patients are experiencing symptoms of **carbon monoxide (CO) poisoning**. CO is **colorless** and **odorless**. Patients often present with mild nonspecific symptoms, including headache, malaise, and fatigue. Severe toxicity manifests as neurologic and cardiac toxicity. Severe cases may manifest as disseminated intravascular coagulation, circulatory shock, multiorgan failure, ischemic cardiac disease, renal failure, or noncardiogenic pulmonary edema. Although there is decreased blood oxygen content, patients will not exhibit cyanosis as there is not enough deoxyhemoglobin present to cause it. Common sources of CO include fossil fuel–burning engines, fumes from coal- or gas-burning stoves, and smoke from accidental fires. CO intoxication is more prevalent during the winter when potentially faulty heating systems are in use or when patients attempt to supplement their home heat using their oven. Initial therapy is aimed at increasing arterial oxygen content by providing supplemental oxygen. Mild intoxication can be managed with supplementary oxygen alone. Elevated carboxyhemoglobin levels require treatment with hyperbaric oxygen.

Respiratory isolation (**a**) is indicated in cases of suspected bacterial meningitis where *N meningitidis* is thought to be the causative organism. Antibiotics and LP (**c**) are appropriate if you suspect meningitis. Triptans and antiemetics (**d**) are first-line treatments for migraine headaches. Transfer to a hyperbaric facility (**e**) is indicated for persistent altered mental status, loss of consciousness, seizure, stroke, myocardial ischemia, or pregnancy with a documented carboxyhemoglobin level greater than 15%.

**307. The answer is a.** *(Rosen, pp 308-311.)* After head trauma, 30% to 90% of patients complain of headache during their convalescence. **Postconcussive headaches** are notable for their **variability** in frequency, location, and associated symptoms. They are often exacerbated by physical activity or changes in position and may be clinically difficult to distinguish from other headache syndromes. In patients with preexisting migraines, increased frequency of their normal migraine syndrome is often noted. Most patients have resolution of their headaches after 4 weeks. In 20% of patients, their postconcussive headache persists for longer than a year. Headache may be one feature of a larger postconcussive syndrome, including nervous system instability. This may include fragmentation of sleep, emotional lability, inability to tolerate crowds, restlessness, inability to concentrate, and anxiety.

Posttraumatic hydrocephalus **(b)** is a rare complication of minor head trauma. It presents with signs and symptoms of increased ICP, including headache, gait instability, dizziness, nausea, and vomiting. It is often transient and may appear as a mild dilatation of the ventricles. Subdural hygromas **(c)** can occur in the weeks following a trauma or may appear as incidental findings. They occasionally increase in size causing symptoms because of mass effect. Cluster headaches **(d)** happen daily at the same time for days or weeks. They are unilateral, short, and boring in quality. The autonomic instability of posttraumatic nervous instability overlaps considerably with posttraumatic stress disorder **(e)**, which has led some researchers to postulate that they share a similar mechanism.

**308. The answer is d.** *(Harrison, Ch 333: Disorders of the Anterior Pituitary and Hypothalamus.)* The patient presents with symptoms consistent with a **prolactin-secreting pituitary adenoma**. The appropriate imaging modality to diagnose a pituitary adenoma is with high-resolution MRI with thin cuts through the sella. Women often present with amenorrhea, infertility, and galactorrhea. Men will present with decreased libido. In both cases, extension beyond the sella may present with visual field defects or other mass-related symptoms.

**(a)** Noncontrast and contrast-enhanced CTs are not particularly sensitive for these lesions that sit in the sella turcica. Bromocriptine **(b)** or other centrally acting dopamine agonists are used to treat pituitary macro- and microadenomas. The presence of RBCs or xanthochromia in the CSF (c) is diagnostic for a SAH. The clinical presentation is inconsistent with SAH. (e) Removing CSF is treatment for IIH.

**309. The answer is a.** *(Scheinfeld, 2009.)* **Anticonvulsant medications** are sometimes used as prophylaxis for migraines. Phenytoin, valproic acid, phenobarbital, and topiramate are among the antiepileptics commonly used to prevent migraines. Phenytoin causes **fetal hydantoin syndrome**, a constellation of birth defects, including growth retardation, cleft palates, hand deformities, and structural cardiac defects. Valproic acid has similar effects with the addition of **neural tube defects**. Phenobarbital, declining in its use for migraine prevention, causes cardiac defects, facial clefts, and urinary tract abnormalities. Early data on topiramate reveal teratogenicity in animal models.

β-Blockers (b) are generally safe during pregnancy. There is significant controversy over the safety of using triptans (c) during pregnancy. The concern is that their vasoconstrictive properties might cause uterine vessels to constrict, limiting fetal blood flow. Most research has shown infants born to mothers taking triptans during pregnancy have rates of birth defects no higher than background. Hypertension and cardiac conditions are primary contraindications to triptan therapy, and the drug should be discontinued if early preeclampsia is suspected. Acetaminophen and antiemetics (d and e) are generally safe to take during pregnancy.

**310. The answer is d.** *(Rosen, pp 1333-1345.)* The patient had a **TIA**, which involves **neurologic deficits that resolve within 24 hours of onset**. TIAs often precede ischemic stroke; up to 50% of patients with a TIA will have a stroke in the next 5 years, with the highest incidence in the first month. It is important to recognize TIAs and to evaluate patients for **cardiac or carotid arterial sources of emboli**. Although the symptoms often resolve, many patients with a TIA will have evidence of infarction on CT/MRI.

The patient did not have a thrombotic (a) stroke. Neurologic deficits are not transient in a cerebral vascular accident. Conversion disorder (b) is a rare disorder that is characterized by the abrupt, dramatic onset of a single symptom. It typically presents as some nonpainful neurologic disorder for which there is no objective data. It is a diagnosis of exclusion. Although migraine auras can include focal neurologic deficits (c), the patient in the vignette does not have a history of migraines and is not complaining of a headache. Todd paralysis (**e**) is a transient focal neurologic deficit that persists after a seizure.

**311. The answer is a.** (*Tintinalli, pp 1144-1152.*) **BPV** is a transient positional vertigo associated with nystagmus. The problem occurs secondary to the creation and movement of canaliths (free-moving densities) in the semicircular canals of the inner ear with a particular head movement. Neurologic deficits are absent in BPV. Note that horizontal, vertical, or rotary **nystagmus** can occur in BPV. It is important to pay special attention to a patient with vertical nystagmus because it may be associated with a brainstem or cerebellum lesion. BPV is treated with the **Epley maneuver** (a series of head and body turns that reposition the canalith), antiemetics, and antihistamines. Key differences between peripheral and central vertigo are seen in the chart.

Food poisoning (**b**) would not cause vertigo. If it is associated with vomiting and diarrhea, it can lead to dehydration and light-headedness but not vertiginous symptoms. Meniere disease (**c**) is an inner ear disease of unclear etiology. It presents with recurrent attacks of vertigo and tinnitus, with deafness of the involved ear between attacks. Labyrinthitis (**d**) presents with hearing loss and sudden, brief positional vertigo attacks. TIAs (**e**) involving the vertebrobasilar system can present with vertigo but is an unlikely diagnosis in this case of recurrent positional vertiginous symptoms.

| | **Peripheral Vertigo** | **Central Vertigo** |
|---|---|---|
| Pathophysiology | Disorder of vestibular nerve (CN VIII) | Disorder of brain stem or cerebellum |
| Severity | Intense | Less intense |
| Onset | Sudden | Slow |
| Pattern | Intermittent | Constant |
| Nausea and vomiting | Usually present | Usually absent |
| Exacerbated by position | Most of the time | Less of the time |
| Hearing abnormalities | May be present | Usually absent |
| Focal neurologic deficits | Usually absent | Usually present |
| Fatigability of symptoms | Yes | No |
| Nystagmus | Horizontal, vertical, rotary | Vertical |

**312. The answer is a.** (*Rosen, pp 88, 1413-1415.*) High clinical suspicion in this case is for **myasthenia gravis**, an autoimmune condition in which **acetylcholine receptor antibodies** block acetylcholine binding and prevent normal neuromuscular conduction. The disease typically affects young women and older men, and presents with **generalized weakness worsening with repetitive muscle use that is usually relieved with rest.** Ptosis and diplopia are usually present. The **edrophonium test** is used to help diagnose myasthenia gravis. It involves administering edrophonium, a short-acting anticholinesterase, which prevents acetylcholine breakdown. With the increased acetylcholine levels at the neuromuscular junction, the patient experiences a subjective and objective improvement of symptoms by preventing rapid breakdown of acetylcholine at the myoneural junction. Serologic testing (**b**) for antibodies to acetylcholine receptors is useful when positive and should be obtained in the workup of this patient. A negative test does not exclude the disorder. The electromyogram is diagnostic. (**c**) You may consider a CT scan to evaluate the patient for possible mass lesion or aneurysm that is causing her ptosis and diplopia. However, the clinical scenario is more consistent with myasthenia gravis. (**d**) An electrolyte panel will likely be normal. (**e**) If the edrophonium test is normal, an LP should be considered.

**313. The answer is b.** *(Rosen, pp 88, 1400-1401.)* The patient has a **progressive ascending peripheral neuropathy**, also known as **Guillain-Barré syndrome**. Patients can usually remember a preceding viral illness, usually gastroenteritis. **Deep tendon reflexes are typically absent.**

Hypokalemic periodic paralysis is part of the heterogeneous group of muscle diseases known as periodic paralyses and is characterized by episodes of flaccid muscle weakness occurring at irregular intervals. Most of the conditions are hereditary and are more episodic than periodic. Peripheral vascular disease (**c**), a common complication of longstanding diabetes, causes paresthesias in the distal lower extremities and not acute paralysis. Tetanus (**d**) manifests as muscular rigidity caused by the *Clostridium tetani* toxin preventing release of inhibitory neurotransmitters. Lockjaw is a common complaint in generalized tetanus. A brain abscess (**e**) typically presents with fever, headache, and focal neurologic findings, and is usually caused by an associated trauma, surgery, or infectious spread from another site.

**314. The answer is c.** *(Rosen, pp 89, 1400-1401.)* Progressive paralysis in Guillain-Barré syndrome can rapidly ascend to the respiratory system and cause **respiratory failure**. Patients need to be monitored and provided ventilator support as necessary.

(**a**) Guillain-Barré syndrome is a transient, not permanent, condition. (**b, d, and e**) are not complications of the syndrome.

**315. The answer is d.** (*Tintinalli, pp 121-122.*) This patient presents with **hypokalemia**, secondary to increased potassium losses through vomiting and diarrhea as well as reduced oral intake. Potassium deficiency results in hyperpolarization of the cell membrane and leads to **muscle weakness, hyporeflexia, intestinal ileus, and respiratory paralysis**. Characteristic ECG findings include flattened T waves, U waves, and prolonged QT and PR intervals.

Hyponatremia (**a**) and hypernatremia (**b**) mainly affect the CNS, resulting in headache, anorexia, lethargy, and confusion. In more severe cases, hyponatremia causes seizures, coma, and respiratory arrest, whereas patients with profound hypernatremia develop ataxia, tremulousness, and spasms. Hyperkalemia (**c**) can lead to cardiac dysrhythmias and typically exhibits distinctive ECG findings, including peaked T waves, prolonged QT and PR intervals, and widened QRS complex that can progress to a sine wave pattern. Signs of hypercalcemia (**e**) include bony and abdominal pain, renal stones, and altered mental status (remembered by: "bones, stones, groans, and psychiatric overtones"). In addition, cardiac effects include bradycardia, heart blocks, and shortened QT interval on ECG.

**316. The answer is d.** (*Rosen, pp 1333-1345.*) The CT image shows a large hypodensity in the right parietal-occipital region representing an **ischemic stroke**. Ischemic strokes comprise **80%** of all strokes, with hemorrhagic strokes accounting for the other 20%. Ischemic events include **thrombotic** (thrombus forming at the site of an ulcerated atherosclerotic plaque), **embolic** (thrombus embolized to a distal site), and **lacunar** (small terminal artery occlusion) strokes. This patient likely had a cardioembolic secondary to atrial fibrillation. Atrial fibrillation is an important risk factor for an embolic stroke, particularly when patients are noncompliant with anticoagulation therapy, as the patient in the vignette. Intracranial bleeding secondary to a hemorrhagic event appears hyperdense on CT scan. The diagram below illustrates the cerebral circulation.

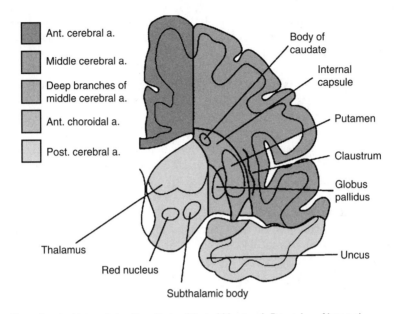

Ant. cerebral a.

Middle cerebral a.

Deep branches of middle cerebral a.

Ant. choroidal a.

Post. cerebral a.

Body of caudate

Internal capsule

Putamen

Claustrum

Globus pallidus

Uncus

Thalamus

Red nucleus

Subthalamic body

*(Reproduced, with permission, from Kasper DL et al.* Harrison's Principles of Internal Medicine. *New York, NY. McGraw-Hill, 2005: 2381.) (Courtesy of CM Fisher, MD.)*

**317. The answer is b.** *(Rosen, pp 1386-1388.)* Consider **MS** as a diagnosis in presentations of various neurologic symptoms that are difficult to explain by a single CNS lesion, particularly those occurring in a woman in her third decade of life. MS is a **multifocal demyelinating CNS disease** that in 30% of cases initially presents with **optic neuritis** (unilateral eye pain and decreased visual acuity).

Myasthenia gravis **(a)** commonly presents with muscle weakness that is exacerbated by activity, sleeplessness, or alcohol intake, and is relieved by rest. The most frequent initial symptoms include ptosis, diplopia, and blurred vision. Vertebrobasilar insufficiency **(c)** presents with cerebellar and brainstem symptoms, such as vertigo, dysphagia, and diplopia, none of which are present in this patient. Encephalitis **(d)** is an infection of brain parenchyma and presents with altered mental status that may be associated with focal neurologic deficits. Patients might present with behavioral and personality changes, seizures, headache, photophobia, and generalized symptoms of fever, nausea, and vomiting. Guillain-Barré syndrome **(e)** is the most common polyneuropathy. It is described as an ascending paralysis that is often preceded by a viral syndrome. Classically it is associated with the loss of deep tendon reflexes.

**318. The answer is e.** *(Rosen, pp 1386-1388.)* Demyelinating MS lesions are often well demonstrated on **MRI** but cannot be visualized on **(d)** CT scan.

The edrophonium test **(a)** is used as an adjunct in the diagnosis of myasthenia gravis. A carotid artery angiogram **(b)** is useful when evaluating the carotid arteries for trauma, dissections, or thrombus. Analyzing CSF **(c)** can help aid you in the diagnosis of MS as it often reveals oligoclonal banding and elevated protein.

**319. The answer is d.** *(Rosen, pp 1341-1343.)* The patient is a good candidate for **fibrinolytic therapy.** She is having an **acute ischemic stroke** (in the distribution of the middle cerebral artery), has no contraindications to the therapy, and is being evaluated within the 4.5-hour therapeutic window from the onset of symptoms. Exclusion criteria for the use of thrombolytics include

- Evidence of intracranial hemorrhage on noncontrast head CT (absolute)
- Minor or rapidly improving stroke symptoms
- Clinical suspicion for subarachnoid hemorrhage
- Active internal bleeding within last 21 days
- Known bleeding diathesis
- Within 3 months of serious head trauma, stroke, or intracranial surgery
- Within 14 days of major surgery or serious trauma
- Recent arterial puncture at noncompressible site
- LP within 7 days
- History of intracranial hemorrhage, A-V malformation
- Witnessed seizure at stroke onset
- Recent myocardial infarction, or systolic BP > 185 mm Hg or diastolic BP > 110 mm Hg

The head CT may initially appear normal and starts to show the extent of injury within 6 to 12 hours after the onset of symptoms.

**(a)** Current guidelines recommend that thrombolytics be administered within 4.5 hours of the patient's symptom onset. Any patient whose symptoms are present upon waking up from sleep is excluded because it cannot be certain when the symptoms began. **(b)** The general consensus in the neurology literature is to *not* treat hypertension in patients with acute ischemic stroke unless they are candidates for thrombolysis and their BP is greater than 185 mm Hg systolic or 100 mm Hg diastolic. Labetalol is often recommended over nitroprusside. Labetalol preserves normal cerebral autoregulation whereas nitroprusside, a vasodilator, may divert blood from the injured tissue, and cause increased ischemia. Heparin therapy (c) has not been shown to reduce stroke-related mortality or disability in the setting of acute stroke. If the patient is not a candidate for thrombolytics, aspirin (e) should be given in the setting of acute ischemic stroke. Maintenance therapy with daily aspirin or another antiplatelet agent has been shown to help reduce stroke recurrence after a TIA.

**320. The answer is e.** (*Rosen, pp 1413-1415.*) **Myasthenia gravis** is an autoimmune disease of the **neuromuscular junction** that is more common in women in their 20s and 30s and men in their 70s and 80s. Myasthenia gravis results from autoantibodies directed against the nicotinic acetylcholine receptor at the neuromuscular junction. This leads to destruction of acetylcholine receptors and competition with acetylcholine for the remaining receptors. **Muscular weakness** and **fatigability** are the hallmarks of myasthenia gravis. Ocular symptoms manifest early and include ptosis, diplopia, and muscle weakness. Symptoms usually worsen as the day progresses. Diagnosis is usually made by the **edrophonium** or **Tensilon test**.

(a) Botulism is a toxin-mediated disease that causes acute weakness by the irreversible binding of botulinum toxin to the presynaptic membrane of nerves subsequently inhibiting the release of acetylcholine. The classic presentation of botulism is a descending, symmetric paralysis. Unlike myasthenia gravis, botulinum toxin decreases cholinergic output, which may lead to anticholinergic signs, such as dilated pupils, dry skin, urinary retention, constipation, and increased temperature. (b) Lambert-Eaton myasthenic syndrome is often associated with small-cell carcinoma of the lung. Autoantibodies cause a decreased release of acetylcholine from presynaptic nerves. However, with repeated stimulation, the amount of acetylcholine in the synaptic cleft increases leading to an improvement of symptoms throughout the day. (c) The third cranial nerve innervates many of the extraocular muscles and the levator palpebrae. In addition, ciliary nerve fibers that run along the third cranial nerve function to constrict the pupil. Damage to the third cranial nerve often results in ptosis, mydriasis, and the classic "down and out" eye. However, these symptoms do not wax and wane as presented in this scenario. (d) Guillain-Barré syndrome is an ascending peripheral neuropathy classically presenting after a history of viral illness. It is associated with loss of deep tendon reflexes and earlier symmetric, distal weakness.

**321. The answer is a.** *(Rosen, pp 1341-1343.)* This patient's BP of 215/118 mm Hg needs to be lowered to **185/110 mm Hg** to make her a good candidate for **thrombolytic therapy**. **Labetalol** is the agent of choice in this case. Other agents to consider include nitroprusside in combination with labetalol, and nicardipine.

Fibrinolytic administration **(b)** at this level of hypertension carries a risk of intracranial bleed. Daily aspirin **(c)** has been shown to reduce the incidence of strokes. However, aspirin should not be administered within 24 hours of fibrinolytic use because it increases the risk of postthrombolytic bleed. Antiseizure prophylaxis with phenytoin **(d)** is not indicated in ischemic strokes although a small percentage of stroke patients will seize within the first 24 hours. Hyperventilation and mannitol **(e)** are used for temporary management of increased intracranial pressure owing to cerebral edema in an ischemic stroke, which peaks at 72 to 96 hours. There is no role for mannitol in acute stroke in a patient without signs of elevated intracranial pressure.

**322. The answer is c.** *(Rosen, pp 2036-2038.)* Patients with initial flu-like symptoms **from the same household** who were exposed to combustion products (ie, from a home generator) are at risk for **carbon monoxide (CO) poisoning**. CO binds to hemoglobin with greater affinity than oxygen and shifts the oxygen-hemoglobin dissociation curve to the left, thus decreasing oxygen release. Clinically, patients with mild CO toxicity present with flu-like symptoms, nausea, and vomiting, which progresses to chest pain, dyspnea, confusion, seizures, dysrhythmias, and coma. CO level can be obtained by a **carboxyhemoglobin level** from blood. CO poisoning is treated with oxygen and, if severe, with **hyperbaric oxygen** therapy.

An important clue to the diagnosis is the development of similar symptoms in the patient and her husband at the same time. While it is important to consider ordering a WBC count **(a)**, a head CT scan **(b)**, and an LP **(d)** for evaluation of the symptoms, think CO poisoning when there are multiple patients with the same symptoms in the setting of exposure to combustible products. It is not appropriate to do nothing **(e)** because the patient is clearly in need of medical attention.

**323. The answer is a.** *(Rosen, pp 1333-1345.)* The middle cerebral artery is the most common site of intracranial cerebral artery thrombosis. Clinical findings can include contralateral hemiplegia, hemianesthesia, and homonymous hemianopsia. The upper-extremity deficit is usually more severe than the lower-extremity deficit. Aphasia occurs if the dominant hemisphere is involved. Gaze preference is in the direction of the lesion.

Choice **(b)** is incorrect because the findings are ipsilateral to the area of injury. Choice **(c)** describes deficits in the anterior cerebral artery (ACA) distribution with greater deficits in lower extremity and altered mentation because of frontal lobe involvement. Crossed deficits such as contralateral motor and ipsilateral cranial nerve findings **(d)** occur in brainstem strokes, which are supplied by the posterior circulation. Pure motor **(e)** or sensory loss occurs in lacunar infarcts, which involve small penetrating arteries.

**324. The answer is e.** *(Rosen, pp 93-100.)* Do not get confused with the multiple signs and symptoms in this case! They involve three distinct areas of the brain: the brainstem (facial droop, dysphagia, vertigo, and vertical nystagmus), cerebellum (ataxia, vertigo, and vertical nystagmus), and visual cortex (diplopia). All of these anatomical areas are supplied by the posterior circulation, specifically the **vertebrobasilar artery**. A mnemonic to help remember the presentation of a vertebrobasilar stroke is the "three Ds": **dizziness (vertigo)**, **dysphagia**, and **diplopia**. There are cerebellar and cranial nerve deficits observed on both sides of the body.

**(a)** Lacunar infarcts are small infarcts that are usually caused by a hypertensive vasculopathy but may occur in diabetics and can affect both the anterior and posterior cerebral vessels. Lacunar strokes involve penetrating cerebral arterial vessels lying deep in the gray matter (internal capsule) or brainstem. BPV **(b)** is a transient positional vertigo associated with nystagmus. Neurologic deficits are absent in BPV. Note that horizontal, vertical, or rotary nystagmus can occur in BPV; however, vertical nystagmus is *always* worrisome as it may indicate a brainstem or cerebellum lesion. Labyrinthitis **(c)**, an infection of the labyrinth, presents with hearing loss and sudden brief positional vertigo attacks and does not involve other neurologic deficits. The posterior cerebral artery **(d)** delivers blood supply to the occipital cortex and upper midbrain. Clinical findings include contralateral homonymous hemianopsia, hemiparesis, hemisensory loss, memory loss, and ipsilateral cranial nerve III palsy that is pupil sparing.

**325. The answer is a.** (*Tintinalli, pp 1148-1150.*) You should suspect **BPV** in this patient. BPV is a transient positional vertigo associated with nystagmus. The problem occurs secondary to the creation and movement of canaliths (free-moving densities) in the semicircular canals of the inner ear that is associated with a particular head movement. The **Dix-Hallpike maneuver** is a diagnostic test designed to reproduce transient vertiginous symptoms and nystagmus of BPV. The maneuver involves having the patient go from sitting to a supine position with eyes open and head rotated to the affected side. The test is positive if the maneuver reproduces vertigo and the patient exhibits latent rotary nystagmus. A negative Dix-Hallpike maneuver does not exclude the condition.

Caloric stimulation testing (**b**) is performed for acoustic nerve evaluation by introducing cold or warm water or air into an ear canal and observing transient nystagmus. It is unnecessary for BPV diagnosis. Orthostatic vital signs (**c**) should be obtained if you suspect orthostatic hypotension. The patient in this case is symptomatic when he lies down, not when he is standing or sitting up, which is not consistent with this diagnosis. Head CT scan (**d**) should be ordered if you suspect central, rather than peripheral, causes of vertigo. ECG (**e**) is necessary if you suspect a cardiac cause of dizziness.

**326. The answer is b.** (*Rosen, pp 1560-1561.*) This woman presents with **iron deficiency anemia** secondary to **menorrhagia**. A history of chronic heavy menses and pale conjunctiva on examination should make you suspicious of this common disorder. About 20% of women and 3% of men are iron deficient. **Complete blood count** provides **hemoglobin and hematocrit** levels to diagnose anemia. Typically, the mean corpuscular volume (MCV) is low in iron deficiency anemia. In addition, the patient usually exhibits low serum iron, low serum ferritin, and a high total iron-binding capacity.

Electrolyte or renal function abnormalities (**a**) are unlikely in a young healthy woman. Except for tachycardia, the ECG (**c**) will be normal unless the patient has underlying cardiac disease, which can lead to ischemia in the setting of anemia. Chest x-ray (**d**) is not useful as an initial diagnostic test. It is appropriate to obtain it if you suspect a lung infiltrate, mass, congestive heart failure, or other cardiopulmonary disease. Chest CT with contrast (**e**) would help to diagnose a pulmonary embolism that may present with weakness, dyspnea on exertion, and tachycardia. In this case, however, the patient has no risk factors and has a better alternative diagnosis based on history and physical examination findings.

**327. The answer is b.** (*Tintinalli, pp 125-126.*) This common presentation of **hypercalcemia** is initially managed with **aggressive isotonic saline IV hydration** to restore volume status. Hypercalcemia impairs renal concentrating ability, and patients typically present with **polyuria, polydipsia,** and **dehydration** and may develop **kidney stones**. Increased calcium levels also cause generalized weakness, bone pain, neurologic symptoms (ataxia, altered mental status), GI dysfunction (abdominal pain, nausea, vomiting, anorexia), and ECG abnormalities (shortened QT interval). A handy mnemonic for symptoms of hypercalcemia is "bones, stones, groans, and psychiatric overtones."

Calcitonin (**a**) decreases calcium levels by reducing bony osteoclast activity and intestinal calcium absorption. It does not produce an immediate effect and is generally not started in the ED. Loop diuretics such as furosemide (**c**) increase renal elimination of calcium but worsen volume depletion. Patients need to be hydrated first. Obtaining a chest radiograph (**d**) is a good idea while the patient is getting IV hydration. This patient has a significant smoking history and recent weight loss, which should raise your suspicion of a neoplastic lung process causing hypercalcemia. Malignancy is an important cause of hypercalcemia; others include endocrine abnormalities (hyperparathyroidism, hyperthyroidism, pheochromocytoma, adrenal insufficiency), granulomatous disease (sarcoidosis, tuberculosis), drugs (thiazides, lithium), and immobilization. The patient's ECG (**e**) may show a shortened QT interval. Very high calcium levels may cause heart block.

**328. The answer is c.** (*Tintinalli, pp 1546-1547.*) Unilateral findings of ptosis and miosis as well as anhidrosis are seen in **Horner syndrome** that results from **interrupted sympathetic nerve supply to the eye**.

Palsy of the oculomotor nerve results in a "down and out" eye because of the dysfunction of the extraocular muscles innervated by the oculomotor nerve. In addition, the pupil appears mydriatic as a result of the loss of function of the ciliary parasympathetic nerves. Ptosis is common because the oculomotor nerve innervates the levator palpebrae. Homan sign (**a**) refers to leg pain with dorsiflexion of the foot sometimes seen in patients with deep venous thrombosis. This sign has poor sensitivity and specificity. Bell palsy (**b**) involves unilateral facial paralysis as a result of peripheral involvement of the facial nerve. In patients with a central facial nerve lesion the forehead is spared. Kehr sign (**d**) refers to left shoulder pain associated with splenic rupture. Nikolsky sign (**e**) is sloughing of the outer epidermal layer with rubbing of the skin seen in dermatologic diseases, such as pemphigus vulgaris and scalded skin syndrome.

**329. The answer is a.** *(Tintinalli, pp 1128-1129.)* This patient has an **ICA dissection** secondary to chiropractic neck manipulation. ICA dissection can occur spontaneously or in minor neck trauma and should be considered in a **young patient with acute stroke**. ICA dissection should also be suspected in patients with **neck pain and Horner syndrome** because of the disruption of ipsilateral oculosympathetic fibers. In this scenario, it presents with ipsilateral Horner syndrome and contralateral ischemic motor deficits. Other causes of acute Horner syndrome include **tumors** (ie, Pancoast tumor), stroke, herpes zoster infection, and trauma.

Cavernous sinus syndrome **(b)** presents with headache, ipsilateral eye findings, and sensory loss in the distribution of cranial nerve V—ophthalmic branch. Eye findings include proptosis, chemosis, Horner syndrome, and ophthalmoplegia caused by the involvement of cranial nerves III, IV, and VI. It does not cause decreased strength in the extremities. MS **(c)** is an inflammatory demyelinating CNS disease, resulting in various neurologic abnormalities, such as optic neuritis, transverse myelitis, and paresthesias. Transverse myelitis **(d)** is a postviral or toxic inflammation of the spinal cord that results in sensory loss and paresis. An isolated spinous process fracture **(e)** typically occurs in the setting of trauma and is considered a stable vertebral fracture. It does not result in motor weakness.

**330. The answer is c.** *(McIntyre, 2009.)* This patient presents with **vertebrobasilar insufficiency** (vertigo) and **claudication** (atypical arm pain with exercise), symptoms consistent with **subclavian steal syndrome**. This phenomenon occurs in patients with subclavian artery occlusion or stenosis proximal to the vertebral artery branch, which causes retrograde blood flow in the vertebral artery with ipsilateral arm exercise. Collateral arteries arising from the subclavian artery distal to the obstruction deliver blood to the arm. During arm exercise these vessels dilate and siphon blood from the head, neck, and shoulder to increase perfusion of ischemic arm muscles. This results in temporary reversal of blood flow in the vertebral artery leading to vertebrobasilar insufficiency and symptoms of vertigo, dizziness, syncope, dysarthria, and diplopia. Arm pain is a result of muscle ischemia.

Superior vena cava syndrome **(a)** is caused by an obstruction of the superior vena cava typically caused by the compression of a tumor. The most common complaints include edema and venous distention of the face and upper extremities. Facial plethora and telangiectasias are also commonly noted. Aortic dissection **(b)** can cause a difference in BP in the extremities. In general, patients complain of tearing chest pain that radiates into their back. If suspicion is high for aortic dissection, a CT scan with contrast or echocardiography should be performed to rule out the diagnosis. Angina pectoris **(d)** refers to myocardial ischemia caused by insufficient coronary blood flow to meet myocardial oxygen demand. It typically presents with symptoms of chest discomfort relieved with rest or nitroglycerin. Patients might complain of arm pain or radiation of pain to the arms, but the presentation does not involve neurologic deficits. Vestibular neuronitis **(e)** refers to acute self-limiting dysfunction of the peripheral vestibular system that causes vertigo.

**331. The answer is c.** *(Tintinalli, p 1912.)* This patient presents with **symmetric proximal muscle weakness** and characteristic **heliotrope rash** of **dermatomyositis**. It is an idiopathic inflammatory myopathy with associated dermatitis. The characteristic of the disease is progressive symmetric proximal muscle weakness with possible dysphagia, symmetric heliotrope rash in the periorbital region or neck, elevated creatinine kinase, and abnormal electromyogram and muscle biopsy. There is also an associated risk of malignancy.

Myasthenia gravis **(a)** is an autoimmune disorder of the neuromuscular junction in which antiacetylcholine receptor antibodies compete with acetylcholine at the nicotinic postsynaptic receptors. The disease causes characteristic progressive reduction in muscle strength with repeated muscle use. Bulbar muscles are most commonly involved, and patients report worsening of symptoms at night and improvement with rest or in the morning. MS **(b)** is an inflammatory demyelinating CNS disease, resulting in various neurologic abnormalities, such as optic neuritis, transverse myelitis, and paresthesias. Rhabdomyolysis **(d)** refers to muscle fiber breakdown because of a variety of etiologies, such as trauma, burns, ischemia, seizures, excessive muscular activities, sepsis, and myopathies. Its complications include hyperkalemia, metabolic acidosis, and acute renal failure. Disseminated gonococcal infection **(e)** is a systemic disease secondary to the presence of *Neisseria gonorrhoeae* in the bloodstream. In the early bacteremic phase patients present with fevers, migratory polyarthritis, and rash; this evolves from disseminated erythematous macules into hemorrhagic pustular lesions. Serious complications may include meningitis, osteomyelitis, and endocarditis.

**332. The answer is b.** *(Tintinalli, pp 1072-1073.)* This patient has **Lyme disease**, the most common vector-borne zoonotic infection in the United States. The spirochete, *Borrelia burgdorferi*, is transmitted to humans by the **deer tick *Ixodes***, and although the risk of infection after a bite is about 3% in highly endemic areas (Northeast and Midwest); it increases to 25% if the tick is attached for longer than 72 hours. This patient presents in the second stage of Lyme disease. The first stage involves the development of **erythema migrans**, a spreading annular erythematous lesion with central clearing occurring commonly at the tick bite site 2 to 20 days after the bite. The second stage typically occurs within 6 months of the initial infection and is characterized by fever, fatigue, arthralgias, neuropathies (ie, Bell palsy), cardiac abnormalities (ie, myocarditis presenting with conduction delay), and multiple annular lesions. Tertiary stage of Lyme disease occurs year after the infection and consists of chronic arthritis, subacute encephalopathy, and polyneuropathy.

Primary and secondary stages of the disease are treated with doxycycline. Tertiary stage is treated with IV ceftriaxone or penicillin.

Some sources refer to any facial nerve palsy as Bell palsy **(a)**, whereas most consider Bell palsy an idiopathic facial nerve paralysis. An easy way to look at it is that facial nerve paralysis may have an identifiable cause or may be idiopathic, in which case it is referred to as Bell palsy. In either case, exclude Lyme disease in patients with facial nerve palsy by sending Lyme titer levels. Ramsay Hunt syndrome **(c)** is a facial nerve palsy secondary to varicella-zoster virus (VZV). VZV causes chicken pox and may remain dormant in nerve ganglia for years. In addition to cranial nerve VII paralysis, the syndrome is characterized by severe ear pain, vertigo, hearing loss, and classic shingles in the ear. A brain tumor **(d)** may cause facial nerve compression centrally and may present with partial facial paralysis with forehead sparing. The forehead is bilaterally innervated, and the intact contralateral branch provides motor function. RMSF **(e)** is a tick-borne *Rickettsia rickettsii* infection. The disease involves constitutional symptoms of high fever, myalgias, severe headache, and a characteristic blanching erythematous macular rash that spreads from distal extremities to the trunk.

**333. The answer is d.** *(Rosen, p 1607.)* This patient is tachypneic, probably as a result of some underlying anxiety, which has resulted in paresthesias, carpal spasm, and tetany. This occurs as a result of an alkalemic environment that decreases ionized calcium levels. The treatment is reassurance, a rebreathing mask allowing for carbon dioxide retention and possibly sedation. The patient's metabolic profile is consistent with a respiratory alkalosis (elevated pH, low carbon dioxide). The blood gas indicates a pure alkalosis; therefore an acidosis is not seen (**a and c**). The bicarbonate level is normal and therefore it is not caused by a metabolic disturbance (**b**). Patients with hyperthyroidism (**e**) may be tachycardic, hyperthermic with an elevated BP. Upon physical examination, these patients may also appear to be underweight; have bulging eyes (exophthalmos); and complain of palpitations, diarrhea, tremors, and generalized anxiety. Hyperthyroidism is not a direct cause of tetany.

# Pediatrics

## Questions

**334.** A 6-month-old girl is brought to the ED because of persistent crying for the past 6 hours. Her teenage father informs you that she has been inconsolable since awaking from her nap. No recent illness, trauma, fever, or other complaints are reported. On physical examination the patient is alert, awake, and crying. You note swelling, deformity, and tenderness of the left femur. When inquired about this finding, the caretaker responds, "Her leg got stuck between the rails of her crib." You obtain the following radiograph as seen below. Which of the following is the next best step in management?

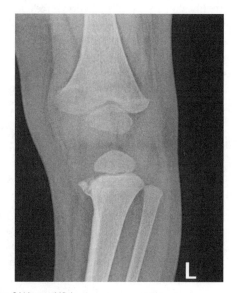

*(Courtesy of Ethan S. Wiener, MD.)*

a. Genetic workup for osteogenesis imperfecta and other bone abnormalities
b. Orthopedic consultation for closed reduction
c. Serum electrolytes including calcium and phosphate
d. Perform skeletal survey and contact Child Protective Services
e. Placement of posterior splint and discharge home with orthopedic follow-up

**335.** A 4-year-old boy is brought to the ED by a concerned mother after she noticed lesions under his nose and around his mouth as seen in the image below. The patient is otherwise well with no change in behavior, fever, or vomiting reported. On physical examination, you note a well-nourished, well-developed male in no acute distress with multiple small round, honey-colored lesions with slightly erythematous centers. What is the predominant organism involved?

a. Group B *Streptococcus*
b. *Staphylococcus aureus*
c. *Streptococcus pyogenes*
d. *Streptococcus pneumoniae*
e. *Salmonella* spp.

**336.** A 3-year-old African American boy with a history of sickle-cell disease presents to the ED after he developed a low-grade fever, runny nose, and an erythematous discoloration of both cheeks. His vital signs are heart rate (HR) 110 beats per minute, respiratory rate (RR) of 24 breaths per minute, and pulse oximetry of 98% on room air. The patient looks well and is in no acute distress. You note a macular lesion in both cheeks. The rash is not pruritic and there is no associated cellulitis or suppuration. What is the most serious complication to consider in this patient?

a. Osteomyelitis
b. Viral encephalitis
c. Pneumonia
d. Aplastic anemia
e. Meningitis

**337.** A 9-month-old boy is brought to the ED with a 2-day history of fever, vomiting, and fussiness. The patient has had multiple episodes of emesis that follow intense periods of fussiness after which the patient seems to relax and go to sleep. He has had no fever or diarrhea. In between these episodes, he has slightly decreased energy but otherwise seems well. Oral intake is decreased and urine output has been decreased since the day of presentation. Which of the following statements is true regarding this condition?

a. The majority present with vomiting, colicky abdominal pain, and currant jelly stools.
b. Air enema is the therapeutic intervention of choice.
c. Plain films of the abdomen can usually confirm the diagnosis.
d. Surgical intervention is often indicated.
e. Most of these have a "lead point" as the underlying pathologic cause.

**338.** A 7-year-old girl with sickle-cell disease and a previous history of admissions for acute painful crises presents with a 1-day history of fever and cough. She is tachypneic on presentation with a temperature of 102°F. Auscultation of the chest reveals rales on the right. A chest radiograph confirms the diagnosis of pneumonia. After initial treatment with antibiotics and intravenous (IV) fluids, patients with this condition are most at risk of developing which complication?

a. Acute chest syndrome
b. Sepsis as a result of the relative immunodeficiency of patients with sickle-cell disease
c. Empyema
d. Stroke
e. Congestive heart failure because of the anemia coupled with infection

**339.** A 2-year-old boy is brought to the ED by his parents stating that he is limping. The mother states that he was fine yesterday but woke up today and would not bear weight. He had a normal active day yesterday with no notable falls. On examination, the patient is in mild distress. His vital signs are a temperature of 101°F, HR 120 beats per minute, RR 24 breaths per minute, and blood pressure (BP) 90/55 mm Hg. He has mild nasal congestion. He is able to move his left lower extremity only a small amount and has discomfort with range of motion of his left hip. He is unable to bear weight. There is no swelling, rash, warmth, or erythema. White blood cell (WBC), C-reactive protein (CRP), and erythrocyte sedimentation rate (ESR) are all normal. Radiograph of the hips bilaterally and left femur and knee are all negative. After high-dose ibuprofen in the ED, the patient is able to bear weight. What is the most appropriate management of this patient?

a. Admit for IV antibiotics for septic arthritis or osteomyelitis.
b. Consult orthopedics after ultrasound for aspiration of hip in the operating room (OR).
c. Bone scan to evaluate for osteomyelitis.
d. Nonsteroidal anti-inflammatory drugs (NSAIDs) and reassurance to parents with follow-up in 24 hours.
e. Splint leg for treatment of occult fracture through growth plate that cannot be visualized on initial radiographs.

**340.** A 21-month-old girl, previously well, presents with 7 days of fever and rash. She has been seen previously during this episode by her primary physician and diagnosed with a "viral illness." On further questioning, the mother indicates that the patient has had red eyes, but no discharge. She has had no vomiting, diarrhea, cough, congestion, or complaints of pain. She has, however, seemed very irritable and fussy throughout the last few days and cannot seem to get comfortable. On examination, the patient is highly irritable and intermittently consolable. Vital signs reveal temperature 101°F rectally, HR 170 beats per minute, RR 22 breaths per minute, and BP 100/60 mm Hg. Her conjunctivae are mildly injected with no purulent discharge. The oropharynx is clear though she has dry, cracked lips. There are two anterior cervical nodes measuring 2.5 cm each. The heart is tachycardic without a murmur. The lungs are clear, and abdomen is soft and nontender with no hepatosplenomegaly. The skin reveals a diffuse, blanching, erythematous, macular rash. The extremities have no swelling or tenderness. Laboratory evaluation reveals WBC 13,500/μL, Hgb 9.5 mg/dL, platelets 870/μL, CRP 89, ESR 85, and normal electrolytes; liver function tests reveal aspartate aminotransferase (AST) 110 U/L and alanine aminotransferase (ALT) 88 U/L. Which of the following is the most appropriate next step in the management of this patient?

a. Consult cardiology for statim (STAT) echocardiogram.
b. Perform additional laboratory tests, including Epstein-Barr viral titers, strep test, antinuclear antibody, and bone marrow biopsy.
c. Reassure the parents that the initial diagnosis was probably accurate.
d. Administer IV antibiotics and perform lumbar puncture.
e. Admit for administration of intravenous immunoglobulin (IVIG) and aspirin.

**341.** A 6-day-old infant is brought to the ED by his mom who describes the newborn as breathing fast, poor feeding, and appearing blue. He has no history of fever or vomiting. The patient was born full term at home to a G4P3 mother with an uncomplicated antenatal course. The mom had prenatal laboratory tests but is unaware of the results. On examination, the patient is lethargic with central and peripheral cyanosis. The rectal temperature is 95.4°F, HR 180 beats per minute, RR 70 breaths per minute, and BP unobtainable in the extremities by automatic pressure meter. The oxygen saturation on room air is 65%, which does not improve with administration of 100% oxygen by face mask. Auscultation reveals a harsh 3/6 systolic murmur with an active precordium. Lungs reveal diffuse, bilateral rales, and wheezes. Liver edge is palpated 3 to 4 cm below right costal margin. Which of the following is the most important next step in the management of this patient?

a. Intubation for administration of 100% oxygen
b. STAT portable chest radiograph and electrocardiogram (ECG)
c. Administration of IV antibiotics and full sepsis workup
d. Administration of prostaglandin bolus followed by continuous drip
e. Immediate surgical intervention and activation of extracorporeal membrane oxygenation (ECMO) team

**342.** A 27-day-old presents to the ED with a complaint of a 2-day history of nonbilious vomiting. The child has had no fever and no diarrhea. He has always been a "spitter," according to mom, but this seems more excessive and "forceful." The patient has had no wet diapers over the course of the previous 12 hours and is fussy in the examination room. There are no other complaints. The mother has just finished feeding the child formula as you walk into the room and you see the child has an episode of projectile vomiting. The examination reveals temperature 99.8°F, HR 180 beats per minute, RR 50 breaths per minute, and pulse oxymetry of 95% on room air. The remainder of the examination is nonfocal and benign except for slightly prolonged capillary refill. You order the appropriate radiographic studies and consult the appropriate services. If you were to check a set of electrolytes in this patient, what would be the most likely result?

a. Na 137, K 3.7, Cl⁻ 112, HCO₃ 22, glucose 110
b. Na 137, K 3.1, Cl⁻ 89, HCO₃ 39, glucose 55
c. Na 145, K 6.2, Cl⁻ 122, HCO₃ 35, glucose 55
d. Na 145, K 3.1, Cl⁻ 89, HCO₃ 16, glucose 80
e. Na 122, K 6.2, Cl⁻ 122, HCO₃ 35, glucose 55

**343.** A 35-year-old G4P3 woman presents to the ED in labor. The mother says that her due date is not for 2 more weeks. She indicates that she ruptured her membranes several hours ago and that her contractions have been within a few minutes for a few hours. She is placed immediately in position to check her progress and the infant's head is seen to be crowning. The baby is then born precipitously in the ED. Which of the following interventions should be immediately instituted for this newborn?

a. Begin resuscitative efforts with positive-pressure ventilation immediately because this is a high-risk infant.

b. Administer two breaths of positive-pressure ventilation to assist movement of fluid out of lungs so that the newborn may begin effective respirations.

c. Call the neonatal ICU to let them know that a premature infant will be coming and will probably need to have a "workup."

d. Assign an Apgar score so that all of the medical personnel may know the status and understand their roles for the next few minutes.

e. Dry the infant, suction the mouth and nose, stimulate semivigorously, and observe for several seconds for respiratory effort before initiation of any other intervention.

**344.** A 15-month-old girl is brought to the ED by EMS secondary to seizure activity noted at home. The patient is a previously well child. Her immunizations are up to date. The patient is reported to have been recently well but was noted to be a little cranky this morning. She has had no cough, congestion, vomiting, diarrhea, or rash. This afternoon, the patient was being observed in the playroom when her eyes rolled back and she began having generalized tonic-clonic activity that lasted for approximately 2 minutes. When emergency medical services (EMS) arrived, the patient was in her mother's arms, tired but arousable, and in no apparent distress. On examination, the temperature is 103.1°F, HR 155 beats per minute, RR 32 breaths per minute, and BP 95/50 mm Hg. She has normal tympanic membranes, oropharynx reveals several tiny erythematous and vesicular appearing lesions posteriorly, lungs and heart examinations are normal, and abdomen is soft and nontender. Skin examination is clear with brisk capillary refill. Over the course of your evaluation, the patient becomes increasingly interactive, well-appearing, and playful. Which of the following is the most appropriate course of action for this patient?

a. Obtain complete blood count (CBC), blood culture, urinalysis, urine culture, chest radiograph, and determine treatment on the basis of the results of these tests.
b. Obtain blood and urine for culture, administer ceftriaxone, and discharge home.
c. Reassure parents that this is a benign condition and that no further testing is indicated at this time.
d. Obtain routine blood work and head computed tomographic (CT) scan and call for neurology consultation for first-time seizure.
e. Obtain head CT scan and perform lumbar puncture secondary to fever and seizure to rule out meningitis.

**345.** A 13-year-old African American boy is brought to the ED by his mother for a complaint of right knee pain over the course of 1 to 2 weeks. The only notable trauma that the patient can recall was jumping on a trampoline 1 to 2 weeks ago with friends that resulted in right lower-extremity pain. On the morning of presentation, the patient complained of increased pain when ambulating and was noted to be limping. He denies fever. No other trauma and no recent illness were noted by the family. On examination, the patient is afebrile with normal vital signs. He has no previous medical problems and is noted to be overweight but is in otherwise good health. The lower-extremity examination reveals no swelling or erythema over any of the joints. His knee has no focal tenderness or pain with range of motion, but the hip is noted to be painful with internal and external rotation. He has a normal neurosensory examination of the distal extremity. A radiograph is performed. Which of the following is the most likely diagnosis?

a. Legg-Calvé-Perthes disease
b. Slipped capital-femoral epiphysis (SCFE)
c. Septic arthritis
d. Osgood-Schlatter disease
e. Transient synovitis of the hip

**346.** A 4-year-old girl is brought to the ED by her mother with a chief complaint of abdominal pain and bloody stool. The patient has a 2-day history of abdominal and leg pain. The leg pain worsened today to where the patient did not want to walk and the abdominal pain is so severe that she is buckled over in pain. There is no significant past medical history, no recent travel, and no family history of inflammatory bowel disease. On examination, the patient has temperature of 37.5°C, HR 122, RR 24, and BP 95/60 mm Hg. She is alert but in moderate painful distress. HEENT (head, eyes, ears, nose, and throat) is normal. Lungs are clear to auscultation. Heart is regular with no murmur. Abdomen is soft but diffusely tender. Extremities reveal bilateral swelling and tenderness of her knees. Skin examination reveals nonblanching purple and red lesions (macules and patches) on the flexural surface of her lower extremities and on buttocks. These lesions are nontender. Which of the following is the most appropriate test to evaluate her current condition?

a. Renal
b. Integument
c. Gastrointestinal (GI)
d. Musculoskeletal
e. Neurologic

**347.** A 4-year-old boy is brought to the ED by his mother with a complaint of ear pain since last night. The patient also complains of mild congestion and cough. He has normal oral intake, activity, and urine output. On examination, the patient is alert, interactive, and playful. His temperature is 100.6°F, HR 128 beats per minute, RR 26 breaths per minute, and pulse oxymetry is 98% on room air. His right tympanic membrane has slight erythema with several bubbles of clear fluid noted inferiorly. His left tympanic membrane is erythematous and bulging with opaque, purulent fluid noted. There is no neck stiffness, mastoid tenderness, or difficulty breathing. The patient has a primary care physician who checks the patient regularly. Which of the following is the best treatment for this patient?

a. Analgesics only.
b. A third-generation cephalosporin.
c. Amoxicillin 40 to 50 mg/kg/d.
d. Treatment with analgesics initially and consideration of oral high-dose amoxicillin in 48 to 72 hours if no resolution of symptoms.
e. No treatment is needed for this viral illness.

**348.** A 3-week-old girl is brought to the ED by her parents after they noticed blood in her stool. The patient is the full-term product of an uncomplicated pregnancy and delivery without any medical issues up to this point. She has been feeding well (breast-feeding primarily) and active without fever, respiratory problems, or fussiness. She has had several episodes of nonforceful, nonbilious emesis after feeds with multiple wet diapers each day. She normally has several soft, seedy stools. In the last day, the parents noticed streaks of blood in her stool and today she had grossly bloody stool. The patient does not seem to be in any distress or discomfort. On examination, the temperature is 98.9°F, HR 155 beats per minute, and RR 44 breaths per minute. The patient is awake, active, and in no apparent distress. Her abdomen is soft and nontender with normal bowel sounds and no masses. Examination of her anus does not reveal a fissure. Which of the following is the most likely diagnosis?

a. Acute gastroenteritis
b. Milk protein colitis
c. *Clostridium difficile* colitis
d. Intestinal malrotation
e. Necrotizing enterocolitis

**349.** A 9-day-old boy is brought to the ED for fever and fussiness. He was born full term. However, the delivery was complicated by prolonged rupture of membranes (PROM) and the mother had a fever for which she was treated with antibiotics before delivery. The baby did well in the nursery, and has been at home and feeding without any difficulties until the day of presentation when he became fussier, less interested in feeding, and the parents noted a temperature of 101.5°F (measured under patient's arm). On presentation, his temperature is 102.4°F, HR 160 beats per minute, RR 48 breaths per minute, and pulse oxymetry of 97% on room air. His anterior fontanelle is open and flat; conjunctivae are clear; neck is supple without masses; and the heart, lung, and abdominal examinations are normal. The skin shows tiny (1-3 mm) pustules with a surrounding rim of erythema on the patient's trunk. No vesicular lesions are noted. Which of the following is the most likely organism responsible for this patient's condition?

a. *Escherichia coli*
b. *Listeria monocytogenes*
c. Group B *Streptococcus*
d. *Staphylococcus aureus*
e. Herpes simplex virus (HSV)

**350.** A 9-year-old boy, who is a recent immigrant from Uzbekistan, presents to the ED complaining of pain and swelling in his right knee, which has been intermittent over the course of several months. The pain sometimes affects his ankles and wrists. His parents, through an interpreter, deny recent fever, vomiting, chest pain, and difficulty breathing. They do indicate that he has had exercise intolerance and dyspnea on exertion. On examination, you note a diastolic murmur at the right upper sternal border. Which of the following findings by itself would establish the diagnosis?

a. Elevated ESR
b. Positive ASO (antistreptolysin O)
c. Choreiform movements
d. Positive strep test
e. Knee aspiration with 25,000 WBC, primarily neutrophils

**351.** A 5-month-old previously healthy girl presents to the ED with a 4- to 5-day history of constipation and decreased feeding. The patient is a full-term product of an uncomplicated antenatal course and delivery. She also had recent congestion and cough that resolved with administration of tea prepared by a family friend. The mother denies any recent fever or vomiting. On examination, the temperature is 99.9°F, HR 165 beats per minute, and RR 22 breaths per minute. The BP was not obtained. The patient has a weak cry, is notably flaccid, and ill-appearing. You note that patient is drooling. Her pupils are poorly responsive and she is not tracking to light or faces. Which of the following is the most likely cause of this condition?

a. Type I spinal muscular atrophy
b. Brain tumor
c. Infant botulism
d. Meningitis
e. Organophosphate poisoning

**352.** A 6-month-old boy is brought to the ED after being found apneic and cyanotic at home. The patient's mother called 911 and began cardio-pulmonary resuscitation (CPR). The patient responded within seconds to minutes. On arrival to the ED, he was noted to be awake and responsive but slightly mottled with mild respiratory distress. Within minutes of arrival, the patient becomes apneic suddenly, cyanotic, and bradycardic. Which of the following is the most important initial response?

a. Administer epinephrine.
b. Provide oxygen via non-rebreather face mask.
c. Jaw thrust, chin lift, and bag-valve-mask ventilation.
d. Endotracheal intubation.
e. Chest compressions.

**353.** A 4-year-old boy is brought to the ED by his parents who state that he is having difficulty breathing. The patient has a 1-week history of fever, congestion, and cough. Over the last 2 days, he has appeared tired with intermittent vomiting and persistently increased RR despite administration of acetaminophen. On presentation, his vital signs are temperature 100.5°F, HR 185 beats per minute, RR 50 breaths per minute, BP 75/40 mm Hg, and pulse oxymetry of 88% on room air. He is ill-appearing and listless. He has diffuse rales noted on auscultation, pulses are weak and thready, and his liver is palpable 3 to 4 cm below the right costal margin. After several attempts at a peripheral IV, the patient becomes increasingly somnolent. Which of the following is the most appropriate method of obtaining access in this patient?

a. Internal jugular central line
b. Femoral vein central line
c. Saphenous vein cutdown
d. Large-bore IV in antecubital fossa
e. Intraosseous needle

**354.** A 3-year-old girl is brought to the ED with acute onset of respiratory distress. She recently emigrated from Africa. Her initial vitals include HR of 115 beats per minute, BP of 110/60 mm Hg, and RR of 28 breaths per minute with oxygen saturation of 88% on room air. She is also febrile to 103.5°F. She is ill- and anxious-appearing, sitting forward in her mother's lap, and drooling. Her mother tells you that she had a sore throat that began 2 days ago and that she was going to see her pediatrician this week for her initial vaccinations. Given this patient's history and presentation, which of the following should be of particular concern?

a. Epiglottitis
b. Retropharyngeal abscess
c. Epstein-Barr virus (EBV) pharyngitis
d. Ludwig angina
e. Peritonsillar abscess

**355.** A 5-month-old boy, ex-34-week preemie, is brought to the ED by his mother who reports that the infant has been breathing with extra effort for the last 2 days. He has no other past medical history and is currently on immunizations having received the full course of vaccines at both 2 and 4 months. The mom reports the child has had rhinorrhea and cough. Upon physical examination, the patient has a temperature of 101.1°F, HR 160 beats per minute, RR 70 breaths per minute, pulse oximetry of 87% on room air. He has copious nasal discharge, audible wheezing with diffuse rhonchi, and rales upon chest auscultation. He also has intercostal retractions and nasal flaring. A chest radiograph shows increased perihilar markings, hyperinflation, and diffuse patchy areas of atelectasis versus infiltrates. Given this patient's history and physical examination, which of the following is the most likely etiology of his symptoms?

a. Foreign body aspiration
b. Asthma
c. Pneumococcal pneumonia
d. Respiratory syncytial virus (RSV)
e. Parvovirus B19

**356.** A 4-year-old girl is brought to the ED after falling from a tree. She hit her head on the ground and has significant temporal swelling on the left side. In transit to the hospital by her parents, the patient had multiple episodes of emesis. On arrival to the ED, the patient is confused and agitated and then becomes acutely unresponsive and apneic. You make the decision to endotracheally intubate the patient. Which of the following is the most appropriate endotracheal tube (ETT) to use in this intubation?

a. 4.0 uncuffed ETT
b. 4.0 cuffed ETT
c. 5.0 cuffed ETT
d. 5.5 uncuffed ETT
e. 4.5 uncuffed ETT

**357.** A 2-year-old boy is brought to the ED shortly after a choking episode. His parents noted he had been playing with coins on the floor just before the episode. There has been no previous history of fever or runny nose in the past few days. The parents tried to feed the patient after the episode, but he has been unwilling to take anything orally. On examination, the patient is calm with stable vital signs and a pulse oximetry of 98% on room air. He spits in a cup every couple of minutes but is otherwise in no apparent distress. His oropharynx is unremarkable and lungs are without wheezes or rales. His radiograph is seen below. Which of the following most likely accounts for the patient's symptoms?

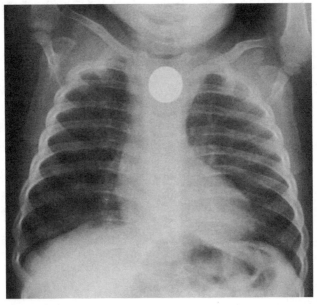

*(Courtesy of Adam J Rosh, MD.)*

a. Foreign body aspiration
b. Bronchospasm
c. Foreign body ingestion
d. Epiglottitis
e. Allergic reaction

**358.** A 2-year-old girl is brought into the ED with 2 days of fever and runny nose. Today she developed a dry, harsh, "barking" cough. Her temperature is 103.3°F, HR 123 beats per minute, RR 25 breaths per minute, and pulse oximetry of 98% on room air. On evaluation you note an alert, responsive but somewhat anxious female, in moderate respiratory distress with stridor and suprasternal retractions at rest. She has nasal congestion, equal air entry bilaterally with no rales or wheezes, and a normal ear and throat examination. After receiving a single treatment of racemic epinephrine, she feels better and her work of breathing improves. Which of the following is the most appropriate next step in management?

a. Chest radiograph
b. CBC and blood culture
c. Soft tissue radiograph of the neck
d. Broad-spectrum antibiotics
e. A dose of steroids

**359.** A 3-month-old boy with decreased feeding over the last 24 hours is brought to the ED by his mother. The patient has been doing well without any prior medical problems until today when the mother noted sweating and irritability, particularly with feeding. In the ED, the patient attempts to feed but within minutes stops and begins to cry. Vital signs include a pulse of 240 beats per minute, RR of 50 breaths per minute, temperature of 98.2°F, and pulse oximetry of 98% on room air. On physical examination, the patient is pale and clammy to touch. Breath sounds are clear on auscultation. Pulses are normal and symmetric in all extremities. An ECG is seen below. Which of the following is the most appropriate next step in management?

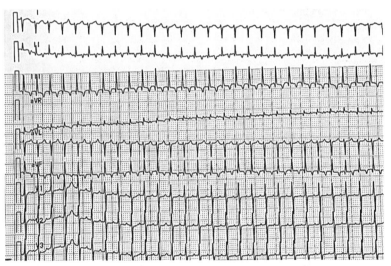

(Reproduced, with permission, from Shah BR, Lucchesi M. Atlas of Pediatric Emergency Medicine. New York, NY: McGraw-Hill; 2006: Figure 5-10.)

a. Synchronized cardioversion at 0.5 J/kg
b. Verapamil 0.1 mg/kg bolus
c. Defibrillation at 2 J/kg
d. Adenosine at 0.1 mg/kg followed by 0.2 mg/kg if first dose is ineffective
e. Carotid massage

**360.** A 4-year-old uncircumcised boy is brought to the ED by his caretaker for an 8-hour history of swelling and redness of the penis. The caretaker states that she retracted the foreskin over the penis to clean it and could not move it back afterward. The patient's vital signs are within normal limits. On examination, he is crying and becomes irritable whenever you try to examine the genital area. The glans is edematous and erythematous. The testicular examination shows bilateral descended testicles with a normal cremasteric reflex. Which of the following is the most appropriate next step in management?

a. Manual reduction of the foreskin over the glans
b. Dorsal slit incision or circumcision
c. Topical lidocaine
d. Catheterization to prevent obstruction and urinary retention
e. Topical steroids to reduce the swelling

**361.** A 10-week-old girl is brought to the ED after 5 hours of abdominal distension and green stained vomiting. The patient is a previously well infant with an uncomplicated antenatal course and normal vaginal delivery. However, she spent an extra day in the neonatal intensive care unit (NICU) when born because of "water on the lungs." On the day of presentation, the patient is unable to hold any fluids down without vomiting. Her vital signs reveal HR of 185 beats per minute, RR of 65 breaths per minute, and temperature of 100.8°F. Abdominal examination reveals a diffusely tender abdomen that is hypertympanic. Which of the following is the definitive study of choice?

a. Upper GI series
b. Abdominal ultrasound
c. Findings on physical examination
d. CBC, electrolytes, and urine analysis
e. Serum lactate

**362.** A 5-year-old boy who fell from the monkey bars and landed on his left elbow is brought into the ED for evaluation. The patient has no significant medical history. On physical examination, you note the patient is holding his left arm in an adducted position. There is obvious swelling around the elbow with decreased range of motion secondary to pain. He complains of hand numbness, but the motor and vascular examination is normal. The radiograph shown below shows posterior displacement of the capitellum with evidence of a dark shadow posterior to the distal humerus. Which of the following is the most serious complication associated with this injury?

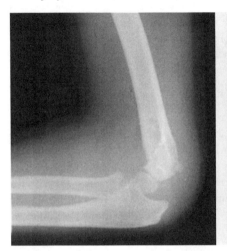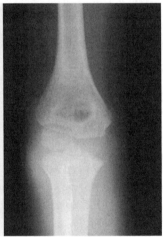

*(Reproduced, with permission, from Simon RR, Sherman SC, Koenigsknecht SJ. Emergency Orthopedics: The Extremities. 5th ed. New York, NY: McGraw-Hill; 2007: Figure 6-18.)*

a. Transection of the brachial artery
b. Malunion of distal humerus
c. Motor deficit from injury to the ulnar nerve
d. Chronic arthritis of the elbow
e. Chronic deformity of the hands and fingers caused by contractures

**363.** A 7-year-old boy presents to the ED 1 hour after slipping and landing on his right outstretched hand. He was evaluated and splinted by emergency medical technicians (EMTs) and brought to the ED. On examination, you note a deformity of his right wrist. There are no neurovascular deficits. A radiograph of the wrist is shown below. Which of the following states is true regarding physeal fractures in children?

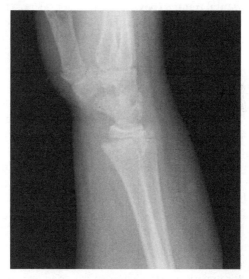

*(Reproduced, with permission, from Shah BR, Lucchesi M.* Atlas of Pediatric Emergency Medicine. *New York, NY: McGraw-Hill; 2006: Figure 19-3.)*

a. Salter-Harris type IV is defined as a crush injury of the growth plate.
b. The most common type of fracture is the Salter-Harris type II.
c. This patient's radiographic findings are consistent with Salter-Harris type V.
d. Fractures through the physis, metaphysis, and epiphysis are classified as Salter-Harris type III.
e. The worse prognosis is seen with Salter-Harris type I fractures.

# Pediatrics

## *Answers*

**334. The answer is d.** *(Fleisher and Ludwig, pp 1341-1342.)* This is a case where **nonaccidental trauma (NAT)** should be considered. This is a classic example of a **"bucket handle" fracture. Metaphyseal corner fractures**, known as bucket handle fractures, are considered **pathognomonic for abuse** and are caused by rapid shearing forces or twisting motion. Spiral fractures in a nonambulating child, fractures of the posterior ribs, sternum scapula or spinous processes, or multiple fractures in various stages of healing are also highly indicative of abuse and may be the only presentation of child abuse. Any type of trauma that does not fit the mechanism should raise the suspicion and alert the physician of the possibility of abuse. In this case, the fracture pattern mandates further workup for NAT. According to the AAP (American Academy of Pediatrics), the **skeletal survey** is the initial test of choice for all children suspected of being abused. Additional workup may be indicated based on the age and presentation of the child. In this case, a head CT scan and ophthalmology consultation should be strongly considered. All states have mandatory reporting of child abuse. It is also mandatory to contact the local **Child Protective Services** to further investigate the situation.

Osteogenesis imperfecta **(a)** is a rare genetic condition caused by mutations of the type I procollagen gene. Children may present with fractures in the setting of little or no trauma. Classic blue sclerae may be present. This type of injury **(e)** should not be simply splinted and discharged home. A simple posterior long leg splint may be adequate treatment for this fracture at this time but not for the overall disposition. Orthopedic surgery **(b)** should be included early in the intervention, but their expertise in not necessarily critical in the immediate treatment algorhythm. Electrolyte abnormalities **(c)** that may be responsible for pathological fractures in children are exceedingly rare when compared to child abuse and should only be considered once NAT is excluded or in the presence of other abnormalities in the physical examination.

**335. The answer is c.** *(Fleisher and Ludwig, p 925.)* This is a case of **impetigo**. It is a superficial skin infection caused most commonly by *S pyogenes* (group A β-hemolytic *Streptococcus*). When large pustules are observed (> 1 cm), the term used to describe this condition is bullous impetigo. The typical presentation if impetigo includes honey-crusted lesions on erythematous skin. These tend to be pruritic and easily spread by the patient. Although possible, systemic infection is uncommon so patients typically are well appearing. Treatment includes either oral or topical antibiotic therapy. Options include erythromycin or cephalexin; linezolid may be used in resistant cases of *Staphylococcus*. Topical therapy with mupirocin is very effective. Hand washing is critical to also limit the spread of infection to other family members. Treatment of the skin lesions does not prevent the development of nephritis.

Group B *Streptococcus* (**a**) does not generally cause impetigo. It is a well-known cause of severe perinatal infection, such as pneumonia and meningitis. *Staphylococcus aureus* (**b**) is commonly associated with impetigo and is usually mixed with *Streptococcus*. *Staphylococcus aureus* is the sole isolate in 10% of cases. Therefore, it is important to treat for both organisms. *Streptococcus pneumoniae* (**d**) is a well-known pathogen involved in many types of infection. It is one of the most common agents found in osteomyelitis, pneumonia, meningitis, pericarditis, peritonitis, and cellulitis. But it does not usually cause impetigo. *Salmonella* (**e**) is known to cause infectious diarrhea, meningitis, and osteomyelitis, particularly in sickle-cell patients.

**336. The answer is d.** *(Fleisher and Ludwig, pp 513, 935-936.)* This is a case of **erythema infectiosum** or **Fifth disease**. Infection by **parvovirus B19** produces this pattern of a **"slapped cheek" appearance**. It is characterized by an eruption that presents initially as an erythematous malar blush followed by an erythematous maculopapular eruption on the extensor surfaces of extremities that evolves into a reticulated, lacy, mottled appearance. Fever and other symptoms may be present but are uncommon. In patients with **chronic hemolytic anemias** like sickle-cell disease, **aplastic anemia** is a serious complication. Pregnant women should avoid exposure to this virus, because it may cause fetal hydrops in 10% of cases.

Sickle-cell patients can develop osteomyelitis (**a**); however, the clinical presentation is inconsistent. Patients with osteomyelitis caused by *Salmonella* species are generally those with sickle-cell disease. However, the most common organism that causes osteomyelitis in patients with sickle-cell disease is *S aureus*. Encephalitis (b) is an inflammation of the brain parenchyma and is not commonly caused by parvovirus. Common etiologic agents include herpes simplex, herpes zoster, varicella-zoster, West Nile virus, and toxoplasmosis. Pneumonia (c) is a common diagnosis in patients of all ages. In children, the most common causative agents are viral. The most commonly found bacterial agent is *S pneumoniae*. Meningitis (e) is an infection of the meninges that surround the brain. It is caused by viral and bacterial entities. The most common bacterial agents include *E coli*; group B *Streptococcus*; and *L monocytogenes* in very young infants and *S pneumoniae*, *N meningitides*, and *H influenzae* in older children.

**337. The answer is b.** *(Fleisher and Ludwig, pp 1520-1522.)* This is a classic story and presentation for **intussusception**, where a **part of intestine telescopes inside of another and causes ischemia**, which can lead to infarction of bowel. This is a **true GI emergency**. The most common type of intussusception is ileo-colic and the most common reason is idiopathic. Ileo-ileal and colo-colonic intussusceptions are possible though rare in comparison. **The most common age group is 3 to 12 months** with greater than 80% occurring within the first 2 years of life. Air enema is both diagnostic and therapeutic and has been widely adopted as the intervention of choice for these patients.

(a) Although the classic triad consists of colicky abdominal pain, vomiting, and currant jelly stools, fewer than 20% of patients will present with all of these findings. (c) Plain films cannot typically confirm or refute the presence of intussusception, though air present in the cecum indicates no ileo-colic intussusception. Radiographs are important, however, to exclude the presence of free air before attempting an enema reduction. From a diagnostic perspective, ultrasound has been employed and demonstrated to have very high sensitivity for intussusception. (d) Although surgical consultation is warranted before reduction in the case that perforation is identified with the enema or for unsuccessful reductions, relatively few patients ultimately require surgical correction. (e) There is a lead point in a small minority of patients in the classic age range. The incidence of pathologic lead points increases as the age of the patient increases beyond the classic age group. Lead points can be hypertrophied Peyer patches, a Meckel diverticulum, a polyp, or a tumor.

**338. The answer is a.** *(Fleisher and Ludwig, pp 869-870.)* **Acute chest syndrome** is characterized **by pneumonia with pulmonary infarction,**

**hypoxia**, and **diffuse pulmonary edema**. This is one of the most serious and life-threatening complications of sickle-cell disease. One must be very cautious with IV fluid hydration because overaggressive fluid administration can lead to pulmonary edema in patients who have pneumonia or previously suffered from acute chest syndrome. Administration of IV antibiotics, transfusions for anemia, and oxygen are the mainstays of therapy.

(**b**) Disseminated infection leading to sepsis and (**c**) empyema are complications of bacterial pneumonia in general. Patients with sickle-cell disease have an inherent immunodeficiency owing to autosplenectomy, but these are not specific complications of this patient's treatment. (**d**) Stroke is another complication of sickle-cell disease, but it is not caused by fluid resuscitation. (**e**) Likewise, patients with long-standing anemia are at risk for congestive heart failure and, indeed, many patients with sickle-cell disease have an enlarged heart. However, this is a chronic complication and not one specifically associated with treatment of pneumonia and acute chest syndrome.

**339. The answer is d.** *(Fleisher and Ludwig, p 1573.)* This is a case of **toxic synovitis**, also called **transient synovitis of the hip**. Despite its name, this is a benign and self-limiting condition that typically responds to rest and NSAIDs. It is thought to be a postinfectious inflammatory process, though the true cause is unknown. The course is usually from several days to a couple of weeks. Though fever is not a typical part of most patients with toxic synovitis, it can be present and low grade or could potentially be unrelated. It is most important to distinguish this condition from a septic arthritis. The main differences are that the joint can often be gently maneuvered in toxic synovitis whereas in true septic joints even the smallest amount of joint motion typically produces intense pain and patients will strongly resist full range of motion.

If this was a septic joint, it would be important to (**a**) admit the child for IV antibiotics, but probably more importantly to (**b**) consult orthopedics for a probable trip to the operating room where the joint would be aspirated and irrigated. This is not a case where a bone scan (**c**) would be indicated to rule out osteomyelitis, especially in light of totally normal inflammatory markers. Further, MRI has mostly replaced bone scan for evaluation of patients with osteomyelitis because it is a highly sensitive and far more specific test. Finally, although we often worry about occult, or Salter-Harris I, type fractures, this patient has no history of trauma and no point tenderness and is weight bearing at the time of discharge making this a very unlikely diagnosis.

**340. The answer is e.** *(Fleisher and Ludwig, pp 1157-1164.)* This is a patient with **Kawasaki disease (KD)**. This entity is defined by the following criteria: **fever lasting for a minimum of 5 days, plus 4 out of 5 of the following: cervical lymphadenopathy of greater than 1.5 cm; dry, cracked lips or other oral mucous membrane involvement (strawberry tongue); truncal, nonvesicular rash; nonpurulent conjunctivitis; swollen or edematous hands and feet.** KD is a systemic inflammatory vasculitis of unknown etiology. The characteristic constellation of symptoms, as this patient meets, requires immediate action to prevent complications of the disease. Another common finding, and one that many practitioners use to help in the diagnosis of "atypical" cases, is intense irritability of the child. The most serious sequelae involve **coronary artery aneurysms**. These occur in approximately 20% to 25% of untreated patients. This number is reduced to 2% to 4% if treatment occurs within the first 10 days of symptom onset. Additional treatment with aspirin is recommended both for its antiplatelet and anti-inflammatory effects.

Although this patient will require a cardiology consultation **(a)**, it is not the next step in management because it is critical not to delay treatment. The absence of coronary artery aneurysms should not dissuade you from initiation of treatment and their presence does not, in the short term, alter therapy. There are no laboratory values that contribute to making the diagnosis, although there are some characteristic findings. Typically these patients have elevated serum markers of inflammation, ESR, and CRP, and can have elevated transaminases, as is present in this case. The other classic finding is a thrombocytosis, which typically doesn't present itself until at least a week into the disease and can reach over 1 million/mm$^3$ in some cases. Additional laboratory tests **(b)** are not required except in cases where the diagnosis is truly in question. Therefore, answer choices **(c)**, reassurance, and **(d)**, continued septic workup, are incorrect. Antibiotics have no role in the treatment of this condition.

**341. The answer is d.** *(Fleisher and Ludwig, pp 699-701.)* The most important next step is administration of **prostaglandin bolus followed by a drip**. This patient is in **severe cardiac failure** due to **impending closure of his ductus arteriosus**. The patient is presenting in a classic time frame, approximately **4 to 7 days after birth**. Ductal-dependent congenital heart lesions that present in this manner typically include transposition of the great arteries, truncus arteriosus, total anomalous pulmonary venous return, left heart hypoplasia, and coarctation. The most important next step is administration of a medication that will assist the ductus to remain open while preparing for surgical intervention.

Oxygen (a) is a stimulant to close the ductus (as is appropriate in normal infants) and should not be administered, though this patient will likely need to be intubated to take away his work of breathing and because prostaglandins can cause apnea. In truth, immediate administration of oxygen for a very brief period is warranted as a diagnostic tool. In lesions with right-to-left mixing, the saturations will not improve. In pulmonary conditions causing this presentation or in cardiac conditions without right-to-left shunting, the saturations will improve. This is a very important piece of diagnostic information. The other choices, (b) chest radiograph and ECG, and (e) cardiology consultation, would need to be done; however, the patient requires immediate intervention with prostaglandin. Antibiotics would likely be administered to this patient early on because sepsis is common, this is a home birth, the patient is hypothermic, and this intervention is critical early therapy for infectious processes. Still, the presentation is classic for closure of the ductus arteriosus and recognition of this condition is critical.

**342. The answer is b.** *(Fleisher and Ludwig, pp 617-622.)* This patient has **pyloric stenosis** and will exhibit a hypochloremic, metabolic alkalosis with hypokalemia. Hypoglycemia is common in children of this age who experience poor intake of calories and who have very poor glycemic reserves. The low chloride and high bicarbonate are the result of hydrochloric acid loss from stomach with repeated episodes of vomiting leading to an alkalemia. As a result, the patient will physiologically try to balance ions and trade intracellular $H^+$ for extracellular $K^+$, thus lowering the serum potassium. Pyloric stenosis typically presents between 3 and 6 weeks of life. It is most common in first-born male patients. If you were looking for the finding of an olive on examination, you will be disappointed in the majority of cases. It can sometimes be felt in the operating room under anesthesia.

(a) is incorrect because these values are physiologically normal. (c) and (e) are incorrect because both the potassium and chloride are elevated and this is not consistent with pyloric stenosis. (d) is incorrect because the bicarbonate is low. Low bicarbonate can be a very late finding in pyloric stenosis and is a sign of severe physiologic disturbance secondary to hypovolemia, resulting in a patient progressive to a hypovolemic shock-like state.

**343. The answer is e.** *(Fleisher and Ludwig, p 599.)* Precipitous deliveries occur in the ED. When they do, it is always a somewhat tension-filled moment waiting to see what the infant will do. But that is exactly what one ought to do. It is important to allow a newborn, especially one who is nearly full term, to demonstrate what he or she will do initially. **Do not get overly aggressive initiating resuscitation efforts in an otherwise normal infant.** The first course of action here, as in any delivery, is to **dry, suction,** and **stimulate the baby** and observe for respiratory response first and then cardiovascular response (in the form of color, respiratory effort, cry, and heart rate).

Beginning resuscitative efforts immediately with positive-pressure ventilation **(a or b)** is premature and may harm the infant by causing a **pneumothorax** if the infant is making efforts against the bag breaths causing increased intrathoracic pressure. Even a couple of breaths to start without first assessing the infant's effort are not indicated. One would likely call the neonatal ICU **(c)** in such a circumstance to accept the newborn, but there is no specific workup indicated and so none would be initiated. APGAR scores **(d)** are typically assigned at 1 minute and 5 minutes and are a universal way to communicate initial status of a newborn. It need not be done immediately at birth or before the initial assessment and any necessary intervention.

**344. The answer is c.** *(Fleisher and Ludwig, pp 569-570, 1017-1018.)* This patient had a **simple febrile seizure**. Approximately 2% to 5% of children will experience a febrile seizure during their lifetimes. Febrile seizures occur between the ages of **3 months and 5 years**, are associated with fever, and are categorized as either simple or complex. Simple febrile seizures are generalized and **last less than 15 minutes.** Complex febrile seizures are prolonged, recur within 24 hours, or are focal. The approach to a patient with a febrile seizure is, for all intents and purposes, identical to that of the same patient who has not had a seizure, so long as the seizure has stopped by the time you are evaluating the patient. If the seizure continues, attend to it as you would any seizure with indicated medications and attention to ABCs. Once the patient is stable, it is important to identify the source of the fever. This patient, having a temperature of 103°F and lesions consistent with Coxsackie virus infection on the posterior pharynx, does not need any testing. If there were no identifiable source of infection with fever in this age female, it would be reasonable to consider obtaining a urine specimen to rule out urinary tract infection (UTI).

In the presence of an otherwise normal examination, other diagnostic tests **(a and b)** are not indicated. CBC and blood cultures in otherwise well appearing, fully immunized children of this age are no longer indicated to evaluate for occult bacteremia. Neither a head CT scan nor a neurology consultation (**d**) is warranted for a first-time febrile seizure. A lumbar puncture to rule out meningitis (**e**) is not indicated in this patient who has regained normal mental status, appears well, and has no neurologic deficit.

**345. The answer is b.** *(Fleisher and Ludwig, pp 1575-1576.)* This is a case of a patient with a **SCFE**. SCFE is a condition of the femur where the **femoral head slips or shears off from the neck of the femur through the physis**. It is more common in boys than in girls, typically in early or mid-adolescence and is more common in African American children than in Caucasian children. Its cause is unknown. SCFE can present either with a complaint of tightness that progresses to more significant pain leading to a limp or more dramatically with extreme pain and inability to bear weight. It is not uncommon for a child to present with a complaint of **knee pain that is referred to the hip**. A careful examination will often better localize the origin of the pain to the hip. It is usually unilateral though it can be bilateral in upward of a quarter of the cases. The diagnosis is made on radiograph. It is classically described as the "ice cream falling off of the cone" appearance. Treatment is surgical.

Legg-Calvé-Perthes (**a**), also known as avascular necrosis of the femoral head, typically affects younger children aged 2 to 6 years and is uncommon in African American as compared with Caucasian children. Septic arthritis (**c**) is typically characterized by fever, intense pain, inability to bear weight, and large effusions with elevated inflammatory markers. Osgood-Schlatter (**d**) disease is the most common cause of knee pain in this age group. It is caused by the patellar tendon pulling on its insertion at the tibial tuberosity. It is characterized by localized tenderness and treatment is conservative. Transient synovitis (**e**) of the hip is typically a postinfectious condition of young, toddler-aged children. It would be unlikely to occur in a 13-year-old.

**346. The answer is a.** *(Fleisher and Ludwig, pp 1117-1118.)* This is a case of **Henoch-Schönlein purpura (HSP)**, also termed anaphylactoid purpura. HSP is an **inflammatory vasculitis** whose cause is unknown. It is thought to be postinflammatory. The organism most frequently associated with HSP is *Campylobacter jejuni*, but this is found in a minority of cases, and many other organisms and factors have been implicated. HSP typically occurs in the spring months and is most common in young children between 2 and 12 years of age, though it can occur at any age. HSP is characterized by its characteristic rash, a **purpuric rash that typically occurs on the buttocks and flexural surface of the lower extremities onto the soles**. Abdominal pain, joint pain and arthritis, and hematuria with renal involvement are also common. Treatment is mostly supportive with NSAIDs for pain control although steroids are used for patients with severe abdominal pain. There is recent evidence to suggest that steroids may benefit a larger percentage of patients. **One feared complication of HSP** that is certainly a consideration in this patient **is intussusception**. Physicians must consider this diagnosis in patients with abdominal pain and HSP, and perform x-rays, ultrasound, and obtain surgical consult where indicated. Unlike most patients with idiopathic intussusception, these patients are far less likely to have successful reductions with air or barium enemas and many require surgical reduction. HSP often affects the kidney causing hematuria. The majority of patients recover from HSP without any complication, but prolonged renal involvement leading to renal failure and hypertension can occur in approximately 1% of patients.

The skin lesions (**b**) resolve, as does the GI involvement (**c**) with the risk of intussusception decreasing to baseline levels with resolution of disease. The arthritis (**d**) is similarly self-limiting and pain control is the best treatment until that time. The neurologic system (**e**) is involved in a small percentage of patients, but this is atypical and does not lead to lasting complications.

**347. The answer is d.** (*Fleisher and Ludwig, pp 900-903, 1545-1548.*) This is a case of a **viral URI** with an **acute otitis media (AOM)**. Treatment for otitis media evolved significantly over the last several years. Otitis has traditionally been treated in the United States with oral antibiotics, but there are now data showing that most of these infections resolve spontaneously, even those caused by bacterial organisms. Bacterial otitis media can present similarly but is more typical to have viral symptoms for several days leading to eustachian tube inflammation and dysfunction, which subsequently predisposes a child to secondary bacterial infection from the fluid that cannot drain from the middle ear. In cases of AOM in children older than 2 years for whom secondary complications are less likely, the recommended treatment is analgesics (can be topical, oral, or a combination of both) with a 48- to 72-hour period of waiting and observing for improvement or persistence of symptoms.

This will avoid unnecessary antibiotics in many children. The remainder should be treated with amoxicillin at a high dose (80-90 mg/kg/d divided into two doses) as first-line therapy.

Analgesics only (a) is a good start, but ignores the fact that the patient has purulent middle ear fluid and may require antibiotics in the near future for resolution. A third-generation cephalosporin (b) has been recommended as second- or third-line treatment for patients with AOM if amoxicillin fails. Amoxicillin at 40 to 50 mg/kg/d (c) is no longer recommended therapy for treatment of AOM because of resistant *S pneumoniae*. The incidence of treatment failure at this dose is high. No treatment (e) for this patient also ignores his discomfort and is not an appropriate choice.

**348. The answer is b.** *(Fleisher and Ludwig, p 823.)* This is a case of **milk protein colitis**, a common cause of **rectal bleeding** in this age group. Some infants have sensitivity to cow's milk protein (which is fundamentally different from human milk proteins) that leads to an allergic antibody response causing a true colitis that results in bloody stools. Approximately a third of these patients will have a similar reaction to soy milk proteins. The resulting symptoms are dramatic but generally without other consequence except in cases where the exposure is long-standing and bleeding is ongoing. This can lead to malnourishment, anemia, and poor growth. Milk protein colitis is more frequently seen in bottle fed infants but can be seen in exclusively breast-fed infants where the proteins are thought to transfer from the mother's milk into the infant, which results in the same symptoms as if the patient were drinking milk directly. Treatment is elimination of offending agent from the diet, typically with total resolution of symptoms. Most patients will grow out of their sensitivity by 2 years of age and milk products can be reintroduced at that time.

Acute gastroenteritis (a) typically presents with multiple episodes of vomiting and diarrhea. It can occur with or without fever. *Clostridium difficile* colitis (c) does cause bloody stool, but it generally follows an antibiotic exposure or is associated with other risk factors. It would be highly unusual in an otherwise healthy 3-week-old without risk factors. Both intestinal malrotation (d) and necrotizing enterocolitis (e) are GI and surgical emergencies that can be associated with blood in stool but occur in ill-appearing infants.

**349. The answer is c.** *(Fleisher and Ludwig, pp 890-892.)* This is a case of **newborn sepsis**. Neonatal sepsis is defined as an invasive bacterial infection occurring during the **first 90 days of life**. The most common cause of newborn sepsis is **group B β-hemolytic** *Streptococcus* **(GBBS)**. Approximately a third of women are carriers of this organism in their vagina and exposure is through the birth canal. There is increased risk with PROM that is thought to result in ascending infection. Increased colony counts result in increased risk for neonatal sepsis and thus the tendency to screen pregnant women and to treat at the time of delivery for either screen-positive women or women with fever or PROM. **Any infant younger than 4 weeks with fever greater than 100.3°F** (and most would say any infant < 8 weeks) **requires a full workup to search for the source of infection.** This workup includes a CBC, blood culture, urinalysis and urine culture, and a lumbar puncture for cell counts and culture. Many people recommend sending the CSF for HSV culture and polymerase chain reaction, particularly if there are any maternal risk factors or suspicious skin lesions, or in any infant who is very ill.

The other organisms listed are all known causes of neonatal sepsis but less likely than GBBS. *Escherichia coli* **(a)** is the second most common pathogen and is the most common of the enteric pathogens that cause this condition. It is the most common cause of UTIs in infants, which can lead to bacteremia as well. *Listeria* **(b)** is a commonly cited source of infection in neonatal sepsis. Exposure is primarily from unprocessed meats and unpasteurized produce. *Staphylococcus aureus* **(d)** is an unlikely pathogen in an immunocompetent patient this age. HSV **(e)** is an important pathogen to consider in neonatal sepsis. Obtaining the maternal history is important to help diagnose this condition, though many patients who ultimately are diagnosed with neonatal HSV have no known maternal history of vaginal herpes. The lesions on this patient's trunk are most consistent with a benign newborn rash called erythema toxicum neonatorum and are unrelated to the fever.

**350. The answer is c.** (*Fleisher and Ludwig, pp 1025-1026*) This patient has **Rheumatic fever**, an inflammatory and autoimmune complication of *S pyogenes* **infections** (typically pharyngeal). Rheumatic fever can be diagnosed on the basis of the **Jones criteria**, which include five major and multiple minor criteria. In order to establish the diagnosis, one must meet at least two major or one major and two minor criteria.

The five major criteria are:
Arthritis

Endocarditis
Subcutaneous nodes (known as Osler nodes)
Erythema marginatum
Sydenham chorea

The exception to having to meet two criteria is the presence of **Syden-ham chorea** in a young child. This alone can establish the diagnosis.

ESR **(a)** is a nonspecific inflammatory marker that may be elevated, as could CRP, in patients with rheumatic fever and it is one of the minor criteria that can be used as supporting evidence. The same is true for evidence of a group A streptococcal infection, be it antistreptolysin (ASO) titer **(b)** or a positive rapid strep test **(d)**. Arthrocentesis on a knee with a large effusion can reveal a lot of important information, but it cannot provide a diagnosis of rheumatic fever. A white blood cell count on the knee aspirate over 50,000 cell/hpf, however, can make one strongly suspicious of a bacterial infection and may prompt further investigation. A count of 25,000 **(e)** is a nonspecific inflammatory effusion and would not, in itself, prompt any specific further activity.

**351. The answer is c.** *(Fleisher and Ludwig, pp 1026-1027.)* This is a classic case of **infant botulism** characterized by generalized weakness, pupillary unresponsiveness, and hypoventilation. Patients often present with an initial complaint of constipation. They are noted to have a particularly weak cry. The condition is caused by release of the **botu-linum toxin** from *Clostridium botulinum*. The toxin prevents release of acetylcholine from the neuromuscular junction. Older children present with complaints of diplopia, dysarthria, and dysphagia. Young infants are particularly susceptible from ingestion of **honey**, which can harbor *C botulinum* spores. The pH in infant stomachs does not destroy the spores. Therefore, honey is not recommended for any infant younger than 1 year.

This is not a case of spinal muscular atrophy (ie, Werdnig-Hoffman disease) **(a)**, which is an autosomal recessive disorder characterized by muscle weakness that can affect every aspect of eating, breathing, and moving and will often be apparent from very early on—even before the age of this child. Brain tumors **(b)** can cause some of these symptoms but would not typically present with generalized weakness and poorly responsive pupils. This child doesn't show particular signs of increased intracranial pressure like vomiting or persistent irritability. Similarly, this patient is not showing signs of meningitis (**d**). She is afebrile and is not irritable. Organophosphate poisoning (**e**) causes increased muscarinic and nicotinic tone from the inhibition of acetylcholinesterase. The symptoms may be similar to this patient with drooling and weakness. In addition, diarrhea, autonomic dysfunction, and CNS disturbances are common. This condition is unlikely in a nonmobile infant and exposures are uncommon in this setting.

**352. The answer is c.** (*Fleisher and Ludwig, pp 7-17.*) This patient has become apneic and **requires assisted ventilation**. The correct approach is to do a **jaw thrust and chin lift** in order to provide optimal airway positioning and begin bag-valve-mask ventilation. This is the most important skill to learn in pediatric resuscitation. In many cases, providing oxygen appropriately is all that is needed to resolve the bradycardia and circulatory issues. **The most common cause of arrest in children is respiratory.** This is a classic case of respiratory arrest causing cyanosis and subsequent bradycardia.

Epinephrine (**a**) is certainly in the algorithm for bradycardia, but the first step in resuscitation is always addressing the airway. Oxygen should be administered to this patient and a non-rebreather face mask (**b**) can provide high oxygen delivery. However, the patient is not respiring so this method is ineffective. Endotracheal intubation (**d**) may be necessary to establish a definitive airway in this patient. However, it will take time to set up and perform. The simplest and quickest intervention is jaw thrust or chin lift with bag-valve-mask ventilation. Chest compressions (**e**) are soon to follow in this patient's resuscitation, but the initial intervention is attention to airway and breathing.

**353. The answer is e.** (*Fleisher and Ludwig, pp 17-19.*) This patient is in **shock**. Attempts at peripheral IV access are acceptable, but should be limited to two attempts within 60 seconds and then intraosseous (IO) insertion should be attempted. **IO lines can be performed quickly and reliably.** The preferred sites for insertion are the **proximal tibia**, followed by the **distal tibia** and **proximal femur**. In adults, there is a sternal IO system that has gained popularity for its ease of placement and use of flexible tubing once in place. All medications can be administered through the IO line and onset of action is similar to venous administration.

Internal jugular central line (**a**), femoral vein central line (**b**), and saphenous cutdown (**c**) are all very good methods of establishing quick IV access in many critically ill adults and some pediatric patients. However,

IO access is proven to be quick and reliable in the pediatric population and should be utilized when peripheral access is difficult to obtain in an unstable patient. A large-bore IV in the antecubital fossa (**d**) is also a good method of vascular access, but peripheral access was not obtained in this individual.

**354. The answer is a.** *(Fleisher and Ludwig, pp 908-911.)* **Epiglottitis** is a life-threatening inflammatory condition of the epiglottis, aryepiglottic, and paraglottic folds. The etiology is usually infectious, with *Haemophilus influenzae* type b as the classic and most common etiology before the introduction of the *H influenzae* type b vaccination. Most cases now appear in **adults** and **nonimmunized children,** and are seen most commonly as secondary infections following viral illnesses (the most notorious was primary varicella before the widespread use of that vaccine). Signs and symptoms include a prodromal period of 1 to 2 days with high fever, dysphagia, secretion pooling, and dyspnea. Patients usually sit in an erect or "tripod" position, leaning forward with neck extended to give maximum airway opening, to improve their symptoms. Radiographs of the neck may show the classic **thumbprint sign** of an enlarged, inflamed epiglottis, although a CT scan of the neck may delineate the condition further. However, these are typically difficult to obtain because of the fact that patients are not stable enough to leave the ED and need continuous monitoring in case of airway compromise, so no radiographic studies are typically performed. The classic approach to a patient with suspected epiglottitis is to leave them in their caretaker's arms, try to avoid agitating them, and call immediately for ENT (ear, nose, throat) and anesthesia assistance in the ED. Direct laryngoscopy is contraindicated because it may induce laryngospasm. These patients require direct visualization, often only in the OR, with the appropriate services prepared for the need to place a surgical airway emergently. IV antibiotics and steroids are indicated to help treat the infection and decrease swelling.

Retropharyngeal abscesses (**b**) may present somewhat similarly but not typically in the same level of extremis as this patient. The classic physical examination finding is an inability to extend the neck because this stretches the inflamed prevertebral soft tissue area. Retropharyngeal abscess is suspected on the basis of a lateral neck film that demonstrates a widened prevertebral soft tissue stripe. EBV pharyngitis (**c**) may present with erythema or exudate of the tonsils, dysphagia, fever, and cough. In addition, patients may be very uncomfortable and moderately ill appearing, but will typically not present with airway compromise and hypoxia. In addition, clinical mononucleosis is usually a condition of older children and adolescents. Ludwig angina (**d**) is an infection of the submandibular space. (**e**) Peritonsillar abscess is often a secondary infection of strep throat and will present with trismus, difficulty swallowing, and fever.

**355. The answer is d.** *(Fleisher and Ludwig, pp 916-917.)* **RSV** is a common cause of respiratory distress in infants, especially younger than 6 months, and the most common cause of the clinical condition known as **bronchiolitis**. Diagnosis is made clinically on the basis of the constellation of symptoms, as this patient demonstrates. Patients who are at risk of increased disease severity are those with chronic lung disease, especially ex-preemies, those with an immunocompromised condition, and those with complex congenital heart disease. These patients are eligible for receiving palivizumab, an injectable antibody that confers passive immunity and can reduce the likelihood of severe lower respiratory tract disease caused by RSV in susceptible individuals. The condition associated with RSV infections overlap with those of other respiratory tract pathogens including rhinovirus, parainfluenza virus, coronavirus, echovirus, and Coxsackie virus. The clinical condition of bronchiolitis is caused by RSV in approximately 70% of cases, especially during the peak months of November to April. The diagnosis is confirmed by a rapid antigen test of a nasal aspirate, but this is typically only useful in patients whose diagnosis is unclear or in whom management may be different based on concomitant conditions. Management is largely supportive. A variety of medications including albuterol, aerosolized epinephrine, and corticosteroids are often administered. However, none have been shown to be consistently beneficial in treating the symptoms or reducing the duration of illness. Respiratory precautions are necessary to limit transmission.

Foreign body aspiration (**a**) can happen in children of this age and, if undetected initially, can cause similar symptoms. Often, a radiograph will show an ingested object or stridor may be present. It is believed that bronchiolitis is a precursor to asthma (**b**) and that infants who develop bronchiolitis are more likely to develop asthma as they get older, though the diagnosis of asthma does not apply to someone with their first wheezing episode at this age. Pneumococcal pneumonia (**c**) is the predominant cause of bacterial pneumonia in this age group although the incidence has declined with the consistent administration of Prevnar (pneumococcal conjugate vaccine), a conjugated vaccine against this pathogen that significantly reduces the incidence of serious (invasive) disease by this pathogen. This patient would have received two doses of the vaccine by this age if he is current on his shots. Pneumococcus can super infect patients as well, but this clinical scenario is classic for bronchiolitis. Parvovirus B19 (e) is the etiologic agent of Fifth disease. Fifth disease is a mild illness that occurs most commonly in children. The child typically has a fever associated with a "slapped-cheek" appearance to the face and a lacy red rash on the trunk and limbs.

**356. The answer is b.** *(Pediatric Advanced Life Support Provider Manual, 2006.)* There were recent changes in the Pediatric Advanced Life Support (PALS) recommendations regarding ETTs. Previously, uncuffed ETTs were recommended for all patients younger than 8 years. This was based on the anatomical consideration that the narrowest part of the airway in children is the subglottic area whereas in adults it is the glottis (larynx) itself. Though this is true, it has become clear through further research that cuffed tubes are preferable for providing a better seal without an increased risk for endothelial damage from overinflation of the balloon and will provide better ventilation in patients with poor lung compliance. With this complication in mind, it is important not to blow the balloon up to a pressure greater than 20 cm $H_2O$. There are two acceptable methods for choosing the appropriate ETT size. One relies on the length-based resuscitation tape that should be available and utilized in the resuscitation of all small children. The formula that has been endorsed by the American Heart Association for calculation of the appropriate tube size for a **cuffed tube** is **ETT size (mm of internal diameter of tube) = (age in years/4) + 3**. This calculation in the above patient would yield a size of **4.0 mm for a cuffed tube**.

To calculate the size of an **uncuffed ETT**, the calculation is as follows: **size (in mm) = (age in years/4) + 4**. That would yield an ETT size of 5.0 mm for an uncuffed tube. This is not one of the choices. That leaves (**a, c, d, and e**) as incorrect choices. Finally, it is worth mentioning the emphasis that PALS has placed on tube placement confirmation. This must be done by a variety of methods. Auscultation over the chest as well as the stomach, bilateral chest wall rise, pulse oxygenation monitor, and perhaps most importantly, end-tidal $CO_2$ monitoring for patients with a perfusing rhythm are all essential methods for confirming placement.

**357. The answer is c.** *(Fleisher and Ludwig, pp 276-282.)* **Foreign body ingestion** and aspiration are common in this age group with peak occurrence between **6 months and 4 years**. In this patient, the position of the coin on the anterior-posterior chest film aids with the diagnosis. When the coin is in the **esophagus, it is seen head-on in the AP projection**. When it is localized in the trachea, it is seen in the sagittal plane because the cartilaginous tracheal rings in children are incomplete and remain open posteriorly, causing the coin to sit sagittal or sideways. After assessing the patient's status (respiratory distress, inability to swallow, etc), it is important to assess characteristics of the foreign body ingested. Ingested foreign bodies usually get obstructed in three common locations: thoracic inlet (60%-80%), at the gastroesophageal junction (10%-20%), and at the aortic arch (5%-20%). A good way to remember this is by their level in the spine: C4-C6, T8, and T4, respectively. Once they pass the pylorus, most foreign bodies pass through the remainder of the GI tract. Objects larger than 2 × 5 cm, sharp objects (needles, tacks), or disc batteries should be considered for removal.

Although foreign body aspiration **(a)** is a possibility, the position of the coin in the radiograph and the absence of respiratory symptoms make this diagnosis unlikely. If there is a suspicion for an aspirated foreign body, the patient should undergo bronchoscopy. Bronchospasm **(b)** occurs as a reaction to aspirated foreign bodies and should always be considered in patients presenting with cough or respiratory symptoms. Although seen infrequently in children since the advent of the *H Influenzae* vaccine, patients with epiglottitis **(d)** classically present with drooling and assume a "tripod position" to assist their breathing and will often show evidence of respiratory distress. Allergic reaction **(e)** is unlikely given the absence of dermatologic or respiratory symptoms.

**358. The answer is e.** *(Fleisher and Ludwig, pp 907-908.)* This is a case of **laryngotracheitis** or **croup**. It is the most common cause of stridor and upper respiratory obstruction in children 6 months to 3 years old. It usually begins with constitutional symptoms and subsequently patients develop the characteristic "seal-like" cough. The etiology is most commonly the **parainfluenza virus**. Diagnosis is usually clinical. Treatment includes racemic epinephrine, particularly when stridor is present. After administration of racemic epinephrine, patients should be observed for 3 to 4 hours to monitor for a rebound effect after the epinephrine wears off. **Steroids** are administered as well to **reduce the swelling of the larynx**. Dexamethasone is the commonly administered steroid. Some home-based treatments, such as taking a child outdoors to breath cool air (as croup presents most typically in the winter) or into the bathroom to breath the steam produced when running hot water in the shower both seem to aid in symptomatic relief.

Radiographs of the chest (a) to evaluate for pneumonia and the soft tissues of the neck (c) are not indicated in patients presenting with classic findings for croup. A CBC and blood culture (b) are of no utility in a patient with this classic viral illness. Antibiotics (d) are not effective in patients with a viral illness.

**359. The answer is d.** *(Fleisher and Ludwig, pp 706-711.)* The ECG shows a **narrow complex tachycardia at 300 beats per minute** with no variability and absent P waves. This is diagnostic of **supraventricular tachycardia (SVT)**. SVT is the **most common pathologic arrhythmia of childhood**. It is sometimes confused with sinus tachycardia, which usually presents at a rate of fewer than 225 beats per minute in infants and fewer than 150 beats per minute in older children and adults. This finding, coupled with variability with respirations and evidence of normal P waves, will prove to be useful in differentiating sinus tachycardia from SVT. This dysrhythmia is typically well tolerated in young children and infants. SVT will often present with a history of pallor, poor feeding, tachypnea, and lethargy, or irritability. Older children will describe palpitations, lightheadedness, and shortness of breath. Signs of congestive heart failure or shock may be present. SVT can occur in children with no structural lesions and is associated with fever, infection, or sympathomimetic drugs (such as cold medicine or bronchodilators), but is most often idiopathic. Stability is the most important factor in managing patients with SVT. Stable patients usually have normal mental status and only mild symptoms. Unstable patients typically present in congestive heart failure or shock. **Adenosine** is safe and effective and has a short half-life. It is the first-line therapy in patients with stable SVT. It must be administered rapidly through a large-bore IV in a vein as close to the heart as possible (antecubital is classic and generally adequate) and followed by a 10- to 20-mL normal saline bolus using the double stopcock method to flush it quickly. Adenosine will block conduction at the atrioventricular (AV) node leading to a brief period of asystole, which can be very disconcerting to those receiving or administering the medication.

Synchronized cardioversion (a) is the treatment for any unstable patient or when other treatment options failed. Carotid massage (e) is not recommended in children owing to the concerns of dislodging plaques or causing an intimal tear. Verapamil (b) should be avoided in infants because it can cause potentially lethal hypotension. Defibrillation (c) is the treatment for patients in ventricular fibrillation or pulseless ventricular tachycardia.

**360. The answer is a.** (*Fleisher and Ludwig, p 1560.*) This is a case of **paraphimosis**. Paraphimosis is a **true emergency**. It occurs when the **foreskin of an uncircumcised male is retracted beyond the glans and not returned to its normal position**. Ensuing congestion and edema make it difficult for it to be retracted back to its normal position. **Manual reduction** is the first-line treatment for paraphimosis. Manual reduction is performed by placing your thumbs over the glans as you attempt to gently pull the engorged foreskin tissue back over the head of the penis. Ice can be applied to the penis to help decrease swelling. In addition, a dorsal penile nerve block can be used for analgesia making it easier to perform a manual reduction.

Dorsal slit or circumcision **(b)** should be considered after the initial attempts at manual reduction have failed and typically in consultation with a urologist. Topical lidocaine **(c)** is not described for treatment of this condition. Topical steroids **(e)** can be considered in the treatment of phimosis, not paraphimosis. Catheterization **(d)** is rarely indicated as most paraphimoses are retractable in the ED and urinary retention is uncommon.

**361. The answer is a.** (*Fleisher and Ludwig, pp 1523-1525.*) The patient's clinical presentation is very concerning for **malrotation with midgut volvulus**. Malrotation occurs when there is an inappropriate fixation of the intestines at the ligament of Treitz during fetal life. Signs and symptoms of malrotation may be nonspecific and include vomiting, which is characteristically bilious, and abdominal distension. Most cases present in the first year of life. The most catastrophic presentation of malrotation occurs when the abnormally fixed mesentery twists around itself and the superior mesenteric artery leading to bowel infarction, shock, sepsis, and death, all of which can all occur within a few hours. The **definitive diagnostic study of choice** is an **upper GI series**. Contrast in the gut will fail to demonstrate the classic "C-loop" of the four parts of the duodenum and instead show the "corkscrew" appearance classic of this condition.

Ultrasound **(b)** is not the imaging modality of choice for malrotation. It is commonly used to diagnose pyloric stenosis. Some physicians begin the workup with a plain film of the abdomen **(c)** looking for air-fluid levels, dilated loops, or pneumatosis coli that can be seen in patients with severe distention. The classic plain film finding is that of the "double bubble."

However, plain films are less sensitive and specific than an upper GI series and couldn't be used as a definitive diagnostic study. CBC, electrolytes, and urine analysis (**d**) will not provide sufficient information to rule this disease out but may show electrolyte abnormalities, dehydration, leukocytosis and elevated specific gravity. Serum lactate (**e**) rises late in the disease process and is an indicator of ischemia.

**362. The answer is e.** *(Fleisher and Ludwig, pp 1349-1350, 1584.)* The patient's presentation and radiographic findings are consistent with a **supracondylar fracture**. Supracondylar fractures are the most common type of elbow fracture in children and important to recognize early because of the risk of injury to the arteries and nerves that pass through this area. Patients typically present with pain, swelling, and decreased range of motion with the arm held in adduction. Most fractures occur after a fall on an outstretched hand with the distal humerus displacing posteriorly. Posterior fractures are classified in three categories. Type I fractures show only an increased anterior fat pad sign and evidence of a posterior fat pad that is always pathologic, although not specific for this condition. Type II fractures have an obvious non displaced fracture. Type III show posterior displacement of the capitellum and have no cortical contact between the fracture fragments. Types II and III require reduction and fixation.

The most serious complication of supracondylar fractures is **Volkmann ischemic contracture**. This occurs when high-pressure builds up in the forearm compartments leading to a compartment syndrome. It can also be caused by kinking of the brachial artery with subsequent ischemia if not repaired. If the condition is not addressed, there is potential for permanent damage to nerves and muscles of the forearm leading to contractures. Patients who develop pain upon passive extension of the fingers, forearm tenderness, or refuse to open the hand have a very high risk of developing this condition.

Ulnar nerve injury (**c**) is rare in supracondylar fractures. The most commonly injured nerve is the anterior interosseous nerve. Brachial artery transection (**a**) is uncommon and generally results in a pulse deficit on examination. Malunion (**b**) and arthritis (**d**) are far less common and less serious sequelae than the contractures.

**363. The answer is b.** *(Fleisher and Ludwig, pp 1335-1336.)* This is a **Salter-Harris type II** fracture that involves the **physis and meta-physis**. The physis or growth plate is a common site of fractures in pediatric patients.

Approximately 20% of fractures involve this area of active bone growth with a peak incidence in early adolescence. The most widely used system of classification for these fractures is the Salter-Harris classification. In this system, there are five classifications of injuries. In general, the higher the Salter-Harris classification, the worse the prognosis and the higher the chance for growth arrest. **Salter-Harris I** occurs when the fracture involves the growth plate. There may be no radiographic evidence of these fractures initially; therefore you must have a high suspicion. This injury should be suspected in any patient who is tender around the physis of a bone even in the absence of obvious radiographic fracture. Treatment for this injury includes early immobilization and referral. Prognosis is usually good. **Salter-Harris II** is the most common type, accounting for approximately 75% of fractures involving the growth plate. The fracture occurs through the growth plate and into the metaphysis. **Salter-Harris III** occurs when a fracture breaks through the growth plate and into the epiphysis. **Salter-Harris IV** involves the metaphysis, physis, and epiphysis. Salter-Harris V is a crush injury to the growth plate and has a high potential for growth arrest.

A crush injury to the growth plate **(a)** is known as a **Salter-Harris type V**. **(c)** The patient's radiograph is consistent with a Salter-Harris type II. Fractures through the metaphysis, physis, and epiphysis **(d)** are known as Salter-Harris type IV. Salter-Harris type I fractures **(e)** have the best prognosis. The worst prognosis and highest incidence of growth arrest is seen with type V fractures.

# Vaginal Bleeding

## Questions

**364.** A 23-year-old woman presents to the emergency department (ED) with irregular menstrual bleeding. She denies any abdominal pain, dizziness, or palpitations. The patient reports that her last menstrual period (LMP) was 2 weeks ago with normal flow and duration. Which of the following ancillary tests is critical in defining the differential diagnosis for this patient?

a. Type and screen.
b. Coagulation panel.
c. β-Human chorionic gonadotropin (β-hCG).
d. Complete blood count (CBC).
e. No ancillary tests are needed.

**365.** A 30-year-old G2P2 with a history of *Chlamydia* presents to the ED with acute onset of severe lower abdominal pain associated with vaginal bleeding that began 2 hours before arrival. She denies any prior medical history but does report having a tubal ligation after the birth of her second child. Her vitals are significant for a heart rate (HR) of 120 beats per minute and a blood pressure (BP) of 90/60 mm Hg. On physical examination, her cervical os is closed and she has right adnexal tenderness with blood in the posterior vaginal vault. Given this patient's history and physical examination, which of the following diagnoses do you most strongly suspect?

a. Heterotopic pregnancy
b. Pelvic inflammatory disease (PID)
c. Placenta previa
d. Ectopic pregnancy
e. Abruptio placentae

**366.** A 28-year-old G1P0 at 36 weeks presents with the sudden onset of severe abdominal pain with distention and vaginal bleeding. She denies contractions. Her vitals are significant for an HR of 120 beats per minute and a BP of 156/80 mm Hg. Upon further history, the patient reports the pain developed immediately after recent cocaine use. Which of the following conditions are you concerned about because of which you call a stat OB-GYN?

a. Uterine rupture
b. Acute cocaine intoxication
c. Placenta accreta
d. Vasa previa
e. Ruptured ovarian cyst

**367.** A 24-year-old G2P0010 in her second trimester presents to the ED with vaginal spotting for the past day. She denies any abdominal pain and is otherwise in her usual state of health. Her vital signs are HR of 76 beats per minute, BP of 120/65 mm Hg, respiratory rate of 16 breaths per minute, and temperature 98.9°F. Which of the following conditions is the most likely cause of this patient's symptoms?

a. Ectopic pregnancy
b. Placenta previa
c. Abruptio placentae
d. Uterine rupture
e. Ovarian torsion

**368.** A 24-year-old G3P1112 presents to the ED with vaginal bleeding and clots. Her vital signs include an HR of 110 beats per minute, BP of 130/70 mm Hg, and RR of 14 breaths per minute with an oxygen saturation of 99% on room air. She is afebrile and in mild distress. Recent medical history is significant for vaginal delivery 2 days ago with prolonged labor. Pelvic examination is significant for a large, boggy uterus, and a normal vaginal wall. What is the most likely diagnosis in this patient?

a. Genital tract trauma
b. Endometritis
c. Uterine atony
d. Ectopic pregnancy
e. Uterine artery rupture

**369.** A 40-year-old G1P0101 presents to the ED with suprapubic pain and general malaise for the last 3 days without improvement. Her vitals are significant for HR of 115 beats per minute, BP of 100/60 mm Hg, and temperature of 101°F. Upon physical examination, her abdomen is soft with significant suprapubic tenderness to light palpation but no rebound or guarding. Her pelvic examination reveals a scant amount of dark red vaginal blood and yellow discharge. Her past medical history is significant for an emergent cesarean section 2 weeks ago without any other gynecologic history. What is the most likely diagnosis in this patient?

a. Uterine atony
b. Retained products of conception
c. Uterine inversion
d. Endometritis
e. Tubo-ovarian torsion

**370.** A 17-year-old girl presents to the ED with worsening nausea and vomiting. She reports her LMP was 9 weeks ago and has had some "morning sickness" over the past several weeks. However, for the past week her nausea and vomiting has been so severe that she is unable to tolerate more than a few sips of water or juice. Her vitals include HR of 96 beats per minute, BP of 190/100 mm Hg, and temperature of 99°F. Her physical examination is significant for a fundal height at the umbilicus. After obtaining a positive β-hCG, sonographic evaluation reveals the following image. What is the most likely underlying condition for this patient's symptoms?

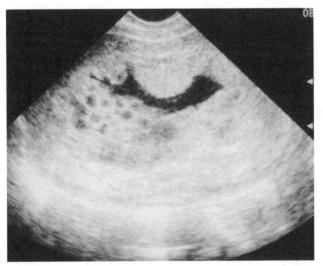

*(Reproduced, with permission, from Knoop KJ, Stack LB, Storrow AB. Atlas of Emergency Medicine. New York, NY: McGraw-Hill, 2002: 272.) (Courtesy of Robin Marshall, MD.)*

a. Ectopic pregnancy
b. Hydatidiform mole
c. Ovarian torsion
d. Abruptio placentae
e. Hyperemesis gravidarum

**371.** A 25-year-old G1P0 presents to the ED with vaginal bleeding. She recently discovered that she was pregnant and has yet to be medically evaluated. She does not know her LMP. Before presentation, the patient was in her usual state of good health with no history of trauma or any other symptoms. She reports using two absorbent pads an hour for the bleeding and does not notice passing fetal tissue. On physical examination, her cervical os is open. Which of the following is the most appropriate diagnosis?

a. Threatened abortion
b. Complete abortion
c. Inevitable abortion
d. Incomplete abortion
e. Missed abortion

**372.** A 36-year-old G4P2103 presents to the ED with vaginal spotting for the past 2 days. She also reports occasional abdominal cramping and low back pain. The patient states that she is 4 months pregnant. She denies any other past medical history or gynecologic problems. Her initial vital signs include HR of 89 beats per minute, BP of 144/70 mm Hg, and RR of 15 breaths per minute with oxygen saturation of 98% on room air. Her pelvic examination reveals a closed os. Upon ultrasound examination, an intrauterine pregnancy is visualized; however, a fetal HR (FHR) is not detected. Given this patient's symptoms and physical examination, which of the following is the most appropriate diagnosis?

a. Threatened abortion
b. Complete abortion
c. Inevitable abortion
d. Incomplete abortion
e. Missed abortion

**373.** A 33-year-old G3P2002 presents to the ED complaining of vaginal bleeding that started earlier in the day. She has gone through two pads over the last 12 hours. She describes mild lower abdominal pain. Her BP is 105/75 mm Hg, HR is 78 beats per minute, temperature is 98.9°F, and RR is 14 breaths per minute. Pelvic examination reveals clotted blood in the vaginal vault with a closed cervical os. Transvaginal ultrasound documents an intrauterine pregnancy. Which of the following is the correct diagnosis?

a. Threatened abortion
b. Complete abortion
c. Inevitable abortion
d. Incomplete abortion
e. Missed abortion

**374.** A 21-year-old G4P1001 presents to the ED because she was unable to find the outpatient laboratory. She states that she was recently diagnosed with a miscarriage and was told to follow up today for repeat blood work. She denies vaginal bleeding, abdominal cramping, and has no other complaints. Her BP is 115/70 mm Hg, HR is 68 beats per minute, temperature is 98.6°F, and RR is 15 breaths per minute. Pelvic examination is normal with a closed cervical os. β-hCG is 125 mIU/mL and old records reveal her blood type to be B+. Which of the following is the correct diagnosis?

a. Threatened abortion
b. Complete abortion
c. Inevitable abortion
d. Incomplete abortion
e. Missed abortion

**375.** A 19-year-old G2P1001 presents to the ED with complaints of severe lower abdominal cramping and vaginal bleeding with the passage of several large clots. She states that she is approximately 10 weeks by LMP but has not followed up with her OB-GYN yet this pregnancy. She denies trauma or injury and has no other complaints. Her BP is 98/50 mm Hg, HR is 88 beats per minute, temperature is 98.6°F, and RR is 18 breaths per minute. Pelvic examination reveals several large clots in the vaginal vault with what appears to be mucinous material emerging from the external os. The internal os is 1 cm on bimanual examination. β-hCG is 100,850 mIU/mL and transabdominal ultrasound reveals an intrauterine pregnancy with an estimated gestational age of 9w5d by crown-rump length (CRL) and an FHR of 80. Her blood type is O+. Which of the following is the correct diagnosis?

a. Threatened abortion
b. Complete abortion
c. Inevitable abortion
d. Incomplete abortion
e. Missed abortion

**376.** A 28-year-old woman presents to the ED with heavy menstrual flow for the last 2 days with clots. She reports using about two pads every hour. The patient states that she has occasional metromenorrhagia in the past and has been treated with oral contraceptives. She reports symptoms of feeling lightheaded but denies any syncope, palpitations, chest pain, abdominal pain, or weakness. Her initial vital signs include HR of 96 beats per minute, BP of 135/70 mm Hg, and RR of 14 breaths per minute with oxygen saturation of 99% on room air. Upon physical examination, the patient is obese and you note a pronounced hairline. Which of the following conditions is most consistent with this patient's presentation?

a. Intrauterine pregnancy
b. Polycystic ovaries
c. Ectopic pregnancy
d. Follicular cyst rupture
e. Corpus luteum cyst rupture

**377.** A 22-year-old woman presents to the ED with diffuse pelvic pain and vaginal bleeding. She reports that it is about the same time when she normally has her menses. She also reports some pain with defecation, dyspareunia, and points of dysmenorrhea in the past. The patient states that she has felt this way before, but that the pain has now worsened and is intolerable. Her physical examination reveals a soft abdomen with normal bowel sounds without rebound tenderness. The patient does not guard and there is no costovertebral tenderness. Her pelvic examination is significant for blood in the posterior vaginal vault, a closed os and no palpable masses or cervical motion tenderness. Given this patient's history and physical examination, which of the following is the most likely diagnosis?

a. Ureteral colic
b. Pregnancy
c. Ruptured ectopic pregnancy
d. Endometriosis
e. Appendicitis

**378.** A 51-year-old woman presents to the ED with heavy vaginal bleeding. She reports that she has bleeding for 12 consecutive days. She also reports missing a period 3 months ago, with an ensuing menses that she states was quite heavy. She denies having any hot flashes, vaginal dryness, night sweats, or changes in weight. The patient further denies any abdominal or back pain, syncope, and palpitations but states that recently she often feels lightheaded and cannot perform her normal activities of daily living. Her initial vital signs include HR of 110 beats per minute, BP of 140/88 mm Hg, and RR of 18 breaths per minute with oxygen saturation of 98% on room air. Upon physical examination, she appears pale with a nontender abdomen and warm skin. Her pelvic examination reveals blood clots in the vaginal vault with a closed os, an enlarged uterus, and no adnexal tenderness. An ultrasound is performed that does not show any abnormalities. Which of the following diagnostic tests is most appropriate for this patient?

a. Endometrial biopsy
b. Hormonal therapy trial
c. Laparoscopic examination
d. Dilation and curettage
e. Hysterectomy and salpingectomy

**379.** A 29-year-old G1P0010 presents to the ED with sharp, right-sided flank pain of acute onset associated with nausea. The pain began approximately 1 hour before arrival. She denies any fever, hematuria, vomiting, change in bowel habit, or sick contacts. She cannot recall her LMP at this time. The patient is afebrile and her vitals are within normal limits when you begin your physical examination, which reveals a soft abdomen with mild diffuse tenderness to palpation without rebound. The patient has exquisite right flank pain. An initial urine dip is negative. Given the information you have so far, which of the following is the most probable diagnosis?

a. Appendicitis
b. PID
c. Ectopic pregnancy
d. Ureteral stone
e. Diverticulitis

**380.** A 23-year-old G1P0 presents to the ED with vaginal spotting that began earlier in the day. She denies any abdominal pain, trauma, dysuria, or back pain. Her initial vital signs include HR of 90 beats per minute, BP of 125/60 mm Hg, and RR of 14 breaths per minute with oxygen saturation of 99% on room air. Her pelvic examination is significant for a scant amount of blood in the posterior vaginal vault and a closed os. The patient has no tenderness upon bimanual examination. She states that she is 6 weeks pregnant. Given this patient's presentation, which of the following ancillary tests must be performed?

a. CBC
b. Basic metabolic panel
c. Coagulation panel
d. Type and screen
e. Urinalysis

**381.** A 22-year-old woman presents to the ED with vaginal bleeding that began earlier in the day. She reports that her LMP was 3 weeks ago. She denies any metromenorrhagia in the past. Upon physical examination, her cervical os is closed with clots in the posterior vaginal vault. There is no adnexal or cervical motion tenderness. She has mild abdominal cramps but no localizing pain. Her pregnancy test is negative. Given this patient's clinical presentation, what is the most likely diagnosis?

a. Threatened abortion
b. Normal menstrual flow
c. Ectopic pregnancy
d. Dysfunctional uterine bleeding
e. PID

**382.** A 26-year-old G1P1001 presents to the ED with vaginal spotting for the last 3 days with occasional left-sided pelvic pain. Her physical examination includes a closed cervical os, scant blood within the vaginal vault with left adnexal tenderness. Given this patient's history and physical examination, you suspect an ectopic pregnancy. In addition to a quantitative β-hCG, which of the following laboratory tests may prove helpful in the evaluation of this patient?

a. Estrogen level
b. Follicle-stimulating hormone (FSH) level
c. Thyrotropin (TSH) level
d. Progesterone level
e. CBC

**383.** A 30-year-old woman with no prior pregnancies presents to the ED with diffuse pelvic pain and vaginal spotting. The following transvaginal ultrasound is performed and shown below. What is the minimum β-hCG level needed to obtain this sonographic image?

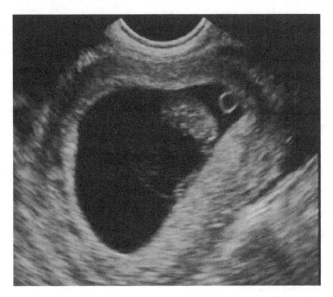

(Reproduced, with permission, from Knoop KJ, Stack LB, Storrow AB. Atlas of Emergency Medicine. New York, NY: McGraw-Hill, 2002: 645.) (Courtesy of Michael J. Lambert, MD, RDMS.)

a. 1000 mIU/mL
b. 950 mIU/mL
c. 1500 mIU/mL
d. 4000 mIU/mL
e. 6500 mIU/mL

**384.** A 32-year-old G2P1001 presents to the ED with severe abdominal pain and vaginal bleeding. She reports that she is currently in her third trimester and that she has been diagnosed and treated for preeclampsia. Her vitals are significant for a BP of 195/100 mm Hg. Upon physical examination, her abdomen is distended and hard to the touch. Given this patient's history and physical examination, what emergent intervention is most appropriate?

a. Ultrasound
b. Pelvic examination
c. Tocolytics
d. Blood transfusion
e. Maternal/fetal monitoring with possible delivery

**385.** A 28-year-old G2P0010 presents to the ED stating that she is pregnant and has vaginal spotting of blood. Pelvic examination reveals blood in the vaginal vault, but no active bleed, and a closed internal os. Transvaginal ultrasound reveals an intrauterine pregnancy consistent with a gestational age of 11 weeks. Her BP is 130/75 mm Hg, HR is 82 beats per minute, temperature is 99.1°F, and RR is 16 breaths per minute. Laboratory results reveal a WBC 10,500/μL, hematocrit 40%, and platelets 225/μL. She is blood type B, Rh-negative. Which of the following is the most appropriate intervention before discharging the patient from the ED?

a. Administer 50 μg of anti-D immune globulin.
b. Administer 2 g of magnesium sulfate to prevent eclampsia.
c. Administer penicillin G to prevent chorioamnionitis.
d. Administer ferrous sulfate to prevent anemia.
e. Administer packed red blood cells to increase blood volume.

**386.** A 4-year-old girl presents to the ED with her mother for a concern that she has been sexually abused. The mother bases this concern on a small amount of vaginal spotting that she noted in the patient's underwear this morning. The patient has no complaints and denies any abuse. Additional history is difficult due to the patient's age. Your physical examination is unremarkable. Regarding this patient, which of the following statements is true?

a. A pelvic examination should never be performed in the ED on a patient this young due to the risk of fistula formation.
b. The patient should immediately be transferred to a certified rape-examination center for evidence collection.
c. The most likely cause of her symptoms is a vaginal foreign body.
d. The patient should be evaluated for a bleeding disorder such as von Willebrand disease.
e. Reassure the mother that this is normal and that no specific intervention is required.

**387.** An 84-year-old woman presents to the ED after she noticed a small amount of vaginal spotting in her underwear over the last several weeks. She states that she is sexually active. She denies shortness of breath and weakness and has not noticed any other bleeding or bruising. Her BP is 130/75 mm Hg, HR is 82 beats per minute, temperature is 98.1°F, and RR is 16 breaths per minute. Her physical examination is unremarkable with the exception of a smooth, shiny, and friable epithelium and introital stenosis of less than 2 cm on pelvic examination. Regarding this patient, which of the following statements is true?

a. She should immediately undergo a complete evaluation, including a CBC, prothrombin time/partial thromboplastin time/international normalized ratio (PT/PTT/INR), type and screen, and CT scan of the abdomen and pelvis for staging.
b. The gynecology service should be consulted for emergent endometrial biopsy.
c. Reassure the patient that vaginal bleeding is part of the normal aging process and that additional evaluation is not required.
d. She should be evaluated for a bleeding disorder such as von Willebrand disease.
e. She should be advised to seek outpatient follow-up for serum hormone levels and Papanicolaou smear.

# Vaginal Bleeding

## *Answers*

**364. The answer is c.** (*Rosen, pp 199-203.*) A **urine or serum β-hCG** should be one of the first ancillary tests considered in any female of reproductive age, especially in a female patient presenting with vaginal bleeding regardless of their sexual, contraceptive, and menstrual history. In addition to the initial and timely urine qualitative test, a follow-up serum quantitative β-hCG is warranted if the urine test was positive. Patients who present with vaginal bleeding or abdominal pain and a positive urine or serum β-hCG need additional evaluation to determine the status of the pregnancy and exclude ectopic pregnancy. Determining if a patient is pregnant may also help distinguish if, for example, the emergent cause of her bleeding is an ectopic pregnancy versus a pathologic cervical lesion.

Although a type and screen **(a)** may be necessary in a patient with severe vaginal bleeding and hemodynamic instability, this patient is currently stable. A type and screen may also be indicated, however, if this patient is found to be pregnant in order to determine her Rh status. A coagulation panel **(b)** may be considered later in determining if the vaginal bleeding is induced by conditions such as von Willebrand disease, a relatively common cause of menorrhagia. A CBC **(d)** may also be helpful in distinguishing such conditions as idiopathic thrombocytopenia purpura. Remember the most important question to answer initially is if this patient is pregnant.

**365. The answer is d.** (*Rosen, pp 199-200.*) This patient has a significant risk factor for having an **ectopic pregnancy**. Tubal ligations raise the likelihood of having an ectopic pregnancy by providing an outlet for improper implantation of an embryo into the abdominal cavity or somewhere outside of the uterus. Extrauterine implantation most commonly occurs in the fallopian tubes, up to 95% of the time. As always, **determining the patient's β-hCG status is crucial in the beginning stages of her workup**. In a normal pregnancy, the β-hCG doubles every 48 to 72 hours but may only increase by two-thirds in this time frame in ectopic pregnancies. In a stable patient, a transvaginal ultrasound is may be warranted to determine the size and location of the ectopic and to determine any associated free fluid indicating rupture. β-hCG levels dictate whether a transvaginal (> 1500 mIU/mL) or transabdominal (> 6500 mIU/mL) approach should be used. Smaller, nonruptured ectopics may be treated with methotrexate. However, this patient is hemodynamically compromised and has most likely ruptured. Surgical intervention is warranted in these cases. Patients with ectopic pregnancies may also present with back or flank pain, syncope or peritonitis in cases with significant abdominal hemorrhage. Risk factors also include previous ectopics, intrauterine devices, PID, sexually transmitted diseases (STDs), in vitro fertilization, and recent elective abortion.

The incidence of a coexisting heterotopic pregnancy (**a**) is about 1/30,000 but increases to 1/8000 in women on fertility drugs. Both gastrointestinal (GI) and gynecological conditions should be included in the differential diagnosis of women presenting with abdominal pain. PID (**b**) often presents with gradual pelvic pain and discharge with other systemic signs of an infectious etiology, such as fever. **Placenta previa (c)** usually presents with **painless** vaginal bleeding in the second trimester. **Abruptio placentae (e)** also presents in the second or third trimester and is **painful**.

**366. The answer is a.** (*Rosen, pp 194-196, 2345-2346.*) **Uterine rupture** presents as uterine pain without contraction and vaginal bleeding. It is most prevalent in women who have had a previous cesarean section, recent cocaine, or prostaglandin use. **Cocaine** use leads to a sympathomimetic state (exhibited as tachycardia, hypertension, dilated pupils, diaphoresis, and change in mental status) and may cause **extreme vasoconstriction**. In the pregnant patient, this vasoconstriction may compromise blood flow to the uterus and fetus causing friable and necrotic tissue, which is prone to rupture. This is an obstetric emergency that necessitates emergent surgical intervention for stabilization of both mother and child.

Placenta accreta (**c**) is usually **painless** and associated with brisk, bright-red vaginal bleeding. It is caused by an indistinct placental cleavage plane and seen in the delivery of the placenta itself. Vaginal bleeding may be seen with ruptured membranes as in vasa previa (**d**); however, this is relatively **painless** and rarely seen in the ED setting. Ruptured ovarian cysts (**e**) should still be considered in the pregnant patient, and, although this may also be painful, it is rarely severe and other more life-threatening causes should be higher up on the differential diagnosis.

**367. The answer is b.** (*Rosen, pp 199-200.*) **Placenta previa**, a condition where the placenta overlies the internal os, is the most probable etiology for this patient's second-trimester **painless vaginal bleeding**. This bleeding is rarely severe and the physical examination is usually unremarkable except for a gravid uterus. It is important to note, however, that manual and speculum pelvic examinations should *not* be done until after placenta previa can be ruled out with an ultrasound, which is often diagnostic. Transvaginal ultrasound can be done because of the wide angle of the probe and low probability of penetrating the cervical os. Vaginal examination may then be performed with awareness that surgical intervention may be necessary to control bleeding.

It is important to emphasize the importance of the patient's presentation regarding **painful** or **painless** vaginal bleeding. Although other factors may alter pain, in general, it is a useful tool in helping to differentiate the diagnosis. Abruptio placentae (**c**), uterine rupture (**d**), and ovarian torsion (**e**) are painful etiologies of vaginal bleeding. Ectopic pregnancy (**a**) is usually more painful after it ruptures but may present as painless vaginal bleeding in the first trimester

**368. The answer is c.** (*Rosen, pp 199-200, 2343-2344.*) Postpartum bleeding is classified as early, if within 24 to 48 hours of delivery, or late, if up to 1 to 2 weeks. Causes of early postpartum bleeding include **uterine atony** (most common cause), genital tract trauma, retained products of conception, and uterine inversion. Late bleeding episodes may be caused by endometritis or retained products of conception. **Uterine atony is common after prolonged labor** and **oxytocin administration**. Physical examination will reveal a soft uterus and blood in the vaginal vault. Treatment consists of bimanual massage and intravenous (IV) oxytocin to stimulate uterine contractions. Ergot alkaloids may be given in refractory cases.

Although genital tract trauma (**a**) is a possible cause of early postpartum bleeding, this patient's physical examination did not reveal any lacerations or mucosal trauma. As explained, endometritis (**b**) is a later manifestation and accompanied with foul-smelling lochia in addition to a tender, swollen uterus. This patient is afebrile and did not exhibit any systemic signs of infection. Ectopic pregnancy (**d**) is extremely unlikely given this patient's recent history of giving birth. Uterine artery rupture (**e**) is also unlikely and most commonly occurs at time of delivery followed by a period of extreme hemodynamic instability.

**369. The answer is d.** (*Rosen, p 2346.*) Postpartum bleeding is classified as early, if within 24 to 48 hours of delivery, or late, up to 1 to 2 weeks.

Causes of early postpartum bleeding include uterine atony, genital tract trauma, retained products of conception, and uterine inversion. Late bleeding episodes may be caused by **endometritis** or retained products of conception. Patients with endometritis most often present with **fever, vaginal discharge, general malaise, and vaginal bleeding**. Upon pelvic examination, the uterus will be soft and tender to the touch. The majority of infections are caused by normal vaginal flora, such as anaerobes, enterococci, and streptococci. Patients who do not respond to initial antibiotic therapy may warrant broader-spectrum coverage and need to be further evaluated for a pelvic abscess or pelvic thrombophlebitis.

Uterine atony (**a**) and uterine inversion (**c**) are earlier causes of postpartum bleeding. Although retained products of conception (**b**) is a possibility in this patient, her presentation is more likely to be infectious given her fever and significant abdominal tenderness. Tubo-ovarian torsion (**e**) is unlikely given that the patient's physical examination did not reveal any peritoneal signs. This patient's clinical picture is consistent with an infectious etiology. If a gynecologic process is not found, other causes of infection must be ruled out including appendicitis.

**370. The answer is b.** *(Rosen, p 2285.)* Patients presenting with a **molar pregnancy** typically have severe nausea and vomiting, a uterus larger than expected for dates, hypertension, and intermittent vaginal bleeding or passage of grape-like contents. Risk factors include a previous history of molar pregnancy, and very young or advanced maternal ages. Typically, laboratory results reveal anemia on a CBC, β-hCG higher than expected, and an ultrasound that shows intrauterine echogenic material. Treatment includes dilation and curettage with future monitoring and evaluation for the development of **choriocarcinoma**.

Ectopic pregnancy (**a**) can be ruled out with the ultrasound evaluation. Ovarian torsion (**c**) can also be ruled out given the sonogram which would show good Doppler flow to both ovaries. Abruptio placentae (**d**) is unlikely given the early stage of this pregnancy. Hyperemesis gravidarum (**e**) is a syndrome of intractable nausea and vomiting that occurs early in pregnancy but is generally not associated with significant changes in vital signs or abnormal findings on ultrasound.

**371. The answer is c.** *(Rosen, pp 2279-2280.)* **Inevitable abortions** are diagnosed in **first-trimester bleeding** with an **open internal cervical os** but **no passage of fetal products**. Determining whether the internal os is open can be difficult and is often confused with the normally distended external os. In inevitable abortions, dilation and curettage with full evacuation of the pregnancy is warranted. Rh immunization may also be needed depending on the status of the patient; therefore, a type and screen should be obtained. First-trimester vaginal bleeding occurs in about 40% of pregnancies with approximately half of them eventually resulting in spontaneous miscarriages.

A threatened abortion (**a**) is defined as any vaginal bleeding with a closed os and no passage of fetal tissue during in the first 20 weeks of gestation. A complete abortion (**b**) is the passage of all fetal products and products of conception with a now closed os. An incomplete abortion (**d**) is the partial passage of fetal products or products of conception but with an open cervical os and some products remaining. A missed abortion (**e**) is when there is a nonliving fetus in the uterus with a closed os.

**372. The answer is e.** *(Rosen, pp 2279-2280.)* This patient presents with **vaginal bleeding** and a **closed os**, which narrows the diagnosis to either a threatened, complete, or missed abortion. The ultrasound examination reveals an **intrauterine pregnancy** that is still present **without a fetal HR**, which confirms the **missed abortion**. A dilation and curettage and Rh prophylaxis is warranted to prevent further infection and coagulopathy.

A threatened abortion (**a**) is defined as any vaginal bleeding with a closed os and no passage of fetal tissue during in the first 20 weeks of gestation. A complete abortion (**b**) is the passage of all fetal products and products of conception with a now closed os. **Inevitable abortions (c)** have an **open internal cervical os** but **no passage of fetal products**. An incomplete abortion (**d**) is the partial passage of fetal products or products of conception but with an open cervical os and some products remaining.

**373. The answer is a.** *(Rosen, pp 199-203.)* In a **threatened abortion**, the patient has vaginal bleeding with a closed internal os in the first 20 weeks of gestation. The risk of miscarriage is approximately 35% to 50%, depending on the patient population and severity of symptoms.

A complete abortion (**b**) is the passage of all fetal products and products of conception with a now closed os. Inevitable abortions (**c**) have an open internal cervical os but no passage of fetal products. An incomplete abortion (**d**) is the partial passage of fetal products or products of conception but with an open cervical os and some products remaining.

**374. The answer is b.** (*Rosen, pp 194-198.*) In a **completed abortion**, the patient has passed all products of conception, including fetal tissue and placenta and now has a closed os. In some patients, β-hCG hormone levels may be followed to ensure that they continue to drop, but this is not necessary in all cases.

A threatened abortion (**a**) is defined as any vaginal bleeding with a closed os and no passage of fetal tissue during in the first 20 weeks of gestation. Inevitable abortions (**c**) have an open internal cervical os but no passage of fetal products. An incomplete abortion (**d**) is the partial passage of fetal products or products of conception but with an open cervical os and some products remaining.

**375. The answer is d.** (*Rosen, pp 1329-1331.*) An incomplete abortion is the partial passage of fetal products or products of conception but with an open cervical os and some products remaining, in this case an age appropriate fetus with an abnormally slow heart rate. In this patient a dilation and curettage or manual vacuum aspiration is warranted.

A threatened abortion (**a**) is defined as any vaginal bleeding with a closed os and no passage of fetal tissue during in the first 20 weeks of gestation. A complete abortion (**b**) is the passage of all fetal products and products of conception with a now closed os. Inevitable abortions (**c**) have an open internal cervical os but no passage of fetal products. A missed abortion (**e**) is when an intrauterine pregnancy is present, but there is no fetal heart rate and the os is closed.

**376. The answer is b.** (*Rosen, pp 193-198, 2281-2285.*) This patient exhibits signs of hyperandrogenism and anovulation as evidenced by her history of irregular, heavy periods and being treated with oral contraceptives. Her physical examination is consistent with hirsutism, which is a result of increased serum testosterone. Many of these patients are also obese. For these reasons, **polycystic ovarian syndrome** is the most probable reason for this patient's symptoms.

Intrauterine and ectopic pregnancy (**a and c**) should always be ruled out with a β-hCG. Follicular cysts (**d**) are very common and usually occur within the first 2 weeks of the menstrual cycle. Pain is secondary to stretching of the capsule and cyst rupture. Follicular cysts usually resolve within 1 to 3 months and do not result in bleeding. Corpus luteum cysts (**e**) occur in the last 2 weeks of the menstrual cycle and are less common. Bleeding into the capsule may occur, but these cysts usually regress at the end of the menstrual cycle. In general, cysts are usually asymptomatic unless they are complicated by rupture, torsion, or hemorrhage. Ultrasound is the preferred mode of imaging.

**377. The answer is d.** *(Rosen, pp 201-202, 2279-2281.)* **Endometriosis** is defined by the presence of endometrial glands and tissue outside the lining of the uterus. This tissue may be present on the ovaries, fallopian tubes, bladder, rectum, appendix, or other GI tissue. There are many different hypotheses as to how this ectopic tissue forms, the most commonly accepted being "retrograde menstruation." Pain most commonly occurs before or at the beginning of menses. Other symptoms that indicate ectopic endometrial implantation and activation include dyspareunia and problems with defecation. Clinical suspicions can only be confirmed with direct visualization through **laparoscopy**. Treatment includes analgesia for acute episodes and hormonal therapy to suppress the normal menstrual cycle so that purely the endometrial tissue may be sloughed during menses. Surgical intervention is taken for those cases that are truly refractory to these treatments.

Ureteral colic **(a)** is unlikely given the lack of flank tenderness, dysuria, and prior history of stones. Obtaining a urinalysis will be complicated by the presence of menstrual blood. Again, pregnancy **(b)** and therefore ectopics **(c)** should always be ruled out with a quick and easy β-hCG. The probability of appendicitis **(e)** is low given that this patient's abdominal examination is unremarkable.

**378. The answer is a.** *(Rosen, pp 2279-2280.)* The menstrual cycle consists of a follicular phase and a luteal phase. The follicular, or proliferative, phase begins on the first day of menses and continues until ovulation whereupon the luteal, or secretory, phase begins. During the follicular phase, endometrial glands form under the influences of estrogen, primarily estradiol. In the luteal phase, estrogen is still present, but progesterone takes over and is mainly responsible for endometrial secretion and prepares the lining of the uterus for implantation. The luteal phase is characterized by an elevated body temperature and stromal edema. When implantation does not occur, menses ensues as a result of falling hormonal levels, which cause coiling and constrict the endometrial arteries. An elevated β-hCG maintains the corpus luteum. **Dysfunctional uterine bleeding (DUB)** is any abnormality in the regular bleeding pattern of the menstrual cycle and anovulation is the usual cause. This is the ovaries' failure to secrete an ovum, which thereby prevents luteinization from occurring. Without progesterone, the endometrium proliferates. This can lead to endometrial hyperplasia, which increases the risk for carcinoma. Other causes of symptoms of DUB include uterine fibroids, uterine polyps, genital tract trauma, exogenous estrogens, endocrine axis dysfunction, and bleeding disorders. Menopause occurs on average at the age of 51 years 6 months. Given that this woman is close to this age, this could also be perimenopausal symptoms. Hormone levels may be checked to see if they are falling. However, endometrial carcinoma may present in a similar way and needs to be ruled out with an **endometrial biopsy**.

Hormonal therapy **(b)** should not be used in this patient given that she is older and this can increase her chances of endometrial hyperplasia. Dilation and curettage **(d)** is not warranted given that she does not have a diagnosis yet. Any surgical intervention, **(c and e)** should be held until a biopsy is performed.

**379. The answer is c.** (*Rosen, pp 199-203.*) It is very important to stress the possibility that any fertile female is pregnant until proven otherwise. Obtaining a urine β-hCG along with an ultrasound could save your patient's life, as other essential tests and consults are being acquired. In this case of a **ruptured ectopic pregnancy**, the presentation is atypical, but it may be said that it is essentially typical of ectopics. These are, by very nature, implantations that can occur anywhere in the abdominal cavity. It is therefore imperative to keep this life-threatening diagnosis at the top of your differential.

Appendicitis **(a)** is unlikely given this patient's examination and temperature. This patient does not have any of the signs for PID **(b)** or any changes in bowel habits that would suggest diverticulitis **(e)**. This clinical scenario is challenging in the sense that the ectopic pregnancy mimics a very painful albeit not life-threatening illness like a ureteral stone **(d)**. It is important to take into account negative tests, as in the urine dip, as well as positive ones to narrow in on the diagnosis. These can be tricky, as some stones are obstructing and do cause hematuria.

**380. The answer is d.** (*Rosen, pp 201, 2282-2284.*) In any patient who is **pregnant** with **vaginal bleeding**, it is imperative to obtain a type and screen in order to identify the **Rh status** of the patient. Rhesus isoimmunization is an immunologic disorder that affects Rh-negative mothers of Rh-positive fetuses. Any transplacental maternal exposure to fetal Rh-positive blood cells can initiate this, whether its origin is traumatic or not. Initial exposure leads to primary sensitization and the production of antibodies. In subsequent pregnancies, these maternal antibodies can then cross the placenta and attack the fetal Rh-positive blood cells. Prevention can be accomplished by giving RhoGAM to all mothers who are Rh-negative. Administration of the immune globulin can be given prophylactically at 28 weeks or at the time of maternal exposure. **(a)** A CBC would be required if the patient described increased bleeding or had signs of anemia or hypovolemia (eg, shortness of breath, dizziness). **(b)** A basic metabolic panel does not add any information regarding this patient's presentation. **(c)** A coagulation panel would be useful if you suspected a bleeding disorder or if the patient was hemorrhaging. **(e)** The patient does not have signs or symptoms of a urinary tract infection.

**381. The answer is b.** *(Rosen, pp 201, 2280-2284.)* It is important to remember that sometimes patients come to the ED with benign or normal conditions in which education and counsel are the treatments of choice.

In this case, it is true that her menstrual flow is early, but a one-time occurrence does not give the diagnoses of dysfunctional uterine bleeding **(d)** or endometriosis. If this patient had a history of bleeding before the day of her presentation, a complete abortion would have to be investigated. Given her negative β-hCG, an ectopic pregnancy **(c)** or threatened abortion **(a)** can be ruled out. PID **(e)** presents with fever, abdominal pain, purulent vaginal discharge, and a positive STD history, not vaginal bleeding.

**382. The answer is d.** *(Rosen, pp 199-200, 2345-2346, 2286-2287.)* **Progesterone levels** may be helpful in distinguishing ectopic pregnancies. A level of less than 5 ng/mL is highly suggestive of an ectopic pregnancy, given that the uterus may not be able to carry the pregnancy. Higher levels indicate that embryo implantation inside the uterus is more likely.

Estrogen levels **(a)** and FSH **(b)** may prove helpful in distinguishing menopausal symptoms or aiding infertile women. TSH levels **(c)** are useful when reaching a diagnosis in women with irregular menstrual flow. A CBC **(e)** is not warranted given that this patient is not hemorrhaging. A type and screen should be performed to determine Rh status.

**383. The answer is c.** *(Rosen, pp 2279-2280.)* Given that this is a transvaginal ultrasound, the threshold for visualizing a pregnancy is lower than the transabdominal approach (β-hCG > 6500 mIU/mL). A transvaginal ultrasound can typically identify a gestational sac when the β-hCG level is greater than 1000 mIU/mL, and the yolk sac when the β-hCG level is greater than 2500 mIU/mL.

**384. The answer is e.** *(Rosen, pp 2280-2281.)* There is a high probability that this patient is suffering from a uterine rupture or abruptio placentae. **Monitoring** should be instilled immediately with **preparation for delivery**. Emergent obstetrical consultation is warranted for repair and possible cesarean section. Risk factors include trauma, hypertension, recreational drug use, smoking, multiparity, and advanced maternal age.

Ultrasound (**a**) is not useful in these cases, given that this is mainly a clinical diagnosis. Tocolytics (**c**) should not be given to prevent delivery, because this is often the treatment of choice. In cases of hemodynamic compromise as a result of excessive blood loss, blood transfusions (**d**) are indicated. A type and crossmatch should be done in this case in preparation for such an intervention. A brief external look to examine for vaginal bleeding may be done, but a complete pelvic examination (**b**) is not warranted because it may worsen bleeding.

**385. The answer is a.** *(Rosen, p 2415.)* **Rh isoimmunization** occurs when an Rh-negative female is exposed to Rh-positive blood during pregnancy or delivery. Initial exposure leads to primary sensitization with production of immunoglobulin M antibodies. A patient with a threatened abortion, who has Rh-negative blood, is at increased risk for Rh isoimmunization and therefore should receive **anti-D immune globulin**. A 50-μg dose is used during the first trimester and a 300-μg dose after the first trimester.

(**b**) Eclampsia is a syndrome of hypertension, proteinuria, generalized edema, and seizures that usually occurs after the second trimester in pregnancy. (**c**) Chorioamnionitis is an infection of the chorioamniotic membrane. Pregnant patients after 16 weeks present with fever and uterine tenderness. (**d**) Ferrous sulfate is used as a supplement to help treat anemia. This patient is not anemic. (**e**) This patient does not require a blood transfusion; her BP is normal and her hematocrit is normal.

**386. The answer is c.** *(Rosen, p 2285.)* Although sexual abuse is possible, **vaginal foreign bodies** are a much **more common** cause of vaginal bleeding in this population. Although pelvic examination may be difficult, it is an essential part of the physical examination (**a**) in this patient and may require sedation to adequately visualize the vaginal vault and remove a foreign body (often a bead or other small object). If there are any signs of genital trauma, the proper authorities should be immediately notified. Transfer to a certified rape-collection center (**b**) should be considered. Abnormally heavy vaginal bleeding may be a presenting symptom of von Willebrand factor (VWF) deficiency (**d**) but would not be expected in a patient this young. Vaginal bleeding is not normal in a 4-year-old (**e**), but most of the causes are benign.

**387. The answer is e.** *(Rosen, p 2281)* Up to 40% of postmenopausal women will develop **atrophic vaginitis**, a condition that may cause vaginal dryness, spotting, itching, dyspareunia, and urinary frequency, urgency, and incontinence. Many postmenopausal patients who develop vaginal bleeding are concerned that they have developed cancer and should be referred for an outpatient endometrial biopsy to evaluate for this. Patients with confirmed atrophic vaginitis may be started on estrogen replacement and treated symptomatically with local moisturizers and lubricants.

# Ultrasound in the Emergency Department

## Questions

**388.** A 35-year-old woman presents to the ED via ambulance after being involved in an automobile collision. EMS reports the patient was a restrained front seat passenger in a car struck on the front passenger door with significant cabin intrusion. The patient was nonambulatory on scene and required prolonged extraction from the vehicle. The vital signs on scene after extrication were blood pressure (BP) 105/80 mm Hg, heart rate (HR) 115 beats per minute, respiratory rate (RR) 22 breaths per minute, and oxygen saturation 100% on a non-rebreather mask. Two larger-bore IVs were established with 2 L of normal saline infused during extrication and transport. On arrival in the emergency department (ED), the patient does not remember what happened. She complains of pain in the right forearm and abdomen. In the ED her vital signs are BP 90/65 mm Hg, HR 140 beats per minute, temperature 98.9°F, RR 35 breaths per minute, and oxygen saturation 100% on a non-rebreather mask. Physical examination reveals a diaphoretic patient who responds to painful stimuli. She answers questions but is confused. On examination, her abdomen is nondistended, soft, and tender along the right upper and lower quadrants on moderate palpation. Her dorsal forearm has a 4-cm laceration with active oozing of blood. She is neurovascularly intact in the right extremity, and no deformities are noted. There is no other evidence of trauma. A second liter of normal saline is started, type O–negative blood is ordered, and the type and cross match is sent to the laboratory. Chest and pelvis radiographs are negative for acute injury. You obtain a focused assessment by sonography for trauma (FAST) examination, shown in the following image. What is the next best step in the management of the patient?

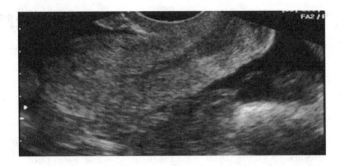

a. Continue intravenous (IV) fluids and obtain a computed tomographic (CT) scan of her head.

b. Continue IV fluids and obtain a CT scan of her abdomen and pelvis.

c. Wait for the hemoglobin result and, if low, administer 2 units of packed red blood cells (RBCs).

d. Transport the patient to the operating room for emergent therapeutic laparotomy.

e. Place interlocking stitches to close the forearm laceration to control bleeding and prevent her BP from dropping even further.

**389.** A 16-year-old girl present to the ED complaining of severe sudden-onset sharp pain located in the right lower quadrant (RLQ). The pain started suddenly 1 hour before presentation. The pain is associated with a single episode of nonbloody emesis; however, no diarrhea, vaginal bleeding, vaginal discharge, frequency, or burning with urination was reported. The patient denies any sexual activity in her past. She states she is G0P0 and her last normal menstrual period was 3 weeks ago. Her BP is 130/75 mm Hg, HR is 115 beats per minute, temperature is 99.3°F, RR is 18 breaths per minute, and oxygen saturation is 100% on room air. Physical examination shows a very uncomfortable appearing patient holding her RLQ. Her abdomen is tender in the RLQ with mild voluntary guarding but no rebound tenderness, Rovsing sign, psoas, or obturator signs. Pelvic examination shows right adnexal tenderness, with no masses, cervical motion tenderness, or discharge. Laboratory results reveal a urinalysis with 1+ leukocyte esterase, negative qualitative β-human chorionic gonadotropin (β-hCG), white blood cell (WBC) count 8000/μL, hematocrit 46%, and platelets 270/μL. Which of the following ultrasound findings helps to rule out ovarian torsion as this patient's diagnosis?

a. Unilateral enlarged ovary secondary to edema
b. Venous and arterial blood flow detected with Doppler sonography of the right ovary
c. Free fluid in the pouch of Douglas
d. Normal-sized ovary with no surrounding ovarian mass
e. Presence of right adnexal mass measuring 5 cm at largest diameter

**390.** A 23-year-old woman presents to the ED with abdominal discomfort located in the left lower quadrant (LLQ) for the past 3 days. The pain is intermittent, nonradiating, with no alleviating or aggravating factors. She denies vomiting, diarrhea, dysuria, vaginal bleeding, or vaginal discharge. The patient states she is sexually active with one partner and her last menstrual period (LMP) was 2 weeks ago. Her BP is 115/70 mm Hg, HR is 75 beats per minute, temperature is 98.6°F, RR is 15 breaths per minute, and oxygen saturation is 100% on room air. Physical examination is unremarkable. Urinalysis shows no evidence of hematuria or infection. Qualitative β-hCG is positive. Bedside transvaginal pelvic ultrasound is obtained as seen below.

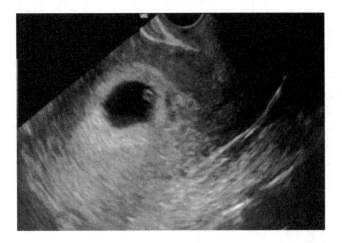

Which of the following is the earliest ultrasound finding confirming intrauterine pregnancy (IUP)?

a. Gestational sac with visualized endometrial stripe
b. Gestational sac containing yolk sack and embryonic pole with visualized endometrial stripe
c. Blighted ovum with visualized endometrial stripe
d. Intradecidual sign with visualized endometrial stripe
e. Gestational sac containing yolk sac with visualized endometrial stripe

**391.** Emergency medical service (EMS) was called to the scene of an unconscious 38-year-old man with labored breathing. EMS intubated the patient, placed two large-bore IVs, and began a normal saline infusion. On arrival in the ED, his BP is 70/30 mm Hg, HR is 140 beats per minute, temperature is 98.9°F, and oxygen saturation is 100% on a non-rebreather. Physical examination reveals a diaphoretic male, moving all four extremities spontaneously, but he is not following commands. The neck examination reveals elevated jugular venous pressure and a midline trachea. A single puncture wound is noted just below the xiphoid process; however, no abdominal distension is appreciated on abdominal examination. Your FAST examination is as shown in the following the ultrasound image. What is the next best step in the patient's management?

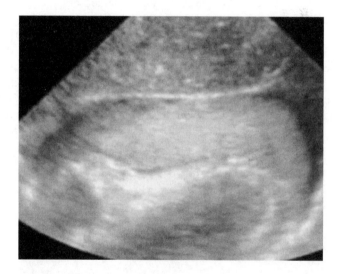

a. ED resuscitative thoracotomy after placement of a chest tube.
b. Immediate transfer to the operating room for emergent laparotomy and pelvic binding.
c. Immediate transfer to operating room for emergent thoracotomy.
d. Stat CT scan of the abdomen and pelvis to evaluate for hollow viscus injury.
e. Perform a stat bedside pericardiocentesis.

**392.** A 42-year-old woman presents to the ED complaining of abdominal pain that is located in her right upper quadrant (RUQ). The pain started 5 hours before presentation after a meal. She describes the pain as sharp, radiating around the right flank and into the back. The pain never completely goes away but waxes and wanes in intensity. This pain is associated with nausea and vomiting, but no diarrhea or fever has been noted. Her review of systems reveals that she has been getting sharp pains in her RUQ after meals for the past year. Her BP is 145/75 mm Hg, HR is 110 beats per minute, temperature is 100.3°F, RR is 16 breaths per minute, and oxygen saturation is 100% on room air. The physical examination shows a non-distended abdomen with tenderness to palpation in the RUQ. There is no rebound or guarding. When the patient tries to inhale during deep palpation of the RUQ, she is forced to pause during inspiration because of extreme pain. Laboratory results reveal WBC 16,000/μL, hematocrit 48%, platelets 250/μL, aspartate aminotransferase (AST) 45 U/L, alanine aminotransferase (ALT) 40 U/L, alkaline phosphatase 75 U/L, amylase 50 U/L, lipase 40 U/L, sodium 140 mEq/L, potassium 3.5 mEq/L, chloride 110 mEq/L, bicarbonate 24 mEq/L, blood urea nitrogen (BUN) 9 mg/dL, creatinine 0.5 mg/dL, and glucose 85 mg/dL. You obtain a bedside ultrasound scan as seen below and find the following image showing a gallbladder wall thickness of 7 mm. Which of the following is a later finding of cholecystitis?

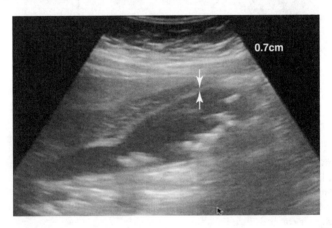

a. Cholelithiasis
b. Sonographic Murphy sign
c. Mucosal sloughing
d. Gallbladder wall thickening
e. Pericholecystic fluid

**393.** A 25-year-old man presents to the ED after being shot in the face with a shotgun at long range. The patient complains of pain generally across his face; however, the pain is greatest around his right eye. He is not sure if he can see out of the eye because the right eyelid is swollen shut. His BP is 140/80 mm Hg, HR is 105 beats per minute, temperature is 98.4°F, RR is 18 breaths per minute, and oxygen saturation is 100% on room air. Physical examination shows multiple pellet marks across the face. The right eyelid has a grouping of pellet marks and is swollen shut with surrounding ecchymosis and edema. The eyelid cannot be pried open secondary to pain limitation and further attempts at direct visualization of the eye where deferred for concern of manually increasing intraocular pressure. The rest of the physical examination was unremarkable. Bedside ocular ultrasound was obtained as seen below. Which of the following is the most likely diagnosis?

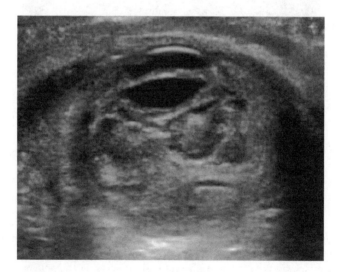

a. Intact globe
b. Retinal detachment
c. Lens dislocation
d. Globe rupture
e. Retrobulbar hematoma

**394.** A 70-year-old man presents to the ED complaining of pain in his left back and flank. He describes the pain as dull and aching. The pain started 1 day before presentation while watching TV. The pain is constant and does not radiate. He has no history of trauma or heavy lifting, and nothing seems to make the pain worse or better. His BP is 170/95 mm Hg, HR is 88 beats per minute, temperature is 97.6°F, RR is 17 breaths per minute, and oxygen saturation is 100% on room air. The physical examination and laboratory studies are unremarkable. A bedside ultrasound is obtained as seen below with the transverse and sagittal views of the aorta. Which of the following is the most accurate way to measure abdominal aortic aneurysm diameter?

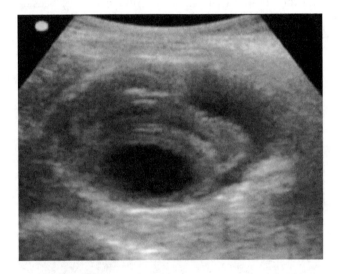

a. While viewing the aorta in a sagittal plane, measure anterior to posterior diameter from inner wall to inner wall.
b. While viewing the aorta in a transverse plane, measure anterior to posterior diameter from inner wall to inner wall.
c. While viewing the aorta in a transverse plane, measure anterior to posterior diameter from outer wall to outer wall.
d. While viewing the aorta in a sagittal plane, measure the anterior posterior diameter from outer wall to outer wall.
e. While viewing the aorta in a transverse plane, measure anterior to posterior diameter from outer wall to inner wall.

**395.** A 55-year-old woman is brought to ED after being struck by an automobile. Per EMS, she was crossing an intersection when an automobile ran a stop sign striking her on the left side. The patient was found lying supine in the street alert and oriented to person, place, and time. Prehospital vital signs were BP 100/85 mm Hg, HR 120 beats per minute, RR 22 breaths per minute, and oxygen saturation 95% on room air. Intravenous access was established with normal saline being infused during transfer to your ED. On arrival in the ED, the patient complains of pain in the left hip and pelvic region. Vital signs in the ED are BP 95/60 mm Hg, HR 135 beats per minute, temperature 97.5°F, RR 28 breaths per minute, and oxygen saturation 100% on a non-rebreather. Physical examination reveals a pale diaphoretic patient. The breath sounds are clear bilaterally and her abdomen is soft and nondistended. Her pelvis appears stable, but exquisite pain is elicited with rocking of the pelvis. Her extremity examination reveals no leg length or temperature discrepancies, and she is neurovascularly intact throughout the lower extremities. The examination of her perineum reveals ecchymosis on the perineum and blood at the urethral meatus. You obtain a FAST examination as seen below and a pelvic radiograph that shows markedly widened view of the pubic symphysis. After pelvic binding is applied, what is the next best step in the management of this patient?

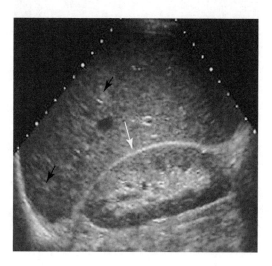

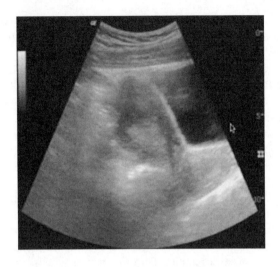

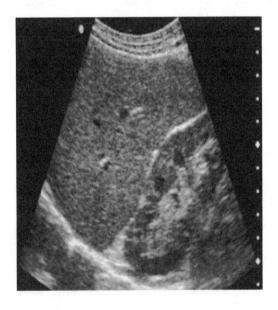

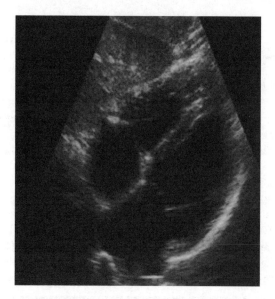

a. CT scan of the abdomen and pelvis with intravenous contrast
b. Transport to operating room for emergent laparotomy
c. Transport to the interventional radiology suite for embolization
d. Foley catheter to evaluate for hematuria
e. CT thorax with intravenous contrast

**396.** A 30-year-old man presents to the ED complaining of severe pain in the left side and back. He states that the pain started suddenly 5 hours before presentation and describes the pain as stabbing. The patient has never experienced the pain previously and states the pain comes and goes in intensity but never completely goes away. The pain radiates to his left groin and denies any alleviating or aggravating factors. The patient denies any hematuria, burning with urination, fever, vomiting, changes in bowel habits, recent trauma, or heavy lifting. His BP is 155/80 mm Hg, HR is 105 beats per minute, temperature is 99.5°F, RR is 18 breaths per minute, and oxygen saturation is 100% on room air. Physical examination shows a patient in obvious pain who cannot seem to find a position of comfort. The only remarkable finding was costovertebral angel tenderness on the left side. Laboratory results reveal sodium 142 mEq/L, potassium 4.0 mEq/L, chloride 110 mEq/L, bicarbonate 24 mEq/L, BUN 12 mg/dL, creatinine 0.7 mg/dL, and glucose 100 mg/dL. Urinalysis shows 2+ blood and RBC 20 to 50/hpf. A bedside renal ultrasound is obtained. Which of the following findings on ultrasound is consistent with severe hydronephrosis?

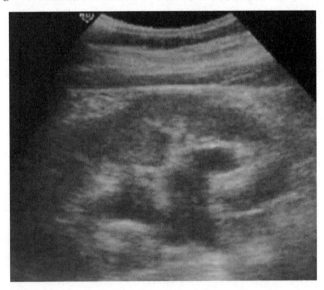

a. Anechoic collections around the renal pelvis with dividing segments of renal cortex
b. Prominent anechoic renal calyces
c. Prominent anechoic renal pelvis and calyces
d. Prominent anechoic renal pelvis and calyces with cortical thinning
e. Prominent renal pelvis and calyces with echogenic structure at ureteropelvic junction casting clean shadowing in the background

**397.** A 48-year-old man was reroofing the second story of his house when he slipped and fell to the ground, landing on his right side. EMS arrived at the scene, placed the patient in spinal precautions, and established an IV. On arrival to the ED, he complains of pain along the right costal margin going to his right lateral chest and in his RUQ. He states it hurts to breathe but has not other complaints. His BP is 130/80 mm Hg, HR is 110 beats per minute, temperature is 98.9°F, RR is 25 breaths per minute and shallow, and oxygen saturation is 100% on room air. Physical examination reveals the patient taking rapid shallow breaths and holding his right hemithorax. His neck examination shows no elevated jugular venous pressure and his trachea is midline. His chest wall is tender down the right lateral wall. You do not palpate crepitus. His breath sounds are equal to auscultation bilateral. His abdominal examination reveals a nondistended abdomen, but there is tenderness in the RUQ. A 2-L bolus of normal saline is started and you obtain a FAST examination, as shown in the following image. What is the next best step in the management of this patient?

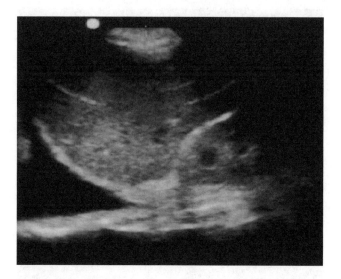

a. Chest tube thoracostomy
b. Rapid sequence intubation
c. CT scan of the thorax with intravenous contrast
d. CT scan of the abdomen and pelvis with intravenous contrast
e. Transport to the operating room for emergent laparotomy

**398.** A 55-year-old man presents to the ED complaining of epigastric abdominal pain. He describes the pain as gradual in onset, burning in nature, and radiates through to his back. It is associated with vomiting and diarrhea. His BP is 180/90 mm Hg, HR is 100 beats per minute, temperature is 98.9°F, RR is 20 breaths per minute, and oxygen saturation is 100% on room air. On physical examination, his abdomen is soft and nondistended, but there is marked tenderness in the epigastrium. The remainder of his examination is normal. Laboratory results reveal WBC 12,000/μL, hematocrit 48%, platelets 250/μL, AST 500 U/L, ALT 600 U/L, alkaline phosphatase 450 U/L, amylase 1500 U/L, lipase 2000 U/L, total bilirubin 3.0 mg/dL, sodium 150 mEq/L, potassium 4.4 mEq/L, chloride 90 mEq/L, bicarbonate 20 mEq/L, BUN 9 mg/dL, creatinine 0.5 mg/dL, and glucose 110 mg/dL. You obtain a bedside ultrasound scan that reveals as shown in the following image. Which of the following findings is consistent with extrahepatic biliary obstruction?

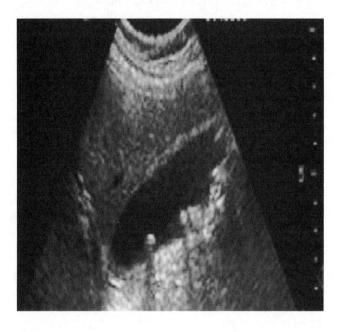

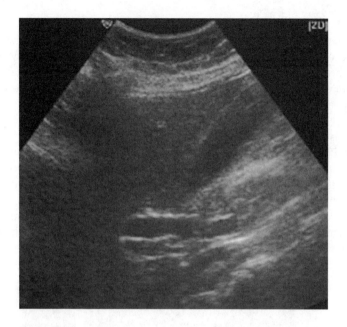

a. Mickey Mouse sign
b. Increased echogenicity with irregular texture of the liver
c. Playboy bunny sign
d. Double barrel shotgun sign or parallel channel sign
e. Antler signs

**399.** A 25-year-old woman with a history of pelvic inflammatory disease presents to the ED with abdominal pain. The pain is located in the RLQ and has been sharp, constant, and nonradiating for the last 2 days. The pain is associated with some vomiting and vaginal spotting. The patient denies fever, change in bowel habits, or vaginal discharge. Her LMP was 4 weeks ago and has been having unprotected sex with two partners. Her BP is 110/75 mm Hg, HR is 80 beats per minute, temperature is 99.1°F, RR is 16 breaths per minute, and oxygen saturation is 100% on room air. Physical examination reveals a tender abdomen in the RLQ with no rebound or guarding. Pelvic examination shows a closed cervical os with scant vaginal bleeding. There was right adnexal tenderness without fullness and no cervical motion tenderness. Urinalysis shows no evidence of hematuria or infection. Qualitative β-hCG is positive. The following ultrasound images are obtained of the uterus and left ovary, respectively. Which of the following confirms an ectopic pregnancy?

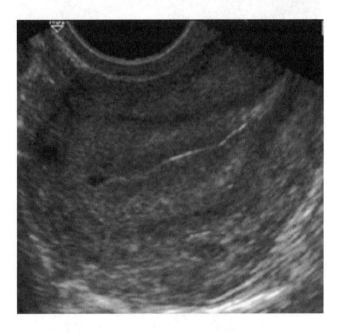

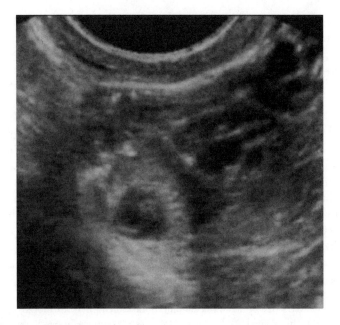

a. Free fluid in the cul-de-sac posterior to the cervix
b. Gestational sac with yolk sac in the adnexa
c. Complex adnexal mass
d. Tubal ring
e. Ring of fire sign

**400.** A 30-year-old, 8 weeks' pregnant woman presents to the ED with vomiting 10 to 20 times a day for the past 5 days. The patient also noticed some vaginal spotting over the last day, with no discharge, no urinary complaints, no abdominal pain, and no diarrhea. Her BP is 135/75 mm Hg, HR is 100 beats per minute, temperature is 97.9°F, RR is 18 breaths per minute, and oxygen saturation is 100% on room air. Physical examination shows dry mucous membranes and a nontender abdomen with a gravid uterus extending half way between the pubic symphysis and umbilicus. Pelvic examination shows scant blood in the vaginal vault with a closed cervical os. Laboratory results reveal serum sodium 143 mEq/L, potassium 3.9 mEq/L, chloride 95 mEq/L, bicarbonate 19 mEq/L, BUN 15 mg/dL, creatinine 1 mg/dL, and glucose 105 mg/dL; urinalysis shows a specific gravity greater than 1.030 g/mL and 3+ ketones; and quantitative β-hCG is 1,500,000 mIU/mL. Which of the following ultrasound findings confirms the diagnosis?

a. Thin-walled unilocular anechoic cystic structure measuring 4 cm in diameter on the ovary
b. Cluster of grapes in the uterine cavity
c. Hypoechoic stripe between the endometrium and chorionic membrane
d. Multiple thin-walled multilocular cystic masses on each ovary measuring approximately 6 cm in diameter
e. Hypoechoic solid spherical mass in the uterine wall

**401.** A 35-year-old man presents to the ED with pain and redness on his left anterior forearm. The patient does have a history of intravenous drug abuse and states he has noticed his symptoms for the last 4 days after injecting heroin in the region. He denies fever, chills, nausea, vomiting, and malaise. His BP is 140/70 mm Hg, HR is 85 beats per minute, temperature is 99.2°F, RR is 16 breaths per minute, and oxygen saturation is 100% on room air. Physical examination shows an area of erythema on the proximal anterior forearm extending 5 × 5 cm. The area is warm and painful to touch, with a central area of induration, but no obvious fluctuance. The patient has full range of motion of his left elbow and is neurovascularly intact in the distal left upper extremity. The rest of the physical examination is unremarkable. A bedside soft tissue ultrasound is performed. Which of the following images is diagnostic of an underlying abscess?

a.

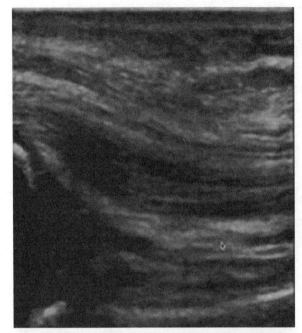

b.

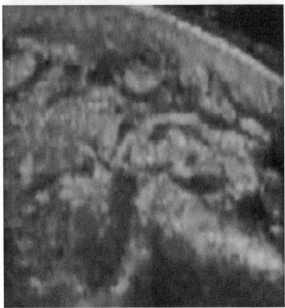

c.

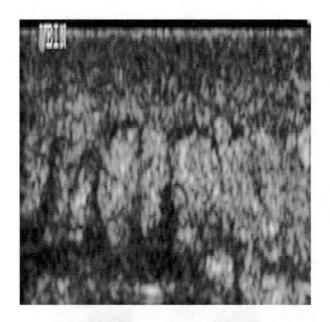

d.

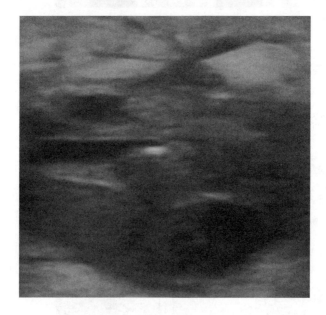

e.

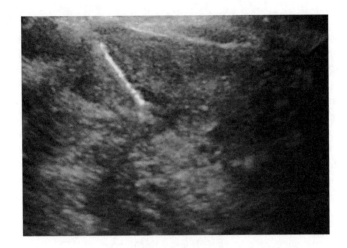

**402.** A 60-year-old woman presents to the ED stating that she is turning yellow. Her husband first noticed her skin turning yellow 2 weeks ago. The patient has no other complaints and is otherwise healthy. Her BP is 130/70 mm Hg, HR is 80 beats per minute, temperature is 97.4°F, RR is 16 breaths per minute, and oxygen saturation is 100% on room air. On physical examination, her abdomen is soft without any tenderness, organomegaly, or masses. Her skin examination reveals jaundice. Laboratory results reveal WBC 10,000/μL, hematocrit 48%, platelets 250/μL, AST 400 U/L, ALT 450 U/L, alkaline phosphatase 500 U/L, amylase 50 U/L, lipase 40 U/L, direct bilirubin 15.2 mg/dL, total bilirubin 16.5 mg/dL, sodium 140 mEq/L, potassium 3.5 mEq/L, chloride 110 mEq/L, bicarbonate 24 mEq/L, BUN 10 mg/dL, creatinine 0.6 mg/dL, and glucose 85 mg/dL. Which of the following is an abnormal common bile duct (CBD) diameter?

a. 40-year-old man postcholecystectomy with 9-mm-diameter CBD
b. 75-year-old woman with 7-mm-diameter CBD
c. 50-year-old man with 4-mm-diameter CBD
d. 40-year-old postcholecystectomy with 10-mm-diameter CBD
e. 60-year-old man with 9-mm-diameter CBD

**403.** A 58-year-old-woman presents to the ED with the complaint of left-sided back pain, fever, vomiting, and fatigue. The patient states all of her symptoms started 15 days ago with low abdominal pain associated with burning on urination that has progressively worsened with migration of pain up her right side. She said that the pain was consistent with her previous urinary tract infections (UTIs), so she tried home remedies before coming to the hospital 4 days ago. Chart review shows the patient was started on ciprofloxacin for pyelonephritis. She has been compliant with her medications since they were started, but she seems to be getting worse. Her history is significant for multiple UTIs and diabetes. Her BP is 150/85 mm Hg, HR is 110 beats per minute, temperature is 100.5°F, RR is 18 breaths per minute, and oxygen saturation is 100% on room air. Physical examination shows a nontoxic-appearing patient with mild left-sided costovertebral angel tenderness and left upper quadrant (LUQ) tenderness. Her examination shows no peritoneal signs or masses. Laboratory results reveal WBC 15,000/μL, hematocrit 48%, platelets 250/μL, sodium 135 mEq/L, potassium 4.5 mEq/L, chloride 110 mEq/L, bicarbonate 23 mEq/L, BUN 20 mg/dL, creatinine 1.2 mg/dL, and glucose 250 mg/dL. Urinalysis shows 1+ leukocyte esterase, 1+ blood, 1+ bacteria, 5 to 10 RBC/hpf, and 5 to 10 WBC/hpf. A bedside left renal ultrasound is obtained as shown in the following image. Which of the following is most suggestive of renal abscess?

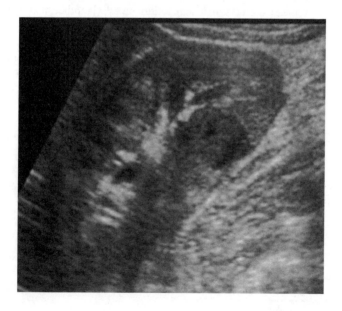

a. Solitary anechoic cystic structure with internal septations and areas of echogenic debris
b. Solitary anechoic smooth cystic structure with no internal echoes
c. Prominent echolucent renal pelvis and calyces
d. Multiple anechoic smooth cystic structures with no internal echoes
e. An irregular heterogeneous solid structure that is hyperechoic relative to surrounding parenchyma

**404.** A 35-year-old man presents to the ED complaining of pain and swelling in his left lower extremity. The patient states the pain started when he woke up this morning. With further questioning, the patient states he was aboard a transatlantic flight from England yesterday. There is no history of trauma, he has never experienced leg pain like this in the past, and currently has no chest pain or shortness of breath. He has no history of medical problems. His BP is 130/75 mm Hg, HR is 75 beats per minute, temperature is 99.3°F, RR is 16 breaths per minute, and oxygen saturation is 98% on room air. Physical examination shows his left leg is larger in circumference compared to his right. The left leg is slightly red and warm to touch with soft compartments, symmetric pulses, and intact sensation. The left calf is tender with palpation and dorsiflexion of the ankle. Which of the following ultrasound findings is consistent with deep venous thrombosis (DVT)?

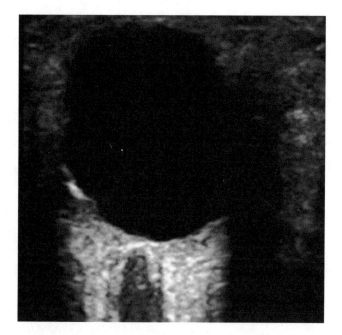

a. Noncompressible anechoic cystic structure in the popliteal fossa
b. Noncompressible superficial femoral vein
c. Noncompressible spherical echogenic structure superficial to femoral artery
d. Noncompressible middle section of the great saphenous vein
e. Semicompressible cystic structure with fluid dissecting into the soft tissue planes of the calf

**405.** A 35-year-old woman presents to the ED complaining of a headache. The patient states the headache has been coming and going for months. The headache is not maximal or sudden in onset and today it is not really different from previous episodes. The patient decided to come to the ED today because she was experiencing periods where her vision seemed dim. With further questioning, the patient states she gets periodic whooshing sound in her ears. Her BP is 145/75 mm Hg, HR is 93 beats per minute, temperature is 97.9°F, RR is 16 breaths per minute, and oxygen saturation is 100% on room air. Her physical examination is unremarkable; however, the fundi were not clearly visualized on funduscopic examination. Ultrasound evaluation of the eye is obtained as shown in the following image. Which of the following further suggests the most likely diagnosis?

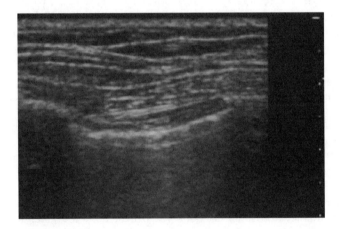

  a. Ribbon-like echogenic structure in the vitreous chamber that is free floating with eye movement
  b. Optic nerve sheath diameter of 6 mm
  c. Loss of globe volume with echogenic matter in the vitreous chamber
  d. Optic nerve sheath diameter of 4 mm
  e. Color Doppler flow of the optic disk showing only blood flow exiting the globe

**406.** A 27-year-old woman, G2P1, currently 20 weeks' gestation, presents to the ED complaining of right-side and back pain. The pain was sudden in onset 2 hours before presentation and described as stabbing in nature. The pain radiates to the right groin and is not associated with any alleviating or aggravating factors. The patient does complain of some vomiting but no other associated symptoms. Her previous pregnancy was uncomplicated. Her BP is 120/70 mm Hg, HR is 90 beats per minute, temperature is 97.9°F, RR is 16 breaths per minute, and oxygen saturation is 100% on room air. Physical examination shows her in pain, and she cannot seem to find a position of comfort. There was mild right-sided costovertebral angle tenderness. The abdominal examination shows a gravid uterus palpable at the level of the umbilicus but no tenderness or peritoneal signs. Laboratory results reveal sodium 138 mEq/L, potassium 4.0 mEq/L, chloride 110 mEq/L, bicarbonate 24 mEq/L, BUN 15 mg/dL, creatinine 0.6 mg/dL, and glucose 105 mg/dL. Urinalysis shows 2+ blood and RBC 20 to 50/hpf. Which of the following ultrasound findings is suggestive of pathologic obstructive hydronephrosis in this patient?

a. Bilateral prominence of the renal collecting system with full bladder
b. Prominence of the right renal collecting system in the supine pregnant patient
c. Bilateral anechoic collections around the renal pelvis with dividing segments of renal cortex
d. Unilateral prominent renal pelvis located outside the medial margin of the renal cortex and no calyceal dilation
e. Prominence of the right renal collecting system while in the left lateral decubitus position

**407.** A 27-year-old man presents to your ED by ambulance after being involved in an automobile accident. The patient was a restrained rear seat passenger in T-bone–style accident striking the patient's rear passenger side door. EMS reports there was significant cabin intrusion of the car. The patient was able to climb out of the other side of the car and was ambulatory on scene. Now, he complains of neck and right chest pain. The chest pain is sharp and worse with breathing. He has no other complaints. His BP is 135/70 mm Hg, HR is 110 beats per minute, temperature is 98.2°F, RR is 20 breaths per minute, and oxygen saturation is 100% on room air. Physical examination reveals clear breath sounds bilaterally and marked tenderness of the right lateral thorax with no crepitus or ecchymosis. The abdomen is soft, nondistended, and nontender. A supine AP chest radiograph is normal. You place the ultrasound on the patient's anterior chest wall and obtain the following images. Which of the following diagnoses does the ultrasound finding support?

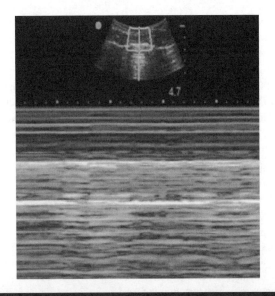

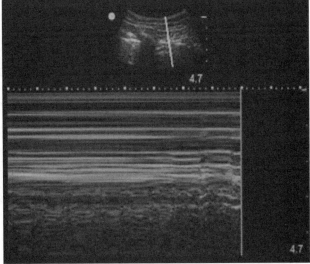

a. Pulmonary contusion
b. Chest wall contusion
c. Rib fracture
d. Pneumothorax
e. Hemothorax

**408.** A 28-year-old woman presents to the ED with vaginal bleeding. The patient found out she was pregnant 7 weeks ago but was never able to follow up in the OB clinic for prenatal care. She is G3P2. The patient says the bleeding started 1 hour before presentation and was not associated with any trauma, abdominal pain, abdominal cramping, or a gush of clear fluid from the vagina. The patient is a smoker but denies using any drugs of abuse. Her BP is 120/70 mm Hg, HR is 85 beats per minute, temperature is 98.2°F, RR is 16 breaths per minute, and oxygen saturation is 100% on room air. Physical examination is only remarkable for a gravid uterus extending approximately 30 cm above the pelvic brim and blood dripping from the introitus. Bedside transabdominal pelvic ultrasound is performed. Which of the following ultrasound findings would make a digital examination of the cervix contraindicated?

a. Placenta implanted in the lower portion of the uterus
b. A cervix 4 cm in length
c. Hyperechoic fluid collection between the placenta and uterine wall
d. Placenta implanted high and posterior on the uterine wall
e. Breach fetus with foot as presenting part

**409.** A 58-year-old woman presents to the ED with abdominal pain. She reports that the pain is in the RUQ and has been getting progressively worse over the last month. The pain is now a sharp, constant, and non-radiating. The pain is worse when she lays on her right side. She denies any urinary complaints. Her BP is 125/75 mm Hg, HR is 75 beats per minute, temperature is 96.9°F, RR is 18 breaths per minute, and oxygen saturation is 98% on room air. On physical examination, her abdomen is nondistended and soft. She does have pinpoint tenderness to palpation under the right costal margin. Laboratory tests are within normal limits. You obtain a bedside ultrasound of the RUQ that revealed the following. Which of the following findings is suggestive of malignancy?

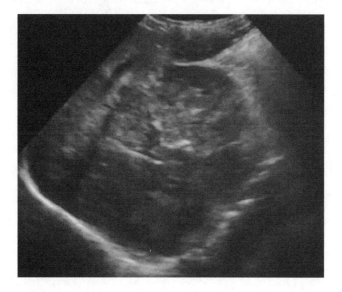

a. Heterogeneous mass with irregular boarders
b. Phrygian cap present in the mass
c. Well-defined smooth mass margins with no internal echoes
d. Homogenous echogenicity throughout the mass
e. Riedel lobe present in the mass

**410.** A 45-year-old man presents to your ED after a fall from standing position. The patient states he was not watching where he was going when he tripped on a rug and fell into the coffee table. The patient hit his left side on the edge of the table. He denies loss of consciousness. He complains of pain in the left flank and pain in his left shoulder when he takes a deep breath. On examination his vital signs include a BP of 140/75 mm Hg, HR of 95 beats per minute, temperature of 98.9°F, RR of 16 breaths per minute, and oxygen saturation of 100% on room air. The lungs are clear to auscultation bilaterally and the abdomen is tender in the LUQ. There is no rebound, guarding, or organomegaly. There is no ecchymosis noted in the left flank. You obtain a bedside FAST examination, shown in the following image. What is the next best step in the management of this patient?

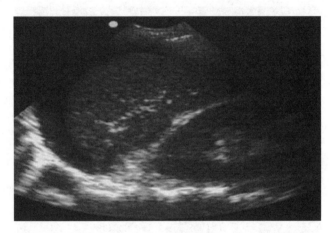

a. Transfuse 2 units of type O-negative blood and start cross-matched blood once available.
b. Perform CT scan of the abdomen and pelvis with intravenous contrast.
c. Perform emergent laparotomy.
d. Upright chest radiograph to rule out free air under the diaphragm.
e. If his pain resolves, prescribe ibuprofen for pain control and have him follow up with his primary care physician in 5 days for a repeat abdominal examination.

# Ultrasound in the Emergency Department

## *Answers*

**388. The answer is d.** (*Cosby, pp 58, 62, 80-82; Ma, pp 79-81, 90.*) The pelvic view of this FAST examination shows an **anechoic collection in the pouch of Douglas** (rectouterine pouch) and vesicouterine pouch representing free fluid in the peritoneal cavity. In the **setting of trauma, free peritoneal fluid is presumed to be blood.** In the supine position the pelvis is the most dependent portion of the peritoneal cavity making it the most sensitive region to find free fluid. In female patients, fluid often collects between the anterior wall of the rectum and posterior wall of the uterus. In male patients the equivalent is the rectovesical pouch. This is anatomically significant because free fluid often collects between the anterior wall of the rectum and posterior wall of the bladder in males.

Obtaining a CT of head (**a**) is a good consideration with the mechanism of injury and depressed mental status. However, the more likely cause of the depressed mental status in this patient is profound shock. Taking the patient for a CT scan will delay definitive management in the operating room. (**b**) Although CT scan of the abdomen and pelvis may provide diagnostic images, it is not recommended in the unstable patient because it delays definitive therapy. Abdominal exploration and hemorrhage control by the trauma surgeon is both diagnostic and therapeutic. (**c**) Following hemoglobin is misleading in the early stages of hemorrhage. Initial hemoglobin studies will be near normal because the concentration of hemoglobin remains the same despite low blood volume. This patient has lost a significant volume of blood and laboratory studies should not delay the initiation of a blood transfusion in an unstable patient. Hemorrhage control (**e**) is paramount; however, the primary source of bleeding for this patient is in the abdomen and nothing should delay transport to the operating room.

**389. The answer is d.** (*Ma, pp 354-355, 362, 369; Cosby, pp 176-177; Lyon, pp 86-87.*) The diagnosis of **ovarian torsion** can be difficult to rule out despite all imaging modalities available to the clinician. The gold standard to ruling out ovarian torsion is laparoscopy; however, this is not practical and reserved for patients with high clinical suspicion for torsion. However, patients with **no ovarian or adnexal masses measuring 3 to 4 cm in diameter** and **normal-sized ovaries are extremely unlikely to have ovarian torsion.**

**Unilateral enlarged ovary secondary to edema (a)** is the **most common ultrasound finding in patients who do have torsion.** Ovarian enlargement, in the case of torsion, results from venous and lymphatic congestion secondary to crimped vascular supply to and from the ovary. Venous and arterial flow detected with Doppler sonography of the right ovary **(b)** does not rule out ovarian torsion. The ovary is a dual-blood-supply organ meaning that blood flow to one area of ovary does not mean that blood flow to other areas of the ovary is adequate. Free fluid in the pouch of Douglas **(c)** is a very nonspecific finding that can often be found in the case of ovarian torsion. Presence of a right adnexal mass measuring 5 cm in diameter **(e)** does not rule out ovarian torsion. In fact, masses greater than 3 to 4 cm are often required to tilt the ovary leading to vascular compromise.

**390. The answer is e.** (*Cosby, pp 136-138; Ma, pp 296-297, 304; Lyon, pp 99, 101.*) The ultrasound (see figure below) reveals a **gestational sac** containing the **yolk sac**, characterized by a **ringlike echogenic structure located at the periphery of the gestational sac.** A **gestational sac surrounding a yolk sac confirms gestational product.** IUP can be confirmed if the endometrial stripe can be visualized with both the gestational and yolk sacs. The yolk sac can be detected by transvaginal ultrasound between 5 and 6 weeks and transabdominal ultrasound at 6 weeks.

An intrauterine gestational sac **(a)** is suggestive of an IUP; however isolated fluid collections in the uterus are not uncommon with ectopic pregnancy. Isolated fluid collections in the uterus are called pseudogestational sacs and can be falsely reassuring of an IUP. An intrauterine gestational sac with yolk sac and embryonic pole **(b)** confirms an IUP, but it is not the earliest finding. An **embryo can be detected on transvaginal ultrasound around 6 weeks** and **transabdominal ultrasound around 7 weeks.** Blighted ovum **(c)** is a consistent with embryonic demise. It is characterized by a gestational sac with a gestational age greater than 7 weeks and absence of embryonic product development inside. Intradecidual sign **(d)** is an embryo completely embedded within the endometrial decidua but does not displace the endometrial stripe. This finding is

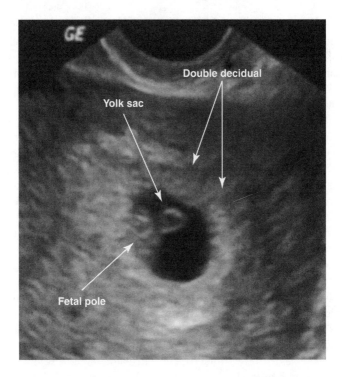

difficult to recognize and easily mimicked by small fluid collections in the uterus. Therefore, the intradecidual sign is not a reliable confirmation of IUP. The **double decidual sign** is another finding **diagnostic of an IUP**. It is characterized as a gestational sac surrounded by two layers: inner layer decidua capsularis and outer layer decidua vera. The decidua capsularis and decidua vera are separated by a thin hypoechoic layer forming the double decidual sign. Some authors list the double decidual sign as the earliest conformational finding of an IUP. However, like the decidual sign it is technically difficult to recognize and small uterine fluid collections can mimic the double decidual sign.

**391. The answer is e.** *(Cosby, pp 82-83, 105-106; Ma, p 94.)* This patient has a **partial anechoic and echogenic** collection between the heart and pericardium consistent with **hemopericardium**. The patient's clinical presentation of hypotension, elevated jugular venous pressure, and hemopericardium is consistent with **pericardial tamponade**, which is a life-threatening condition. **Pericardiocentesis** should be attempted, in addition to fluid resuscitation, as a temporizing measure so the patient can be transferred to the operating room for definitive repair of his injuries. The classic presentation of pericardial tamponade is associated with Beck triad: low arterial BP, jugular venous distention, and muffled or distant heart sounds. However, when the classic presentation is not appreciated clinically, ultrasound provides valuable information that can rapidly guide management.

There are multiple findings on ultrasound that suggest cardiac tamponade. The **earliest finding** is usually the **collapse of the right atrium during atrial diastole**, then collapse of the right ventricle during ventricular diastole. During end ventricular diastole both ventricles should be maximally dilated. The last finding, and the most difficult to appreciate on bedside ultrasound, is flattening or deviation of the interventricular septum toward the left ventricular cavity.

Another **ultrasonographic finding** that supports the diagnosis of **cardiac tamponade** is a **plethoric inferior vena cava**. Normally, the inferior vena cava transiently narrows during inspiration when blood is pulled into the thoracic cavity during inspiration. This occurs secondary to negative pressure in the thoracic cavity that is generated by respiration and creates a gradient for blood to flow across the diaphragm between the abdomen and thorax. In cardiac tamponade, the inferior vena cava will appear plethoric and have no respiratory variation as blood flow into the heart is blocked by the tamponade. However, if the patient's circulatory volume is low secondary to hemorrhage elsewhere, respiratory variation may still be present.

ED resuscitative thoracotomy (**a**) is not indicated in this case. The most widely accepted indication for ED thoracotomy is in a penetrating trauma patient with a loss of vital signs in or near the ED. Taking the patient to the operating room for laparotomy (**b**) is not the best choice, because the patient has no evidence of hemoperitoneum. Transfer to the operating room for thoracotomy (**c**) should occur after a temporizing pericardiocentesis is performed. If the tamponade is not immediately addressed, the patient is at risk of deteriorating into pulseless electrical activity. A CT scan (**d**) is not indicated because a diagnosis of pericardial tamponade was made by ultrasound.

**392. The answer is c.** (*Lyon, pp 61-62; Cosby, pp 201-204; Ma, pp 174-180.*) This patient's RUQ study reveals (figure below) a **thickened gallbladder wall**, **pericholecystic fluid**, **cholelithiasis**, and **a sonographic Murphy sign**. Considering the history, physical examination findings, and bedside ultrasound images, **cholecystitis** is the most likely diagnosis. **Mucosal**

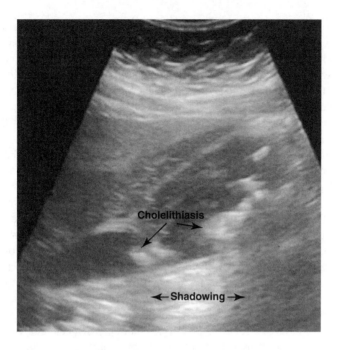

sloughing occurs as a result of **prolonged ischemia** to the mucosal surface of the gallbladder wall. Characterized by **debris floating in the gallbladder lumen**, mucosal sloughing is evidence of **advanced disease**.

There are numerous ultrasound findings that suggest cholecystitis. However, no ultrasound finding alone is enough to make the diagnosis of cholecystitis and must be considered with the entire clinical picture. The presence of a sonographic Murphy sign and cholelithiasis (**a and b**) alone has a sensitivity of 91% and specificity of 66% for cholecystitis. The **sonographic Murphy sign** is considered **more specific for cholecystitis** than hand palpation because the gallbladder is compressed under direct visualization as the patient inhales. The presence of cholelithiasis does not mean cholecystitis, but their presence supports the diagnosis. At least 95% of patients found to have cholecystitis have gallstones present. Gallbladder wall thickening (**d**) is another finding suggestive of cholecystitis. **Measurement of the anterior gallbladder wall** should be **less than 3 mm**. A wall thickness of 3 to 5 mm is indeterminate particularly after a meal, as the post-prandial gallbladder contracts giving a thickness up to 5 mm. A **gallbladder** wall greater than 5 mm is abnormal. However, congestive heart failure (CHF) and chronic liver disease are known to cause thickened gallbladder walls without the presence of cholecystitis. **Gallbladder distension is a sign of gallbladder obstruction.** The normal gallbladder is often less than 10 cm in length and 5 cm in diameter. However, this is a very nonspecific finding. Pericholecystic fluid (e) is a later finding of cholecystitis characterized by a collection of fluid around the gallbladder wall. Of all the ultrasound findings, pericholecystic fluid is the most specific finding for cholecystitis. However, similar to gallbladder wall thickening, CHF and chronic liver disease can lead to pericholecystic fluid without the presence of cholecystitis.

**393. The answer is d.** (*Ma, pp 449-452, 454-458.*) The globe is a fluid-filled structure that is easily evaluated by ultrasound. Serious ocular injury can be easily missed, as the patient may not be able to report vision loss secondary to lid edema or altered mental status. Lid edema also makes a complete evaluation of the eye difficult for the physician and repeated evaluations can be deleterious to the patient. The normal anterior and posterior chamber is typically anechoic as seen in the figure. The image provided in this case reveals a **posterior chamber with echogenic matter** occupying most of the volume of the vitreous chamber consistent with a **vitreous hemorrhage**. In the setting **of penetrating trauma a vitreous hemorrhage is highly suggestive of globe perforation**. Other ultrasound findings suggestive of globe perforation or rupture are **decreased size of globe** and **buckling of the sclera posteriorly** secondary to vitreous matter leaking. When evaluating the eye with ultrasound, particularly in the case of potential globe rupture, care must be taken to minimize pressure exerted on the eye by the ultrasound probe itself. Proper technique consists of liberal application of ultrasound gel over the closed eye lid with the sonographers hand rested on the patient's forehead or nasal bridge. The ultrasound probe only requires contact with the gel to obtain adequate images of the globe and therefore does not need to rest on the closed eyelid itself.

A completely anechoic anterior and posterior chamber (a) would be highly suggestive of a globe without major injury. However, the image provided shows obvious vitreous hemorrhage. Retinal detachment (b) is characterized by a highly echoic membrane that floats freely in the vitreous matter with eye movement. Retinal detachment is often associated with blunt trauma and typically does not lead to large vitreous hemorrhage. Significant lens dislocation (c) can be characterized as either partial or complete.

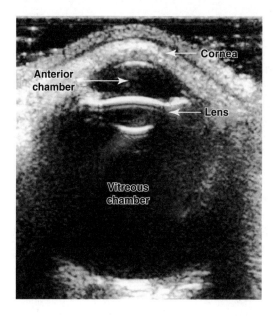

A partial dislocation on ultrasound shows a lens positioned in its usual location just posterior to the iris; however, with ocular movements the lens appears to move independently of the surrounding structures. With complete lens, dislocation the lens is completely out of normal position relative to the iris. Vitreous hemorrhage is not associated with lens dislocation. A retrobulbar hematoma (**e**) is characterized by hypoechoic stripe posterior to the globe. The ultrasound in this case shows bleeding in the vitreous chamber. If the bleeding had been outside the eye between the orbital wall and globe, retrobulbar hematoma would be the correct answer.

**394. The answer is c.** *(Lyon, pp 48-50; Ma, pp 154-156; Cosby, pp 228-230.)* In the case of an unstable patient many clinicians may go directly to the **distal aorta** to evaluate for abdominal aortic aneurysm because it is the **most common location for aneurysmal development**. The distal aorta can usually be identified with the probe placed just superior to the umbilicus. In the stable patient, however, a systematic approach is used to evaluate the abdominal aorta for pathology. The abdominal aorta is broken into a proximal, middle, and distal segment. The proximal segment is defined by the aorta visualized just below the xiphoid process to the takeoff of the superior mesenteric artery. The middle segment is the area just distal to the superior mesenteric artery. The anatomic significance of the middle segment is any aneurysm within 1 to 2 cm of the superior mesenteric artery that is highly likely to include the renal arteries. The distal segment of the aorta is just proximal to the aortic bifurcation into the common iliac arteries. While imaging, each segment in transverse orientation anterior to posterior diameter is taken measuring from **outer wall to outer wall**. This ensures accurate measurements by including any mural thrombus that would be excluded if the measurements were taken from (**b**) inner wall to inner wall. The aorta tapers from proximal to distal with the upper limit of normal 2.5 cm in the proximal segment and 1.8 cm in the distal segment. The diagnosis of abdominal **aortic aneurysm** can be made when a measurement **greater than or equal to 3 cm** is recorded in any one of the three segments. Sagittal sections of the aorta can also be obtained to further evaluate the contour of the aorta and assess for luminal irregularities, such as thrombus, or intimal flaps that would suggest aortic dissection. (**a and d**) However, caution should be used when measuring anterior to posterior diameter on sagittal sections because of cylinder tangent effect. A longitudinal beam slice through the center of the vessel will show an accurate maximal diameter. However, caution should be used as an off-center slice of the sidewall of the vessel will give a falsely reduced AP diameter. Measuring outer wall to inner wall (**e**) is not an accurate measurement because it could potentially miss mural thrombus.

**395. The answer is c.** (*Cosby, p 81; Ma, p 103.*) This patient has a **negative FAST examination**. This patient's examination and radiograph reveals an **open book pelvis fracture**. Pelvic fractures have a high association with **retroperitoneal hemorrhage**. **Ultrasound is not sensitive or specific for evaluating the retroperitoneal space**. The optimal management choice is transport to interventional radiology for embolization of the bleeding retroperitoneal vessels from the pelvic fracture.

A CT scan of the thorax, abdomen, and pelvis with intravenous contrast (**a and e**) would be ideal if the patient was stable. CT scan is very sensitive and specific for solid-organ injury, hollow viscous injury, and retroperitoneal injury. However, considering this patient's injuries and instability, CT scan is not the best answer. Emergent exploratory laparotomy (**b**) is a reasonable answer for this patient as other peritoneal injuries can be evaluated and managed. In addition, the pelvis can be packed in an effort to limit hemorrhage. However, the patient may still need vascular embolization despite the surgeon's effort. Therefore, laparotomy delays definitive management of the bleeding. Evaluating for hematuria (**d**) is not priority at this time as the patient is not stable. There is already high suspicion for urogenital injury given her pelvic fracture and finding of blood at the urethral meatus. Once stabilized, the patient should get a retrograde cystourethrogram to evaluate for severity of urogenital injury before Foley placement.

**396. The answer is d.** (*Ma, pp 229-231, 240-243, 246; Cosby, pp 237, 245-248; Middelton, pp 104, 106-107.*) This patient's presentation, examination, and laboratory studies are classic for **nephrolithiasis**. The gold standard for evaluation for nephrolithiasis is spiral CT scan of the abdomen and pelvis without intravenous contrast; however, this requires exposure to ionizing radiation. In young patients with classic presentation of nephrolithiasis and microscopic hematuria or young patients with repeat visits for similar to previous episodes of nephrolithiasis, ultrasound is a great alternative to CT scan. Identification of severe hydronephrosis on ultrasound is an indication of further imaging and admission for urology evaluation. **Severe hydronephrosis** is defined by the presence of dilation of both the renal pelvis and calyces leading to thinning of the renal cortex.

Prominent anechoic renal calyces and prominent anechoic renal pelvis and calyces (**b and c**) are descriptive of minor and moderate hydronephrosis, respectively. Grading mild to moderate hydronephrosis is subjective and of little clinical significance; however, the key feature of no cortical thinning is absent in both cases. Comparing the affected kidney to the unaffected kidney is often required to fully appreciate mild hydronephrosis. Patients with mild to moderate unilateral hydronephrosis, no UTI, and are low risk for abdominal aortic aneurysm, ovarian tumors, and retroperitoneal masses can follow up with urology on an outpatient basis if their pain is controlled and are tolerating oral intake.

Anechoic collections around the renal pelvis with dividing segments of renal cortex (**a**) are consistent with sonolucent renal pyramids. Sonolucent renal pyramids are normal variants. They can be differentiated from dilated renal calyces by the presence of renal cortex separating each sonolucent triangle. Prominent renal pelvis and calyces with echogenic structure at ureteropelvic junction are casting clean shadow in the background. (**e**) The dilated renal pelvis and calyces are consistent with moderate hydronephrosis. There is no mention of cortical thinning that goes against severe hydronephrosis. The echogenic structure with clean shadowing is consistent with a renal stone lodged at the ureteropelvic junction; in this case it is likely the source of obstruction. Detecting obstructing renal stones in between the ureteropelvic and ureterovesicular junction is uncommon secondary to shadowing from bowel gas. Stones located in the renal pelvis are non-obstructive and of little clinical significance.

**397. The answer is a.** (*Cosby, pp 72, 83; Ma, pp 89, 94.*) This patient's FAST examination shows an **anechoic fluid collection above the right hemi-diaphragm** as seen in figure below. In addition, there is loss of normal mirror artifact and continuation of the spinous shadow beyond the diaphragm. Mirror artifact around the diaphragm is a normal finding and, when absent, raises suspicion for underlying pathology. The liver is a highly reflective organ and therefore easily interrogated with ultrasound. The aerated lung tissue, on the other hand, reflects very little sound, and therefore lung is not easily evaluated by ultrasound. Physical properties beyond the scope of this text lead to near 100% reflection of sound waves at the tissue-air interface of the diaphragm. The reflected sound waves then cross-back through the liver where they are again reflected in various angles before they either completely attenuate or make it back to the ultrasound probe. The ultrasound machine assumes the signal has traveled in a straight line and incorrectly interprets these signals as if they had originated far beyond the diaphragm. Therefore, a liver-like image is projected superior to the diaphragm almost as if the diaphragm is a mirror of the true liver. Because almost all of the sound waves are reflected at the diaphragm, the hyper-echoic surface of the spine is not visible superior to the diaphragm. However, with hemothorax or pleural effusions the tissue-fluid interface is less reflective of sound. As more sound waves now pass through to the highly reflective thoracic vertebral bodies, an image of the spinal column can be scene superior to the diaphragm.

In the setting of trauma, a fluid collection above the diaphragm is presumed to be a hemothorax. Chest tube thoracostomy is required to prevent further accumulation of blood from compromising respiratory status and monitor loss of blood. An immediate output of greater than 20 mL/kg of blood or continued bleeding of greater than 3 mL/kg/h is generally viewed as an indication for thoracotomy in the operating room. Rapid sequence intubation **(b)** is not indicated at this time. The patient is having difficulty breathing because of pain limitation; however, his saturation is acceptable and his normal mental status suggests he is ventilating well. Should the patient become hemodynamically unstable, develop hypercapnia from

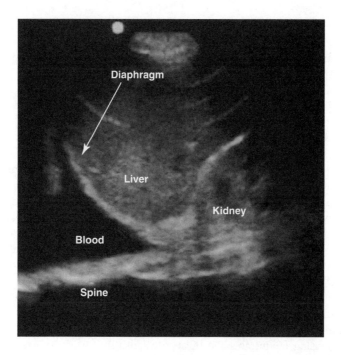

Diaphragm

Liver

Kidney

Blood

Spine

hypoventilation, or become hypoxic refractory noninvasive oxygen supplementation, intubation would be indicated. CT thorax, abdomen, and pelvis with intravenous contrast (**c and d**) should be done after the hemothorax is addressed. Emergent laparotomy (**e**) is not indicated in this case as the patient has no free fluid in the abdomen and the patient's vital signs are acceptable.

**398. The answer is d.** (*Cosby, pp 187-188, 207; Ma, pp 176-177, 180-181; Lyon, pp 62-63.*) This patient's history and physical examination is nonspecific; however, the laboratory values suggest **biliary tract obstruction with pancreatitis**. On ultrasound the CBD is normally much smaller than the portal vein. When dilated, it becomes similar in size to the neighboring portal vein that gives the appearance of a "**double barrel shotgun**" or "**parallel channel.**" Suspicion of biliary obstruction requires an evaluation of the CBD to assess for dilation. The CBD is most easily seen at the portal triad consisting of the portal vein, CBD, and hepatic artery. The three come together to make the "**Mickey Mouse sign**" (**a**) with the head being the portal vein, the right ear the CBD, and the left ear the hepatic artery. The Mickey Mouse sign is a normal anatomic finding. The main lobar fissure tracks to the gallbladder and excellent landmark for locating a contracted gallbladder. A CBD that appears similar in size to the portal vein highly suggests CBD obstruction. In most people a CBD width of less than 7 mm is considered normal. However, instances exist where a CBD diameter greater than 7 mm is normal. The CBD dilates with age and after cholecystectomy. Postcholecystectomy patients have a normal CBD diameter up to 1 cm. Age can be accounted for by adding 1 mm for every decade greater than age 40. For example, an 8-mm-diameter CBD in a patient aged 80 years is normal.

Increased liver echogenicity with irregular texture (**b**) is a finding of liver cirrhosis. **The playboy bunny sign (c)** is another normal anatomic finding. When the hepatic veins converge on the inferior vena cava, they often give the appearance of the playboy bunny emblem. The hepatic veins can be important structures because they divide the liver into its anatomic lobes. The middle hepatic vein travels in the median longitudinal fissure (MLF). The anatomic significance of this is that the gallbladder often lies near the MLF. Thus, the middle hepatic vein is a good reference point to find the MLF and in turn the gallbladder. **The antler sign (e)** is a pathologic finding for intrahepatic biliary duct dilation. It is characterized as irregular dilated tubules radiating outward from the porta hepatis, giving the appearance of dear antlers. The antler sign is indicative of biliary obstruction; however, the sonographer cannot differentiate intrahepatic from extrahepatic obstruction with this finding alone. Common causes of intrahepatic obstruction are biliary duct cancer and hepatic masses.

**399. The answer is b.** (*Cosby, pp 141-148; Ma, pp 300-304; Lyon, pp 99-101.*) Figure below shows an **endometrial stripe** with a **tiny psuedogestational sac** showing there is **no obvious IUP**. Figure below shows **gestational sack with yolk sack in the left adnexa confirming ectopic pregnancy**. There is also a fetal pole present; however, this is not required to make the definitive diagnosis of ectopic pregnancy. The other options provided are suspicious for ectopic pregnancy and depending on the clinical scenario still require laparoscopy. However, (**a, c, d, and e**) are only suspicious for ectopic pregnancy and not definitive findings.

Free fluid in the pelvis (**a**) of a pregnant patient is concerning for ectopic pregnancy, however, nonspecific. One-third of patients with an ectopic pregnancy have no free fluid in the pelvis. Small volumes of free fluid in

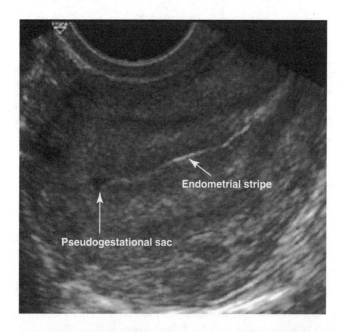

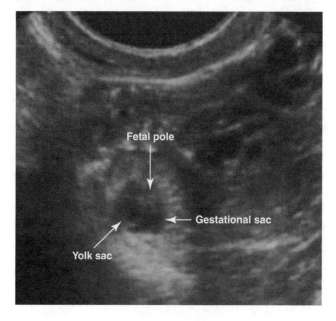

the cul-de-sac from ruptured ovarian cyst are not uncommon. However, the larger the volume of free fluid, the more suspicion there is for ectopic pregnancy. **A complex adnexal mass (c) is the most common sonographic finding in ectopic pregnancy.** The mass typically represents a tubal hematoma, ectopic trophoblastic tissue, or distorted contents of an ectopic gestational sac. Pelvic ultrasound of the pregnant patient that finds an empty uterus with a complex adnexal mass is highly suspicious for ectopic pregnancy. However, the presence of an adnexal mass does not confirm that an ectopic pregnant as surrounding bowel, abscess, and ovarian tissue can be similar in appearance. ED detection of a complex adnexal mass in the pregnant patient always warrants obstetrical consultation for possible laparoscopy or further imaging. A tubal ring **(d)** is a concentric hyperechoic (white) structure found in the adnexa; it is effectively a gestational sac outside of the uterus. It sometimes takes the appearance of ovarian cyst but has thicker and more echogenic margins. The presence of a tubal ring is associated with a greater than 95% chance of ectopic pregnancy. The ring of fire sign **(e)** describes the appearance of trophoblastic blood flow around an adnexal mass when color Doppler is applied to the image. Sonographers use this finding to differentiate adnexal mass from surrounding tissue. However, like an adnexal mass or tubal ring, it does not make the definitive diagnosis of an ectopic pregnancy.

**400. The answer is b.** (*Cosby, pp 148, 155-157; Ma, pp 286-297, 308-309.*) This patient presents with vaginal bleeding, uterus to large for dates, and hyperemesis gravidarum. Her metabolic and urine analysis are consistent with vomiting and dehydration. The **quantitative β-hCG is extremely high**. The β-hCG in normal pregnancies usually levels off at 10 weeks around 100,000 mIU/mL. The most likely diagnosis in this case is a **molar pregnancy**. A molar pregnancy can be confirmed by direct visualization of the hydatidiform mole with pelvic ultrasound. The classic appearance of a **hydatidiform** is a **cluster of grapes** or **snowstorm appearance** in the intrauterine cavity.

A thin-walled unilocular anechoic cystic structure 4 cm in diameter on the ovary **(a)** is consistent with a corpus luteum cyst. The corpus luteum cyst is a simple cyst greater than 3 cm in diameter and typically a benign finding in pregnancy. The corpus luteum cyst is usually unilateral. If the patient has multiple large multilocular anechoic cystic masses on each ovary **(d)**, it is suggestive of theca lutein cyst. Theca lutein cysts are exacerbated corpus luteum and have an association with very high β-hCG levels. They are commonly seen in patients with gestational trophoblastic disease and with ovarian hyperstimulation from fertility medications. Though this patient likely has theca lutein cyst, it is a result of the gestational trophoblastic disease and not the primary problem. Both corpus luteum cyst and theca lutein cyst usually resolve spontaneously. A hyperechoic stripe between the endometrium and chorionic membrane (c) is consistent with a subchorionic hemorrhage. This is common finding in patients who present with vaginal bleeding in the first trimester. Pregnant patients with subchorionic hemorrhage are believed to have a higher incidence of embryonic demise. This finding, however, does not explain a uterus to large for dates, hyperemesis, and elevated quantitative β-hCG. Hypoechoic solid spherical mass in the uterine wall (e) is consistent with uterine fibroids. Uterine fibroids can create problems with dysfunctional uterine bleeding and pelvic pain; however, they are generally considered a benign finding. They are often palpable and can mislead the examiner for a uterus to large for dates; however, they do not explain the hyperemesis and elevated β-hCG.

**401. The answer is d.** (*Cosby, pp 331-332, 343, 348; Ma, pp 440-444.*) A subcutaneous abscess has a variety of sonographic appearances. The abscess cavity itself can have a spherical or lobulated appearance. The **fluid content of an abscess is usually very dark** in appearance relative to surrounding soft tissue; however, in some cases the abscess cavity may be isoechoic to surrounding soft tissue.

The sonographic appearance of **cellulitis (c)** is primarily related to the presence of edema. Differentiating inflammatory edema from chronic dependent edema can be challenging. Classically cellulitis is described as a cobblestone-like and characterized by thickened and abnormally bright subcutaneous tissues traversed by a lattice of broad dark bands of edema. Cellulitic tissue is often found neighboring abscess cavities. **Normal soft tissue (a)** ultrasound findings from superficial to deep are as follows. Normal skin is typically thin and homogeneous with a bright layer of connective tissue separating the skin from the subcutaneous tissues. The subcutaneous tissues are primarily fat appearing dark relative to surrounding soft tissue. Intertwined in the fat are bright layers of connective tissue breaking the fat layer into fat lobules. Mixed in the subcutaneous layer are veins, which are thin-walled tubular structures that easily compress and are not pulsatile. Arteries are much thicker-walled tubular structures that are pulsatile. Nerve tissue is often described as honeycomb-like when viewed in cross section. Between the subcutaneous tissue and muscle is the bright layer of fascia. Muscle appears relatively dark with a regular pattern of internal striations in long axis and speckled in appearance in short axis. Bone is characterized by the very bright outer cortex with clean acoustic shadowing in the far field. **Chronic lymphedema, (b)** like cellulitis, has thickened skin and subcutaneous tissues. However, chronic edema is not as echogenic as acute inflammatory edema. Chronic edema also collects in horizontal bands as opposed to the cobblestone pattern of acute inflammatory edema. **Retained foreign bodies (e)** are an important potential source of soft tissue infection and often easily overlooked. Radiography works well for radiopaque objects such as metal, glass, and gravel. However, radiolucent matter such as wood, plastic, and organic compounds like cactus spines or thorns are frequently missed. If historical clues suggest a foreign body could be present, ultrasound is an excellent adjunct to radiography when evaluating for retained foreign bodies. Depending on the composition and size of the foreign body, variable degrees of acoustic shadowing are created. Gravel and wood cast an acoustic shadow similar to that of gallstones. Wood fragments, depending on size, cast a brightly echogenic anterior surface similar to bone. Foreign bodies retained for longer than 24 to 48 hours are frequently surrounded by an echolucent halo, resulting from reactive hyperemia, edema, abscess, or granulation tissue, which may be helpful in locating retained foreign bodies.

**402. The answer is e.** (*Cosby, p 207; Ma, pp 176-177, 180-181; Lyon, pp 62-63.*) In the jaundiced patient initial workup consists of determining obstructive from nonobstructive jaundice. Ultrasound images diagnostic of a **dilated CBD confirm obstructive jaundice.** Once the CBD is identified either in long axis or in short axis, the diameter from inside wall to inside wall is obtained.

**Normal CBD diameter is usually less than 7 mm.** However, patients who have had a cholecystectomy may have a diameter greater than 7 mm. Once the gallbladder has been removed, the reservoir for bile storage, after ampulla of Vater closure, is no longer present. Upon closure of the ampulla of Vater, the bile backs up the CBD normally dilating it up to 1 cm. Age is also a normal contributor to CBD dilation. The rule of thumb for CBD assessment in the elderly is addition of 1 mm for each decade of age greater than 40. For example, an 80-year-old patient with a CBD diameter of 8 mm is normal.

**403. The answer is a.** (*Ma, pp 233-234, 241, 247; Cosby, pp 250-252; Middelton, pp 131-132, 117-123.*) This patient's history is concerning for the development of **a renal abscess.** Ultrasound evaluation is **excellent screening tool for renal or perinephric abscess** development. The sonographic appearance of an abscess, regardless of the location, is variable in terms of the cavity shape and degree of internal echo. Classically an abscess cavity appears as a spherical cystic structure. The purulent matter in the cavity is represented by internal septations and echogenic debris, either floating or collecting in dependent portions of the cavity. **A renal abscess is contained within the renal cortex, while a perinephric abscess extends beyond the renal cortex into the perinephric fat.**

Smooth cystic structures with no internal echoes are consistent with renal cyst. Simple renal cysts **(b)** are common and, when present in small numbers, they have little clinical significance. However, when the surface area of both kidneys is occupied by an abundance of renal cyst **(d)**, the suspicion for polycystic kidney disease is high. Patients with polycystic kidney disease are prone to renal insufficiency and cerebral aneurysm. Prominent echolucent renal pelvis and calyces **(c)** are consistent with a mild to moderate hydronephrosis. Hydronephrosis indicates renal outflow obstruction, and with coexisting infection it requires admission for urgent urology evaluation to prevent abscess formation. However, the presence of hydronephrosis alone is not consistent with renal abscess. Irregular heterogeneous solid structure that is hyperechoic relative to surrounding parenchyma **(e)** is concerning for renal malignancy. The most common malignancy of the kidney is renal cell carcinoma, which carries a poor prognosis if not detected early. Any solid mass or cystic mass with internal septations requires further imaging with CT scan or MRI for further evaluation to help differentiate benign from malignant mass. Though a solid appearing mass could represent an abscess, it is more suggestive of renal malignancy.

**404. The answer is b.** (*Ma, pp 374-382, 385-388; Cosby, pp 256-262.*) Emergency ultrasound evaluation of the lower extremity for DVT requires sequential compression of the major deep veins from the common femoral vein to trifurcation of the popliteal vein. The common femoral vein bifurcates into the superficial and deep femoral veins. The superficial vein travels through obturator canal to the popliteal fossa where it becomes the popliteal vein. The popliteal vein further divides into the peroneal, anterior, and posterior vein known as the trifurcation. **Normal deep veins collapse under moderate pressure applied by the sonographer.** A study is **positive for DVT when the deep vein under interrogation does not collapse fully when pressure is applied to the skin with the ultrasound**

**probe**. An artery is differentiated from the vein by its thicker wall and pulsatile nature.

An anechoic cystic structure in the popliteal fossa (**a**) is consistent with a **Baker cyst**. A Baker cyst develops from a communication between the synovium of the knee and semimembranosus bursa. Chronic inflammation of the knee leads to increased synovial fluid production that tracks into the cyst causing cyst enlargement. The Baker cyst can be differentiated from a DVT on ultrasound by noting that the cyst has a spherical structure as opposed to the tubular shape of a vein. The Baker cyst can enlarge and rupture leading to intense pain and swelling of the calf. The fluid of a ruptured Baker cyst tracks trough the tissue planes of the calf. The volume loss of the cyst makes it somewhat compressible when pressure is applied to the cyst. (**e**) A noncompressible spherical structure superficial to the femoral artery is consistent with a lymph node. Lymph nodes are differentiated from DVT by the spherical shape of the lymph node compared to the tubular structure of the vein. Lymph nodes also tend to lie superficial to the vasculature. The sonographer can also apply Doppler to the lymph node showing blood flow in and out of the node hilum as well as throughout the node itself. The great saphenous vein (**d**) is a superficial vein. Thrombosis of the saphenous vein is not associated with embolic disease. However, thrombosis of the proximal segment, when it enters the common femoral vein, is often treated as a DVT because of the high frequency of proximal extension into the common femoral.

**405. The answer is b.** (*Ma, pp 449-453, 456-460.*) The most likely diagnosis in this case is **idiopathic intracranial hypertension (previously pseudotumor cerebri)**. If adequate funduscopic examination could be obtained, it would show **bilateral papilledema**. Ultrasound evaluation of the optic nerve sheath can be helpful in suggesting **elevated intracranial pressure**. The image provided shows a normal globe with the optic nerve and sheath in the plane of view posterior to the globe. The optic nerve exits the globe posteriorly and is characterized as a homogenous structure with low internal echogenicity surrounded by the echogenic nerve sheath. A measurement of the optic nerve sheath diameter is taken 3 mm posterior to the optic disk. Normal measurements vary by age from 5 mm or less in adults (**d**), 4.5 mm in children age 1 to 15 years, and 4 mm in children younger than 1 year. Optic nerve sheath diameters typically plateau at approximately 7.5 mm even in significantly increased intracranial pressures.

Ribbon-like echogenic structure in the vitreous chamber that is free floating with eye movement (a) suggests retinal detachment. Retinal detachment is often associated with scotomas and floaters followed by unilateral vision loss classically in a curtain closing like manner. Loss of globe volume with echogenic matter in the vitreous chamber (c) suggests globe rupture with vitreous hemorrhage. Globe rupture would be extremely unlikely without a history of trauma and no physical examination findings. Color Doppler flow of the optic disk showing only blood flow exiting the globe (e) suggests central retinal artery occlusion. When using color Doppler, two colors are displayed: red indicating blood flow in the direction of the probe and blue indicating blood flow away from the probe. If color Doppler is applied to an image of the optic disk, a normal image will consist of red and blue flow correlating with arterial blood flowing toward the retina and ultrasound probe and blue flowing away from the retina and ultrasound probe. Loss of the red color flow suggests there is obstruction of the retinal artery. Central retinal artery occlusion is characterized by painless unilateral vision loss.

**406. The answer is e.** (*Ma, pp 240-241, 246-247, 250; Cosby, pp 248-252.*) In the patient with **renal outflow obstruction**, bedside ultrasound is used to evaluate primarily for **hydronephrosis**. There are multiple instances where hydronephrosis may not be pathologic. The pregnant patient with a large gravid uterus can normally have mild to moderate hydronephrosis, secondary to ureter compression by the uterus. Classically the right kidney is involved over the left kidney (b); however, hydronephrosis associated with pregnancy may be bilateral. The presence of right-sided hydronephrosis in a pregnant patient can be better evaluated by having the patient void and lay in the left lateral decubitus position for reevaluation. If the hydronephrosis does not resolve within a short period of time, it is much more suspicious for pathologic hydronephrosis.

Bilateral prominent renal collecting system with a full bladder (a) is a common benign finding. In the well-hydrated patient with a full bladder, mild bilateral hydronephrosis can develop. Rescanning the both kidneys after emptying the bladder should show resolution of the hydronephrosis. Conversely, the dehydrated patient with urinary obstruction can have normal appearing kidneys. If there is a high clinical suspicion for renal outflow obstruction, reevaluation with ultrasound should be performed after intravenous or oral hydration. Bilateral anechoic collections around the renal pelvis with dividing segments of renal cortex (c) are consistent with sonolucent renal pyramids. Sonolucent renal pyramids are normal variants and easily mistaken for dilated renal calyces consistent with hydronephrosis. They can be differentiated from dilated renal calyces by the presence of renal cortex separating each sonolucent triangle. Unilateral prominent renal pelvis located outside the medial margin of the renal cortex and no calycle dilation (d) describes an extrarenal pelvis. An extrarenal pelvis is a benign congenital variant that is easily mistaken for hydronephrosis. The key features of an extrarenal pelvis are no surrounding renal cortex and no dilated renal calyces.

**407. The answer is d.** (*Cosby, pp 56-57, 73; Ma, pp 83-84, 91-92, 96.*) This is an example of a **stratosphere sign** (see figure below) with a lung point diagnostic of a **pneumothorax**. The "B" in B mode stands for brightness. B mode is the mode of ultrasonography used with routine imaging. When a sound wave returns to the transducer, it is converted to a gray-scale pixel that corresponds to the amplitude or "loudness" of that reflected sound wave. The different shades of gray pixels represent the amount of reflected sound based on the acoustic impedance of the tissues scanned. From these pixels an image is generated and displayed on the monitor for interpretation.

The "M" in M mode stands for motion. When the machine is switched to M mode, a line will appear on the B-mode image that is simultaneously displayed. This line corresponds to a single piezoelectric channel that can be focused on an area of interest. In this case the line is focused through the lung-chest wall interface. Once the line is focused on an area of interest, the channel is plotted in a graph with time on the horizontal axis and depth on the vertical axis. By plotting this single channel of ultrasound waves over time, the movement of tissue relative to the ultrasound probe can be interpreted.

When scanning a normal thorax in M mode, the soft tissues of the chest wall generate a series of horizontal lines, while the aerated lung sliding deep to the chest wall gives a grainy appearance. This is called the **seashore sign** (see figure below). If air gets between the visceral and parietal pleura, the movement of the visceral pleura is no longer appreciated. Instead of the grainy beach-like image, a series of horizontal lines in projected. These horizontal lines look like a continuation of the horizontal lines from the chest wall giving a stratosphere sign.

Once the stratosphere sign is appreciated, the probe is positioned posterolaterally in an effort to find where the visceral and parietal pleura contact. The site where the pneumothorax ends and normal lung starts is called the lung point. At the lung point, the screen will show stratosphere sign with brief periods of seashore sign as the visceral pleura slides into view with respiratory cycles. Visualizing the lung point is 100% specific for the diagnosis of pneumothorax.

Another finding suggestive of pneumothorax is a sliding lung sign. With real-time imaging the parietal and visceral pleura are visualized as an echogenic surface deep to the chest wall. During a normal respiratory cycle, the mobile visceral pleura slides over the fixed parietal pleura. The presence of a sliding lung sign virtually rules out a pneumothorax. The absence of a sliding lung sign is highly sensitive for pneumothorax. However, false positives can be caused by pulmonary contusions, bullous emphysema, or acute respiratory distress syndrome (ARDS).

Pulmonary contusion (**a**) is less likely with a normal chest radiograph and the presence of a stratosphere sign with lung point. If real-time imaging showed the loss of a sliding lung sign and a lung point was not shown, pulmonary

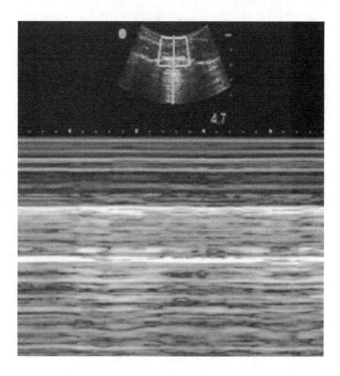

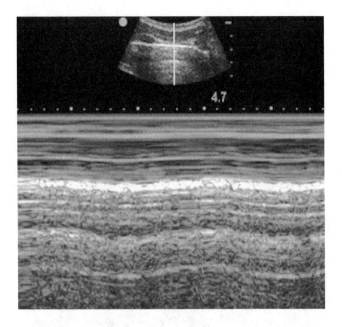

contusion would be more likely. The patient may have chest wall contusions (b) and rib fractures (c), but these are not responsible for the ultrasound findings seen in the question. A hemothorax (e) would be represented by an anechoic fluid collection in the dependent portions of the thorax.

**408. The answer is a.** *(Ma, pp 324-327, 337-340, 343-346.)* **Placenta previa** is a **contraindication to digital examination of the cervix** as placental trauma from the examination itself can lead to profuse vaginal bleeding. **Any patient presenting to ED in the second or third trimester of pregnancy with bleeding should have ultrasound performed before pelvic examination to rule out placenta previa.** Late in pregnancy, presenting fetal parts obscure the cervix from transabdominal ultrasonography making it difficult to determine the exact proximity of the placental edge to the internal cervical os. Thus, if the placenta is implanted in the lower uterine segment, the pelvic examination should be deferred until translabial or transvaginal ultrasound can be obtained to pinpoint the placental location in relation to the cervix.

A cervical length of 4 cm (b) can be reassuring indicating the bleeding is not secondary to changes in labor. The normal cervical length is 3 to

5 cm. As the cervix shortens with effacement and dilation, a cervical length less than 3 cm is concerning for labor or risk of preterm labor. In this case the exact gestation age is not obvious; however, based on physical examination it is clearly a third-trimester pregnancy. Various fetal ultrasound measurements can be conducted to determine an estimated fetal weight, which would offer some correlation to appropriate gestational age such as biparietal diameter, femur length, and abdominal circumference. A hyperechoic fluid collection between the placenta and uterine wall (c) is suggestive of placental abruption. Ultrasound will show evidence of placental hemorrhage in only 50% of cases; thus it is not a reliable test to rule out abruption. Abruption is difficult to detect because the normal architecture of the placenta often mimics abruption on ultrasound. In addition depending on the age of the hemorrhage, abruption can be hyperechoic (early), hypoechoic, or anechoic (late).

Whether evidence of abruption is detected or not cardiotocographic monitoring is required to determine next step in management. Placental abruption is not a contraindication to pelvic examination in pregnancy. A placenta implanted high and posterior in the uterus (d) is normal and rules out placenta previa; thus digital examination of the cervix is not contraindicated in this instance. Ultrasound is an excellent way to detect a breech fetus. (e) When a breech fetus is detected and the patient is in labor, digital examination is warranted.

**409. The answer is a.** (*Cosby, pp 209-211; Ma, pp 184-186.*) Hepatic masses are a common incidental finding. Distinguishing benign from serious lesions by ultrasound can be difficult given the overlap in the sonographic appearance. Thus, most incidental lesions in the liver require further imaging. Normal liver tissue on ultrasound has a salt and pepper heterogeneous appearance. **Solid heterogeneous or cystic lesions with soft internal echoes that contain irregular boarders are concerning for neoplastic or infectious lesions.** When numerous heterogeneous lesions are present, the suspicion for metastatic disease is very high.

Phrygian cap (b) is an incidental finding on the gallbladder. A mucosal fold in the fundus of the gallbladder giving a tortuous fundus characterizes it. This finding is not pathologic; however, it should be carefully evaluated as gallstones in the phrygian cap are often missed. Well-defined masses with smooth margins that are anechoic or homogenous internally (c and d) are usually associated with benign masses. Riedel lobe (e) is an accessory lobe off the right lobe extending inferiorly toward the pelvis. It is normal hepatic tissue and will have the same salt and pepper echogenicity as the rest of the liver. The clinical significance of this is that it can be mistaken for hepatomegaly.

**410. The answer is b.** *(Cosby, pp 60, 80-81; Ma, pp 79-81, 89.)* The perisplenic view of this FAST examination shows an **anechoic stripe** in the **subphrenic space** representing **free fluid in the peritoneal cavity**. In the **setting of trauma** free peritoneal fluid is presumed to be **blood**. Blood in the perisplenic region most commonly collects in the subphrenic space.

In this case the patient gives a classic **Kehr sign** for **splenic rupture**. Blood in the left subphrenic space irritates the diaphragm giving referred pain to the left shoulder. Many low to moderate grade liver and spleen injuries can be managed nonoperatively or with interventional radiology by embolizing bleeding vessels. Because this patient is **clinically stable**, further imaging with a **CT scan is the next best step** in management.

If the patient had been hemodynamically unstable, it would be appropriate to begin a blood transfusion and (**a**) bring the patient to the operating room (**c**) for definitive management. Solid organ injury does not lead to pneumoperitoneum (**d**); thus upright chest radiography would not be helpful. Further imaging and observation is required to ensure that the patient does not deteriorate. Discharging the patient home directly from the ED (**e**) is inappropriate in the setting of an intraperitoneal bleed.

# Environmental Exposures

## Questions

**411.** A 58-year-old man presents to the emergency department (ED) with reported blister formation over both feet that initially began 2 days ago. He denies any past medical history, medications, or allergies. His social history is significant for alcohol dependence and recently becoming undomiciled. He denies any sick contacts or recent travel. Upon physical examination, these lesions are fluid-filled and his feet are grossly cyanotic and tender to the touch. His foot is shown below. What is the most likely diagnosis in this patient?

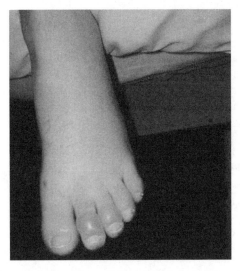

*(Reproduced, with permission, from Knoop KJ, Stack LB, Storrow AB.* Atlas of Emergency Medicine. *New York, NY: McGraw-Hill, 2002: 517.)*

a. Chilblains
b. Frostbite
c. Trench foot
d. Thermal burn
e. Herpes

**412.** A 43-year-old insulin-dependent diabetic woman presents with an intensely pruritic rash across her back for the last several days. She reports a recent trip to the Caribbean with her family last week, none of whom has similar symptoms. She denies any insect bites, new detergents, soaps, or clothes, and has otherwise been at her baseline of health with no constitutional symptoms. The patient is on insulin glargine for her diabetes and reports a hemoglobin $A_{1C}$ of less than 7 mg/dL. Upon physical examination, the patient has small vesicular lesions on an erythematous base with no visible purulence. The rash does not follow a dermatome distribution and is clustered across her back. Which of the following is the most appropriate treatment choice for this patient?

a. Calamine lotion
b. Acyclovir
c. Chlorhexidine lotion
d. Diphenhydramine (Benadryl)
e. Parenteral antibiotics

**413.** A 32-year-old otherwise healthy man develops dizziness, nausea, and confusion after running a race. Emergency medical services (EMS) are available on-site and the patient is given intravenous (IV) fluids. He is oriented to person and time but not place. He appears generally confused and it is difficult to obtain contact information from him. The patient is brought to the ED whereupon his symptoms generally resolve, except for diffuse muscle fatigue. Laboratory tests are drawn at this time, which are essentially normal, except for minimally elevated hepatic transaminases. Given this patient's symptoms and laboratory evaluation, what is the most likely diagnosis?

a. Heat syncope
b. Heat edema
c. Rhabdomyolysis
d. Heat stroke
e. Heat exhaustion

**414.** A 42-year-old man presents to the ED after sustaining an electric shock when he was changing a wall outlet. The patient complains of pain in the finger that was shocked. Visual inspection reveals localized erythema at the distal tip but good capillary refill, 2+ radial, and ulnar pulses and full range of motion of that hand and extremity. Chest auscultation reveals a normal $S_1$ and $S_2$ with clear and equal breath sounds bilaterally. There are no other signs of trauma. What diagnostic test should be performed next in the complete evaluation of this patient?

a. Urinalysis
b. Basic metabolic panel
c. Chest radiograph
d. Electrocardiogram (ECG)
e. Arterial Doppler

**415.** An 18-year-old man presents to the ED with right leg pain and swelling after swimming at a local beach. He reports swimming in the ocean, whereupon he felt a sharp sting in his right leg. Upon physical examination, there is no gross deformity of the right lower extremity and there is a palpable dorsalis pedis and posterior tibial pulse. There is tenderness to palpation over the lateral calf with many punctuate, erythematous lesions as seen below. Which of the following is the most appropriate treatment of choice for this patient?

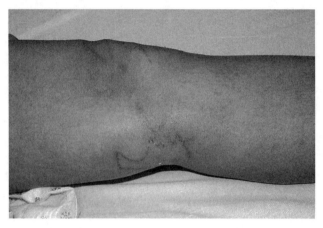

*(Courtesy of Corey Long, MD.)*

a. Fresh water
b. Vegetable oil
c. Vinegar
d. Toothpaste
e. Household window cleaner

**416.** A 49-year-old man presents to the ED with pain, erythema, and swelling to his left forearm after a chemical spill sustained at work. He irrigated the area with water and applied a cold packet before arriving but states that the burning sensation in his arm is now worse. The patient works in a glass factory and reports using a rust-removing agent. What tissue-saving treatment must be administered emergently?

a. Limb tourniquet
b. Calcium gluconate
c. Alkalinization of urine
d. Silver sulfadiazine ointment
e. Surgical debridement

**417.** A 23-year-old construction worker is brought by ambulance to the ED with bilateral knee pain. He reports mixing cement the day before and kneeling in the process. The patient states that his jeans were soaked through most of the day but did not attempt to wash the cement off. Upon physical examination, you see marked tissue necrosis of both knees extending to the bone in some places. Which chemical was this patient most likely exposed to?

a. Hydrocarbon
b. Phenol
c. Ammonia
d. Formic acid
e. Lime

**418.** A 40-year-old veterinary assistant presents to the ED with puncture wounds over her right upper extremity and neck. She reports being bitten multiple times by a cat in her care, and also states that the cat's immunizations were up to date. The injury was sustained 2 days ago with minimal initial symptoms. However, today the patient noticed redness and pain in that area. She denies any fever, chills, nausea, vomiting, or any other constitutional symptoms. Her initial vitals include an oral temperature of 99.7°F, a heart rate (HR) of 90 beats per minute, blood pressure (BP) of 125/75 mm Hg, respiratory rate (RR) of 14 breaths per minute, and an oxygen saturation of 99% on room air. Multiple punctate wounds may be seen over her right lateral neck extending down to her deltoid with surrounding erythema and edema. Which antibiotic coverage for the specific organism involved in this type of injury would be most appropriate?

a. A first-generation cephalosporin/*Staphylococcus aureus*
b. Amoxicillin/clavulanate (Augmentin)/*Pasteurella multocida*
c. Clindamycin/*Streptococcus* sp.
d. Vancomycin/methicillin-resistant *S aureus*
e. Bacitracin ointment/*S aureus*

**419.** A 26-year-old woman presents to the ED with a history of spilling hot soup over her left arm earlier in the day. She states that she immediately put her hand under cold water and applied ice. Upon physical examination, the involved area covers the dorsum of her hand and extends up to the middle of her forearm with no circumferential or digital involvement. She can freely flex and extend all joints of that upper extremity. In addition, two large fluid-filled bullae are noted in the area of the forearm. What is the burn degree and relative area of involvement in this patient?

a. First-degree/9%
b. Second-degree/9%
c. Second-degree/2.25%
d. Third-degree/9%
e. Third-degree/4.5%

**420.** A 60-year-old male cook reports spilling hot oil over his left thigh while attempting to pull a pan off of the stove. He presents to the ED with erythema extending over his left thigh without any blister formation or circumferential involvement. The patient reports that he was wearing thick pants at the time of the accident that he removed quickly and promptly irrigated the area with water. There are no other signs of injury. What is the burn degree and relative area of involvement in this patient?

a. First-degree/9%
b. First-degree/4.5%
c. Second-degree/2.25%
d. Second-degree/9%
e. Third-degree/4.5%

**421.** You are the physician staffing a clinic in the Rocky Mountains when 29-year-old male mountain-climber presents with nausea, vomiting, and dizziness. Upon review of systems, he denies fever, cough, abdominal pain, or dysuria but does report anorexia and some ankle swelling. What diuretic is the drug of choice in this patient?

a. Furosemide
b. Hydrochlorothiazide
c. Bumetanide
d. Fosinopril
e. Acetazolamide

**422.** A 25-year-old female scuba diver presents to the ED with multiple areas of periarticular joint pain and red, itchy skin. Her initial vitals include an oral temperature of 98°F, BP of 110/65 mm Hg, HR of 88 beats per minute, RR of 14 breaths per minute, and oxygen saturation of 97% on room air. Upon physical examination, the patient has pain upon palpation of bilateral knees and ankles with full range of motion in these joints. Areas of erythema that do not follow a specific dermatomal pattern cover most of the lower extremities, torso, and back with areas of excoriation where patient reports scratching. There are no other lesions. Which of the following is the most likely diagnosis?

a. Sexually transmitted disease (STD)
b. Decompression sickness
c. Descent barotrauma
d. Ascent barotrauma
e. Nitrogen narcosis

**423.** A 19-year-old rookie Navy Seal presents to the ED with a history of syncope upon ascent from a dive. The length and depth of the dive was within decompression regulation. He currently complains of feeling light-headed with a moderate frontal headache. Vital signs include HR of 86 beats per minute, BP of 130/65 mm Hg, and RR of 16 breaths per minute with oxygen saturation of 93% on room air. Upon physical examination, he appears somewhat confused and is oriented only to person and place. He has no focal neurologic deficits. What underlying event is the cause for this patient's symptoms?

a. Pulmonary embolism
b. Cardiac ischemia
c. Transient ischemic attack
d. Dysbaric air embolism
e. Nitrogen narcosis

**424.** A farmer in Texas presents to the ED with right leg numbness, localized edema, and tremors. He reports being out in the field when the symptoms began. He denies contact with insecticides and reports being at his baseline of health prior to the event. His initial vitals include HR of 105 beats per minute, BP of 175/90 mm Hg, and RR of 22 breaths per minute with oxygen saturation of 97% on room air. Which of the following is the most appropriate initial treatment of choice in this patient?

a. Antivenin
b. Tetanus prophylaxis
c. Antibiotic prophylaxis
d. Sedation
e. Atropine

**425.** A 23-year-old man presents to the ED after sustaining a bee sting. The patient points to his left arm when asked where the pain is. Upon physical examination, you see a single puncture wound with surrounding erythema and swelling. The patient is in no respiratory distress and is phonating well. Chest auscultation reveals clear breath sounds bilaterally with no wheezing. The oropharynx is patent without any tonsillar or uvular displacement. Which of the following is the most appropriate next step in management?

a. Subcutaneous epinephrine 0.01 mL/kg
b. IV epinephrine 0.01 mL/kg
c. Steroids
d. Observation
e. Antihistamines

**426.** An 18-year-old man is brought into the ED and reports that a stray dog at the park bit him. The patient complains of right forearm pain, where he was bitten. Upon physical examination, you note a superficial macerated laceration on the dorsal surface of the distal forearm with no active bleeding. The patient is able to freely flex and extend all joints in the right upper extremity. In addition to localized wound care, antibiotics, and tetanus prophylaxis, what other expeditious measures should be taken in the care of this patient?

a. Reporting the incident to local authorities
b. Rabies immunization
c. Tight suturing of the laceration
d. Antihistamines
e. Irrigation with povidone-iodine solution

**427.** A 31-year-old man presents to the ED with left calf pain. He reports general malaise, nausea, and myalgias since a recent trip to Arkansas. His initial vitals include oral temperature of 99°F, HR of 76 beats per minute, BP of 128/70 mm Hg, RR of 16 breaths per minute, and oxygen saturation of 98% on room air. Upon physical examination, there are diffuse petechiae of the left lower extremity from the anterior distal tibia to the mid-thigh. Closer examination reveals a small necrotic lesion at the level of the lateral mid-calf with surrounding edema as seen below. The patient's calf is tender to the touch and upon dorsiflexion. Which of the following is the most likely cause of this patient's clinical symptoms?

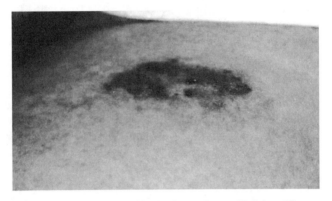

(Reproduced, with permission, from Knoop KJ, Stack LB, Storrow AB. Atlas of Emergency Medicine. New York, NY: McGraw-Hill, 2002: 531.)

a. Deep venous thrombosis (DVT)
b. Scorpion sting
c. Brown recluse spider bite
d. Black widow spider bite
e. Thrombocytopenia

**428.** A 23-year-old avid high-altitude skier presents to the ED with intense pain, tearing, and bilateral ocular foreign body sensation. He denies any trauma, past medical problems or contact lens use. His physical examination is significant for bilateral decreased visual acuity, injected conjunctiva, and diffuse punctuate corneal lesions with a discrete inferior border. His pupils are equal, round, and reactive to light. Given this patient's history and physical examination, which of the following is the most likely diagnosis?

a. Corneal abrasion
b. Iritis
c. Ultraviolet keratitis
d. Corneal foreign body
e. Corneal laceration

**429.** A 44-year-old woman returns from a mountain excursion with headache symptoms, nausea, and vomiting that are improving. Her initial vital signs in the ED are HR of 93 beats per minute, BP of 120/60 mm Hg, RR of 18 breaths per minute, and oxygen saturation of 96% on 2-L nasal cannula. Her chest examination is clear to auscultation with no palpable overlying crepitus and there are no signs of peripheral edema. Which of the following medications is indicated in this patient?

a. Acetazolamide
b. Dexamethasone
c. Nifedipine
d. Furosemide
e. Morphine

**430.** A 20-year-old college student presents to the ED with a cutaneous lesion as depicted below. He is brought in by friends who report being out in an open field during stormy weather when the injury occurred. The patient denies any recent travel or sick contacts. He also denies any symptoms except for some generalized confusion. Which aspect of the physical examination of this patient is initially most pertinent to the nature of this type of injury?

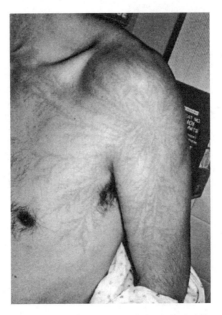

*(Reproduced, with permission, from Tintinalli J, Kelen G, Stapczynski J. Emergency Medicine: A Comprehensive Study Guide. New York, NY: McGraw-Hill, 2004: 1238.)*

a. Testing of cranial nerves
b. Otoscopic evaluation of tympanic membranes
c. Evaluation of gait cadence
d. Testing of cerebellar deficits
e. Palpating the cervical spine for tenderness

**431.** A 24-year-old man presents to the ED with diffuse facial pain, pruritus, erythema, and dizziness after reportedly falling on to an anthill. His initial vital signs include HR of 102 beats per minute, BP of 118/75 mm Hg, and RR of 18 breaths per minute with oxygen saturation of 98% on room air. What is the initial appropriate assessment in this clinical scenario?

a. Give tetanus prophylaxis.
b. Begin local wound care.
c. Assess airway, breathing, and circulation.
d. Start IV fluid administration.
e. Give oral antihistamines.

**432.** An undomiciled man of unknown age presents to the ED unresponsive. His ECG is shown below. What is the most appropriate next step in treatment?

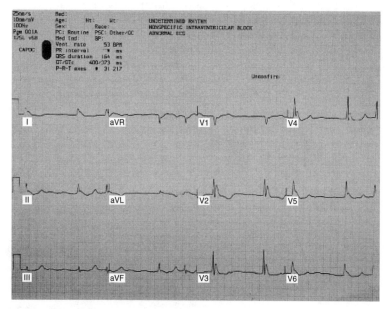

*(Reproduced, with permission, from Knoop KJ, Stack LB, Storrow AB. Atlas of Emergency Medicine. New York, NY: McGraw-Hill, 2002: 516.)*

a. Defibrillation
b. Cardiac pacing
c. Advanced cardiac life support
d. Advanced cardiac life support and rewarming
e. Cardiopulmonary bypass

**433.** A 26-year-old man presents to the ED in agony with a Gila monster still attached to his arm after being bitten. He reports that he is the animal's main handler, with no prior biting incidents. He reports localized pain but denies weakness, nausea, or feeling light-headed. The animal bite occurred about 45 minutes ago. After the animal is carefully removed, what should be done next in the care of this patient?

a. Check for any remaining embedded teeth and begin wound care.
b. Administer antivenin.
c. Give tetanus prophylaxis.
d. Administer broad-spectrum antibiotics.
e. Apply suction device.

**434.** An anxious college student presents to the ED at 2 AM stating a bat woke him up. He heard something flying around his bedroom and, when he turned the lights on, he saw a bat fly into his closet. He is unsure if he was bit by the bat but noticed bat droppings in his bed. Which is the most appropriate management for the patient?

a. Reassure him that there is nothing to do and discharge him.
b. Immunoprophylax with human rabies immune globulin and human diploid cell vaccine.
c. Administer ciprofloxacin 500 mg.
d. Admit him to the hospital for 24 hours of observation.
e. Immunoprophylax with human diploid cell vaccine.

# Environmental Exposures

## Answers

**411. The answer is b.** *(Rosen, pp 1861-1867.)* Frostbite usually occurs when temperatures fall below 0°C (32°F). There are essentially three phases to the freezing injury cascade. Phase 1 (prefreeze) includes initial skin cooling, increased blood viscosity, and microvascular leakage that causes localized edema formation. Phase 2 (freeze-thaw) is when extracellular crystal formation begins, thereby causing intracellular shrinkage and essentially collapse of the cellular network. Finally, phase 3 (vascular stasis/progressive ischemia) involves further coagulation, interstitial leakage, and cell death, thus resulting in blister formation, cyanosis, and ultimately mummification of the tissue. The bullae formed may also have a hemorrhagic appearance. It is important to note that wind and moisture may increase the freezing rate. Management includes rapid rewarming with water at a temperature of 37°C to 40°C (98.6°F-104°F) with care in preventing refreezing. Friction massage, which furthers tissue loss, should be avoided. Rewarming is a painful procedure that requires parenteral analgesia. Patients may also have a degree of dehydration and benefit from crystalloid administration.

(**a**) Chilblains, also known as pernio, are a condition commonly seen in the homeless population as a result of chronic dry-cold exposure and mostly affect the face, hands, and pretibial areas. Trench foot (**c**), also known as immersion injury, is common in this population; however, it usually presents as a loss of sensation with pallor and mottling. (**d**) Thermal burns may present with bullae formation but do not elicit cyanosis. (**e**) Herpes is also unlikely given the distribution and lack of contacts with similar lesions.

**412. The answer is c.** *(Rosen, p 1887.)* This patient is suffering from **miliaria rubra**, more commonly known as **prickly heat** or **heat rash**. This is an acute inflammatory disorder of the skin that occurs in tropical climates, also lending the term "lichen tropicus." It occurs because of sweat gland blockage and staphylococcal infection. The acute phase is noted by vesicular lesions that are caused by obstruction of the sweat glands, which subsequently rupture. The rash is confined to *clothed areas* and may progress to a profunda stage, in which the obstruction delves deeper into the skin and produces larger vesicles that may become infected. These, however, are not pruritic and may resemble a chronic dermatitis. The antibacterial treatment of choice is **chlorhexidine**, which is to be used in the acute phase. Salicylic acid may also be used to assist in desquamation but should not be used on large areas because of possible salicylate intoxication. **(a and d)** Although calamine and diphenhydramine (Benadryl) may assist in symptomatic relief, they do not offer treatment. **(b)** Acyclovir is to treat herpes infection. **(e)** Treatment is especially important in this patient with insulin-dependent diabetes mellitus (IDDM) to prevent further infectious complications that necessitate parenteral antibiotics.

**413. The answer is e.** *(Rosen, pp 1886-1890.)* The diagnosis of **heat exhaustion** is initially made upon clinical presentation. Patients may have general malaise, fatigue, frontal headache, impaired judgment, diaphoresis, and nausea, and show signs of dehydration with tachycardia and orthostatic hypotension. Heat exhaustion may progress to heat stroke and lies along a spectrum in which intermediate cases may often be difficult to delineate; however, the treatment is essentially the same. It is important to bring the patient to a cool location and start fluid replacement slowly as to prevent cerebral edema, especially in younger patients. To help distinguish between heat exhaustion and heat stroke, hepatic transaminases are helpful. Elevations to several thousand units may be seen in heat exhaustion or healthy runners after a marathon, whereas in heat stroke the levels are elevated to tens of thousands. **(a)** Heat syncope results from the dilatation of cutaneous vessels to assist in the delivery of heat to the skin's surface, thereby pooling the blood to the periphery and causing syncope. Elderly patients and those who stand for long periods are especially prone to this. **(b)** Heat edema occurs in patients who are not acclimated to warmer temperatures and thereby develop swollen feet and ankles. This is not a central process and altered mental states do not occur. **(c)** Rhabdomyolysis may result in any case where there is muscle breakdown caused by dehydration, stress, or exogenous factors. The patient may have mild rhabdomyolysis; however, it alone does not explain this patient's symptoms. **(d)** Neurologic dysfunctions, including seizures and coma, are a hallmark of heat stroke, which result when treatment is not initiated and thermoregulatory responses fail. These patients often have dry, hot skin with core temperatures above 105°F.

**414. The answer is d.** (*Rosen, pp 1893-1902.*) The patient sustained a low-voltage (< 1000 V) electrical injury from the wall socket. All patients sustaining such an injury warrant an ECG and cardiac monitoring in the ED. In the United States, household wiring has 120 V of alternating current with a frequency (number of switches from positive to negative) of 60 Hz. Alternating current causes continuous muscle contraction and stimulation that may cause ventricular fibrillation. Direct current usually just causes a single muscle spasm and is the less dangerous of the two, depending on the voltage. The current is equal to the voltage over the resistance (Ohm law). This patient sustained a superficial thermal burn and most likely did not become part of the circuit given that there were not any clear entry or exit wounds as seen in direct-contact injuries. Disposition of this patient should include localized wound care, close follow-up, and instructions to return if there are any worsening symptoms.

(**a and b**) Although a urinalysis to screen for myoglobin and a basic metabolic panel to check renal function might be performed, it is not necessary given the nature of this patient's injury. (**c and e**) A chest x-ray and arterial Doppler will not prove efficacious given the clinical examination.

**415. The answer is c.** (*Rosen, pp 756-757.*) This patient sustained an injury from a venomous marine animal. Approximately 50,000 such incidents occur yearly. Marine animals may be divided into two classes: stingers and nematocysts. Stingers include sea urchins, stingrays, catfish, cone shells, and starfish. Radiographs may be useful in delineating the calciferous material deposited in the skin for removal. Nematocysts are much more prevalent and account for the majority of envenomations and most likely account for this patient's distress. This class includes jellyfish, fire corals, Portuguese man-o-war, and anemones. These creatures have spring-loaded venomous glands that discharge upon mechanical or chemical stimulation. The number of nematocysts on a tentacle can number in the thousands. These stinging cells can remain activated after weeks of the animal being beached. The venom contains various peptides and enzymes that may cause progression of symptoms, including nausea, muscle cramps, dyspnea, angioedema, and anaphylaxis. The preferred treatment is *vinegar*, which deactivates the nematocyst. In cases where medical attention cannot be sought in a timely manner, urine has been shown to be just as efficacious. An attempt may be made to shave off nematocysts after proper analgesia. Patient should be given tetanus prophylaxis and antihistamines as needed.

(a) Fresh water activates the nematocyst and should be avoided. (b, d, and e) Vegetable oil, toothpaste, and household window cleaners should also be avoided as they might cause further irritation and pain.

**416. The answer is b.** (*Rosen, pp 769-770.*) Chemical burns are a common occupational hazard and can be caused by a variety of solvents containing acidic or alkali mixtures. Initially, it is important to remove the patient from the offending chemical and irrigate with copious amounts of water to dilute the agent. It is important to assess the affected area, size, and depth of the burn, as some patients will need transfer to a burn center. This patient was chemically burned by a rust-removing agent, which commonly contains **hydrofluoric acid (HF)**. Other solvents include high-octane gas and germicides. **Pain out of proportion to sustained injury** is usually seen in these cases. As HF is a relatively weak acid, its extreme electronegativity, however, makes it very dangerous. Fluoride avidly binds to available cations, such as calcium and magnesium, thereby causing cell death. Profound **hypocalcemia** has been demonstrated in HF exposure. ECG monitoring and administration of exogenous cations, such as topical **calcium gluconate gel**, can act as chelating agents to the fluoride ions. IV or intradermal calcium gluconate may also be used. Calcium chloride should be avoided given its ability to cause tissue necrosis upon extravasation.

(a) Placing a tourniquet upon the limb may cause ischemia and further cell death. (c) Alkalinization of urine would not be of benefit in this type of exposure. (d) Silver sulfadiazine may be applied later on for wound care. (e) The extent of this injury at this time does not warrant surgical debridement; however, close wound-care monitoring should be instilled to recognize cases when tissue necrosis progresses.

**417. The answer is e.** (*Rosen, pp 770-773.*) This patient was exposed to **lime**, which is present in **cement**. When water interacts with dry **cement**, hydrolysis occurs forming an alkali with a pH of 10 to 12. **Alkali burns form a liquefaction necrosis**, causing quick dissolution of involved tissue. Acid burns form a coagulation necrosis, which is somewhat slower in nature. The best treatment is **intense irrigation** upon initial contact, a ritual performed by the more experienced individuals who work with lime. This patient will need further debridement and wound care because of his exposure.

(a) Hydrocarbons are present in mainly gasoline and paint thinners. (b) Phenol is found in dyes, deodorants, disinfectants, and agriculture solvents, which causes cell denaturing upon contact. Ammonia (c) is present in many household cleaners, as a cooling agent in refrigerator units and as a fertilizer owing to its high nitrogen content and may act differently depending on what form it is in. For example, it may freeze skin on contact or affect breathing because of its vapors. Formic acid (d) is a caustic organic acid used in many industries that causes a coagulation necrosis. Treatment for exposure to all of these chemicals includes copious irrigation and observation for systemic side effects.

**418. The answer is b.** *(Rosen, pp 734-735.)* **Cat bites** involve **puncture wounds** often extending down through skin into tendons and bones owing to the nature of the animals' sharp teeth. The reported incidence of infection from these bites may be as high as 30% to 50%, with many patients presenting only after an infection has incurred. It is important to note that cat bites have a higher infection rate compared to dog bites, given the typical puncture wound that inoculates bacteria down the track deep into tissue and becomes enclosed. *Pasteurella multocida* is a strong gram-negative, facultative anaerobic rod found in the oral cavity of the majority of healthy cats and may cause severe systemic infection, especially in the immunocompromised. Patients need to be followed closely as these infections may seed deep into joints and tissue requiring debridement.
(a) First-generation cephalosporins have proven to be only minimally effective. The organism is resistant to (d) vancomycin and (c) clindamycin. (e) Antibiotic topicals, such as bacitracin, would be inappropriate given the high virulence of this organism.

**419. The answer is c.** *(Rosen, pp 759-761.)* This patient sustained a **second-degree burn involving 2.25% of her body surface area (BSA)**, according to the rule of nines. The rule of nines aids in estimating the area of involvement as seen below. In the adult, each anterior or posterior surface of the upper extremity and head is equal to 4.5%. Each surface of the lower extremity is equal to 9%. Each surface of the chest and torso is equal to 18%. Perineal areas account for 1% of BSA. Children and infants have increased total BSA relative to their weight, thereby requiring different fluid requirements and area estimation. More percentage is dedicated to the head given their larger head-to-body ratios (7% in children and 9% in infants). The **treatment for this patient involves silver sulfadiazine dressings and close follow-up.** Prophylactic antibiotics are not warranted in these cases, given the chance of increased future resistance rates. For areas of

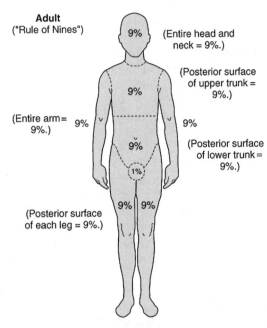

Adult
("Rule of Nines")

9%    (Entire head and
neck = 9%.)

(Posterior surface
of upper trunk =
9%.)

9%

(Entire arm =    9%
9%.)

9%

(Posterior surface
of lower trunk =
9%.)

9%

1%

(Posterior surface
of each leg = 9%.)

9%  9%

*(Reproduced, with permission, from Tierney LM, McPhee SJ, Papadakis MA. Current Medical Diagnosis & Treatment. New York, NY: McGraw-Hill, 2006.)*

greater involvement and inhalation burns, fluid resuscitation may become necessary to account for losses. This is done using the **Parkland formula**: 4 mL/kg/%TBSA (total BSA), one-half to be given over first 8 hours and the remaining half to be given over the next 16 hours. Ringer lactate is the fluid of choice. It is also important to protect against hypothermia and provide adequate analgesia. Depending on the extent and area of the burn, some patients may need transfer to a burn facility where further escharotomy and debridement may be performed.

First-degree burns (**a**) are characterized primarily by erythema, having the appearance of a simple sunburn. It involves the epidermis only and usually heals without scar formation. Second-degree burns (**b and c**) are superficial partial thickness burns involving the epidermis and part of the dermis, resulting in painful erythema and blister formation. Follicles and glands may or may not be involved. These blisters are best left intact. Third-degree burns (**d and e**) are full-thickness burns involving the epidermis, dermis, and subcutaneous fat that results in pale, charred skin. Surgical debridement and grafting are necessary in these cases. Fourth-degree burns extend through the skin, fat, muscle, and bone, and are often limb and life-threatening.

**420. The answer is b.** (*Rosen, pp 759-761.*) Please see explanation in previous question.

**421. The answer is e.** (*Rosen, pp 1921-1923.*) This patient is an otherwise healthy male with no reason to have congestive heart failure (CHF), renal failure, hepatic failure, or cardiomyopathy. Instead, he is an avid **mountain-climber**, which should hint at **acute mountain sickness (AMS)** in this clinical scenario. Early on, symptoms may mimic an acute viral syndrome with nausea, vomiting, headache, and anorexia. However, these symptoms progress to include **peripheral edema, oliguria, retinal hemorrhages, and finally high-altitude pulmonary or cerebral edema**. The initial treatment for all of these conditions across the spectrum of AMS includes **gradual descent**. A descent of 1500 to 3000 ft reverses high-altitude sickness in most cases. Supplemental **oxygen** is indicated in all cases. Diuretics, such as *acetazolamide* have been proven effective not only for treatment but for prophylaxis. Symptomatic treatment for vomiting and headache may also be indicated. Hyperbaric oxygen therapy is indicated in severe cases. Risk factors for AMS include, but are not limited to, rapid ascent, chronic obstructive pulmonary disease (COPD), sickle-cell disease, cold exposure, heavy exertion, and sleeping at higher altitudes.

Furosemide (**a**) and hydrochlorothiazide (**b**) are indicated in CHF and hypertension. Bumetanide (**c**) is a more potent loop diuretic, also not indicated. Fosinopril (**d**) is an angiotensin-converting enzyme (ACE) inhibitor.

**422. The answer is b.** (*Rosen, pp 1908-1910.*) This patient is suffering from **decompression sickness**, more commonly known as "the bends." This term refers to a spectrum of states whereupon bubbles of nitrogen gas collect in the blood and tissues. To help illustrate, picture a bottle of soda being opened, allowing the bubbles to rapidly come out of the solution to the top. Clinically, the degree of collection is a result of the depth and length of the dive. Other risk factors include inherent fatigue, heavy exertion, dehydration, and flying after a dive. A patent foramen ovale may also prove to be dangerous in causing gas bubbles to embolize to the arterial system. Decompression sickness can progress from its initial musculoskeletal involvement to include the cardiovascular, respiratory, and central nervous system (CNS). Divers should ascend in a slow, gradual manner to avoid to collection of nitrogen gas in these tissues. Transport to the nearest **hyperbaric chamber** is the treatment of choice. IV fluid hydration and supplemental oxygen may also be warranted.

An STD (a) is unlikely. Descent barotrauma (c) includes sinus, ear, and skin squeeze. Divers who hold their breath upon descent may also develop lung squeeze. Ascent barotrauma (d) involves similar conditions in addition to pneumomediastinum and pneumothorax. Nitrogen narcosis (e), also known as "rapture of the deep," is an interesting phenomenon in which prolonged dives produce a euphoric effect upon the diver because of the collection of nitrogen gas in the tissues. This may prove dangerous in the face of an emergency, given a false sense of security and impaired motor skills.

**423. The answer is d.** (*Rosen, p 1909.*) Being a rookie diver, this patient ascended to the surface too quickly. As in decompression sickness, nitrogen gas bubbles form and subsequently travel to the arterial system through the pulmonary veins into the cardiac chambers. **Arterial gas embolism** may also occur in patients with an underlying patent foramen ovale. Symptoms are usually sudden and dramatic. Divers, who may have been thought to drown, actually passed out during ascent because of an underlying embolism. Treatment includes hyperbaric oxygen therapy and the avoidance of air transport.

Although cardiac ischemia (b) may occur because of this, it is not the precipitating event. Pulmonary embolism (a) in otherwise healthy individuals with no risk factors is low probability as the inciting event. Transient ischemic attacks (c) may present in a variety of ways, but given this clinical scenario, a serious diving-related cause must be investigated first. (e) Nitrogen narcosis occurs secondary to breathing gasses at higher-than-normal atmospheric pressure. It occurs as the diver descends to depths greater than 70 ft. Clinically, patients appear as if they are ethanol intoxicated. The condition clears with resurfacing.

**424. The answer is a.** (*Rosen, pp 743-750.*) This patient suffered a **venomous snakebite**. Pit vipers, such as rattlesnakes, copperheads, and water moccasins, are the most prevalent and are present in all states except Alaska, Maine, and Hawaii. Coral snakes are the second most prevalent and are present mainly in the southern states. **Red on yellow, kill a fellow; red on black, venom lack** is a commonly used phrase to help remember which snakes are dangerous. Venomous snakes can also be recognized by their triangular heads, elliptical pupils, fangs, and the presence of a pit between the eye and nostril—characteristics that may not be noticed by the victim initially. Therefore, there is a snakebite grading system, which requires antivenin with progressive symptoms of edema, coagulopathy, and neurologic manifestations. The amount of antivenin is dependent on the severity of these symptoms. Venom itself has a number of substances including proteolytic enzymes and polypeptides, which promote coagulation, neuromuscular blockage, cell lysis, and death. Anaphylaxis may also occur. Airway, breathing, and circulation (ABCs) must always be initially assessed.

Tetanus prophylaxis (**b**) should be given at some point in treatment, but it is not the initial treatment of choice. Antibiotic prophylaxis (**c**) is not clinically indicated in these cases. Sedation (**d**) with benzodiazepines may be used in other venomous bites, such as scorpions, as a result of the extreme pain and neurologic manifestations but is not clinically indicated here. Atropine (**e**) and pralidoxime are used in cases of organophosphate exposure.

**425. The answer is d.** (*Rosen, pp 750-752.*) History-taking should include prior bee stings in this child, as each successive sting increases the possibility of anaphylaxis given sensitization. The ABCs must be initially addressed. Stings most commonly present with localized burning, erythema, and edema at the sting site lasting for about 24 hours. The patient is asymptomatic and only warrants **observation** at this time. Toxicity and anaphylaxis are evident soon after the sting and include vomiting, diarrhea, fever, and neurologic manifestations, such as seizures and altered mental status. This child most likely sustained a sting from a honeybee or bumblebee, given the single puncture wound. Aphids contain retroserrate-barbed stingers, which are removed upon stinging, thereby eviscerating and killing the insect. Vespids, such as wasps, hornets, and yellow jackets, do not contain this mechanism and may sting many times. "Killer bees," as popularized by the film industry, contain the same amount of venom as other species. The difference is that they are more aggressive, not more toxic.

Our patient's condition at this time does not warrant epinephrine (**a and b**) in any form. Steroids (**c**) and antihistamines (**e**) are usually given in patients with systemic signs. $\beta_2$-Agonists (eg, albuterol) may also be given for respiratory symptoms.

**426. The answer is b.** (*Rosen, pp 733-734, 737-738.*) Given that the bite was sustained by an **unknown stray dog** that may be difficult to locate, **rabies immunization** should be given promptly. If the dog could be found, quarantining the animal for 10 days for observation may be a valid option and could save the patient from the rigorous postexposure prophylaxis schedule. It is important to note the powerful effects of **water and soap irrigation** in these cases, as it has been proven as the most effective means of lowering the virulence of the organism and should be initiated quickly. For immunizing against the rabies virus, it is important to give the **immunoglobulin** in addition to the **cell vaccine**. As much of the initial dose should be infiltrated around the wound site as possible and then be given intramuscularly. Pregnancy is not a contraindication to giving the vaccine. All patients should be monitored for an antibody response. In the United States, the predominant threat to humans is **bats**, which most commonly carry the virus. This should be considered in individuals who are cave spelunkers and present with hydrophobia and neurologic symptoms. Small rodents (squirrels, rats, chipmunks) and lagomorphs are herbivores and do not carry the virus.

(a) Reporting the incident to local health officials is also warranted, but may be done later. Suturing the sustained lacerations in these types of injuries is controversial, but should never be tight (c). Head and neck lacerations may be sutured for cosmetic reasons. Given the adequate blood supply to these areas, infection rates are low. Antihistamines (d) are not usually indicated in cases of dog bites. Irrigation of the wound with Betadine (povidone-iodine) solution (e) should never be performed as it causes further maceration of the skin edges and tissue necrosis.

**427. The answer is c.** (*Rosen, pp 752-755.*) This patient's **necrotic lesion** and travel to the **south-central states** is classic for a **brown recluse spider bite**. These injuries may present with systemic symptoms of fever, chills, myalgias, hemolysis, petechiae, and eventually seizure, renal failure, and death. The brown recluse spider can be distinguished by its **violin-shaped cephalothorax**. Its venom contains hemolytic enzymes and substances that cause vasoconstriction. Initial lesions may appear targetoid, as blood supply to the central area is diminished and becomes necrotic. Lesions have been shown to cause significant scarring and infection. Initial treatment should include the ABCs, wound care, analgesia, and tetanus prophylaxis. Patients may be observed in the ED for a period of 6 hours to see if envenomation occurred. Antibiotics may become warranted if infection ensues. Loxosceles reclusa antivenin is manufactured in Brazil but is not currently available in the United States.

Although these bites may cause a coagulopathy, a DVT (a) and thrombocytopenia (e) are not the underlying causes but rather a manifestation of envenomation. Scorpion stings (b) are not so subtle. Patients feel immediate localized pain followed by neurologic symptoms that may include salivation, fasciculations, and blurred vision. The venom of Black widow spiders **(d)** causes pseudoperitoneal symptoms because of painful muscle spasm. Spasms may resolve spontaneously or progress to hypertension and cardiovascular failure. Black widow spiders have a signature hourglass bright-red marking on the underside of the abdomen. The Brown recluse spider typically has a violin-like marking on its abdomen.

**428. The answer is c.** *(Rosen, pp 860-862.)* This patient has **ultraviolet keratitis**, also known as **snow blindness**. This is essentially a radiation burn when an individual comes in close contact with an **ultraviolet-ray–containing light source**. It may be caused by sun lamps, tanning booths, or high-altitude environments. Patients usually present about 6 to 10 hours postexposure complaining of eye pain, blepharospasm, tearing, photophobia, and foreign body sensation. Physical examination reveals an injected eye with decreased visual acuity. Corneal examination reveals punctuate lesions that are clearly demarcated by a protective covering from the ultraviolet rays, such as the inferior conjunctiva. Treatment consists of a short-acting cycloplegic agent for pain management and broad-spectrum ophthalmologic antibiotics. Treatment is guided to assist in the quick, natural healing capacity of the cornea, in which the patient should feel better in a couple of days.

Although a corneal abrasion **(a)** is possible, given the patients' symptoms, his history and lack of trauma or contact lens use suggest otherwise. Regardless, the treatment is the same. Iritis **(b)** usually is an injury of blunt trauma, resulting in ciliary spasm. Patients complain of photophobia and eye pain. Physical examination reveals ciliary flush, cells and flare in the anterior chamber, and a small, poorly dilating pupil. Corneal foreign bodies **(d)** and corneal lacerations **(e)** are usually traumatic injuries in which the patient can recall a specific event. Corneal foreign bodies can be visualized upon physical examination using fluorescent dye and may present with an abrasion or ulceration. Small corneal lacerations may be difficult to diagnose. A positive Seidel test, in which fluorescent dye streams from a corneal wound indicate leaking aqueous humor, can be diagnostic. This is an ophthalmologic emergency that may warrant surgical repair.

**429. The answer is a.** *(Rosen, pp 1918-1922.)* This patient is recovering from **acute mountain sickness** with no signs of CHF or pulmonary edema. The first-line treatment is descent and oxygen supplementation, which is already accomplished in this patient. Other treatment considerations include hyperbaric oxygen therapy, which improves hypoxemia for all altitude illnesses. As for medication regimens, **acetazolamide** is indicated even in patients with a history of altitude illness as prophylaxis. It works to decrease the formation of bicarbonate by inhibiting carbonic anhydrase. This diuretic action counters the fluid retention in acute mountain illness. It also decreases bicarbonate absorption in the kidney, causing a metabolic acidosis, which stimulates hyperventilation. This compensatory mechanism is turned off when the pH is close to the physiologic range of 7.4. It is this hyperventilation that counters the altitude-induced hypoxemia, thereby relieving symptoms.

Dexamethasone (b) works to decrease vasogenic edema and intracranial pressure. It is generally used as adjunctive therapy in high-altitude cerebral edema. Nifedipine (c) works by decreasing pulmonary artery pressure in high-altitude pulmonary edema as does the diuresis resulting from (d) furosemide. Morphine (e) is thought to reduce pulmonary blood flow and decrease hydrostatic forces in pulmonary edema.

**430. The answer is b.** *(Rosen, pp 1896-1902.)* This patient sustained a **direct lightning injury**, as evidenced by the typical **fern-like pattern** exhibited. These injuries may inflict fractures, cardiovascular collapse, burns, blunt abdominal injuries, and neurologic damage. **Tympanic membrane ruptures** are a common associated injury caused by the outflow tract of the lightning strike, and it is important to check for blood in the ear canals of these patients. It is important to quickly assess the ABCs of these patients and establish an airway. Immobilization of the cervical spine is often indicated as well as close ECG monitoring. Patients should be admitted for observation after obtaining a complete blood count (CBC), creatinine kinase with MB fraction, basic metabolic panel, and appropriate radiographs of involved areas. Although 50 to 300 people die of lightning strikes each year in the United States, most injuries sustained are not lethal.

**431. The answer is c.** *(Rosen, pp 751-752.)* **Fire ants** have proven to be a real threat to humans. Ninety-five percent of clinical cases result from the *Solenopsis invicta* species, another member of the Hymenoptera, which was imported from Brazil in the 1930s. This ant is found in many of the southern states given that it cannot survive long winters and is slowly replacing the less dangerous species native to North America. It is small and light-reddish to dark brown and its venom is 99% alkaloid, which is unique to the animal kingdom. This causes hemolysis, membrane depolarization, local tissue destruction, and activation of the complement pathway, all of which could be especially dangerous in this patient with facial injuries. The sting usually produces a pustule within 24 hours. Local burning, erythema, and pruritus are common. About 10% of cases have progressive, systemic symptoms including nausea, vomiting, dizziness, respiratory distress, and further hypersensitivity. Therefore, assessment of this patient's airway and circulation are imperative. Continuous monitoring is indicated to detect hemodynamic instability.

Local wound care (**b**) may be performed after the patient is deemed stable. Beginning IV fluids (**d**) may be done if the patient becomes hemo-dynamically unstable but is not initially warranted. Tetanus prophylaxis (**a**) may be administered after the initial assessment. IV antihistamines, not oral (**e**), may be given as indicated. It is unclear as to whether this patient's symptoms of dizziness are a result of trauma or initial systemic effects of the envenomation and therefore continuous monitoring is warranted.

**432. The answer is d.** (*Rosen, pp 1868-1881.*) In all critically ill patients, it is important to remove clothing, obtain a rectal temperature, and initiate continuous monitoring, including an ECG, while assessing the ABC status of the patient. The clinician must initiate **advanced cardiac life support** and **rewarm** the patient once a rectal temperature has confirmed **hypothermia**. A tympanic temperature is not accurate below 94°F. It is important to remember that severely hypothermic patients who appear dead have a good chance of a normal neurologic outcome with continued resuscitation and rewarming. Remember that a **patient is not dead until they're warm and dead!** Those at extremes of age, users of sedative hypnotics, undomiciled individuals, and those with chronic illness, altered mental status, or sepsis are at most risk for hypothermia. Rewarming should begin with removing all wet clothing and placing warm blankets over the patient with progressive attempts made to rewarm the patient: mechanical warming blanket, warm IV fluids, gastric lavage/peritoneal warming, and lastly cardiopulmonary bypass.

Defibrillation (**a**) and cardiac pacing (**b**) are not currently indicated in this patient. Osborne (J) waves are indicative of a junctional rhythm, as seen in this patient, and are consistent with hypothermia. Prolongation of any interval, bradycardia, asystole, atrial fibrillation/flutter, and ventricular tachycardias may also be seen.

**433. The answer is a.** *(Rosen, pp 745, 747, 750.)* Only two venomous lizards are found in the world, whose natural habitat is in the southwestern United States and Mexico. These animals are usually not aggressive, despite the Gila monster's name, and bites are usually a result of direct handling as in this case. Both the Gila monster and the Mexican-beaded lizard are easily identified by their thick bodies and beaded scales with either white and black or pink and black configuration. Envenomation from these bites occurs from the glands along the lower jaw and introduced into the victim through grooved teeth, which the animal uses to continuously chew after it has bitten down. These teeth may become embedded in the victim, thereby distributing more venom.

Antivenin **(b)** is not available for these bites, as they are rarely fatal. Broad-spectrum antibiotics **(d)** and tetanus prophylaxis **(c)** should be administered at a later interval. Applying a suction device **(e)** as in snakebites is not warranted. The patient should be observed for at least 6 hours for systemic effects.

**434. The answer is b.** *(Rosen, pp 1723-1731.)* The patient should receive **full immunoprophylaxis** for the **rabies virus**. The Centers for Disease Control and Prevention (CDC) recommends postexposure prophylaxis when a bat is found indoors in the same room as a person who might be unaware that a bite or direct contact had occurred and rabies cannot be ruled out by testing the bat. Full prophylaxis in the United States includes passive immunization with human rabies immune globulin and active immunization with human diploid cell vaccine. Immune globulin is administered in and around a bite wound if visualized. Human diploid cell vaccine is administered at a distant site from the immunoglobulin, usually in the deltoid, to avoid cross reactivity. Human diploid cell vaccine is subsequently administered on days 3, 7, 14, and 28.

**(a)** The patient should not be sent home without full immunoprophylaxis. Ciprofloxacin **(c)** has no role in this patient or in rabies treatment. Rabies is caused by a virus. Admitting the patient for observation **(d)** is incorrect because rabies virus incubation ranges from 30 to 90 days with some reporting up to 7 years. The patient should receive immunoprophylaxis and be sent home. **(e)** The patient should receive both active and passive immunoprophylaxis unless they already received it in the past. In that case, they only receive the vaccine.

# Eye Pain and Visual Change

## Questions

**435.** A 24-year-old woman presents to the emergency department (ED) complaining of right eye pain and blurry vision since waking up this morning. She states that the pain began after taking out contact lenses that were in her eyes for over 1 week. Her blood pressure (BP) is 120/75 mm Hg, heart rate (HR) is 75 beats per minute, temperature is 99.1°F, and respiratory rate (RR) is 16 breaths per minute. Her right and left eye visual acuity is 20/60 and 20/20, respectively. Her conjunctivae are injected. The slit-lamp examination reveals a large area of fluorescein uptake over the visual axis. Which of the following is the most appropriate therapy?

a. Call the ophthalmology consult for an emergent corneal transplant.
b. Prescribe a systemic analgesic for pain control and advise the patient to not wear her contact lenses for the next week.
c. Prescribe ciprofloxacin eye drops, oral analgesia, update tetanus prophylaxis, and arrange for ophthalmology follow-up.
d. Prescribe oral amoxicillin, a topical anesthetic, such as tetracaine, and have patient follow-up with an ophthalmologist.
e. Prescribe ciprofloxacin eye drops and have patient strictly wear an eye patch until her pain resolves.

**436.** A 60-year-old woman presents to the ED complaining of pain in her right eye and burning sensation over half of her forehead and scalp. On physical examination, you notice a patch of grouped vesicles on an erythematous base located in a dermatomal distribution on her scalp and forehead. There are also a few vesicles located at the tip of the patient's nose. Her visual acuity is 20/20 bilaterally, heart is without murmurs, lungs are clear, abdomen is soft, and there are no gross findings on neurologic examination. Which of the following is the most concerning complication of this patient's clinical presentation?

a. Central nervous system (CNS) involvement leading to meningitis
b. Ophthalmic involvement leading to anterior uveitis or corneal scarring
c. Cardiac involvement leading to endocarditis
d. Permanent scarring of her face
e. Nasopalatine involvement leading to epistaxis

**437.** A 31-year-old nurse in your hospital has noticed a lesion in her left eye. She denies change in vision, pain, fevers, or discharge. A picture of her eye is shown below. Which of the following is the most likely diagnosis?

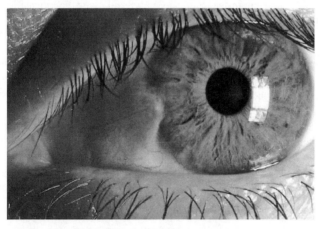

*(Reproduced, with permission, from Knoop KJ, Stack LB, Storrow AB. Atlas of Emergency Medicine. New York, NY: McGraw-Hill, 2002: 43.)*

a. Hordeolum
b. Chalazion
c. Dacryocystitis
d. Pinguecula
e. Pterygium

**438.** A 72-year-old man presents with right eye pain for 1 day. The patient has a history of diabetes, hypertension, and "some type of eye problem." He does not recall the name of his eye problem or the name of his ophthalmic medication. However, he does remember that the eye drop has a yellow cap. Which class of ophthalmic medication is the patient taking?

a. Antibiotic
b. β-Blocker
c. Mydriatic/cycloplegic agent
d. Miotic
e. Anesthetic

**439.** A 35-year-old woman presents with a right-sided red eye for 3 days. She denies pain and notes that she has watery discharge from the eye. She has been coughing and congested for the past 5 days. On examination, the patient has a temperature of 98.4°F, HR of 72 beats per minute, BP of 110/70 mm Hg, and RR of 14 breaths per minute. Her visual acuity is 20/20. On inspection, the conjunctiva is erythematous with minimal chemosis and clear discharge. The slit-lamp, fluorescein, and funduscopic examinations are otherwise unremarkable. The patient has a nontender, preauricular lymph node and enlarged tonsils, without exudates. What is the most likely diagnosis?

a. Gonococcal conjunctivitis
b. Bacterial conjunctivitis
c. Viral conjunctivitis
d. Allergic conjunctivitis
e. Pseudomonal conjunctivitis

**440.** A 24-year-old woman presents to the ED at 4 AM with severe left eye pain that woke her up from sleep. She wears soft contact lenses and does not routinely take them out to sleep. She is in severe pain and wearing sunglasses in the examination room. You give her a drop of proparacaine to treat her pain prior to your examination. On examination, her vision is at baseline and she has no afferent pupillary defect. There is some perilimbic conjunctival erythema. On fluorescein examination, a linear area on the left side of the cornea is highlighted when cobalt blue light is applied. No underlying white infiltrate is visualized. No white cells or flare are visualized in the anterior chamber. What is the most appropriate treatment for this condition?

a. Immediate ophthalmology consult
b. Tobramycin ophthalmic ointment
c. Erythromycin ophthalmic ointment
d. Eye patch
e. Proparacaine ophthalmic drops

**441.** A 45-year-old woman presents with right eye pain and redness for 1 day. She has photophobia and watery discharge from the eye. She does not wear glasses or contact lenses and has no prior eye problems. On examination, the patient's visual acuity is 20/20 in the left eye and 20/70 in the right eye. She has conjunctival injection around the cornea and clear watery discharge. On slit-lamp examination, the lids, lashes, and anterior chamber are normal. When fluorescein is applied, a branching, white-colored epithelial defect is seen. The remainder of the head examination is normal and the patient has no cutaneous lesions. Which of the following is the most appropriate treatment for this patient?

a. Admission for intravenous (IV) antibiotics
b. Admission for IV antiviral agents
c. Topical steroids
d. Topical antiviral medication
e. Immediate ophthalmology consultation

**442.** A 21-year-old man presents to the ED with a red eye. The patient complains of rhinorrhea and a nonproductive cough but has no eye pain or discharge. He also has no associated ecchymosis, bony tenderness of the orbit, or pain on extraocular eye movement. His vision is normal, extraocular movements are intact, and intraocular pressure (IOP) is 12. A picture of his eye is shown below. What is the most appropriate management of this condition?

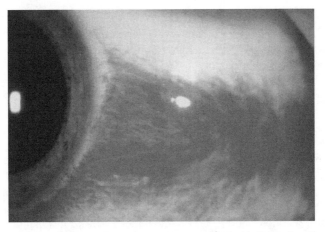

*(Reproduced, with permission, from Riordan-Eva P, Asbury T, Whitcher JP. Vaughan & Asbury's General Ophthalmology. New York, NY: McGraw-Hill, 2004: 124.)*

a. Call ophthalmology immediately.
b. Administer 1% atropine.
c. Elevate patient's head.
d. Administer ophthalmic timolol.
e. Reassurance only.

**443.** A 28-year-old mechanic with no past medical history presents to the ED after a small amount of battery acid was splashed in his right eye. He is complaining of extreme pain and tearing from his eye. Which of the following is the most appropriate next step in management?

a. Call ophthalmology now.
b. Check visual acuity.
c. Check the pH of the tears.
d. Irrigate with normal saline.
e. Apply erythromycin ointment.

**444.** A 45-year-old man lacerated his right forehead after an altercation in a local bar. Instead of seeking medical attention, the patient applied super glue to his wound. He successfully stopped the bleeding, but some of the glue got into his right eye and now he comes to the ED with difficulty opening his right eye. What is the most appropriate treatment of this patient?

a. Call ophthalmology immediately.
b. Wash eye with acetone.
c. Wash eye with normal saline.
d. Use forceps to remove all the glue from the eye.
e. Apply erythromycin ointment.

**445.** The local sorority house recently installed a sun-tanning station. Two days later three sorority girls present to the ED with bilateral eye pain, tearing, and photophobia. After ophthalmic anesthesia instillation, a complete eye examination is performed. Visual acuity is normal. Extraocular eye movements are intact and pupils are equal, round, and reactive to light. IOP is normal. Slit-lamp examination is normal, but fluorescein examination under cobalt blue light illuminates small dots throughout the cornea. What is the most likely diagnosis?

a. Ultraviolet keratitis
b. Anterior uveitis
c. Herpes simplex keratitis
d. Allergic conjunctivitis
e. Corneal ulcer

**446.** A 12-year-old girl presents to the ED for left eye pain and swelling for 2 days. The patient has had cough, congestion, and rhinorrhea for the last week that is improving. On examination, her temperature is 100.8°F, HR 115 beats per minute, RR 12 breaths per minute, and BP 110/70 mm Hg. On eye examination, there is purple-red swelling of both upper and lower eyelids with injection of the conjunctiva. Pupils are equal and reactive to light. There is restricted lateral gaze. Visual acuity is 20/70 in the left eye and 20/25 in the right eye. The rest of the physical examination is normal. What is the most appropriate next step in management?

a. Administer diphenhydramine.
b. Administer amoxicillin/clavulanate.
c. Administer vancomycin IV.
d. Perform computed tomographic (CT) scan of orbits and sinuses.
e. Administer artificial tears.

**447.** A 60-year-old man with a history of hypertension and migraine headaches presents to the ED with a headache. He describes left-sided headache and eye pain that is associated with nausea and vomiting. The patient has a long history of migraines, but says his migraines do not usually include eye pain. On examination, his temperature is 97.6°F, HR 84 beats per minute, RR 12 breaths per minute, and BP 134/80 mm Hg. His neurologic examination is normal. His left eye is mid-dilated and nonreactive. His cornea is cloudy. His corrected visual acuity is 20/50 in the left eye and 20/20 in the right eye. What is the most appropriate next step in management?

a. Administer hydromorphone.
b. Perform head CT scan.
c. Check IOP.
d. Check erythrocyte sedimentation rate (ESR).
e. Discharge patient.

**448.** A 22-year-old man presents to the ED for left eye pain. He was in an altercation yesterday and was punched in the left eye. On examination, his left eye is ecchymotic and the eyelids are swollen shut. He has tenderness over the infraorbital rim but no step-offs. You use an eyelid speculum to examine his eye. His pupils are equal and reactive to light. His visual acuity is normal. On testing extraocular movements, you find he is unable to look upward with his left eye. He also complains of diplopia when looking upward. Funduscopic examination is normal. What is the most likely diagnosis?

a. Orbital blowout fracture
b. Ruptured globe
c. Retinal detachment
d. Cranial nerve III palsy
e. Traumatic retrobulbar hematoma

**449.** You are examining the pupils of a patient. On inspection, the pupils are 3 mm and equal bilaterally. You shine a flashlight into the right pupil and both pupils constrict to 1 mm. You then shine the flashlight into the left pupil and both pupils slightly dilate. What is this condition called?

a. Anisocoria
b. Argyll Robertson pupil
c. Afferent pupillary defect
d. Horner syndrome
e. Normal pupil reaction

**450.** A 65-year-old man with a history of diabetes, hypertension, coronary artery disease, and atrial fibrillation presents with loss of vision in his left eye since he awoke 6 hours ago. The patient denies fever, eye pain, or eye discharge. On physical examination of the left eye, vision is limited to counting fingers. His pupil is 3 mm and reactive. Extraocular movements are intact. Slit-lamp examination is also normal. The dilated funduscopic examination is shown below. Which of the following is the most likely diagnosis?

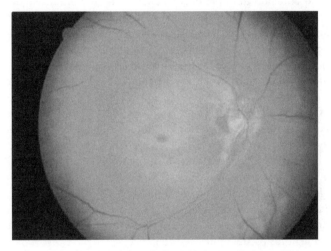

*(Reproduced, with permission, from Knoop KJ, Stack LB, Storrow AB.* Atlas of Emergency Medicine. *New York, NY: McGraw-Hill, 2002: 82.)*

a. Retinal detachment
b. Central retinal artery occlusion
c. Central retinal vein occlusion
d. Vitreous hemorrhage
e. Acute angle-closure glaucoma

# Eye Pain and Visual Change

## Answers

**435. The answer is c.** (*Rosen, pp 860-862.*) The patient most likely sustained a **corneal abrasion** from prolonged **contact lens** use. Epithelial defects of the cornea are diagnosed by slit-lamp examination by observing **fluorescein uptake** in the area of the defect. Treatment usually consists of cycloplegia and topical or oral pain medications. Patients wearing contact lens should be treated with topical antibiotics with **antipseudomonal** coverage. Patients should not wear their contact lens until complete healing of the corneal epithelium. All patients should follow up with an ophthalmologist.

(**a**) Corneal abrasions usually heal well with appropriate care and do not require a transplant. (**b**) A topical antibiotic should also be prescribed to prevent secondary infection. (**d**) Amoxicillin is not an appropriate antibiotic because it is not topical and not antipseudomonal. In addition, tetracaine, if used frequently, can decompose the cornea and cause permanent damage. (**e**) Eye patching should be avoided, particularly with injuries involving contact lens. Data suggest that eye patching confers no benefit in healing small, uncomplicated corneal abrasions and may provide a better environment for pseudomonas to proliferate.

**436. The answer is b.** (*Rosen, p 868.*) The patient has **herpes zoster**, or **shingles**, an infection caused by the **varicella-zoster virus**. The patient's rash most likely involves the **ophthalmic division** of the **trigeminal nerve**. In addition, the vesicles found on the tip of the patient's nose correlate strongly with viral involvement of the eye. **Hutchinson sign** is used to denote vesicles on the tip of a patient's nose in the setting of herpes zoster. When there is ocular involvement, the infection is called **herpes zoster ophthalmicus. Ocular complications** occur in 20% to 70% of the cases involving the ophthalmic division of the trigeminal nerve. Severity varies from mild conjunctivitis to panophthalmitis. In addition, the patient is at risk for anterior uveitis, secondary glaucoma, and corneal scarring.

(a) Complications of zoster include CNS involvement that can lead to meningoencephalitis, myelitis, and peripheral neuropathy; however, the patient's current neurologic examination is unremarkable. (c) Although zoster can disseminate to the visceral organs, like the brain, no cases of endocarditis have ever been reported. (d) The rash of zoster usually heals within a month and do not leave a permanent scar. (e) Epistaxis is not a complication of zoster.

**437. The answer is e.** *(Knoop et al, p 35.)* This patient has a **pterygium**, a triangular growth of tissue from the bulbar conjunctiva to the periphery of the cornea. It is more common on the nasal side of the cornea and may affect one or both eyes. Pterygium is associated with exposure to wind, dust, and sunlight. Most cases are asymptomatic and can be followed by an ophthalmologist. In cases where the pterygium grows into the visual axis or restricts extraocular motion, surgical excision is indicated.

Pinguecula (d) is a yellow-whitish, fatty lesion of the bulbar conjunctiva that may be on either side of the cornea but is more commonly seen on the nasal side. Dacryocystitis (c) is an inflammation of the lacrimal sac that is characterized by pain, swelling, and erythema of the lacrimal sac on the extreme nasal aspect of the lower lid. Pressure on the lacrimal sac in a patient with dacryocystitis may express pus. Hordeolum (a) or stye is an acute infection and abscess of the glands within the eyelids. Chalazions (b) are granulomatous inflammations of meibomian glands in the eyelids. In contrast to the erythematous, edematous, and painful hordeolums, chalazions are usually hard and nontender swellings.

**438. The answer is b.** *(Riordan-Eva et al, chapter 3.)* **Ophthalmic medications** are **color-coded**. While this question may seem esoteric, it can be clinically useful to know the colors of eye medications. In this case, knowing that yellow caps are β-**blockers** suggests that this patient may be currently treated for glaucoma. Medication color knowledge can also help you rapidly locate a specific medication from a large group of eye medications.

Antibiotics (a) are usually tan, mydriatics and cycloplegics (c) are red, miotics (d) are green, and anesthetics (e) are white. Mydriatics and cycloplegics are medications that cause ciliary muscle paralysis and pupil dilation. Miotics are medications that cause pupillary constriction.

**439. The answer is c.** *(Tintinalli, pp 1530-1531.)* This patient has classic **viral conjunctivitis** that is associated with a viral upper respiratory infection.

Patients with viral conjunctivitis typically have **reddened conjunctiva** and **watery discharge**. Preauricular adenopathy is also associated with viral etiology. Treatment includes cool compresses and an antihistamine/α-adrenergic combination medication—naphazoline/pheniramine—for symptomatic care.

Patients with bacterial conjunctivitis (**b**) have thick mucopurulent discharge and often wake up with their eyelids stuck together. These patients are treated with broad-spectrum antibiotics. Bacterial and viral conjunctivitis do not always present classically and they can be difficult to distinguish clinically. Many physicians will therefore treat conjunctivitis patients with antibiotic eye drops until they can be reexamined by an ophthalmologist. Patients who wear contact lenses are at risk for pseudomonal conjunctivitis (**e**). They should be treated with an antibiotic that covers *Pseudomonas*, such as a fluoroquinolone or aminoglycoside. It is very important to always consider gonococcal conjunctivitis (**a**) in sexually active individuals, because this infection can cause permanent visual loss if not rapidly identified and treated. Patients with gonococcal conjunctivitis have a severe conjunctivitis with copious mucopurulent drainage and erythematous conjunctiva. Inpatient IV antibiotics should be started while waiting for results of ocular Gram stain and culture. Allergic conjunctivitis (**d**) presents with watery discharge and eye redness, but itching is the most prominent symptom. Cyclical exacerbations associated with allergen exposure may be clues to the diagnosis of allergic conjunctivitis.

**440. The answer is b.** (*Tintinalli, pp 1535-1536.*) This patient has a **corneal abrasion** from prolonged contact lens use. The abrasion **lights up** after fluorescein staining and cobalt blue illumination of the cornea. Contact lens wearers with abrasions are at high risk for pseudomonal infection and should be treated with an antipseudomonal agent (ie, tobramycin ophthalmic ointment) or fluoroquinolone drops. It is critical to distinguish an abrasion from a corneal ulcer. Ulcers are deeper infections of the cornea that develop from corneal epithelial defects (ie, abrasions). Contact lens wearers are also at high risk for corneal ulcers. The hallmark of a corneal ulcer is a shaggy, white infiltrate within the corneal epithelial defect.

(**c**) Uncomplicated corneal abrasions may be treated with erythromycin ointment. Corneal ulcers are treated aggressively with antipseudomonal antibiotics and immediate ophthalmology consultation (**a**). Some ophthalmologists will see the patient in the ED to perform corneal Gram stain and cultures; while other ophthalmologists will examine the patient in

12 hours in the office setting. Eye patches (d) are controversial but should not be given to patients at risk for fungal infections or pseudomonal infections as they are at risk for rapid corneal melting and perforation. Topical anesthetic agents, such as proparacaine (e), may be helpful to facilitate the examination in the ED but should never be dispensed to patients. Repeated use of these agents can cause corneal injury and vision loss.

**441. The answer is d.** *(Tintinalli, pp 1531-1533.)* This patient has a **corneal epithelial disease** caused by the **herpes simplex virus**. The hallmark of this disease is the branching or **dendritic** ulcer. Patients may also present without corneal involvement but will have typical herpetic skin lesions in the eyelids and conjunctiva. Patients should be treated with topical antivirals, such as trifluridine, with topical antibiotics added to prevent secondary bacterial infection.

IV antibiotics (a) are not indicated for herpes simplex keratitis. Corticosteroids (c) must be avoided as steroids may enhance viral replication and worsen infection. Patients should follow up with ophthalmology in 1 to 2 days. If there is evidence for herpes zoster ophthalmicus, an infection involving the trigeminal nerve with ocular involvement, ophthalmology should be consulted immediately (e) and the patient should be admitted for IV antivirals (b).

**442. The answer is e.** *(Tintinalli, pp 1534-1539.)* This patient has **subconjunctival hemorrhage** caused by conjunctival vessel rupture from coughing. This common ED complaint can result spontaneously or from Valsalva-induced pressure spikes (such as coughing or bearing down), trauma, and hypertension.

Patients can be reassured that subconjunctival hemorrhages spontaneously resolve in 1 to 2 weeks (e). Subconjunctival hemorrhage is sometimes confused with hyphema or blood in the anterior chamber. Hyphemas can be traumatic from a ruptured iris vessel or spontaneous, usually associated with sickle-cell disease. Bleeding within the anterior chamber can cause elevated IOP and must be treated aggressively with β-blockers (d) and mannitol. Carbonic anhydrase inhibitors (Diamox) should be avoided in sickle-cell patients as these medications lower anterior chamber pH, ultimately enhancing RBC sickling and increasing IOP. Pupillary activity stretches the iris vessels and exacerbates bleeding with hyphema; therefore, mydriatic agents, such as atropine (b) are used to keep the pupil dilated. The head of the bed can be elevated (c) to minimize elevations of

IOP. Many ophthalmologists will admit all patients with hyphemas. This is because 30% of hyphemas rebleed in 3 to 5 days, resulting in dangerously high elevations in IOP necessitating surgical therapy. Some ophthalmologists will follow patients with hyphemas less than one-third of the anterior chamber as outpatients. However, ophthalmology should be urgently consulted while the patient is in the ED and individual decisions can be discussed (a).

**443. The answer is d.** *(Tintinalli, p 1542.)* **Chemical injuries** to the eye must be **irrigated** with a minimum of 1 to 2 L of normal saline as soon as they arrive in the ED. Topical anesthesia and the use of a Morgan lens (a special device to provide large volume irrigation to the eye) can help facilitate this procedure.

(b) Irreversible eye damage can occur if irrigation is withheld for a physical examination and visual acuity testing. Checking the pH of the tears (c) helps determine the effectiveness of irrigation, but should be checked after irrigation has begun. When the ocular pH returns to 7.5 to 8.0, irrigation can be stopped and a complete eye examination should be performed. Remember to check visual acuity and pay special attention to corneal clouding or corneal epithelial defects. (e) Patients with epithelial defects or corneal clouding should receive an ophthalmic antibiotic. Patients without corneal or anterior chamber involvement only need erythromycin ointment. The ophthalmologist (a) should be notified, after initial stabilization, of all patients with chemical injury to the eye and follow-up should be arranged within 12 to 24 hours in consultation with the ophthalmologist.

**444. The answer is e.** *(Tintinalli, p 1543.)* Fortunately, super glue or crazy glue (cyanoacrylate) exposure to the eye is usually not permanently damaging to the eye. Corneal irritation can occur from the hard, irregularly shaped glue. To prevent this abrasive effect, large amounts of erythromycin ointment should be applied to the eye and eyelids as a lubricant. Large clumps of glue can be removed manually.

Instrumentation to remove all glue products (d) is not necessary in the ED. The glue will loosen over time and be easier to remove in several days. Washing the eye with normal saline (c) will not be helpful unless there are large free clumps that will be washed away. (b) While applying acetone may help remove cyanoacrylate from clothing and surfaces, acetone (or any other chemical) should never be infused into the eye. (a) These patients should follow up with ophthalmology in 1 to 2 days.

**445. The answer is a.** *(Tintinalli, p 1536.)* These girls forgot to wear eye protection while using the sun-tanning lights and have **ultraviolet keratitis**. History of exposure to sun-tanning lamps, welding, or the sun suggests the diagnosis and fluorescein staining showing **superficial punctate keratitis** confirms the diagnosis. Treatment consists of analgesia, cycloplegics to reduce ciliary spasm and pain, erythromycin ointment, and ophthalmology follow-up in 1 to 2 days. Fortunately, most patients with ultraviolet keratitis make a full recovery with supportive care alone.

Iritis or anterior uveitis **(b)** can also cause eye redness and pain. It is an intraocular inflammation of the anterior uveal tract with numerous possible infectious and inflammatory etiologies. Iritis is diagnosed by history and visualization of cells and flare in the anterior chamber on slit-lamp examination. Consistent with an infectious or inflammatory etiology, cells represent leukocytes floating in the aqueous humor and flare represents a hazy protein accumulation. Herpes simplex keratitis **(c)** has the hallmark dendritic epithelial defect on fluorescein examination. Patients with allergic conjunctivitis **(d)** present with ocular discharge, itching, and dry eyes. While a punctate keratitis may be seen on fluorescein examination, a history of exquisite ocular pain is not consistent with allergic conjunctivitis. Corneal ulcers **(e)** may present with erythema and ocular pain but show white, hazy infiltrates on fluorescein examination.

**446. The answer is c.** *(Tintinalli, pp 1528-1530.)* This patient has **orbital cellulitis**, an infection deep to the orbital septum. The patient had a recent upper respiratory infection and sinusitis, which likely resulted in orbital extension of the infection. *Staphylococcus aureus* and *Haemophilus influenzae* are common etiologies, and mucormycosis must be considered in diabetics and immunocompromised patients.

Distinctive clinical findings of orbital cellulitis are eye pain, fever, **impaired eye motility**, decreased visual acuity, and proptosis. Patients should be treated with IV antibiotics, such as cefuroxime, a combination of penicillin and nafcillin, or vancomycin, and admitted to the hospital. In this case, the diagnosis is clear from the history and physical examination and treatment should be started promptly. Orbital cellulitis must be differentiated from preseptal cellulitis and allergic reactions. Preseptal cellulitis is a superficial cellulitis that does not penetrate the orbital septum. Patients present with swollen, red eyelids, but no vision change, pupil changes, or changes in eye motility.

Orbital and sinus CT scans **(d)** may be performed after antibiotics are started to rule out an abscess. CT scans are also useful when the diagnosis of orbital cellulitis is in consideration but not clinically clear. Patients older than 5 years with preseptal cellulitis may be treated with amoxicillin/clavulanate orally (**b**) and close follow-up with their regular doctor. Children younger than 5 years are at risk for systemic bacteremia and should be admitted for IV antibiotics. Patients with allergic reactions have swelling and erythema of the eyelids but no fever or tenderness to palpation. These patients may be treated with artificial tears (**e**) and antihistamines, such as (**a**) diphenhydramine.

**447. The answer is c.** (*Tintinalli, pp 1543-1544.*) This patient has **acute angle-closure glaucoma**, when the aqueous humor production in the posterior chamber of the eye is unable to drain through the anterior chamber and the resultant obstruction causes **increased IOP**. On examination, patients with increased IOP have a mid-dilated, nonreactive pupil with **corneal clouding** and decreased vision. The diagnosis is clenched by checking the IOP with a tonopen or tonometer. Normal IOP is 10 to 21 mm Hg. Patients with increased IOP should be treated with medications to decrease production of aqueous humor. Checking IOP is a simple, rapid test that should be performed on all patients with headache and orbital pain. If this test is negative, other causes of headache and eye pain should be investigated.

This patient is not experiencing his typical migraine headache and he has abnormalities on his physical examination. Discharging the patient without further investigation is therefore inappropriate (**e**). Pain control is appropriate for this patient, but given his nausea and vomiting, he is not likely to tolerate oral hydromorphone (**a**). Checking an ESR (**d**) is helpful if you suspect temporal arteritis. Head CT scan (**b**) can be considered in the workup of an atypical headache, but simpler tests, such as tonometry, should be performed first.

**448. The answer is a.** (*Tintinalli, pp 1539-1542, 1545-15468; Vassallo, pp 251-256.*) This patient has an **orbital blowout fracture** of the inferior wall causing **entrapment of the inferior rectus muscle** and **restricted eye motility** with diplopia. A CT scan with thin cuts through the orbits can confirm the diagnosis. Patients with this injury are generally started on oral antibiotics because of the risk of infection with sinus wall fractures and may follow up with the institution's appropriate surgical service in 3 to 10 days. These injuries are associated with other eye problems and a careful eye examination must be performed to rule out abrasions, lacerations, foreign bodies, hyphema, iritis, retinal detachment, and lens dislocation.

The patient has no evidence of a retinal detachment (c) given his normal visual acuity and funduscopic examination. However, even with a normal examination in the ED, patients with orbital blowout fractures should be referred to an ophthalmologist for a repeat examination to rule out a traumatic retinal detachment. Ruptured globes (b) are more common with penetrating trauma and clues to this diagnosis are shallow anterior chamber, hyphema, irregular pupil, significant decrease in vision. If a ruptured globe is suspected, a hard eye shield should be applied and ophthalmology consulted. Do not check IOP in patients with suspected ruptured globes as this can worsen the injury. Cranial nerve III palsy (d) presents with problems with medial gaze, upward gaze, downward gaze as well as ptosis. This patient only has difficulty with upward gaze suggesting that cranial nerve III is intact. Traumatic retrobulbar hemorrhage (e) is a displacement of the globe and septum anteriorly caused by bleeding into the orbit. Because the globe has limited capacity for expansion, continued bleeding puts pressure on ocular structures. Optic nerve compression leads to decreased visual acuity and continued globe pressure leads to proptosis. Patients with a traumatic history and clinical signs suggestive of retrobulbar hemorrhage require emergency orbital decompression via lateral cantholysis.

**449. The answer is c.** (*Knoop et al, pp 50-51; Tintinalli, pp 1522-1523.*) This patient has an **afferent pupillary defect (APD)**, also known as a **Marcus Gunn pupil**. In patients with an APD, light shined into the affected pupil causes a small dilation with no constriction. APD is a result of a lesion in the anterior visual pathway of the retina, optic nerve, or optic chiasm preventing reception of the light in the affected eye. Neither pupil constricts since constriction is centrally mediated in the midbrain. APDs are sensitive for disease but not specific. The differential diagnosis for an APD includes central retinal artery or vein occlusion, optic nerve disorders, such as optic neuritis, tumor or glaucoma, and lesions in the optic chiasm or tract.

Anisocoria (a) is unequal pupil size. Under normal room lighting, normal pupils may be 1 to 2 mm different in size. An Argyll Robertson pupil (b) constricts during accommodation (as expected) but does not constrict in response to light. This is usually seen in both eyes and is associated with neurosyphilis. Horner syndrome (d) is decreased sympathetic innervation of the eye from interruption of the sympathetic chain at any point from the brainstem to the sympathetic plexus around the carotid artery. Clinically, patients with Horner syndrome have ptosis, miosis, and anhidrosis.

(e) Normal pupil response to light is pupil constriction followed by a small amount of dilatation.

**450. The answer is b.** *(Tintinalli, pp 1544-1545.)* The differential diagnosis for acute painless loss of vision includes retinal detachment, central retinal artery and vein occlusions, vitreous hemorrhage, and transient ischemic attack. An ophthalmologist should be called immediately when entertaining these diagnoses because a thorough funduscopic examination and prompt treatment is essential. On funduscopic examination, the patient has a **macular cherry-red spot** with a **pale retina** and less pronounced arteries. This is diagnostic of **central retinal artery occlusion**. Occlusion of the central retinal blood supply is commonly caused by emboli, thrombi, vasculitis, or trauma. Treatment aims to dislodge the clot from the main artery to one of its branches and includes digital massage, vasodilation, and lowering IOP.

Acute angle-closure glaucoma **(e)** usually causes painful loss of vision. Central retinal vein occlusion **(c)** presents similarly to retinal artery occlusion but is caused by thrombosis of the central retinal vein from stasis, edema, and hemorrhage. Funduscopic examination shows diffuse retinal hemorrhages and optic disc edema, also called the "blood and thunder" fundus. Treatment involves aspirin and prompt ophthalmology referral. Retinal detachment **(a)** occurs when vitreous fluid accumulates behind a retinal tear displacing the retina. On funduscopy, the retina will be hanging in the vitreous. Clinically, retinal detachment may be heralded by blurry vision or floaters followed by painless vision loss. Vitreous hemorrhage **(d)** is bleeding within the posterior chamber. On funduscopic examination, these patients have blood obstructing the view of the fundus. There are many causes of vitreous hemorrhage, including diabetic retinopathy, retinal detachment, trauma, and age-related macular degeneration.

# Prehospital, Disaster, Administration

## Questions

**451.** You are on an emergency medical services (EMS) ride along when your team receives a call for multiple injured pedestrians after a device is detonated in a downtown building. When you arrive at the scene, there is an incident commander who instructs you that there are dozens of injured casualties and delegates you to triaging the wounded. You are directed to a secure area where the fire department EMS at the scene has brought out dozens of injured office workers. You approach a patient who has several abrasions on his torso, face, and extremities. He has no spontaneous respirations. You perform a chin lift and note chest wall movement and audible respirations. He has a palpable radial pulse and the patient can squeeze your hand on command. He is able to maintain his respiratory effort and you count a respiratory rate (RR) of 24 breaths per minute. Using the simple triage and rapid treatment (START) system, what color would you assign this patient?

a. Green
b. Yellow
c. Red
d. Blue
e. Black

**452.** You take a dispatch call while working a shift in the ED from EMS regarding a 38-year-old woman who developed acute severe respiratory distress while eating a peanut-soy–based dish at a Chinese restaurant. You are also told that she has erythematous wheals all over her body and has diffuse wheezes on auscultation. Her blood pressure (BP) is 92/55 mm Hg, heart rate (HR) 115 beats per minute, RR 28 breaths per minute, pulse oximeter 98% on room air, and she is afebrile. EMS informs you that they are a basic unit. What are the most appropriate initial orders for the EMS unit given their level of training?

a. Perform no procedures in the field, administer supplemental oxygen, and proceed to the ED as quickly as safely possible.
b. Establish an intravenous (IV) and administer IV epinephrine and a normal saline bolus.
c. Establish an IV and administer a normal saline bolus.
d. Administer intramuscular (IM) epinephrine.
e. Perform orotracheal intubation for impending respiratory failure; then establish an IV and administer IV epinephrine.

**453.** While a couple are hiking up a mountain in a large national park, the husband slips and falls down a steep hill, hits his chest wall on a tree trunk, and a branch impales his left flank. He also hears a "pop" from his left knee and cannot move his lower leg. The injured husband is conscious and tells his wife to go for help because he cannot move and is having difficulty breathing. The wife hikes back to the park ranger's headquarters for assistance who then calls report over the radio requesting assistance with getting the patient to your ED, which is located approximately 50 miles away. The hiking terrain has a service road, which is adjacent to their hiking trail and it is a clear, sunny day. What is the most appropriate transfer modality to send to the scene?

a. Send an EMS van via the service road to extricate the patient and transfer him to your emergency department (ED).
b. Send the park ranger in his mountain terrain–equipped vehicle to extricate the patient and bring him back to his headquarters where EMS personnel will be awaiting for further transfer.
c. Send a rotary-wing helicopter and have the park ranger mobilize ground transport to the scene for assistance if necessary.
d. Send an EMS pickup chassis with an integrated modular patient care compartment as the patient may need advanced monitoring during transfer.
e. Send a fixed-wing EMS aircraft and mobilize the park ranger's mountain terrain–equipped vehicle to extricate the patient and transport him to the aircraft.

**454.** A railroad freight car is overturned while traveling through a suburban area, and hundreds of gallons of chemical waste are spilled at the scene. Several of the crew were heavily exposed to the spilled chemicals and are reported to be in critical condition. Some of the crew have already died from the exposure. The incident commander sets up a hot-zone perimeter and has designated decontamination zones. You receive a call from a HAZMAT (hazardous material) paramedic unit with a patient in distress who they believe will not survive long. Under what circumstances is it acceptable to take the patient directly from the hot zone without going through decontamination?

a. If it is reasonably certain that the patient will not survive long enough for the decontamination process.
b. If the toxic chemical is identified and the EMS personnel have adequate equipment to reasonably ensure their safety.
c. If the incident commander orders EMS to bypass the decontamination zone due to the patient's impending deterioration.
d. If the resources at the incident site are overwhelmed by the number of contaminated people and decontamination cannot be performed rapidly.
e. It is never acceptable to bypass the decontamination process after a toxic exposure, especially if the toxin is unknown.

**455.** EMS arrives to your ED with a 60-year-old man in cardiopulmonary arrest. He has a history of three prior heart attacks and cardiac stents due to severe coronary artery disease. EMS tells you that he has been pulseless for 10 minutes. You immediately continue resuscitative efforts via advanced cardiac life support (ACLS) guidelines. After several administrations of ACLS drugs and several rounds of cardiopulmonary resuscitation (CPR), you are contemplating terminating the code due to medical futility. Which of the following factors would lead you to continue your resuscitative efforts?

a. The patient's arrest witnessed by a bystander or EMS who immediately began CPR.
b. Before the cardiac arrest, the patient has been compliant with taking his cardiac medications.
c. The patient has an automated implantable cardioverter-defibrillator (AICD).
d. The patient has previously survived an out-of-hospital cardiorespiratory arrest.
e. The patient's initial out-of-hospital rhythm was asystole.

**456.** In 1966, the National Academy of Sciences published a report entitled "Accidental Death and Disability: The Neglected Disease of Modern Society." This report quantified the magnitude of traffic-related death and disability while describing the deficiencies in prehospital care in the United States. They made a number of recommendations regarding ambulance systems, including a need for ambulance standards, state-level policies and regulations, and adopting a system for providing consistent ambulance services at the local level. As a result of this report, which of the following legislations authorized the US Department of Transportation (DOT) to develop prehospital systems?

a. Highway Safety Act
b. Emergency Medicine Services Act
c. Emergency Medical Treatment and Active Labor Act (EMTALA)
d. Trauma Care Systems Planning and Development Act
e. Joint Commission on Accreditation of Health Care Organizations (JCAHO)

**457.** A patient is brought in by EMS after sustaining injuries from a motor vehicle accident. The police arrive with the patient and inform you that he is in their custody. Your patient's vital signs are stable. You send basic blood work, including a blood alcohol level, a chest radiograph, and a urinalysis. The blood alcohol level comes back above the legal limit for operating a motor vehicle. The rest of the workup is unremarkable. The police officer requests a copy of the patient's medical record. What is the proper response to his request?

a. Because the patient is in police custody, he does not have the same right to privacy as nonincarcerated citizens; hence you are obliged to give the officer the records.
b. Refusal to give the officer the records is considered obstruction of justice and you can be found criminally liable if you do not comply with his request.
c. Unless the patient consents, you are obligated to refuse the officer's request for a copy of the medical records as this violates the patient's rights to privacy under Health Insurance Portability and Accountability Act (HIPAA) laws.
d. As a licensed physician you are allowed to use your best judgment in a case-by-case basis regarding the release of medical records of incarcerated patients to law enforcement officers. You also must document your rationale in the medical record.
e. You may release all pertinent medical information but can withhold certain data from your workup, which can incriminate the patient in order to protect their rights in a subsequent trial.

**458.** A 67-year-old man is brought to the ED by EMS with a chief complaint of chest pain. He is found to be short of breath and diaphoretic. He reports that he vomited 1 hour ago and subsequently feels better. He describes substernal chest pressure that started while doing yard work. He has a history of coronary artery disease and hypertension. He has regularly scheduled appointments with a cardiologist at a neighboring hospital. He requested to be taken to that hospital, but EMS refused and brought him to your ED because it was only 5 minutes away. The patient is angry and requests a transfer to his cardiologist's hospital, which is 20 minutes away. What is the best course of action?

a. You must politely refuse his request and work the patient up for acute coronary syndrome and admit him to your hospital if indicated.
b. Contact the neighboring hospital and speak to the patient's cardiologist. If he agrees to accept the transfer, authorize an ambulance transfer for continuity of care.
c. Transfer the patient only if he has stable vital signs and his cardiologist is on-call at the neighboring hospital.
d. Transfer the patient immediately and inform EMS that they should have respected the patient's wishes in the prehospital setting.
e. Perform the appropriate medical screening examination (MSE), in this case at least an electrocardiogram (ECG) and basic laboratory tests including a troponin, before considering a transfer.

**459.** EMS responds to a call for a suicide attempt. The patient is a 58-year-old man who was recently diagnosed with pancreatic cancer and, according to the family, has been extremely depressed. The patient tried to hang himself in his room in a suicide attempt, and, when family found him still gasping for air, they cut him down. He has a weak, thready pulse, sonorous respirations with stridor and poor air entry. He also has crepitus over the soft tissue of his neck and he appears pale. The family informs EMS that he recently signed a DNR and they have the proper documentation. EMS calls in for your advice on how to proceed. Which of the following is the most appropriate response?

a. The patient has a DNR order; therefore EMS must abide by his advance directive and take no intervention.
b. Take no intervention but bring the patient to the ED as quickly as possible and provide supportive care.
c. Secure the patient's airway but inform EMS that they cannot proceed with CPR if the patient loses his pulse.
d. Secure the patients airway and provide full supportive care, disregarding the patient's DNR directive due to the circumstance of a suicide attempt.
e. Tell EMS to stand by and contact your hospitals medical ethics board for counsel immediately.

**460.** You are working as an ED physician in a small, single-coverage community ED in a level-5 trauma center. Which of the following scenarios can safely be managed at your facility and should not prompt a transfer?

a. A 33-year-old man involved in a high-speed motorcycle accident with multiple traumatic injuries. You have stabilized his vitals and there is no in-house trauma surgeon, but you have a general surgeon.

b. An 11-day-old girl's sepsis and your lumbar puncture results are consistent with bacterial meningitis. You have initiated the proper treatment, including antibiotics and the patient has secure IV access and airway.

c. A 75-year-old man with a history of atrial fibrillation and heart failure comes in with shortness of breath. He has an implanted pacemaker. He reports palpitations and weakness. His initial troponin is negative and his ECG does not reveal any ST elevations. Other than a heart rate of 55 beats per minute, his vitals are stable, the lung sounds are clear, and he has no dependent edema. You do not have an in-house cardiologist, but one can be called in within an hour.

d. A 42-year-old man who fell 20 ft from his roof. Computed tomographic (CT) scan reveals an epidural hematoma. He is intubated and his vital signs are stabilized.

e. A 22-year-old woman is 29 weeks pregnant and has abdominal pain and vaginal bleeding after being involved in a motor vehicle collision. She has a bruise over her lower abdomen where the seatbelt was applied.

**461.** EMS receives a call from dispatch regarding a potential domestic disturbance. Upon arrival, the neighbors tell EMS that they heard a woman screaming in the house and this prompted them to call EMS. When EMS approached the house, an angry man answered the door and said that the call was a mistake, the screams came from the television, and his wife is uninjured. He asks EMS to respect their privacy and asks them to leave. EMS has not seen the wife to corroborate the story. EMS calls you to ask how to proceed. Which of the following is the most appropriate response?

a. Tell EMS to return to their ambulance and leave the scene as the homeowner has refused their care and assured them that there is no need for their intervention.

b. Tell EMS to return to their ambulance, drive a safe distance away, and call the police for help.

c. Ask EMS to politely reason with the husband and explain to him that they are required to perform a quick assessment of the wife based on the nature of their dispatched call.

d. Instruct EMS not to enter the house without permission, but tell them to explain to the husband that they will wait outside but cannot leave the scene until they are allowed to interview the wife.

e. Tell EMS that they cannot leave the scene until they have reasonably ensured the wife's safety and ruled out any imminent danger to her.

**462.** EMS is responding to a call at a local high school football game. One of the high school football players is not responsive to verbal stimuli after a helmet-to-helmet collision with another football player. His RR is 12 breaths per minute, BP 100/65 mm Hg, and a strong pulse is palpated at 60 beats per minute. There is a small crack at the top of the helmet, but it is otherwise intact and strapped tightly to the patient's head. EMS wants to remove the helmet to assess for head trauma, but they call you for permission. What is the most appropriate prehospital management of this patient?

a. Do not attempt to remove the helmet. Maintain cervical spine precautions and transfer the patient on a backboard to the hospital.

b. While maintaining cervical spine precautions, carefully remove the helmet and assess for head injury.

c. Check the patient's pupils if there is asymmetry, remove the helmet with cervical spine precautions, and assess for head injury.

d. Wait at the scene for a physician to arrive with an electric saw for removal of the helmet and further on-scene assessment.

e. Do not remove the helmet but assess the cervical spine for step-off or any signs of obvious injury before transfer.

**463.** EMS calls you for assistance regarding a 42-year-old woman with Hodgkin lymphoma who is hypotensive and displaying rapid, shallow respirations. They are calling from the oncologist's office and he has ordered the EMS personnel to administer IV fluids with dextrose and 3 ampules of sodium bicarbonate because he thinks the patient has severe acidosis from tumor lysis syndrome. The oncologist wants this done en route to the ED as he cannot accompany EMS to the hospital because he has other patients to see in his clinic. This is a deviation from the EMS standard of care protocol; hence they call you as the online medical oversight physician for instruction. What is the most appropriate instruction to give EMS in this situation?

a. They cannot deviate from their prehospital protocols. Tell them to give normal saline and proceed with transfer.

b. The oncologist cannot assume care for the patient without accompanying EMS to the hospital.

c. Although the oncologist cannot accompany EMS to the hospital as the online medical oversight physician, you may authorize EMS to deviate from their prehospital protocols if doing so is in the patient's best interest.

d. Once EMS arrives and begins treatment on the patient, they have established a relationship with the patient and the oncologist's orders cannot supersede prehospital protocols.

e. As the physician on-scene, the oncologist's clinical evaluation and orders supersede both EMS and the online medical oversight physician and EMS is obligated to abide by his orders.

# Prehospital, Disaster, Administration

## *Answers*

**451. The answer is b.** (*National Highway Transportation Safety Administration, 2011.*) In mass-casualty incidents one of the most vital components of triage is to assign the **appropriate acuity level of injury** in a standard, efficient manner that is easy to implement.
Common triage categories include

**Red—immediate care and removal necessary**
**Yellow—delayed care until "reds" are cleared**
**Green— "walking wounded," lowest priority**
**Black—dead at the scene or not survivable injuries**

The most widely used triage system is the START system that focuses on assessing four parameters:

1. Ability to walk
2. Respiratory effort
3. Pulses/perfusion
4. Neurologic status

Patients who are wounded but are able to walk will be given a "green" tag **(a)** signifying a low priority and are attended to or transferred last. Next, patients are assessed for ability to breathe. If they are not breathing, open the airway. If breathing resumes, they are labeled "red" **(c)**; if no breathing resumes, **(e)** they are labeled "black." Also, if the RR is greater than 30, they are assigned "red" **(c)**. For patients with an RR below 30, assess perfusion by checking a radial pulse and capillary refill. If there is no radial pulse or if the capillary refill is greater than 2 to 3 seconds, they are assigned a "red." For those with a radial pulse and RR below 30, the next step is a brief mental status and motor examination in which they are asked to squeeze the examiner's hands. If they cannot do this, they are a "red"; if they can, a "yellow." Significant bleeding should be controlled during any step of the triage process.

In this case, the patient has no spontaneous respirations; therefore he cannot be a "green." After performing a chin lift, he has audible respirations; hence he is not a "black." The next system to assess is pulses/perfusion in which he has a palpable radial pulse. Finally, the patient is able to squeeze the examiner's hand; hence he is tagged as a "yellow." There is no "blue" (**d**) in the START system.

**452. The answer is d.** (*Sytkowski et al, 1983.*) The National Highway Traffic and Safety Administration Act of 1966 set recommendations for first responder and EMT training courses. Because prehospital personnel are covered by state and sometimes local funds, the State Board of Emergency Medical Services is authorized to modify recommended course lengths leading to some discrepancies from state to state. There are **four major levels of EMS training and credentialing**:

1. **First responders** include mandatory training given to firefighters, police officers, and community EMS responders. These are often the first people to arrive on scene. They are trained in CPR, basic life support (BLS), and basic trauma care. Current recommendations are approximately 40 hours of training.
2. **EMT-B (emergency medical technician basic)** is the lowest EMT level. They can perform BLS, automated external defibrillation (AED), basic assessments, and assist in medical administration. They cannot establish IV access; however, in almost all states they can administer IM medications based on predefined protocols or via a verbal order from an online medical physician. The recommended curriculum is a course length of 110 hours.
3. **EMT-Is (emergency medical technician intermediates)** are personnel who have completed EMT-B requirements and are trained in procedures such as establishing IV access, endotracheal (ET) intubation, and manual defibrillation. Current recommendations are approximately 300 to 400 hours of training.
4. **EMT-P (emergency medical technician paramedic**, sometimes abbreviated as "paramedics") is the most advanced EMT level. They receive all EMT-I training in addition to training to perform advanced airway procedures, needle decompression of the chest, ECG interpretation, external pacing, and advanced drug therapy within predefined standardized protocols. Recommendations for their training curriculum range from 1000 to 1200 hours.

In this case the patient is having an **anaphylactic reaction** secondary to a peanut allergy. The best initial treatment is IM epinephrine. **EMT-B units** are trained to administer **IM medications**; in some states they may require an order from the online medical physician before administration.

**453. The answer is c.** *(Tintinalli, pp 11-14.)* There are **three modes of transportation** available to most EMS systems: ground transportation, rotary-wing air (helicopter) transportation, or fixed-wing air (small plane) transportation. Ground transportation is used for the vast majority of acutely ill or injured patients. **Air transport is only indicated when air transport time would be significantly less than ground transport time.** Some **common indications for air transport** are severe injury in which rapid transport is essential; unstable vital signs; significant trauma in patients younger than 12 years; patients older than 55 years or pregnant; multisystem injuries; ejection from a vehicle; pedestrian struck or motorcyclist struck; death in same passenger compartment; penetrating trauma to the abdomen, pelvis, chest, neck, or head; crush injury to the abdomen, chest, or head; and fall from significant height. This is not an exhaustive list and the specific scenario and clinical assessment must always be factored into every individual case.

Once the decision to use air transportation has been made, the next decision is to employ a rotary-wing or a fixed-wing aircraft. A rotary-wing aircraft has a range of 50 to 150 miles and is indicated in scenarios with entrapped trauma patients with extrication time expected to exceed 20 minutes or locations in a topographically difficult to reach by surface areas. Keep in mind that rotary-wing air transportation is limited by poor weather and both modes of air transport carry an inherent risk of crashing that must be considered by the physician. A fixed-wing aircraft is indicated for distances longer than 100 miles when rapid transport is essential. This mode of transportation is also limited by weather, lack of runways, and refueling. One must also consider possible altitude problems for the patient such as pneumothorax, ET cuff, and balloon catheters. However, there are no absolute contraindications to fixed-wing air transport.

In this case, even though there is a service road adjacent to the hiking trail ground, transportation (**a, b, and d**) would not be appropriate. This is due to several factors, including prolonged travel time (the nearest hospital is 50 miles away), a topographically difficult-to-reach surface area, and a prolonged extrication time. In this scenario a rotary-winged aircraft (helicopter) would be ideal because it could assist in the extrication process as the hiker fell down a steep hill and cannot move. A fixed-wing aircraft (e) is not the best choice because ground transportation would still be needed and the patient would have to endure a prolonged extrication time. Additionally, the patient has difficulty breathing secondary to blunt chest trauma suggestive of a pneumothorax, which could be significantly worsened by the altitude required by fixed-wing transport.

**454. The answer is e.** *(Tintinalli, pp 42-46.)* The most important rule of disaster management for chemical agents is **the contaminated patient should never be allowed to enter the ED before being decontaminated.** Each state has a standard operating procedure for mass casualty decontamination. The following are critical steps in the management of chemical mass casualty exposures:

- Recognition of a toxic chemical exposure
- Rapid identification of the agents involved
- Information retrieval on the toxicity and secondary contamination potential of the agent
- Proper protection of self, hospital personnel, already-hospitalized patients, and the facility itself from secondary contamination or loss of serviceability to other patients
- Decontamination and triage of victims
- Stabilization and medical treatment of victims
- Protection of the community-at-large from secondary contamination

This question pertains to the decontamination step of a toxic chemical exposure, which is clearly of imminent risk to the surrounding community because some of the crew of the freight car has died. Patient decontamination should occur outside the hospital. Hot, warm, and cold zones should be established and cordoned off with brightly colored tape. The **hot zone** is the **area of the toxic substance exposure** or **may be the hospital area where arriving patients with no prior decontamination are held.** The **warm zone** is an area where thorough decontamination and further medical stabilization occur. This area should be arranged so that there is no risk of primary contamination, but secondary contamination (transfer of the toxic substance from the victim to personnel or equipment) may occur. Hence, only trained personnel with the proper personal protective equipment (PPE) are allowed in the hot and warm zones. The **cold zone** is the area to which fully decontaminated patients are transferred. The warm and cold zones should be established upwind, uphill, or upstream of the hot

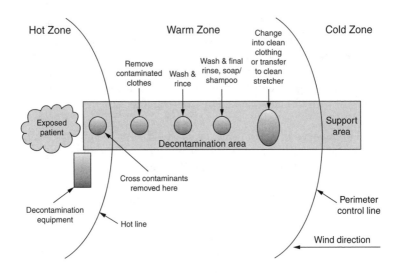

Hot Zone

Warm Zone

Change into clean clothing or transfer to clean stretcher

Cold Zone

Remove contaminated clothes

Wash & rince

Wash & final rinse, soap/ shampoo

Exposed patient

Decontamination area

Support area

Cross contaminants removed here

Decontamination equipment

Hot line

Perimeter control line

Wind direction

*(Courtesy of Shareaf Walid, MD.)*

zone to minimize extension of the hot zone into other decontamination areas. There is no personnel flow between the different zones. The figure below is a schematic representation of a hazardous material incident area.

There are no circumstances when a hot- and warm-zone decontamination can be bypassed, especially in the event that other exposed victims have already died from exposure. Bypassing contamination zones (**a, b, c, and d**) would put the public-at-large, including the ED, at risk, which is never acceptable. Some salient points to remember are that **clothing should be removed quickly** because this is thought to accomplish 80% of the decontamination.

**455. The answer is a.** *(Sasson, 2010.)* In 2010, a meta-analysis from 79 studies during 1950-2008 involving 142,740 patients with presumed out-of-hospital cardiac arrest found parameters that **predicted increased survival to hospital discharge**. EMS should be queried about the presence or absence of these factors to help the physician gauge the utility in continuing resuscitative efforts. Survival was more likely among those cardiac arrests that were **witnessed by a bystander** (13.5%-6.4%), **witnessed by EMS**

(18.2%-4.9%), **who received bystander CPR** (16.1%-3.9%), were **found in ventricular fibrillation/ventricular tachycardia** (23.0%-14.8%), **or achieved return of spontaneous circulation** (33.6%-15.5%).

Patients who have a witnessed arrest tend to have EMS arrive quicker and usually have CPR begin sooner. Hence a witnessed arrest, although not the cause of increased survival, correlates with other factors that lead to improved survival. Medication complince (b) is not an independent predictor of out-of-hospital cardiac arrest survival to hospital discharge. Patients who present in cardiorespiratory arrest with AICDs (c) are already refractory to cardioversion or defibrillation. Survival of a prior arrest (d) has not been shown to favor survival in future arrests. An initial rhythm of asystole (e) is actually a poor prognostic indicator for survival.

**456. The answer is a.** (*National Highway Traffic Safety Administration, 2006.*) A need for an extension of emergency care in the community grew into what is now known as the EMS system, which was established in the 1960s. **The Highway Safety Act** (1966) authorized the US Department of Transportation (DOT) to develop prehospital services. This act also established the National Highway Traffic Safety Administration (NHTSA) to help carry out and distribute government funding to ensure highway safety. This act is vitally important because it established the initial government funding for prehospital services. The **Emergency Medicine Services Act** (1973) (b) provided government funding and training for states to develop regional, county, and local EMS systems. The **EMTALA** (1985) (c) was part of the Consolidated Omnibus Budget Reconciliation Act (COBRA) that penalized EDs that refused care. The **Trauma Care Systems Planning and Development Act** (1990) (d) authorized government funds to states for development of trauma systems. The **JCAHO** (e) is an organization made up of individuals from the private medical sector whose role is to develop and maintain standards of quality in medical facilities in the United States. Medical facilities such as hospitals rely on JCAHO accreditation to indicate to the public that their particular institution meets quality standards.

**457. The answer is c.** (*US Department of Health and Human Services, 2003.*) The **HIPAA** (1996) was created to **protect patient's privacy rights** by establishing rules for disclosures of confidential health information. The act was intended to standardize health information transfers; require identification numbers for providers, health plans, and employers; and to protect confidential protected health information (PHI). The inclusion of PHI protection resulted from fears that electronic transfers and ID numbers could be misused. Hence, the law penalizes disclosures of confidential health information that are not authorized in writing by the patient and violate the privacy rule. The secretary of health and human services imposes civil monetary penalties for violation of any HIPAA requirement, up to $25,000 per disclosure.

Police officers do not have automatic access to a patient's medical record, even if the patient is in their custody. Only if the police serve you with a subpoena for court-ordered medical records are you obligated to share them without the patient's written consent.

Answer choice (a) is incorrect because incarcerated patients are still protected by HIPAA regulations. Answer choice (b) is incorrect because you have no legal ramifications by abiding by HIPAA rules; in fact, both you and your institution are liable for monetary and potentially civil penalties if HIPAA rules are broken. Answer choice (d) is incorrect because HIPAA privacy regulations are not subject to case-by-case discretionary judgments but must be followed with some special exceptions, such as psychotherapy notes and disclosures for billing issues, which are outside the physician's scope of practice. Answer choice (e) is incorrect because it violates the HIPAA law.

**458. The answer is e.** (*US Department of Health and Human Services, 2003.*) The **EMTALA** mandates that **unstable patients cannot be discharged or transferred except for medical necessity**. The purpose of EMTALA was to discourage low-income and high-risk patients from being transferred from one ED to another for financial advantage. Under EMTALA any patient presenting to an ED has the right to an MSE to determine if an emergency medical condition (EMC) exists without regard to the patient's ability or willingness to pay for services rendered. If an EMC exists, the hospital must stabilize the condition within its capacity. If the hospital cannot stabilize the condition, the staff is further obligated to transfer the patient to a facility that can. It is important to understand that an MSE is not a triage but requires any indicated workup, including consultations if necessary, to determine if an EMC exists. If an EMC is not yet stabilized, a transfer cannot be made unless the transferring physician certifies that the benefits outweigh the risks and the transfer is medically appropriate. Additionally, the transferring hospital must do everything in its capacity to minimize the risk of transfer and the receiving hospital must have available space and personnel and agree to take the case. Any hospital that negligently violates an EMTALA policy can be penalized up to $50,000 per violation and physicians who negligently violate may also have to pay up to $50,000 per violation. Civil money penalties such as EMTALA are not covered by malpractice insurance.

In this vignette, the patient has a history of coronary artery disease and presents with shortness of breath, diaphoresis, chest pressure, and vomiting. Given his history, presentation, age, and risk factors, it is clear that the patient is at high risk for a myocardial infarction. Hence, the proper MSE is an ECG and troponin in order to rule out an MI, the EMC, before transfer **(a, b, c, and d)**. If the patient is having an MI and the current facility has the capability of providing effective management based on standard-of-care protocols, they are obliged to admit the patient to their facility. If the current facility does not have the capacity to effectively treat the patient (eg, a cardiac catheterization suite), they can transfer the patient if a receiving hospital agrees to accept him and he is deemed stable for transfer.

**459. The answer is d.** *(Hall, 2003; Cook et al, 2010.)* The EMS-DNR order was created to allow individuals to provide an advance directive to emergency medical technicians regarding their desire for or against resuscitative treatment. This vignette evokes a dilemma where the ethical wishes of rescuers to act for the good of their patient (ie, beneficence) runs counter to the individual's autonomous wishes expressed in the EMS-DNR order. **In the case of a suicide**, especially within the context of the patient's depression at the news of his recent diagnosis of pancreatic cancer, **treatment is necessary**. The patient must be returned to a level of functioning where it is possible to demonstrate that the decision to end life is truly an autonomous decision. In clinically depressed patients, there is legal precedent that judgment is clouded by disease and the respect for patient autonomy is superseded by beneficence or malfeasance. EMTs are usually not in a position to determine if a patient is autonomous; thus they should treat the patient by stabilizing them and transporting them to a facility where a definitive evaluation can be performed.

Answer choices **(a, b, and c)** place the patient's autonomy before beneficence based on his EMS-DNR order, which is not appropriate considering the patient's reported depression and suicidal gesture. Answer choice **(e)** is incorrect because the situation does not afford the time allotment to seek counsel from a medical ethics board. Additionally, it is appropriate to override autonomy in suicidal cases without contacting a medical ethics board.

**460. The answer is c.** *(Tintinalli, p 2; ACEP, 2009; National Highway Traffic Safety Administration, 2006.)* Critically ill patients are often transported initially to a local hospital for assessment and subsequent stabilization. The ED physician must then determine whether their institution has the necessary resources, including access to specialists and personnel, to safely manage the patient. If their facility does not, it is incumbent upon the physician to stabilize the patient and arrange for a transfer to a facility that can adequately manage the patient. The most common reasons for transfers from EDs include trauma, the need for neonatal intensive care, high-risk obstetrics, burns, spinal cord injury, and neurosurgical and cardiac care.

The 75-year-old patient with shortness of breath and pacemaker capture failure has symptomatic bradycardia. Acute myocardial infarction is less likely but not definitively ruled out with a single negative troponin. Other than bradycardia, the patient has stable vital signs and no physical examination findings suggesting fluid overload. It is reasonable to provide supportive care and wait for the cardiologist to arrive. Answer choices **(a, b, d, and e)** are all examples of the most common reasons for ED transfers.

**461. The answer is b.** *(Krebs et al. Federal Emergency Management Agency, 1994.)* The cardinal rule guiding EMS interaction in the field is **safety first**. EMTs are trained to "size up" a scene upon arrival, which is the initial quick analysis vital to safe and efficient operations. The initial size-up provides safety for the emergency crew and validates the information provided during dispatch for other arriving rescuers. If people on the scene require medical attention and a perceived threatening perpetrator is still present, **EMS should leave the scene and drive a safe distance away**. They are even trained to reduce the volume of radios and cut off the ambulance's warning devices, headlights, and interior lights to eliminate them as targets. Once a safe distance is away, they should **call the police or request dispatch to call the police who will then secure the scene for a safe assessment**.

As long as there is no percieved threat of danger, **(a)** EMS is required to make an assessment of a potentially injured person. EMTs should not put themselves at risk **(c, d, and e)** at an unsafe scene.

**462. The answer is a.** *(Tintinalli, p 9.)* A properly fitted football helmet with shoulder pads holds the head in position of neutral spinal alignment; **field removal of these devices is not recommended**. Instead, the helmet and shoulder pads should remain on as the athlete is immobilized and transported on a rigid backboard. Simultaneous removal of the helmet and shoulder pads should be done after clinical assessment and radiographs at the hospital. Radiographs can be repeated after removal of the helmet as clinically indicated.

Answer (**b**) is incorrect because the proper removal of a football helmet requires four people and should not be attempted out of hospital. Answer (**c**) is incorrect because even with pupil asymmetry the EMT's best course of action is to expeditiously transport the patient to the ED for definitive care. EMTs are not trained to perform any techniques to relieve impending uncal herniation. Answer (**d**) is incorrect because the use of an electric saw is not indicated and unnecessary prehospital delays should be avoided. Answer (**e**) is incorrect because adequate cervical spine assessment is unreliable and potentially dangerous in the prehospital setting and would also unnecessarily delay transport.

**463. The answer is c.** *(National Highway Traffic Safety Administration, 2006; Department of Health and Senior Services, http://www.nj.gov/health/ems/ emtbqa.shtml.)* When EMS personnel begin assessment and treatment of a patient, they establish a physician-patient relationship between the medical oversight physician and the patient. Therefore, a physician at the scene should not assume responsibility (**d and e**) unless the online medical oversight physician has given authorization. In general, EMS personnel cannot deviate from the standard-of-care protocols and should document all interactions and exchanges made between the physicians. Under selected circumstances, the on-scene physician (**a**) may control medical care and then give the patient to EMS personnel for transfer. If the on-scene physician who does not follow the EMS protocol directs the medical care of the patient, he or she should accompany (**b**) the patient to the hospital. If the physician-on-scene does not assume control and assists with care that conforms to EMS protocol, he or she is not required to accompany the unit to the hospital.

# Wound Care

## Questions

**464.** A 25-year-old man presents to the emergency department (ED) with a right forearm laceration that he sustained from a piece of glass during a bar fight. He complains of pain at the laceration site but denies a foreign body sensation. On examination, the laceration is superficial and 4 cm long. The patient demonstrates intact strength and sensation distally. Which of the following statements regarding imaging this patient is true?

a. Imaging can be omitted because he does not have a foreign body sensation.
b. Imaging is not indicated because retained glass does not cause an inflammatory reaction.
c. Plain film is the next best step in the management of this patient.
d. Computed tomographic (CT) scan is the most commonly used modality to rule out a foreign body.
e. Plain film cannot rule out bone, teeth, or glass in soft tissue.

**465.** A 30-year-old woman presents to the ED with a left hand laceration. She reports cutting herself while attempting to slice a bagel. She has a superficial 2-cm laceration over the left thenar eminence. No deeper structures are involved. What is the best way to clean the wound?

a. Punch holes in a normal saline bag or bottle and irrigate the wound.
b. Use a high-pressure syringe and irrigate with water.
c. Wound cleaning is unnecessary because wound was sustained from a clean knife.
d. Soak her hand in normal saline for 30 minutes.
e. Apply povidone-iodine to the wound.

**466.** A 40-year-old man presents to the ED with a left foot puncture wound from stepping on a rusty nail. His last tetanus vaccine was during childhood, which resulted in a severe allergic reaction and a prolonged hospital stay. Which of the following is true regarding tetanus immunization in this patient?

a. Give tetanus toxoid.
b. Give tetanus immunoglobulin.
c. Give tetanus immunoglobulin and toxoid.
d. Give neither tetanus toxoid nor immunoglobulin because he has had an allergic reaction in the past.
e. Give tetanus toxoid and immunoglobulin with diphenhydramine.

**467.** A 5-year-old boy is brought to the ED by his mom for a forehead laceration. She reports that he slipped on ice and hit his head. There was no loss of consciousness. The child is alert and active. He has a 3-cm-forehead laceration that crosses the hairline. What is the most appropriate method of wound closure in this patient?

a. Shave the hair surrounding the laceration and close with interrupted sutures.
b. Shave the hair surrounding the laceration and close with topical skin adhesive (Dermabond).
c. Close with staples.
d. Close with Steri-Strips.
e. Close with interrupted sutures.

**468.** A 12-year-old girl presents to the ED with a left index finger laceration. She sustained the injury when her friend accidentally closed the car door on her finger. She has a semicircular laceration distal to the distal interphalangeal (DIP) joint on the volar surface of the left second digit. Sensation distal to the laceration is intact. Range of motion at the DIP joint is intact. The patient hopes to be a hand model in the future and is extremely anxious about the cosmetic result. Which of the following is the best method to provide anesthesia in this patient?

a. Application of a tourniquet to control bleeding and irrigation of the wound with 3 cc of lidocaine
b. Local infiltration through the wound margins with 3 cc of lidocaine
c. Local infiltration through the wound margins with 3 cc of lidocaine with epinephrine
d. A digital block at the base of the proximal phalanx with 3 cc of lidocaine
e. A digital block at the base of the proximal phalanx with 3 cc of lidocaine with epinephrine

**469.** An 18-year-old woman presents to the ED with a lower lip laceration secondary to a fall. The patient reports she fell forward after her heel caught in a storm drain. In addition to small facial abrasions, she has a 3-cm-deep laceration on the inner aspect of the lower lip. You plan to close the laceration to control bleeding and prevent food impaction. Which of the following suture material is the best choice in this patient?

a. 2-0 nylon
b. 6-0 nylon
c. 3-0 monofilament absorbable
d. 1-0 absorbable chromic gut
e. 5-0 absorbable chromic gut

**470.** A 50-year-old man presents to the ED for suture removal. When he was on vacation in Jamaica 2 days ago, he sustained a 4-cm right calf laceration from a piece of glass. At that time, the laceration was irrigated, radiographed to rule out a foreign body, and repaired. Currently, there is good wound edge approximation and no surrounding erythema or discharge from the wound. What is the next best step in management?

a. Have the patient return in 3 days for suture removal.
b. Have the patient return in 8 days for suture removal.
c. Have the patient return in 14 days for suture removal.
d. Remove the sutures.
e. Remove the sutures then replace them to prevent infection.

**471.** A 27-year-old man presents to the ED with the laceration shown below after an altercation. There are no dental fractures and his tetanus immunization is up to date. What are the most appropriate next steps in management?

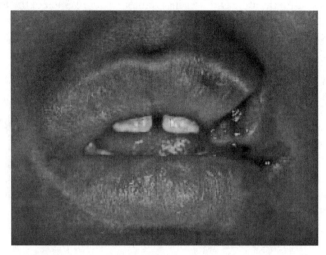

*(Reproduced, with permission, from Knoop KJ, Stack LB, Storrow AB.* Atlas of Emergency Medicine. *NewYork, NY: McGraw-Hill, 2002: 162.)*

a. Infraorbital nerve block and then approximation of the vermilion border
b. Infiltration of local anesthesia into the lip and then approximation of the vermilion border
c. Infraorbital nerve block and closure of mucosal defects before the approximation of the vermilion border
d. Infiltration of the lip with local anesthesia, closure of dermis and mucosal defects, and then approximation of the vermilion border
e. Closure with a commercially available tissue adhesive and Steri-Strips to avoid distorting tissue architecture

**472.** A 44-year-old woman presents to the ED with a deep puncture wound to her left forearm from a dog bite. The dog is appropriately vaccinated. Which of the following statements regarding management of animal bite wounds is true?

a. Infection after dog and cat bites is rare.
b. Irrigate the wound thoroughly and place deep sutures to prevent infection.
c. Delayed primary closure can be used for bite wounds.
d. Dog-bite infections are most commonly secondary to *Pasteurella multocida.*
e. Clindamycin is the most commonly used antibiotic for dog bites.

**473.** A 23-year-old man presents to the ED complaining of a wound to his left lower extremity. He states he was pulling branches out of a flooded creek in his backyard when he punctured his left calf. He states that his legs were in the water when the wound occurred. On examination, the puncture wound is 1 cm in diameter, several centimeters deep, and demonstrates surrounding erythema. After irrigating the wound, you discover a splinter within the wound. What is the most appropriate next step in management?

a. Radiograph to map the exact location of the foreign body.
b. Close the wound with 4-0 nylon.
c. Dress the wound with a sterile bandage and treat with a fluoroquinolone.
d. Remove the splinter.
e. Remove the splinter, close the wound, and treat with fluoroquinolone.

**474.** A 21-year-old woman presents to the ED with a superficial 2-cm mid-forehead laceration sustained from a fall. You irrigate and close the wound. The patient is an aspiring actress and concerned about her long-term cosmetic outcome. She requests detailed wound care instructions. Which of the following statements would be an appropriate wound care instruction to give?

a. Avoid direct sun exposure while the wound is healing.
b. The wound should not be washed until sutures are removed.
c. Sutures should be removed in 7 to 10 days.
d. Appearance of the scar at suture removal will be the final cosmetic outcome.
e. Good suturing technique and meticulous wound care guarantee no scar formation.

**475.** A 17-year-old adolescent presents to the ED with a lip laceration. He sustained the laceration during an altercation. On examination, he has a horizontal, 2-cm laceration of the right lower lip crossing the midline. There is significant swelling of the lower lip. The attending asks you, the intern, to perform a mental block for anesthesia. Which of the following statements regarding mental blocks is correct?

a. A mental block is performed by injecting lidocaine into the mental nerve foramen.
b. The patient requires a right-sided mental block.
c. A mental block is not appropriate in this patient because it will lead to worsened swelling of the lower lip swelling.
d. A mental block anesthetizes the mental nerve, which innervates the lower lip.
e. A mental block is performed with a 3-cc syringe attached to an 18-gauge needle.

**476.** A 9-year-old girl is brought to the ED by her parents after sustaining a forehead laceration. Her dad reports that the patient hit her forehead against a doorknob. On examination, the patient is cooperative but anxious about the upcoming anesthetic injection. She has a 0.5-cm laceration on the mid-forehead with clean edges. Her parents inquire about "skin glue" they heard about on TV. Which of the following statements is true regarding cyanoacrylate tissue adhesives?

a. It cannot be applied to mucous membranes and areas with thick hair.
b. Tissue adhesives have a higher rate of infection and tissue dehiscence than sutures.
c. Tissue adhesives are best suited for forehead lacerations between 5 and 10 cm in length.
d. Tissue adhesives are applied inside the wound to pull skin edges together.
e. Tissue adhesives must be covered with topical antibiotics and bandages to prevent sloughing.

**477.** A 45-year-old woman presents to the ED with multiple facial lacerations. She was sitting by her window when the neighbor's kid hit a baseball through her window. The shattered glass caused multiple superficial lacerations. The most notable laceration is 1 cm on the right eyelid. You rule out the presence of a foreign body and give her a tetanus shot. Which of the following statements regarding eyelid trauma is correct?

a. A slit-lamp examination is unnecessary because it does not help evaluate the eyelid.
b. Tissue adhesives can be used to close eyelid laceration because they are usually small.
c. Lacerations causing ptosis require ophthalmology consultation.
d. Ptosis after an eyelid laceration is common.
e. A lacrimal duct injury should be suspected in a laceration to the lateral canthus.

**478.** A 30-year-old chef presents to the ED with a complete fingertip amputation. She says her knife slipped while chopping vegetables. She brought the amputated pulp in a plastic bag. On examination, the patient has a clean, 5-mm-diameter dermal slice on the distal volar tip of the second digit. There is profuse nonpulsatile bleeding. There is no trauma to the DIP joint, proximal interphalangeal (PIP) joint, or the nail. Her most recent tetanus booster was 1 year ago. Which of the following is the most appropriate next step in management?

a. Consult hand surgery for replantation of the pulp in the operating room.
b. Irrigate the hand and replant distal tip in the ED as soon as possible.
c. Perform a digital block with lidocaine and epinephrine to control bleeding.
d. Immediately place the amputated tip on ice to prevent cell death.
e. Discharge the patient with a pressure dressing and splint after the wound is irrigated and the bleeding is controlled.

# Wound Care

## Answers

**464. The answer is c.** (*Tintinalli, pp 336-342.*) On plain films 80% to 90% of foreign bodies can be seen. Glass larger than 2 mm is visible on plain film.

(**a**) A foreign body sensation has a sensitivity of 43% and specificity of 83%. Therefore, lack of a foreign body sensation cannot be used to rule out a foreign body. (**b**) Retained foreign bodies may lead to a local granulomatous inflammatory response or to local and systemic infection. (**d**) CT is capable of detecting more types of foreign bodies than plain film, but it is not commonly used given the time needed and expense. (**e**) Plain film can usually locate metal, bone, teeth, pencil graphite, gravel, sand, and aluminum. Plain film cannot detect wood, thorns, some plastics, and other organic matter.

**465. The answer is b.** (*Tintinalli, p 305.*) To achieve low bacterial counts through irrigation, a **pressure of 5 to 8 psi is recommended.** This pressure can be generated with an irrigation syringe or a 35-mL syringe and a 19-gauge needle. Water (sterile or tap) is as efficacious as sterile normal saline.

The common recommendation for the amount of irrigant used is **60 to 100 cc per 1-cm wound length.** Using normal saline bottles or bags with holes (**a**) may not generate adequate pressure. Soaking (**d**) is ineffective in cleansing wounds. Disinfectants (**e**) such as povidone-iodine should not be used on an open wound because they can impair host defenses and promote bacterial growth. Last, irrigation is necessary (**c**) regardless of the method of the sustained injury.

**466. The answer is b.** (*Tintinalli, pp 357-358.*) Tetanus toxoid is contraindicated in patients who have had a severe allergic reaction, including respiratory distress or cardiovascular collapse. **Tetanus immunoglobulin can be used in these patients.** Local reaction at injection site resulting in redness, pain, and swelling is not considered a contraindication.

**467. The answer is e.** *(Tintinalli, pp 321-322.)* **Facial lacerations** should be closed with a **6-0 nylon suture** in interrupted fashion. Staples **(c)** do not give the desired cosmesis for a facial wound repair. Staples are more appropriate for scalp laceration. Steri-Strips **(d)** can be used in very small skin openings with minimal tension. They will not provide the tensile strength required for this patient's wound closure. **(b)** Dermabond would be inadequate for use in this laceration that crosses the hairline. Last, shaving surrounding hair **(a)** increases the risk of infection and therefore not recommended. Of note, eyebrows should not be shaved because of the high likelihood that eyebrows will not regrow.

**468. The answer is d.** *(Rosen, p 701.)* Application of a **lidocaine digital block** at the base of the finger will block the digital nerves allowing for appropriate anesthesia. The needle is inserted into the web space on either side and anesthesia is deposited anteriorly and posteriorly. This is repeated on the opposite side of the affected digit.

Local infiltration and digital block **(c and e)** with lidocaine and epinephrine are incorrect as epinephrine is contraindicated in areas of end-organ circulation (tip of nose, glans penis, scrotum, ears, nose, and fingers). Irrigating **(a)** a wound with anesthetic does not provide adequate anesthesia. Although local infiltration **(b)** will provide adequate anesthesia, it may interfere with good wound approximation and therefore may lead to a poor cosmetic result.

**469. The answer is e.** *(Tintinalli, pp 317, 320-321.)* Choosing a suture material is based on tissue type, tissue tension, and whether or not sutures will require removal. Oral mucosa is rapidly healing and under moderate tension. Additionally, because the inner lip mucosa does not require a cosmetic result, absorbable sutures should be used. Therefore, **absorbable chromic gut** is the best suture choice. A **5-0 chromic gut** will provide sufficient tensile strength to match that of the oral mucosa.

**(d)** A 1-0 chromic gut is unnecessarily large. Oral mucosa does not require the tensile strength provided by a 1-0 suture and would leave an uncomfortably large knot mass. **(c)** Absorbable monofilament sutures provide more tensile strength than necessary in this case and are preferred for closure of deep structures (eg, fascia). Nylon sutures **(a and b)** are not the best choice for oral cavity repairs because they would require the patient to return for removal.

**470. The answer is b.** *(Tintinalli, pp 356-359.)* Suture removal is a balance between cosmetic outcome and adequate wound closure. Increasing suture time improves wound strength at the expense of cosmetic outcome. Most sutures can be removed 7 days after placement. Sutures on the **face should be removed in 3 to 5 days** to prevent unsightly hatch markings. Sutures in areas of **high tension, such as arms, legs, hands, and feet require approximately 10 days.** This patient's laceration is large and in a high-tension area; therefore, removing the sutures 10 days after placement is the best management.

Having this patient return in 3 days **(a)** would be too soon and 14 days **(c)** would be too late. **(d and e)** There is no need to remove the sutures 2 days after placement, especially because there are no signs of infection. Only if there were signs of wound infection would suture removal be the appropriate management.

**471. The answer is a.** *(Knoop et al, p 162; Singer and Hollander, pp 35-37.)* This is a laceration of the face crossing the vermilion border (demarcation of the lip mucosa and facial skin). The goal of repair in this case is **approximation of the vermilion border** with less than 2 mm of displacement because significant displacement is cosmetically unappealing. A **nerve block** is required because local anesthesia would distort tissue anatomy, thereby limiting appropriate approximation. The first stitch should focus on approximating the border before closing the other aspects of the wound.

**(b and d)** Infiltration with local anesthesia will distort the tissue anatomy and may make proper alignment unreliable. It should only be used if the patient fails nerve block. Initial alignment of the dermis or mucosal aspects of the laceration **(c and d)** may make approximation of the vermilion border difficult. Tissue adhesive and Steri-Strips **(e)** should not be used to close the lip as it is subject to pulling forces of facial movement. Wound separation in this case could result in a cosmetically unappealing outcome.

**472. The answer is c.** *(Tintinalli, pp 353-355.)* Puncture wounds owing to their depth cannot be cleaned adequately. **Delayed primary closure** in these wounds decreases the risk of abscess formation and wound infection.

**(a)** Approximately 5% of dog bites and 40% of cat bites become infected. Copious irrigation is crucial in preventing wound infections. Most bite wounds can be repaired with primary closure. **(b)** Puncture wounds, small lacerations, and hand and foot wounds carry higher risks of infection and therefore are best managed with delayed primary closure. Placing deep sutures in this patient's puncture wound would increase the risk of wound infection. **(d)** *Pasteurella* is the most common organism in cat bites. Dog bites are often polymicrobial and include aerobes and anaerobes. Antibiotics should be considered in all high-infection-risk patients (ie, elderly, diabetics, immunocompromised patients, puncture wounds, and wounds of the hands and feet). **(e)** The most commonly used antibiotic for dog and cat bites is amoxicillin/clavulanate. Clindamycin with a fluoroquinolone can be used for dog bites in penicillin-allergic patients. Doxycycline can be used for cat bites in penicillin-allergic patients.

**473. The answer is d.** *(Singer and Hollander, pp 196-197; Tintinalli, pp 336-349.)* Foreign bodies with potential to cause infection and inflammatory response **require immediate removal** (examples include thorns, splinters, spines, teeth, soil-covered objects). These materials may cause intense and excessive inflammatory responses. If the foreign body cannot be removed by the ED physician, an appropriate specialist should be consulted.

**(a)** Because organic materials are radiolucent, radiographs will not assist in locating organic foreign bodies. Thorough direct visual inspection is necessary to locate and remove all organic foreign bodies. **(c)** Treating with antibiotics is necessary but less important than the removal of the foreign body. After the splinter is removed, the patient should be treated with an outpatient fluoroquinolone. Wounds with stagnant freshwater exposure are at high risk of infection with gram positive, *Pseudomonas*, and *Aeromonas* species, and require empiric antibiotic coverage. **(b and e)** Closing a puncture wound, especially with a retained foreign body, will lead to an inflammatory response and likely infection. Closing this patient's wound would not be appropriate management.

**474. The answer is a.** *(Tintinalli, pp 356-359.)* Direct sun exposure during healing can lead to permanent hyperpigmentation. Therefore, **avoiding direct sun exposure** and using sunblock for up to 12 months can improve cosmetic outcome.

**(b)** Patients should be instructed to wash the wound with gentle soap and water as early as 8 hours after sutures are placed. Although the wound should be kept dry, instructing against washing is inappropriate. Healing wounds should be patted dry to avoid dehiscence from forceful wiping. **(e)** The patient should be informed that all lacerations scar. Good repair and wound care will improve the appearance of the scar but will not inhibit scar formation. Wounds that heal by delayed closure have the poorest cosmetic outcome. Good edge approximation, using appropriate suture material, and early suture removal all lead to better cosmetic outcomes. (**d**) The early appearance of the scar is not reflective of the long-term outcome. (**c**) Facial sutures should be removed in 3 to 5 days. Leaving sutures in for 7 to 10 days lead to a poorer outcome.

**475. The answer is d.** (*Roberts and Hedges, pp 509-510.*) The **mental nerve** is a continuation of the inferior alveolar nerve. It emerges from the mental foramen below the second premolar and **innervates the mucosa and skin of the lower lip**. A mental nerve block is the most appropriate way to anesthetize this patient given his lip swelling.

(**c**) Local injection with lidocaine will cause further swelling and distort the anatomy further. A mental block will provide anesthesia without distorting the lip anatomy. (**e**) The block should be performed with a 25- or 27-gauge needle. An 18-gauge needle is too large for the procedure. The mental foramen should be palpated with a gloved finger. It is located 1 cm inferior and anterior to the second premolar. Lidocaine should be injected around the foramen. (**a**) Injecting directly into the foramen should be avoided because it can cause neurovascular damage. (**b**) This patient will require bilateral mental blocks because his laceration crosses the midline.

**476. The answer is a.** (*Tintinalli, pp 313-315.*) **Tissue adhesives** close wounds by forming an adhesive layer that brings the edges of the laceration together. They cannot be used on mucosal membranes and areas with thick hair. For optimal results, it should be applied in three to four layers in a dry, bloodless field.

(**b**) Tissue adhesive rate of infection and dehiscence are comparable to sutures when used appropriately. (**c**) They are best suited for small (< 5 cm), clean, straight wounds in low tensile areas. (**d**) It is applied as a layer on the intact epithelium while holding close approximation of the wound edges. It cannot be used inside the wound because it leads to an intense inflammatory reaction. (**e**) After application the wound must be left open to air. Applying topical antibiotics and bandages would cause prolonged exposure to moisture leading to weakening of the adhesive layer. Patients should be instructed not to pick at the edges of the layer and allow it to slough off naturally in 5 to 10 days.

**477. The answer is c.** (*Roberts and Hedges, pp 6618-620; Tintinalli, pp 317-318.*) **Ptosis** results from a laceration through the **levator palpebrae**

**muscle or its tendinous attachment to the tarsal plate.** Repair requires reattachment of the muscle. If the emergency physician is unable to recognize and repair the muscular defect, an ophthalmology consult is warranted.
(a) A complete eye examination should be performed to detect any injuries to the lacrimal duct, supra- and infraorbital nerves, or the globe. (b) Tissue adhesives are contraindicated near the eye and other mucosal surfaces. Even when using tissue adhesives to close nonperiocular lacerations, extra care should be taken to avoid runoffs into the eye. Positioning the patient parallel to the ground, applying small amounts of tissue adhesive, and circumscribing the laceration with petroleum jelly will all prevent runoff into mucosal surfaces. If eyes are exposed to tissue adhesives, irrigate thoroughly.
(d) Ptosis is not common after an eyelid laceration. (e) Lacerations to the upper or lower eyelid medial to the punctum can involve the lacrimal duct. Improper repair of the lacrimal duct can result in chronic tearing.

**478. The answer is e.** *(Roberts and Hedges, pp 843-845).* This patient has a less than 10-mm dermal slice that is generally managed with **bleeding control, nonadherent dressing, and a finger splint to prevent reinjury and decrease pain.** Dressing changes have to be performed every 24 to 48 hours. Fingertip amputation greater than 10 mm, exposure of the bone, or involvement of the nail may require a hand surgeon consultation. However, this patient's dermal slice is 5 mm and does not involve the phalanx or nail; therefore, it can be managed conservatively. Pressure dressing is typically sufficient to control bleeding in dermal tip amputations. If hemostasis is not achieved with direct pressure, commercial hemostatic agents can be used.

Management of fingertip amputations is controversial. For amputations involving a significant amount of the distal digit, various techniques, such as partial-thickness skin grafts and full-thickness skin grafts, exist. Most of these are performed in the operating room by a hand surgeon. (a, b, and d) However, replantation of a less than 10-mm dermal tip is not indicated. Despite replantation, the amputated tip is most likely to necrose and slough off. Using the amputated piece as a natural dressing is unnecessary given the small size of the wound. (c) Digital blocks are helpful for pain relief while the patient irrigates the distal tip. Epinephrine is not recommended for use in digits. The most appropriate way to achieve hemostasis is with direct pressure.

# Endocrine Emergencies

## Questions

**479.** A 30-year-old man with type 1 diabetes presents to the emergency department (ED). His blood pressure (BP) is 100/70 mm Hg and heart rate (HR) is 140 beats per minute. His blood glucose is 750 mg/dL, potassium level is 5.9 mEq/L, bicarbonate is 5 mEq/L, and arterial pH 7.1. His urine is positive for ketones. Which of the following is the best initial therapy for this patient?

a. Give normal saline as a 2-L bolus; then administer 20 units of regular insulin subcutaneously.

b. Bolus 2 ampules of bicarbonate and administer 10 units of insulin intravenously.

c. Give him 5 mg of metoprolol to slow down his heart, start intravenous (IV) hydration, and then give 10 units of regular insulin intravenously.

d. Give normal saline in 2 L bolus and then administer 10 units of insulin intravenously followed by an insulin drip and continued hydration.

e. Give normal saline in 2 L bolus with 20 mEq/L potassium chloride (KCl) in each bag.

**480.** A 39-year-old woman, brought into the ED by her family, states that she has had 4 days of diarrhea and has now started acting "crazy" with mood swings and confusion. The family states that she usually takes a medication for a problem with her neck. Her BP is 130/45 mm Hg, HR is 140 beats per minute, temperature is 101.5°F, and her respiratory rate (RR) is 22 breaths per minute. An electrocardiogram (ECG) reveals atrial fibrillation with a normal QRS complex. After you address the airway, breathing, and circulation (ABCs), which of the following is the most appropriate next step in management?

a. Administer 2 ampules of bicarbonate to treat for tricyclic antidepressant overdose.

b. Administer chlordiazepoxide, thiamine, and folate.

c. Administer ceftriaxone and prepare for a lumbar puncture.

d. Administer propranolol and propylthiouracil (PTU); then wait an hour to give Lugol iodine solution.

e. Administer ciprofloxacin and give a 2-L bolus of normal saline for treatment of dehydration secondary to infectious diarrhea.

**481.** A 65-year-old woman, brought into the ED by her family, states that she has been weak, lethargic, and saying "crazy things" over the last 2 days. Her family also states that her medical history is significant only for a disease of her thyroid. Her BP is 120/90 mm Hg, HR is 51 beats per minute, temperature is 94°F rectally, and RR is 12 breaths per minute. On examination, the patient is overweight, her skin is dry, and you notice periorbital nonpitting edema. On neurologic examination, the patient does not respond to stimulation. Which of the following is the most likely diagnosis?

a. Apathetic thyrotoxicosis
b. Myxedema coma
c. Graves disease
d. Acute stroke
e. Schizophrenia

**482.** A 74-year-old woman who is a known diabetic is brought to the ED by emergency medical service (EMS) with altered mental status. The home health aide states that the patient ran out of her medications 4 days ago. Her BP is 130/85 mm Hg, HR is 110 beats per minute, temperature is 99.8°F, and RR is 18 breaths per minute. On examination, she cannot follow commands but responds to stimuli. Laboratory results reveal white blood cell (WBC) count of 14,000/L, hematocrit 49%, platelets 325/L, sodium 128 mEq/L, potassium 3.0 mEq/L, chloride 95 mEq/L, bicarbonate 22 mEq/L, blood urea nitrogen (BUN) 40 mg/dL, creatinine 1.8 mg/dL, and glucose 850 mg/dL. Urinalysis shows 3+ glucose, 1+ protein, and no blood or ketones. After addressing the ABCs, which of the following is the most appropriate next step in management?

a. Begin fluid resuscitation with a 2- to 3-L bolus of normal saline; then administer 10 units of regular insulin intravenously.
b. Begin fluid resuscitation with a 2- to 3-L bolus of normal saline; then administer 10 units of regular insulin intravenously and begin phenytoin for seizure prophylaxis.
c. Administer 10 units of regular insulin intravenously; then begin fluid resuscitation with a 2- to 3-L bolus of normal saline.
d. Order a computed tomographic (CT) scan of the brain; if negative for acute stroke, begin fluid resuscitation with a 2- to 3-L bolus of normal saline.
e. Arrange for urgent hemodialysis.

**483.** A 21-year-old man presents to the ED. He has a known history of type 1 diabetes. He is hypotensive with BP of 95/65 mm Hg, tachycardic at 120 beats per minute, and tachypneic at 30 breaths per minute. Laboratory results reveal a WBC 20,000/μL, hematocrit 45%, platelets 225/μL, sodium 131 mEq/L, potassium 5.3 mEq/L, chloride 95 mEq/L, bicarbonate 5 mEq/L, BUN 20 mg/dL, creatinine 0.9 mg/dL, and glucose 425 mg/dL. Arterial blood gas reveals a pH of 7.2. Urinalysis reveals glucosuria and ketosis. There is a fruity odor to his breath. Which of the following provides the strongest evidence for the diagnosis?

a. Hypotension, tachycardia, and tachypnea
b. Glucose of 425 mg/dL, ketosis, and leukocytosis
c. Glucose of 425 mg/dL, ketosis, pH 7.2, and bicarbonate of 5 mEq/L
d. Glucose of 425 mg/dL, hypotension, and fruity odor to breath
e. Glucosuria, hypotension, and leukocytosis

**484.** A 21-year-old man presents to the ED complaining of abdominal pain, nausea, and vomiting for 1 day and increased weakness for the last 2 to 3 days. He states that he is using the bathroom to urinate frequently and is drinking large amounts of water. He has no previous medical problems and is not taking any medications. His BP is 110/72 mm Hg, HR is 119 beats per minute, temperature is 98.8°F, and RR is 14 breaths per minute. On examination, he appears mildly confused, is pale, diaphoretic, and has unusually deep respirations and a fruity odor to his breath. Which of the following is the next best step?

a. Check fingerstick glucose.
b. Administer antiemetics.
c. Administer analgesics.
d. Send basic metabolic panel.

**485.** A 32-year-old man is brought to the ED by EMS for confusion. EMS reports that the patient was at a local pharmacy filing his prescriptions when the pharmacist noticed the patient sweating and having difficulty answering questions. In the ED, the patient's BP is 130/68 mm Hg, HR is 120 beats per minute, temperature is 98.9°F, and RR is 12 breaths per minute. The patient is unable to explain what happened. His fingerstick glucose is 410 mg/dL and his urine is positive for ketones. An electrolyte panel reveals Na$^+$ 131 mEq/L, K$^+$ 4 mEq/L, Cl$^-$ 91 mEq/L, and Ca$^{2+}$ 11 mEq/L. Which of the following electrolytes are most important to supplement during the management of his medical condition?

a. Sodium, potassium, and calcium
b. Sodium
c. Potassium
d. Calcium
e. Sodium and calcium

**486.** A 36-year-old immigrant woman is brought to the ED from her workplace. She was found to be agitated and behaving bizarrely. The patient's past medical history and medications are unknown. Her BP is 162/92 mm Hg, HR is 140 beats per minute, temperature is 101.8°F, and RR is 18 breaths per minute. On examination, the patient is delirious, tremulous, and has a large goiter. Which of the following is the most appropriate management of this patient?

a. Administer dantrolene.
b. Administer acetaminophen and broad-coverage antibiotics.
c. Protect airway; administer iodine.
d. Administer diazepam.
e. Protect airway; administer acetaminophen, propranolol, and PTU.

**487.** A 75-year-old woman is brought to the ED by EMS after she had a witnessed seizure on the street. A bystander reports that the patient fell to the ground, had tonic-clonic activity, and was drooling. Her BP is 162/85 mm Hg, HR is 95 beats per minute, temperature is 99.4°F, and RR is 16 breaths per minute. On examination, the patient is unresponsive and has a bleeding superficial scalp laceration. Which of the following electrolyte disturbances is *least likely* to cause a seizure?

a. Hypoglycemia
b. Hyperglycemia
c. Hyponatremia
d. Hypernatremia
e. Hypokalemia

**488.** A 53-year-old woman is brought to the ED by her husband. He states that his wife is feeling very weak over the last 2 days, is nauseated, and vomiting at least three times. The husband states that she was taking a high-dose medication for her joint pain but ran out of her pills last week. Her vital signs are BP of 90/50 mm Hg, HR 87 beats per minute, RR 16 breaths per minute, and temperature 98.1°F. You place her on the monitor, begin IV fluids, and send her blood to the laboratory. Thirty minutes later the metabolic panel results are back and reveal the following:

| | |
|---|---|
| $Na^+$ | 126 mEq/L |
| $K^+$ | 5 mEq/L |
| $Cl^-$ | 99 mEq/L |
| $HCO_3$ | 21 mEq/L |
| BUN | 24 mg/dL |
| Creatinine | 1.6 mg/dL |
| Glucose | 69 mg/dL |
| $Ca^+$ | 11 mEq/L |

What is the most likely diagnosis?

a. Myxedema coma
b. Thyroid storm
c. Hyperaldosteronism
d. Adrenal insufficiency
e. Diabetic ketoacidosis (DKA)

**489.** A 44-year-old agitated woman is brought to the ED by her husband. He states that she has had fevers to 101°F and a productive cough at home for the last 3 days. Today she became labile, agitated, and complained of abdominal pain. She was recently diagnosed with Graves disease and started on PTU. Her BP is 156/87 mm Hg, HR is 145 beats per minute, temperature is 102.4°F, and RR is 20 breaths per minute. On examination, the patient is agitated, confused, and has rales on auscultation bilaterally. Which of the following is the most likely diagnosis?

a. Pheochromocytoma
b. Cocaine ingestion
c. Heat stroke
d. Thyroid storm
e. Neuroleptic malignant syndrome

# Endocrine Emergencies

## Answers

**479. The answer is d.** *(Rosen, pp 1639-1644.)* The mainstay of treatment for **DKA** is **aggressive fluid resuscitation** and **insulin** therapy. The patient should receive 2 L of normal saline within 2 hours of presentation followed by 4 to 6 L over the next 8 to 12 hours depending on the patient's fluid status. In DKA, the average adult has a water deficit of 5 to 10 L. After the first 2 L of fluid, regular insulin is administered, usually first as a 10-U bolus intravenously and then at a rate of 0.1 U/kg/h. Insulin must be administered for ketosis and acidosis to resolve.

(a) Intramuscular and subcutaneous insulin administration is avoided in DKA as absorption may be erratic secondary to volume depletion and poor perfusion. (b) Currently, no study shows a benefit of using bicarbonate in DKA. Bicarbonate administration can cause worsening hypokalemia, paradoxical central nervous system (CNS) acidosis, impaired oxyhemoglobin dissociation, hypertonicity, and sodium over load. (c) Metoprolol, a β-blocker, is not indicated in DKA. The tachycardia in DKA is secondary to volume depletion and acidosis. Correcting the underlying cause will treat the tachycardia. (e) Potassium replacement may be necessary later in therapy because of an overall loss of potassium, but should not be included in the initial fluid boluses. Rapid administration of potassium has potential to precipitate fatal dysrhythmias.

**480. The answer is d.** *(Rosen, pp 1660-1666.)* **Thyroid storm** is a **medical emergency** that will lead to death if not treated in time. The manifestations of thyroid storm include temperature greater than 100°F, tachycardia out of proportion to fever, widened pulse pressure, and dysfunction of the CNS (eg, confusion, agitation), cardiovascular system (eg, high-output congestive heart failure, atrial fibrillation), or gastrointestinal (GI) system (eg, diarrhea, abdominal pain). Thyroid storm is a **clinical diagnosis** because no confirmatory tests are immediately available. The most important factor in reducing mortality is blocking peripheral adrenergic hyperactivity with **propranolol**, a β-blocker. **PTU** is used to inhibit new hormone synthesis in the thyroid and has a small effect on inhibiting peripheral conversion of

$T_4$ to $T_3$. **Iodine** is administered to block hormone release from the thyroid but should be given 1 hour after PTU to prevent organification of the iodine.

**(a)** Tricyclic antidepressant overdose can present with altered mental status and tachycardia. Bicarbonate is administered for a widened QRS on ECG. **(b)** Chlordiazepoxide is given to patients to prevent alcohol withdrawal, which can also present with confusion and tachycardia. **(c)** Ceftriaxone is commonly used to treat meningitis, which can present with confusion, tachycardia, and fever. **(e)** The patient's diarrhea is not caused by an infectious etiology and therefore ciprofloxacin is not required. She may require fluid resuscitation, but for now her BP is stable.

**481. The answer is b.** *(Rosen, pp 1668-1671.)* **Myxedema coma** is a syndrome that represents **extreme hypothyroidism**. It is a life-threatening condition that has a mortality of up to 50%. Signs and symptoms of hypothyroidism are usually present including dry skin, delayed deep tendon reflexes, coarse hair, and generalized nonpitting edema. Myxedema coma, however, is better characterized by profound **lethargy or coma** and **hypothermia**. Hypothermia is present in approximately 80% of patients. In addition, patients may present with respiratory depression and sinus bradycardia.

**(a)** Apathetic thyrotoxicosis is an atypical presentation of hyperthyroidism seen commonly in the elderly but noted in all ages. Signs and symptoms are few and subtle. Patients usually have multinodular goiter. The diagnosis should be considered in elderly patients with chronic weight loss, proximal muscle weakness, depressed affect, new-onset atrial fibrillation, or congestive heart failure. **(c)** Graves disease is secondary to autoimmune stimulation of thyrotropin (TSH) receptors leading to elevated levels of thyroid hormones. **(d)** An acute stroke should not cause periorbital edema and hypothermia. **(e)** Schizophrenia may be mistakenly diagnosed in patients with thyroid abnormalities. It is not a correct diagnosis in this scenario when the patient is unconscious and hypothermic.

**482. The answer is a.** *(Rosen, pp 1644-1646.)* **Hyperglycemic hyperosmolar nonketotic coma (HHNC)** is a syndrome representing marked **hyperglycemia** (serum glucose > 600 mg/dL), **hyperosmolarity** (plasma osmolarity > 350 mOsm/L), considerable **dehydration** (9 L in 70-kg patient), and **decreased mental functioning** that may progress to coma. HHNC may be the initial presentation of previously unrecognized diabetes in an adult with **type 2 diabetes mellitus**. Elderly diabetics are at greater risk for this illness. Osmotic diuresis is even more pronounced than in DKA. Rapid correction of hyperosmolar state may lead to cerebral edema. Unlike DKA, acidosis and ketosis are usually absent or minimal. The mainstay to treatment is fluid resuscitation, insulin administration, electrolyte repletion, and searching for an underlying precipitant.

**(b)** Phenytoin is contraindicated for seizures in HHNC because it is often ineffective and may impair endogenous insulin release. **(c)** Fluid resuscitation is the mainstay of treatment and should always be administered before insulin. **(d)** Although the patient may ultimately receive a CT scan, fluid resuscitation is priority because of the profound dehydration in these patients. **(e)** If a patient has functioning kidneys, hemodialysis is not necessary. However, if the patient has end-stage renal disease, hemodialysis may be necessary to treat over hydration.

**483. The answer is c.** *(Rosen, pp 1639-1644.)* The triad of **hyperglycemia**, **ketosis**, and **acidosis** is diagnostic for **DKA**. All abnormalities in DKA are connected and are based on insulin deficiency. When hyperglycemia surpasses the renal threshold for resorption, glucose is excreted in the urine. This causes an osmotic diuresis that in combination with decreased oral intake and vomiting leads to dehydration and electrolyte abnormalities. Cells, unable to receive glucose from the circulation, switch to starvation mode by increasing proteolysis. The liver starts producing ketoacid subsequently causing acidemia. The acidotic patient increases RR, in an attempt to blow off excess carbon dioxide, and bicarbonate is used up in the process.

**(a)** Hypotension, tachycardia, and tachypnea are commonly seen in DKA but are not specific for the condition. **(b)** Leukocytosis is seen in many other conditions other than DKA. **(d)** Although a fruity odor to breath may suggest acetone, a product of ketone production, it is not reliably present and difficult to distinguish. **(e)** Glucosuria is present with hyperglycemia. Ketones are required for DKA.

**484. The answer is a.** *(Tintinalli, p 1434.)* You should be suspicious for **DKA** as the initial presentation of diabetes mellitus in this patient. Glucose levels are elevated, typically greater than 200 mg/dL. DKA is an acute, life-threatening disorder occurring in patients with **insulin insufficiency** (more common in type 1 diabetes) and results in **hyperglycemia**, **ketosis**, and **acidosis** from osmotic diuresis leading to dehydration and acidosis. This patient exhibits classic signs and symptoms of DKA, such as tachycardia, GI distress, polyuria, polydipsia, fatigue, and confusion. Very deep breathing **(Kussmaul respirations)** reflects respiratory compensation for metabolic acidosis. **Fruity breath odor** in this patient is the result of acetoacetate acid conversion to acetone, which is eliminated during respiration.

Administering antiemetics and analgesics **(b and c)** will temporarily treat the symptoms without addressing the underlying problem. A basic metabolic panel **(d)** is necessary to check for electrolyte abnormalities. Abdominal radiographs **(e)** might be appropriate if you suspect abdominal pathology. In this case, GI distress is a symptom of a metabolic disturbance.

**485. The answer is c.** *(Tintinalli, pp 1435-1437.)* **Potassium** is the most important electrolyte to follow in DKA therapy. Renal losses and vomiting in DKA cause profound **total body potassium deficit**. The measured potassium levels, however, are often **falsely normal or elevated** because of acidosis and total body fluid deficit. Acidemia causes extracellular shift of potassium in exchange for hydrogen ions. With initiation of DKA therapy, potassium levels will quickly fall to true levels causing **significant hypokalemia**, if not closely monitored and replaced.

Although sodium and calcium levels **(a, b, d, and e)** should be monitored, they are not affected as much as potassium. Hyperglycemia-related osmotic diuresis leads to renal losses of sodium chloride in urine. The measured sodium level is artificially lowered further by the hyperglycemia. For every 100 mg of glucose over 100 mg/dL, 1.6 mEq should be added to the measured serum sodium level. In treating DKA, normal saline infusion replaces lost sodium. Hypertonic saline should not be used for sodium replacement in DKA. Osmotic diuresis also causes renal losses of calcium, magnesium, and phosphorus. Initially their levels might be elevated owing to hemoconcentration. These electrolytes should be monitored and restored appropriately during treatment.

**486. The answer is e.** *(Tintinalli, pp 1448-1451.)* This patient presents in a **hyperadrenergic state**, **altered mental status**, **and a large goiter**, placing the diagnosis of **thyroid storm** on top of the differential. The patient is likely to have undiagnosed hyperthyroidism. This is a clinical diagnosis and has to be treated empirically and rapidly since mortality is high despite treatment. The management of thyroid storm involves supportive care (airway protection, oxygenation, IV hydration) and specific therapy to treat adrenergic symptoms and to decrease synthesis and release of thyroid hormone. β-**Adrenergic blockers** are given to reverse adrenergic hyperactivity. **PTU** blocks de novo synthesis of thyroid hormone. **Iodine** blocks release of the preformed hormone but can be given only after PTU has taken effect; otherwise it will promote further hormone production.

Dantrolene (**a**) is used in the management of malignant hyperthermia and neuroleptic malignant syndrome. Administering acetaminophen and broad-coverage antibiotics (**b**) or diazepam (**d**) will not address the underlying etiology of the patient's illness. Iodine (**c**) should not be administered before PTU.

**487. The answer is e.** *(Tintinalli, pp 118, 121-122, 877, 1441.)* **Hypokalemia** presents with **muscle weakness** and characteristic **ECG changes**, such as flat T waves and U waves, and is not associated with seizures or altered mental status.

Glucose level can be rapidly obtained from a fingerstick glucose check. Hypoglycemia (**a**) is a known reversible cause of seizures and is corrected with administration of dextrose. Significant hyperglycemia (**b**) occurs in DKA (glucose usually is 200-800 mg/dL) or nonketotic hyperosmolar crisis (glucose usually is > 800 mg/dL) and is treated with IV fluids and insulin. Hyper- and hyponatremia (**c and d**) are known causes of seizures.

**488. The answer is d.** *(Rosen, pp 1671-1675.)* **Adrenal cortical insufficiency** is an uncommon, potentially life-threatening condition that, if recognized early, is readily treatable. The most common cause of adrenal insufficiency is hypothalamic-pituitary-adrenal axis suppression from **long-term exogenous glucocorticoid administration**. This patient abruptly stopped her high-dose steroids. The clinical presentation of adrenal insufficiency is vague but typically includes weakness, fatigue, nausea, vomiting, **hypotension**, and **hypoglycemia**. Electrolyte abnormalities are common. **Hyponatremia** and **hyperkalemia** are present in more than two-thirds of cases. Management includes supportive care with administration of glucocorticoids and electrolyte correction.

(**a and b**) Myxedema coma is a syndrome of extreme hypothyroidism, whereas thyroid storm is extreme hyperthyroidism. (**c**) Hyperaldosteronism is characterized by hypertension and hypokalemia. (**e**) DKA typically presents with elevated glucose, an anion-gap metabolic acidosis, and ketone production.

**489. The answer is d.** *(Tintinalli, pp 1417-1451.)* This patient presents with a rare but life-threatening hypermetabolic state of **thyroid storm**. It occurs in patients with known or undiagnosed hyperthyroidism and is usually triggered by infection, trauma, myocardial infarction, stroke, or noncompliance with antihyperthyroid medications. Thyroid storm is a clinical diagnosis. The signs and symptoms of this disorder reflect an overactive sympathetic system and include fever, tachycardia out of the proportion to the fever, GI symptoms, and altered mental status. Patients may also develop high-output heart failure. The clue to the diagnosis in this case is the patient's known hyperthyroidism.

Pheochromocytoma **(a)** presents with a similar hyperadrenergic state caused by a catecholamine-secreting tumor but does not result in altered mentation. The hallmark of this disease is hypertension associated with headache, palpitations, and diaphoresis. Cocaine **(b)** acts as a CNS stimulant by blocking reuptake of excitatory neurotransmitters norepinephrine, dopamine, and serotonin. It is, however, less likely than thyroid storm in this patient given her underlying hyperthyroidism and pulmonary infection. Heat stroke **(c)** should be suspected in patients with core body temperature of greater than 104°F (> 40°C) and altered mental status. Neuroleptic malignant syndrome **(e)** is a rare life-threatening reaction to a medication with dopamine receptor antagonism. Such medications include neuroleptics, such as haloperidol, clozapine, and risperidone; lithium; and many antiemetics, such as prochlorperazine, promethazine, and metoclopramide. The syndrome presents as fever, altered mental status, and muscular rigidity.

# Psychosocial Disorders

## Questions

**490.** A 31-year-old woman presents to the emergency department (ED) 20 minutes after the sudden onset of chest pain; palpitations; shortness of breath; and numbness of her mouth, fingers, and toes. She tells you that it feels like she has a lump in her throat. Her medical history includes multiple visits to the ED over a period of 6 months with a similar presentation. Her only medication is an oral contraceptive. She occasionally drinks a glass of wine after a busy day of work when she feels stressed. She tells you that her mom takes medication for anxiety. Her blood pressure (BP) is 125/75 mm Hg, heart rate (HR) 88 beats per minute, and oxygen saturation 99% on room air. An electrocardiogram (ECG) shows a sinus rhythm. Her symptoms resolve while in the ED. Which of the following is the most likely diagnosis?

a. Paroxysmal atrial tachycardia
b. Hyperthyroidism
c. Major depressive disorder
d. Panic disorder
e. Posttraumatic stress disorder

**491.** A 23-year-old woman is brought to the ED for vision loss in her left eye that began shortly after waking up in the morning. She states that she is very depressed since her father was diagnosed with terminal cancer. She was supposed to visit her father today in the hospital but is now in your ED because of her vision loss. Your physical examination is unremarkable. An evaluation by the ophthalmologist is also normal. A head computed tomographic (CT) scan is normal. Which of the following is the most likely diagnosis?

a. Somatization disorder
b. Conversion disorder
c. Hypochondriasis
d. Retinal detachment
e. Anxiety disorder

**492.** Which of the following clinical presentation requires hospitalization?

a. A 37-year-old man with paranoid schizophrenia who has been off his medications for a week and is hearing voices with no apparent violence in his thought content.

b. A 19-year-old woman who ingested 10 multivitamin pills after an argument with her boyfriend.

c. A 39-year-old man with no previous psychiatric history presents with pressured speech, no sleep for 4 days, and is feeling "great."

d. A 22-year-old woman who is having visual hallucinations after ingesting D-lysergic acid diethylamide (LSD).

e. A 43-year-old homeless man with a history of schizophrenia who was recently discharged from the psychiatric ward being managed on antipsychotic medications.

**493.** A 35-year-old woman is eating dinner at a restaurant. Approximately 1 hour after finishing the main course of lamb, red wine, and a fine selection of cheese, the patient experiences a severe occipital headache, diaphoresis, mydriasis, neck stiffness, and palpitations. Which of the following medications is this patient most likely taking?

a. Paroxetine
b. Alprazolam
c. Tranylcypromine
d. Citalopram
e. Amitriptyline

**494.** You walk into the examining room to interview a patient. He refused giving vital signs at the triage station until he saw a doctor because he was afraid that the nurse would inject poison into him. He appears agitated and starts raising his voice as soon as you are in the room. You ask him in a calm voice if you could help him and he replies by shouting obscenities and throwing a box of gloves at you. You start to walk toward him, but he says he will kill you if you get any closer. Which of the following is the most appropriate next step in management?

a. Tell the patient he is being uncooperative and is to leave the ED immediately.

b. Have the nurse go into the room alone to try to calm the patient.

c. Let the patient sit in the room for another hour and see if he calms down.

d. Ask the nurse to prepare an injection of lorazepam that you will give to sedate the patient.

e. Alert hospital security that there is a violent patient and prepare to place the patient in physical restraints.

**495.** A 42-year-old man with a history of schizophrenia is brought into the ED by a friend who states that the patient has not taken his medication for over 2 weeks and is now behaving bizarrely. His BP is 130/70 mm Hg, HR 89 beats per minute, respiratory rate (RR) 15 breaths per minute, and oxygen saturation 99% on room air. On examination he appears agitated and is shouting, "the aliens are about to get me." He is cooperative enough that you decide to use pharmacologic sedation. Which of the following is the most appropriate choice for sedating this patient?

a. Haloperidol and lorazepam
b. Etomidate and succinylcholine
c. Chlorpromazine and lorazepam
d. Ketamine and lorazepam
e. Clozapine

**496.** A 48-year-old man is brought to the ED by family members who state that the patient has remained home-bound for weeks, sleeping for many hours, and appears disheveled. The patient states that he is "fine" and denies any medical symptoms. Initial vitals include HR of 77 beats per minute, BP of 118/55 mm Hg, and RR of 12 breaths per minute with oxygen saturation of 97% on room air. The patient is afebrile with an unremarkable physical examination. He denies any chest discomfort, difficulty breathing, constipation, cold intolerance, weakness, weight changes, or pain. The patient reports that he has had difficulty concentrating, a decreased appetite, and excessive sleeping patterns. The family reports that this has happened before, but that his symptoms self-resolved and were not nearly as severe. Given this patient's presentation, which of the following is the most likely etiology of this patient's symptoms?

a. Hypothyroidism
b. Major depressive episode
c. Diabetes mellitus
d. Subdural hematoma
e. Cushing syndrome

**497.** A 32-year-old woman presents to the ED after an aggressive outburst at work where her behavior was deemed a threat to others. Her coworkers state that she is normally very dependable, kind, and gracious, but that over the course of the week they noticed that she was especially reserved and at times found her conversing with herself. Her initial vitals include HR of 89 beats per minute, RR of 15 breaths per minute, and BP of 130/75 mm Hg with oxygen saturation of 99% on room air. She tells you that she was recently started on a new medication. Which of the following types of medications may be responsible for this patient's behavior?

a. β-Blockers
b. Oral contraceptives
c. Corticosteroids
d. Nonsteroidal anti-inflammatory drugs (NSAIDs)
e. Calcium channel blockers

**498.** A 23-year-old woman is brought to the ED by police officials who state that they found the patient in the middle of a busy intersection screaming. Upon arrival, you see a disheveled woman who is yelling, "You can't get away with this! I'm the Queen of England!" She does not allow for the triage nurse to obtain her vitals, but you can see a young woman who is of normal habitus without any signs of trauma. Her speech is pressured, she is easily distracted by the commotion of the ED, and begins to answer your questions but then continues to describe grandiose ideas about her social status. Given this patient's acute presentation, what is the most likely etiology of her symptoms?

a. Hypothyroid disorder
b. Manic episode
c. Benzodiazepine overdose
d. Anticonvulsant overdose
e. Barbiturate overdose

**499.** A mother brings her 7-year-old daughter to the ED with a reported illness of 3 days where the child has been weak and not eating her usual amount. The mother also reports that she noticed her daughter's urine to be of a reddish color and that her stools have been smaller in caliber. She brings a specimen of her daughter's urine with her. She reports that her daughter has been hospitalized multiple times before for similar reasons and dehydration. Upon physical examination, the patient is without distress, quiet, and states that she feels tired. Her chest is clear to auscultation, her abdomen is benign and her neurologic examination nonfocal. A urinalysis performed fails to show any blood or myoglobin in the child's urine. Which of the following should be included in the differential diagnosis of this child?

a. Malingering
b. Factitious disorder
c. Munchausen syndrome
d. Munchausen syndrome by proxy
e. Conversion disorder

**500.** A 62-year-old man presents to the ED after he was found talking to himself by witnesses on a nearby street. Upon arrival, the patient appears confused and is actively hallucinating. His initial vitals include an irregular HR of 80 to 110 beats per minute, an RR of 14 breaths per minute, and a BP of 160/80 mm Hg with an oxygen saturation of 97% on room air. An ECG indicates atrial fibrillation. The patient can be redirected but states that he is distracted by colorful, floating images in the room. Given this patient's presentation, what is the most likely etiology of his symptoms?

a. Acute psychotic disorder
b. Malingering
c. Conversion disorder
d. Digoxin overdose
e. Antidepressant overdose

**501.** An 18-year-old man presents to the ED after telling a school counselor that he wanted to harm himself. His physical examination is unremarkable without any signs of trauma. He reports occasional excessive alcohol use. He states that his parents recently separated and that he has been living with either parent on a rotating schedule. Overall, he feels supported by family and friends but continues to feel hopeless despite this. Which of the following factors in this patient is most likely to increase his risk of an actual suicidal attempt?

a. Sex
b. Age
c. Hopelessness
d. Alcohol use
e. Parent separation

**502.** A thin 16-year-old girl is brought in the ED after collapsing at home. Her initial vitals include an HR of 110 beats per minute, BP of 80/55 mm Hg, and an RR of 18 breaths per minute with an oxygen saturation of 98% on room air. Upon physical examination, you note a cachectic female in mild distress. Her chest is clear to auscultation; her sunken-in abdomen is soft and nontender. Upon inspecting her extremities, you notice small areas of erythema over the dorsum of her right hand distally. Given this patient's presentation and physical examination, which of the following etiologies must be further explored in this patient?

a. Bulimia
b. Gastroenteritis
c. Malingering
d. Factitious disorder
e. Suicidality

**503.** A 55-year-old woman presents to the ED after a reported syncopal event. Her initial vitals include an HR of 105 beats per minute, an RR of 16 breaths per minute, a BP of 125/60 mm Hg, and an oxygen saturation of 98% on room air. Her ECG is shown below. Which of the following substances is responsible for this patient's ECG findings?

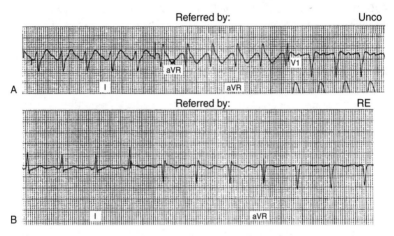

*(Reproduced, with permission, from Tintinalli J, Kelen G, Stapczynski J.* Emergency Medicine: A Comprehensive Study Guide. *New York, NY: McGraw-Hill, 2004: 1031.)*

a. Benzodiazepine
b. Alcohol
c. Tricyclic antidepressant (TCA)
d. Insulin
e. Valproic acid

**504.** A 28-year-old presents to the ED with depressive symptoms and feelings of hopelessness. She denies any active suicidal ideation but has had increasing feelings of guilt over the last few weeks. The patient denies any past medical history except for giving birth 8 weeks ago. Her initial vitals are within normal limits. Given this patient's presentation, which of the following etiologies is most likely?

a. Dysthymic disorder
b. Bipolar disorder
c. Postpartum depression
d. Major depressive disorder
e. Cyclothymic disorder

# Psychosocial Disorders

## *Answers*

**490. The answer is d.** (*Tintinalli, pp 1962-1963.*) A person with **panic attacks** will often present to multiple EDs and be discharged after a workup is normal. A panic attack is a discrete period of intense fear or discomfort in which four or more of the following symptoms develop acutely and peak within 10 minutes: accelerated HR, palpitations, pounding heart, diaphoresis, trembling or shaking, sensation of shortness of breath or a choking feeling, chest pain, nausea, dizziness, lightheadedness, paresthesias, fear of dying, chills, or hot flushes.

(**a**) Paroxysmal atrial tachycardia is a conduction defect of the heart characterized by random episodes of tachycardia. This disorder is seen on an ECG. This patient's ECG is normal. (**b**) Hyperthyroidism can mimic a panic attack, but there is usually greater autonomic hyperactivity. In addition, thyroid hormone levels are increased. (**c**) There are no symptoms of depression described in the patient's presentation. Nonetheless, panic attacks can occur with major depressive disorder. (**e**) The diagnosis of posttraumatic stress disorder cannot be made with the patient's history.

**491. The answer is b.** (*Tintinalli, pp 1965-1967.*) The diagnosis of **conversion disorder** is made by fulfilling the following five criteria:

- A symptom is expressed as a change or loss of physical function.
- Recent psychologic stressor or conflict.
- The patient unconsciously produces the symptom.
- The symptom cannot be explained by any known organic etiology.
- The symptom is not limited to pain or sexual dysfunction.

Conversion disorders generally involve neurologic or orthopedic manifestations. The disorder usually presents as a **single symptom** with a **sudden onset** related to a **severe stress**. In this case, the stress is the diagnosis of terminal cancer in the patient's father. Classic symptoms of conversion disorder include paralysis, aphonia, seizures, coordination disturbances, blindness, tunnel vision, and numbness. The diagnosis cannot be made until all possible organic etiologies are ruled out. Treatment involves identifying the stressor and addressing the issue.

(a) Somatization disorder involves patients with many complaints with no organic cause. (c) Hypochondriasis involves the preoccupation of serious illness despite appropriate medical evaluation and reassurance. (d) Retinal detachment can cause unilateral vision loss and generally presents with progressively worsening vision loss with patients complaining of "floaters." (e) Anxiety disorders involve excessive fear and apprehension that dominates the psychologic life of a person.

**492. The answer is c.** *(Tintinalli, pp 1949-1951.)* This patient presents with a first manic episode. It is necessary to admit these patients in order to prevent behavior that is impulsive and dangerous. A full manic syndrome is one of the most striking and distinctive conditions in clinical practice. The main disturbance in mood is one of elation or irritability.

(a) This man is not a threat to him or others and can be treated as an outpatient. (b) This is a suicidal gesture and the patient should be evaluated by a psychiatrist. She may be able to be managed as an outpatient if reliable family and social support systems are in place and appropriate psychiatric follow-up is arranged. (d) This patient can be safely discharged once her visual hallucinations resolve. (e) This man is appropriately treated.

**493. The answer is c.** *(Tintinalli, pp 1203-1205, 1956-1957.)* **Tranylcypromine** is a **monoamine oxidase inhibitor (MAOI)** that is used in the treatment of depression. Patients who take this medication should avoid eating or drinking foods that contain **tyramine** (similar structure to amphetamine). Tyramine is found in many foods such as aged cheese, wine, certain fish, meats, and sauerkraut. The combination of a MAOI and tyramine can lead to a **sympathomimetic reaction** called a **tyramine reaction**. It occurs within 15 to 90 minutes of ingestion of tyramine. The hallmark symptoms include headache, hypertension, diaphoresis, mydriasis, neck stiffness, pallor, neuromuscular excitation, palpitations, and chest pain. Most symptoms gradually resolve over 6 hours; however, deaths have been reported secondary to intracranial hemorrhage and myocardial infarction. Patients who take a MAOI should be instructed to avoid all tyramine-containing foods.

All of the other answer choices do not cause a tyramine reaction—it is limited only to MAOIs. (a and d) These are serotonin reuptake inhibitors, (b) is a benzodiazepine, (e) is a TCA.

**494. The answer is e.** *(Tintinalli, pp 1939-1940.)* **Violent behavior requires immediate restraint.** Hospital security and the police are best trained to subdue violent patients with the least chance of staff or patient injury. Patients who are threatening or who demonstrate violent behavior should be disrobed, gowned, and searched for weapons. Patients whose behavior suggests the potential for violence should be approached cautiously with adequate security force nearby. The physician should stand in a location that neither threatens the patient nor blocks the exit of the patient or the physician from the room. Physical restraints are frequently required for the violent or severely agitated psychotic, delirious, or intoxicated patient who is a danger to themselves or others. Pharmacologic restraints (haloperidol, lorazepam) are also useful in obtaining behavior control and should be considered once the initial evaluation has been completed.

(a) The patient should not be allowed to leave the hospital before a medical and psychiatric evaluation. (b) No staff member should be alone with a patient who is violent or threatens violence. (c) Although using calming techniques are useful to assuage many patients, it is important not to delay the medical evaluation and prolong detection of a life-threatening process. (d) Giving the patient a sedating medication is useful; however, you should try to first medically evaluate the patient. In addition, you should not enter the patient's room alone with a needle in your hand.

**495. The answer is a.** *(Tintinalli, pp 1952-1953.)* Rapid tranquilization is a method of pharmacologic management of acute agitation or psychosis using high-potency neuroleptics and benzodiazepines. The most common regimen used is the combination of **haloperidol** and **lorazepam**, which can be administered via parenteral, intramuscular, or oral routes. There is a synergistic effect between the two medications. Moreover, the benzodiazepine may prevent the potential extrapyramidal affects that occasionally occur with neuroleptic use.

(b) Etomidate and succinylcholine are used for rapid sequence intubation, which is not indicated in this patient. (c) Chlorpromazine is a low-potency antipsychotic that may cause significant hypotension and is rarely used in the ED setting. (d) Ketamine is a dissociative agent that is not typically used in psychotic patients. (e) Clozapine is an atypical antipsychotic that is used in schizophrenics when other neuroleptics are ineffective. It is not an agent of choice for acute sedation or psychosis.

**496. The answer is b.** *(Rosen, pp 1438-1441.)* A **major depressive episode** is characterized by two or more of the following symptoms over a

2-week period: loss of interest in usual activities, depressed or irritable mood, changes in weight or appetite, insomnia or hypersomnia, psychomotor agitation or retardation, loss of energy, difficulty concentrating, recurrent thoughts of death, and suicidal ideation. This particular patient has three of these symptoms, including excessive sleeping patterns, difficulty concentrating, and a decreased appetite. The danger is that the patient's feelings may be so intensely painful that suicide may be seen as the only way to cope. Some patients may also complain of generalized physical pain, without any clear medical diagnosis able to be made. The cardinal symptom of depression is a **sad or dysphoric mood**.

Hypothyroidism (a) and Cushing syndrome (e) may also be exhibited in patients who appear to be depressed. A simple thyroid-stimulating hormone and cortisol level may be drawn to differentiate a medical etiology for these symptoms. Hyperthyroidism also presents as generalized sluggishness, difficulty concentrating, constipation, cold intolerance, hair loss of the distal one-third of both eyebrows, dysphagia, and myalgias. Fingerstick glucose should also be performed to evaluate for diabetes mellitus (c), which may present as sluggishness, paresthesias, and general malaise. It is also important to keep in mind traumatic causes to this patient's symptoms, given that he lives alone without witnesses to report a fall that may result in a subdural hematoma (d). Intracerebral bleeding may present with sluggishness, especially in subdurals where there is a relatively slower bleed of the bridging veins.

**497. The answer is c.** *(Rosen, pp 1431-1432.)* **Steroid psychosis** is described as a constellation of psychiatric symptoms within the first 5 days of treatment with a corticosteroid. Studies indicate that the amount needed to produce this effect is greater than 40 mg of prednisone, or its equivalent, prescribed daily. Symptoms include emotional lability, anxiety, distractibility, pressured speech, sensory flooding, insomnia, depression, agitation, auditory and visual hallucinations, intermittent memory impairment, mutism, disturbances of body image, and delusions and hypomania. It is important to note that previous history of psychologic difficulties does not predict the development of steroid psychosis. Symptoms can be very severe and should be taken into account when prescribing this medication to patients. Three percent of patients with steroid psychosis commit suicide.

The most common side effect of β-blockers (a) is a depressed mood, owing to its sympatholytic effects; however, these are generally mild and do not require treatment. Oral contraceptives (b), although hormonal in nature, are not thought to produce psychiatric symptoms. Calcium channel blockers (e) and NSAIDs (d) have not been shown to cause psychosis.

**498. The answer is b.** (*Rosen, pp 1440-1444.*) This is a typical **manic episode** whose cardinal features are an elevated mood, grandiosity, flight of ideas, distractibility, and psychomotor agitation. Other medical conditions, such as hyperthyroidism, antidepressant, or stimulant abuse, may cause similar symptoms and must be ruled out with laboratory testing. Certain frontal lobe release syndromes that impair executive functioning must also be investigated as a cause of this patient's symptoms. These patients are usually combative, display impaired judgment and impulsivity, and may need to be chemically or physically restrained.

Hypothyroid disorder (a), benzodiazepines (c), anticonvulsants (d), and barbiturates (e) may all cause depressive symptoms.

**499. The answer is d.** (*Rosen, pp 1458-1461.*) Given that this is an apparent illness or health-related abnormality produced by a parent or caregiver upon another, the **by-proxy** title is given. This is a psychiatric illness defined by the *Diagnostic and Statistical Manual of Mental Disorders* (Fourth Edition) (DSM-IV) as an apparent illness concocted by a caregiver upon a child who presents for medical aid multiple times without ever being given a true diagnosis. There is a failure by the perpetrator to acknowledge the true etiology and a cessation of symptoms in the child once they are separated from the perpetrator. Simulated illness, without producing direct harm upon the child, is commonly seen. As seen in this example, placing tincture in the child's urine to mimic blood. Sadly, produced illness in which the child is harmed is most commonly seen (50% of cases). The most common presentations include bleeding, seizures, vomiting, diarrhea, fever, and rash. Ninety-eight percent of perpetrators are biologic mothers from all socioeconomic backgrounds. Many have a background in health professions or have features of **Munchausen syndrome** in themselves. Most of these mothers have had an abusive experience early in life and use the health care system as a means to satisfy personal nurturing demands. They are said to gain a sense of purpose and meaning when their child is in the hospital, as well as an outlet for pity and comfort. These children may display incidental characteristics that cannot be linked to the presenting complaints. These children may also suffer from learning difficulties or clinical depression caused by many hospitalizations that are incurred upon them.

Malingering (**a**) is frequently found in connection with antisocial personality disorder. These patients are often vague about prior hospitalizations or treatments. In contrast to those with a factitious disorder (**b**), these patients prefer to counterfeit mental illness given the difficulty in objectively verifying or disproving the etiology of the patient's reported symptoms. Amnesia, paranoia, depression, and suicidal ideation are commonly seen. The idea of an external gain motivates these individuals to fabricate medical symptoms. Conversely, factitious disorders are characterized by symptoms or signs that are intentionally produced or feigned by the patient in the absence of external incentives. Munchausen syndrome (**c**) is one of the most dramatic of the factitious disorders. Its name is derived from a Baron Karl F. von Munchausen who amused his friends with fantastic and incredible tales about his personal life. Conversion disorder (**e**) is a rare disorder that is characterized by the abrupt, dramatic onset of a single symptom. It typically presents as some nonpainful neurologic disorder for which there are no objective data.

**500. The answer is d.** (*Rosen, pp 1431, 1978-1980.*) This patient is experiencing a **visual hallucination**, most typical of a medical rather than psychiatric etiology. **Digoxin** is a common precipitant of these symptoms and may begin with yellow-blue changes in vision, known as van Gogh vision. Digoxin directly binds the Na-K ATPase that increases sodium and calcium levels, increasing the contractility of the heart. Hallucinations are often an early symptom of digoxin overdose. Treatment for this includes a protein fragment that binds this medication.

(**a**) Auditory hallucinations are usually seen in psychiatric illness or an acute psychotic episode. Antidepressants (**e**) typically do not produce changes in vision or hallucinations. His symptoms are also not typical of malingering (**b**), given that he was not brought in of his own accord without secondary gain, or of conversion disorder (**c**).

**501. The answer is c.** (*Rosen, pp 1463-1471.*) In the psychiatric literature, there exists a "SADPERSONS" scale that enumerates risk factors. Two points are given for factors that are considered higher risk. These include depression or **hopelessness**, rational thinking loss, organized or serious attempt, and stated future intent. Lower-risk factors, given one point, are male sex, age younger than 19 years or older than 45 years, previous attempts or psychiatric care, excessive alcohol or drug use, separation, divorce or widowed status, and no social supports. Firearms in the household, family violence, abuse, and chronic illness also increase risk.

| | |
|---|---|
| Sex (male) | 1 |
| Age (< 19 or > 45 years) | 1 |
| Depression or hopelessness | 2 |
| Previous attempts/psychiatric care | 1 |
| Excessive alcohol or drug use | 1 |
| Rational thinking loss | 2 |
| Separated, divorced, or widowed | 1 |
| Organized or serious attempt | 2 |
| No social support | 1 |
| Stated future attempt | 2 |

**502. The answer is a.** (*Rosen, pp 1959-1962.*) The physical examination in this patient reveals hand abrasions, indicative of self-purging. Her general appearance suggests either inadequate food intake or excessive calorie burning. **Bulimics** generally consume an adequate amount of food, albeit low calorie, but purge their intake with the goal of weight loss. Other eating disorders, such as anorexia nervosa, can take the form of starvation, diuretic or laxative use, or excessive exercise. These patients generally suffer from a false visualization of their body, believing that their physical form weighs more than what it does in reality. Social pressures, history of abuse or violence, and other eating disorders may factor in to this patient's presentation.

Gastroenteritis (**b**) is unlikely given the lack of history or symptoms. Suicidality (**e**) should be examined in all patients, as their actions may represent a form of occult or hidden self-harm. This patient does not exhibit signs of malingering (**c**) or factitious disorder (**d**).

**503. The answer is c.** (*Rosen, pp 1964-1969.*) **TCAs** are responsible for more drug-related deaths than any other prescription medication. This ECG shows QRS interval prolongation, a common finding with this medication. The mechanism of toxicity is multifold and includes blocking the reuptake of dopamine, serotonin, and norepinephrine. It also binds to the γ-aminobutyric acid (GABA) receptor, thereby lowering seizure threshold. Sodium channel blockade produces the widened QRS interval. There are also anticholinergic and antihistamine effects. Sodium bicarbonate is a first-line intervention for dysrhythmias, acting as alkalizing binder for the acidic TCA. This treatment has been shown to improve conduction and contractility with the goal of preserving a narrow QRS.

Benzodiazepines (a), alcohol (b), ethanol  (d), and valproic acid (e) have not been shown to exhibit any ECG abnormalities.

**504. The answer is c.** *(Rosen, pp 1440, 2346-2347.)* This patient recently gave birth and presents with symptoms of hopelessness and guilt in the subsequent weeks, typical of symptoms seen in this postpartum period. Over half of mothers report depressed mood after childbirth, also known as the "baby blues." This may be linked to rapid decreases in estrogen and progesterone immediately after childbirth. About 40% mothers report that these symptoms last a few days with about half of those having continuing symptoms into weeks. About 2% express suicidal ideation. **Postpartum depression** is more prevalent in those who are unemployed, do not have help with childcare, or have a mood disorder. Treatment varies from cognitive management to antidepressants.

Dysthymic disorder (a) is described as a long-standing, fluctuating, low-grade depression with times of acute episodes. Affected individuals are able to carry out daily routines but gain little pleasure from leisure activities. Cyclothymic disorder (e) is characterized by a life of mood swings, with insufficient severity to meet bipolar disorder criteria. (b) The patient does not exhibit a lifetime history to be given a diagnosis of either of these or the severe mood swings of bipolar disorder. (d) This patient also does not meet the criteria for a major depressive episode.

# Bibliography

2010 American Heart Association Guidelines for Cardiopulmonary Resuscitation and Emergency Cardiovascular Care. *Circulation.* 2010; 122.

American Heart Association Pediatric Advanced Life Support Provider Manual, 2006.

Aminoff MJ, Simon RR, Greenberg D. *Clinical Neurology.* 6th ed. New York, NY: McGraw-Hill; 2005. http://www.accessmedicine.com/content. aspx? aID=2080615.

"Appropriate Interhospital Patient Transfer." ACEP Board of Directors position statement. Feb 2009. http://www.acep.org/Content. aspx?id=29114&terms=transfer.

Beinart SC. Synchronized electrical cardioversion. *eMedicine Journal.* May 2011; http://www.emedicine.com/med/topic2968.htm. Accessed June 30, 2011.

Burnett, LB. Cocaine toxicity in emergency medicine. *eMedicine Journal.* 2010; http://emedicine.medscape.com/article/813959-overview. Accessed June 2011.

Center for Disease Control Treatment Guidelines 2010, Sexually Transmitted Diseases; http://www.cdc.gov/std/treatment/2010/default.htm.

Centor RM, Witherspoon JM, Dalton HP, et al. The diagnosis of strep throat in adults in the emergency room. *Med Decis Making.* 1981;1:239-246.

Cook R, Pan P, Silverman R, Soltys SM. Do-not-resuscitate orders in suicidal patients: clinical, ethical, and legal dilemmas. *Psychosomatics.* 2010 July-Aug;51(4):277-282.

Department of Health and Senior Services, State of New Jersey; Office of Emergency Medical Services website: http://www.nj.gov/health/ems/ emtbqa.shtml.

Draper JC. Teratology and drug use during pregnancy. *eMedicine Journal.* 2006; http://www.emedicine.com/med/topic3242.htm. Accessed January 2012.

Fauci AS, Braunwald E, Kasper DL, et al. *Harrison's: Principles of Internal Medicine.* 17th ed. New York, NY: McGraw-Hill; 2008.

Federal Emergency Management Agency. "EMS Safety: Techniques and Applications." U.S. Government Printing Office, 1994.

Fleisher G, Ludwig S, eds. *The Textbook of Pediatric Emergency Medicine.* 6th ed. Philadelphia, PA: Lippincott Williams & Wilkins; 2011.

Flowers, LK. Costochondritis. *eMedicine Journal.* 2009; http://emedicine. medscape.com/article/808554-overview. Accessed June 2011.

Goldfrank L, Flomenbaum N, Lewin N, et al. *Goldfrank's Toxicologic Emergencies.* 9th ed. New York, NY: McGraw-Hill; 2010.

Goldman L, Ausiello D. *Cecil Textbook of Medicine.* 22nd ed. Philadelphia, PA: Saunders; 2003.

"Guide for Interfacility Patient Transfer." National Highway Traffic Safety Administration. DOT HS 810 599. April 2006.

Hall SA. An analysis of dilemmas posed by prehospital DNR orders. *J Emerg Med.* 1997;15(1):109-111.

Hamilton GC, Sanders AB, Strange GR, et al. *Emergency Medicine: An Approach to Clinical Problem-Solving.* 2nd ed. Philadelphia, PA: Saunders; 2003.

Harvey RA, Champe PC. *Pharmacology.* 4th ed. Philadelphia PA: Lippincott Williams & Wilkins; 2009.

Hasbun R. Computed tomography of the head before lumbar puncture in adults with suspected meningitis. *N Engl J Med.* 2001;345:1727-1733.

"Interim Guidance for EMTALA Final Rule." Department of Health and Human Services branch of the Centers of Medicare and Medicaid Services. Ref: S&C-04-10; Nov 7, 2003. http://www.acep.org/emtala/.

Knoop KJ, Stack LB, Storrow AB. *Atlas of Emergency Medicine.* 3rd ed. New York, NY: McGraw-Hill; 2010.

Krebs DR, Henry KC, Mark B. *When Violence Erupts: A Guide for Emergency Responders.* Baltimore, MD: Mosby; 1990.

Laoteppitaks C. Emergent treatment of alcoholic ketoacidosis. *Medicine Medscape Reference.* 2011; http://emedicine.medscape.com/article/765856-overview.

Lee S. Otitis externa in emergency medicine. *eMedicine Journal.* 2010; http://emedicine.medscape.com/article/763918-overview. Accessed June 2011.

Manno EM. Subarachnoid hemorrhage. *Neurol Clin.* 2004;(22):347-366.

Marx JA, Hockberger RS, Walls RM, et al, eds. *Rosen's Emergency Medicine Concepts and Clinical Practice.* 7th ed. St. Louis, MO: Mosby; 2010.

McIntyre KE. Subclavian steal syndrome. *eMedicine Journal.* October 2009; http://www.emedicine.com/med/topic2771.htm. Accessed June 30, 2011.

McPhee SJ, Papadakis MA, Rabow M, et al. *Lange 2010 Current Medical Diagnosis and Treatment.* 49th ed. New York, NY: McGraw-Hill; 2010.

Moore EE, Feliciano DV, Mattox KL. *Trauma.* 5th ed. New York, NY: McGraw-Hill; 2004.

"National EMS Scope of Practice Model." The National Highway Traffic Safety Administration. DOT HS 810 657; Sept 2006.

"National Standard Curriculum." National Highway Transportation Safety Administration. Retrieved 2011-06-23.

Omori MS. Herpetic whitlow. *eMedicine Journal.* May 2010; http://www.emedicine.com/emerg/topic754.htm. Assessed June 30, 2011.

Ouellette, DR. Pulmonary embolism. *eMedicine Journal.* 2011; http://emedicine.medscape.com/article/300901-overview. Accessed June 2011.

Pinsky MR. Septic shock. *eMedicine Journal.* 2011; http://emedicine.medscape.com/article/168402-overview. Accessed June 2011.

Riordan-Eva P, Asbury T, Whitcher JP. *Vaughn & Asbury's General Ophthalmology.* 17th ed. New York: NY, McGraw-Hill; 2007.

Riviello RJ. Evaluating and treating sexual assault in the emergency department. *Emerg Med Rep.* 2005;26(19).

Roberts JR, Hedges JR. *Clinical Procedures in Emergency Medicine.* 4th ed. Philadelphia, PA: Saunders; 2010.

Ross MG. Eclampsia. *eMedicine Medscape Reference.* 2011; http://emedicine.medscape.com/article/253960-overview. Accessed July 2011.

Sasson C, Rogers MA, Dahl J, Kellermann AL. Predictors of survival from out-of-hospital cardiac arrest: a systematic review and meta-analysis. *Circ Cardiovasc Qual Outcomes.* 2010;3:63-81.

Simon RR, Sherman SC. *Emergency Orthopedics.* 6th ed. New York, NY: McGraw-Hill; 2011.

Singer AJ, Hollander JE. *Lacerations and Acute Wounds.* Philadelphia, PA: F.A. Davis Company; 2003.

Sovari, AA. Long QT syndrome. *eMedicine Journal.* 2011; http://emedicine.medscape.com/article/157826-overview. Accessed June 2011.

"Summary of the HIPAA Privacy Rule." OCR Privacy Brief written by the United States Department of Health and Human Services. Revised edition 05/03. http://www.hhs.gov/ocr/privacy/hipaa/understanding/summary/index.html.

Sytkowski PA, Jacobs LM, Bennett B. Emergency medical personnel training: II. Components of training. *Emerg Health Serv Rev.* 1983 Fall;2(1):11-19.

Tintinalli JE. *Emergency Medicine: A Comprehensive Study Guide.* 7th ed. New York, NY: McGraw-Hill; 2011.

Townsend CM, Beauchamp RD, Evers BM, Mattox KM. *Sabiston Textbook of Surgery: The Biological Basis of Modern Surgical Practice.* 18th ed. Philadelphia, PA: Saunders; 2008.

Vassallo S. Traumatic retrobulbar hemorrhage: emergency decompression by lateral canthotomy and cantholysis. *J Emerg Med.* 2002;22(3): 251-256.

Wang SS. Coronary artery vasospasm. *eMedicine Journal.* 2011; http://emedicine.medscape.com/article/153943-overview. Accessed June 2011.

Young CC. Ankle sprain. *eMedicine Journal.* June 2011; http://www.emedicine.com/emerg/topic30.htm. Accessed June 30, 2011.

# Index

## A

AAP (American Academy of Pediatrics), 392
ABCDE model, 145
Abdominal aortic aneurysm (AAA), 89–90, 94, 101, 103, 158, 280, 473–474
Abdominal radiographs, 282
Abortion, 426, 428–429, 430, 434
Abruptio placentae, 426, 427, 428, 434
Abscess draining, 96–97
Absence seizures, 264–265
Absorbable monofilament sutures, 563
Acarbose, 220
Acetaminophen, 216, 217–218, 226, 229, 234, 257, 260, 261, 343, 345, 346, 348, 350, 352, 357, 578
Acetazolamide, 347, 351, 354, 511, 516
Acetone, 225, 228, 532, 576, 577
Acetylcholine, 216, 359, 363, 369, 403
Acetylcholinesterase, 216, 404
Achilles tendon rupture, 306
Acid burns, 508
Acquired immunodeficiency syndrome (AIDS), 58, 61, 65, 96, 220
Acromioclavicular joint sprain, 307–308
Activated charcoal, 219, 222, 225, 229, 234, 255
Acute chest syndrome, 394–395
Acute coronary syndrome (ACS), 21, 25, 27, 31, 35, 36, 42

Acute iron poisoning, 230
Acute mitral valve regurgitation, 40
Acute mountain sickness (AMS), 511, 515–516
Acute otitis media (AOM), 400–401
Acute pulmonary edema (APE), 31
Acute respiratory distress syndrome (ARDS), 58, 65
Acyclovir, 352, 506
Adenocarcinoma, 35, 281, 287
Adenosine, 33, 42, 161, 409–410
Adenovirus, 37
Adhesion, 90, 100, 287
Adnexal mass, 480
Adnexal tenderness, 99
Adrenal cortical insufficiency, 578
Adrenal crisis, 167
Advanced cardiac life support (ACLS) drugs, 136, 517
Advanced trauma life support (ATLS), 144
Afferent pupillary defect (APD), 535
Agitation, 191, 217, 223, 224, 233, 235, 250, 251, 261, 574, 590, 591, 592
Air enema, 394
Air transportation, 546–547
Airway, breathing, and circulation (ABCs), 35, 41, 140–141, 143, 154, 157, 158, 165, 218, 232, 251, 276, 398, 513, 514, 516, 517
Albuterol, 62
Alcohol, 24, 41, 65, 87–88, 90, 225, 230, 235, 255, 257, 260, 279–280, 353, 593, 594
Alcohol ketoacidosis, 87–88